6TH EDITION

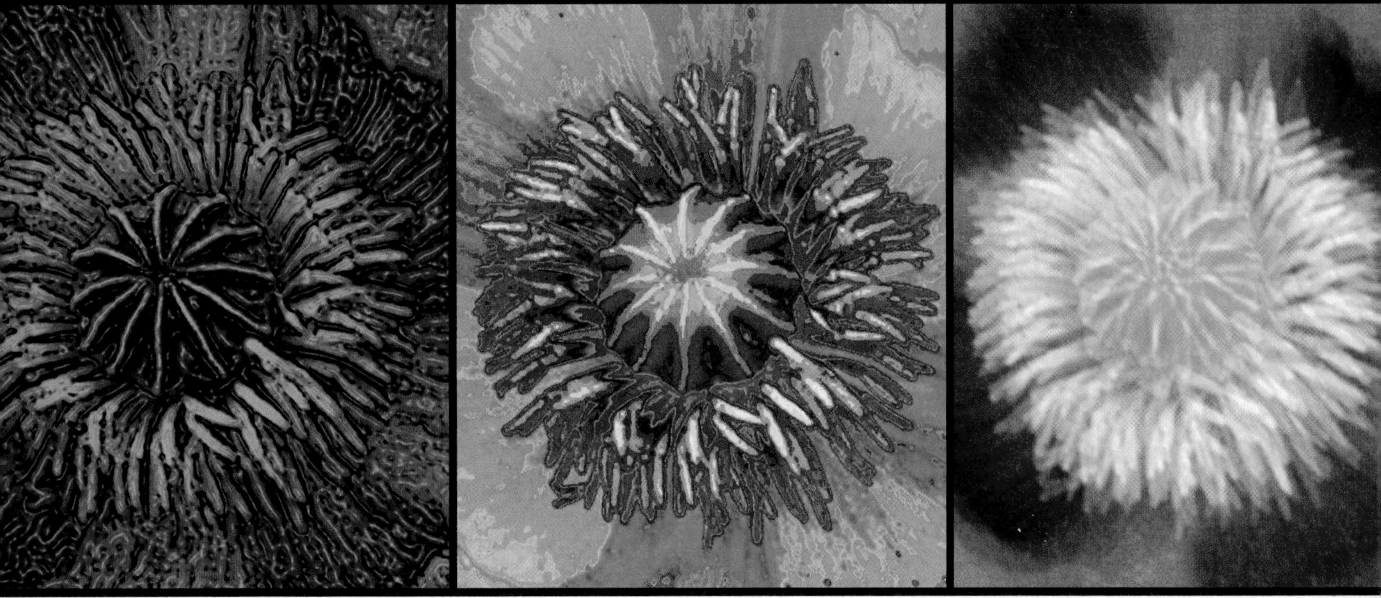

Drug Use and Abuse

Stephen A. Maisto
Syracuse University

Mark Galizio
University of North Carolina at Wilmington

Gerard J. Connors
Research Institute on Addictions, University at Buffalo

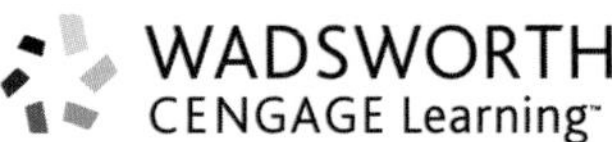

Australia • Brazil • Japan • Korea • Mexico • Singapore • Spain • United Kingdom • United States

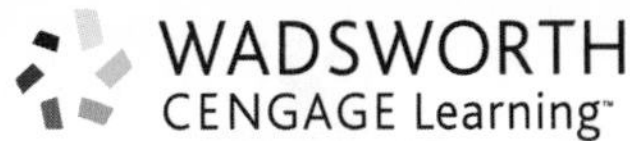

Drug Use and Abuse, **Sixth Edition**
Stephen A. Maisto, Mark Galizio, and Gerard J. Connors

Senior Publisher: Linda Schreiber-Ganster
Executive Editor: Jon-David Hague
Assistant Editor: Paige Leeds
Editorial Assistant: Kelly Miller
Media Editor: Mary Noel
Marketing Manager: Elisabeth Rhoden
Executive Marketing/Communications Manager: Talia Wise
Senior Content Project Manager: Pat Waldo
Creative Director: Rob Hugel
Art Director: Vernon Boes
Print Buyer: Judy Inouye
Rights Acquisitions Account Manager, Text: Bobbie Broyer
Rights Acquisitions Account Manager, Image: Dean Dauphinais
Production Service: Jill Traut/MPS Limited, A Macmillan Company
Text Designer: Lisa Henry
Photo Researcher: Jaime Jankowski, Pre-PressPMG
Copy Editor: Heather McElwain
Illustrator: MPS Limited, A Macmillan Company
Cover Designer: Larry Didona
Cover Image: Gail Smith/Getty Images
Compositor: MPS Limited, A Macmillan Company

Library of Congress Control Number: 2010922548

ISBN-13: 978-0-495-81441-2

ISBN-10: 0-495-81441-5

Wadsworth
20 Davis Drive
Belmont, CA 94002-3098
USA

Cengage Learning is a leading provider of customized learning solutions with office locations around the globe, including Singapore, the United Kingdom, Australia, Mexico, Brazil, and Japan. Locate your local office at **www.cengage.com/global.**

Cengage Learning products are represented in Canada by Nelson Education, Ltd.

To learn more about Wadsworth, visit **www.cengage.com/Wadsworth**

Purchase any of our products at your local college store or at our preferred online store **www.CengageBrain.com.**

Printed in the United States of America
1 2 3 4 5 6 7 14 13 12 11 10

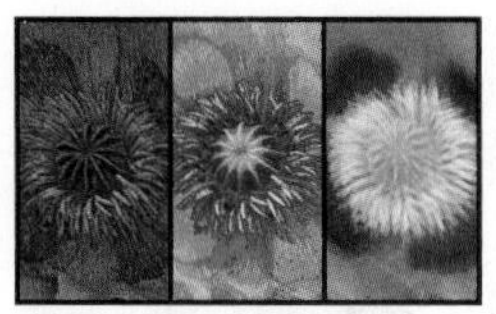

To Sam
S.A.M.

To my parents, Joe and Audrienne,
and to my wife, Kate,
and to my daughter, Annie
M.G.

To Lana and Marissa
G.J.C.

ABOUT THE AUTHORS

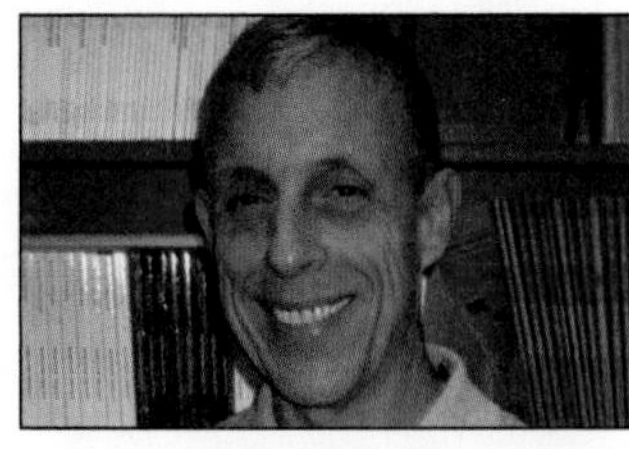

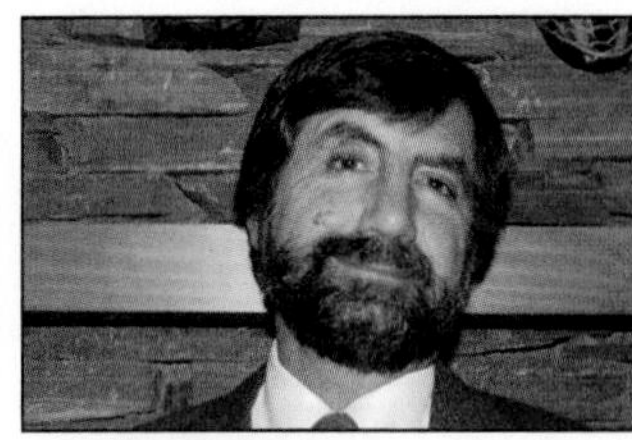

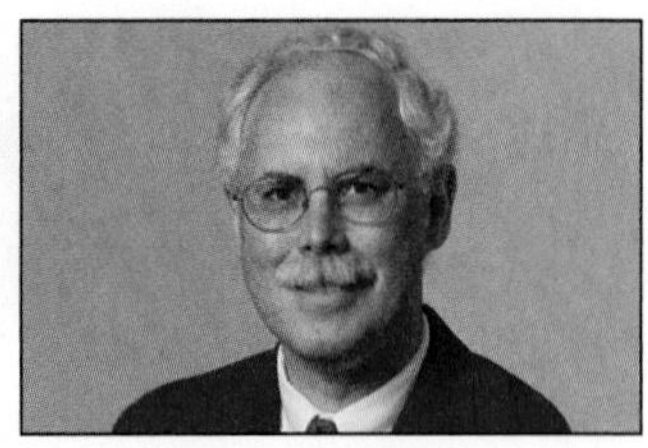

Stephen A. Maisto received a PhD in experimental psychology from the University of Wisconsin—Milwaukee and completed a postdoctoral respecialization in clinical psychology from George Peabody College of Vanderbilt University. He is a professor of psychology at Syracuse University. He has been engaged in research, teaching, clinical practice, and clinical training in the assessment and treatment of the substance-use disorders for 30 years. Dr. Maisto has published over 150 articles, 25 book chapters, and several books on substance use and the substance-use disorders. His current research is supported by the National Institute on Alcohol Abuse and Alcoholism and the Department of Veterans Affairs. Dr. Maisto is a member of the American Psychological Association (Fellow, Divisions of Clinical Psychology and Addictive Behaviors), Association for Psychological Science, Research Society on Alcoholism, and the Association for Behavioral and Cognitive Therapies.

Mark Galizio received his PhD in experimental psychology in 1976, from the University of Wisconsin—Milwaukee, where he served as a research assistant at the Midwest Institute on Drug Abuse. He is chair and professor of psychology at the University of North Carolina at Wilmington, where he has taught and conducted research for over 30 years. He has published extensively in the areas of behavioral pharmacology and behavior analysis and has served as associate editor of the *Journal of the Experimental Analysis of Behavior*. His research has been supported by grants from the National Institute on Drug Abuse, the National Institute of Neurological Disorders and Stroke, and the National Science Foundation. He is a fellow of the American Psychological Association (Divisions of Psychopharmacology and Substance Abuse, Behavior Analysis, Behavioral Neuroscience and Comparative Psychology, and Experimental Psychology) and is past president of the Division of Behavior Analysis.

Gerard J. Connors is director of the Research Institute on Addictions at the University at Buffalo. He earned his doctoral degree in clinical psychology from Vanderbilt University in 1980. Dr. Connors's research interests include substance use and abuse, relapse prevention, self-help group involvement, early interventions with heavy drinkers, and treatment evaluation. He is a fellow of the American Psychological Association (Divisions of Clinical Psychology and Addictions). Dr. Connors has authored or coauthored numerous scientific articles, books, and book chapters. His current research activities are funded by grants from the National Institute on Alcohol Abuse and Alcoholism.

BRIEF CONTENTS

CONTENTS

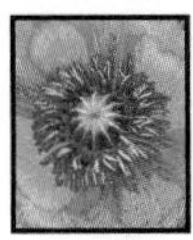

CHAPTER 5 Psychopharmacology and New Drug Development 91

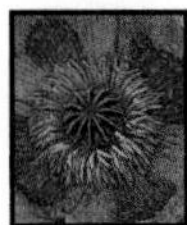

CHAPTER 6 Cocaine, Amphetamines, and Related Stimulants 115

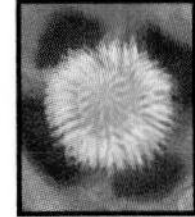

CHAPTER 7 Nicotine 141

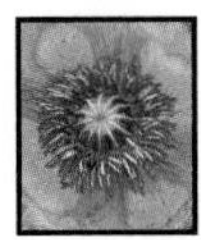

CHAPTER 8 Caffeine 170

We began writing the first edition of this text in the late 1980s. At that time, drug use and related problems were of major interest and concern in the United States and in other countries. Awareness, interest, and concern about drug use have not abated since that time, nor has the need for a general undergraduate text to educate college students on the biological, psychological, and social factors that influence drug use and its effects. Therefore, we have completed this sixth edition, which retains many features of previous editions but also reflects changes that have occurred in this very dynamic area of study since the fifth edition was published in 2008.

As in all of the text's previous editions, the central theme of this edition is that a drug's effects are determined not only by its chemical structure and interaction in the body but also by the drug users' biological and psychological characteristics and the setting in which they use the drug. This central theme is reflected in the inclusion of chapters on pharmacology and psychopharmacology, and is continued throughout the presentation of individual drugs or drug classes and in the discussion of prevention and treatment. The text examines the complexity of human drug consumption on biological, psychological, and social levels. Although the text is scholarly, it is understandable to students with little background in the biological, behavioral, or social sciences.

The text also retains a number of pedagogical features designed to increase students' interest and learning. **Diagnostic pretests** at the beginning of each chapter challenge students to test their knowledge of drugs while drawing their attention to important concepts or facts that follow in the chapter. Pretest answers and explanations at the end of each chapter provide an important review of the main concepts. The **margin glossary** helps students identify and define important terms within the text. **Margin quotes** help bring abstract concepts to life through personal accounts, comments, and quips about drug use and its ramifications. **Drugs and Culture boxes** explore variations in drug use and its consequences. They highlight the importance of differences in drug use that are associated with factors such as a person's sex, race, and ethnic background. Finally, **Contemporary Issue boxes** discuss current controversies involving drugs or drug use, as well as events related to such controversies.

New in This Edition

As mentioned earlier, drugs and drug use are popular and dynamic areas of study. Accordingly, a number of changes have occurred in the field since publication of the fifth edition. Each chapter of the sixth edition has been updated to represent findings from the latest research, as well as to reflect social and legal changes related to drugs. Among the many revisions, we present the latest survey data available at this writing on patterns of drug use in the United States and in other countries worldwide.

Chapter 2, Drug Use: Yesterday and Today, includes new information of the movement to legalize the use of marijuana for medical reasons, updated material on drug legislation, including the 2009 Family Smoking Prevention and Tobacco Control Act, and new coverage of salvia divinorum, which is a candidate for upcoming control legislation.

Chapter 3, Drugs and the Nervous System, contains a restructured neurotransmitter section, with separate sections for amino acid transmitters, as well as a new section on brain changes following chronic drug use.

Chapter 4, Pharmacology, has an updated and more complete section on drug testing, and Chapter 5, Psychopharmacology and New Drug Development, features an expanded discussion of the use of placebo control groups in research on the effectiveness of new medications, along with updated data on the use and importance of generic drugs.

Chapter 6, Cocaine, Amphetamines, and Related Stimulants, adds new sections on the crack sentencing law controversy and on regulations on methamphetamine and the effects of such regulation on the production and availability of methamphetamine. Chapter 6 also contains a new Drugs and Culture Box on the current use of coca in Latin America, as well as updates on the epidemiology of cocaine and methamphetamine use.

Chapter 7, Nicotine, includes a new discussion of the increased use of a water pipe or "hookah" as a means of smoking tobacco among college students. The chapter also has updated National Survey on Drug Use and Health (NSDUH) data on the epidemiology of nicotine use in the United States, along with an expanded and updated section on the treatment of nicotine addiction. Furthermore, Chapter 7 has information on the 2009 legislation in the United States that gives the Federal Drug Administration the authority to regulate tobacco products. Finally, Chapter 7 also features expanded and updated material on the harm-reduction approach to cigarette smoking, including discussion of products billed as "safer" alternatives to traditional cigarettes, such as the electronic cigarette and smokeless tobacco products.

Chapter 8, Caffeine, has the latest epidemiological data on per capita consumption of caffeine in a variety of countries, including children's consumption, and a detailed listing of the caffeine concentration of a variety of beverages, including energy drinks, foods, and medications. Chapter 8 adds an extensive Contemporary Issue Box on energy drinks and the use of energy drinks in combination with alcohol. The chapter also covers the contribution of caffeine to athletic performance, and the latest data on the positive and negative effects of caffeine on health.

Chapter 9, Alcohol, has new epidemiological data on alcohol consumption in the United States and around the world, as well as the health "benefits" of moderate alcohol consumption. Chapter 9 also contains updated data on the effects of a pregnant woman's moderate alcohol use on the health of the fetus that she is carrying.

Chapter 10, Opiates, has expanded coverage of prescription opiate use, including epidemiological trends, abuse patterns, and overdose.

The chapter on marijuana (Chapter 11) includes the latest epidemiological data on marijuana use around the world, including use among youth, and coverage of the latest trends in vehicles of marijuana intake, including blunts and bongs. Chapter 11 also contains the latest information on the therapeutic uses of marijuana, and the latest updates on the relationship between cannabis use and various mental health outcomes.

Chapter 12, on the hallucinogens, has a new section on Salvia—Salvinorin A.

Chapter 13, Psychotherapeutic Medications, includes information on newly prescribed psychotherapeutic medications, with discussion of their benefits and side effects. Chapter 13 also includes new developments in antipsychotic medications, particularly those that focus on glutamate, along with updates on Internet pharmacies, including the Ryan Haight Online Pharmacy Consumer Protection Act of 2008.

Chapter 14, Other Prescription and Over-the-Counter Drugs, has dropped coverage of the compound salvia that, as noted earlier, is now covered in Chapter 12. In addition, Chapter 14 covers the new continuous birth control pill and includes an update on the health risks associated with acetaminophen.

Chapter 15, Treatment of Substance-Use Disorders, includes new information on Internet-based outpatient treatment for alcohol use, as well as updated information on FDA-approved pharmacotherapies for alcohol and other drug use disorders.

Chapter 16, Prevention of Substance Abuse, covers emerging attention to the role of parents in prevention interventions designed for incoming college freshmen students, examples of the latest prevention efforts, such as the Montana Meth Project, and a description of the Amethyst Initiative, along with a presentation of the arguments put forth in support of and against lowering the legal drinking age in the United States.

Accompanying the sixth edition are both new and expanded supplements that will help instructors with class preparation and help students by providing opportunities for review. In the Instructor's Manual with Test Bank, we provide chapter outlines, learning objectives, InfoTrac® College Edition key terms, glossary terms and definitions, useful web links, and test items in three formats (multiple choice, true/false, and essay).

The test bank is also available in ExamView electronic format, which allows instructors to customize and build their own tests. The new companion website offers text-specific, interactive review and enrichment materials for students, including tutorial quizzes, flash cards, and useful web links. Electronic transparencies on CD-ROM provide figures and tables from the sixth edition uploaded into Microsoft PowerPoint that instructors can use as is or modify to create their own presentations. Each new copy of the sixth edition comes with a pass code to the InfoTrac College Edition full-text periodical database. With this database, students will have access to thousands of journal articles from a wide variety of publications.

Acknowledgments

This text could not have been completed without the help of a number of people. Foremost among these individuals are Jon-David Hague, executive editor; Kelly Miller, editorial assistant; Paige Leeds, assistant editor; Pat Waldo, senior content project manager; Vernon Boes, senior art director; and Talia Wise, executive marketing manager. Thanks also go to the production team, including Heather McElwain, copyeditor; Heather Mann, proofreader; David Luljak, indexer; and Jill Traut, production editor at MPS Limited. Thank you as well to the composition team at MPS Limited, led by K. Narayanan.

Many thanks also go to those who contributed time and energy to reviewing our manuscript. The following reviewers offered outstanding suggestions that helped us to produce a better book: Deborah A. Carroll, Southern Connecticut State University; Bradley Donohue, University of Nevada—Las Vegas; Yousef Fahoum, MAP, University of Arkansas at Little Rock/Benton; Charles R. Geist, University of the Virgin Islands; Marc Gellman, University of Miami; Barry Goetz, Western Michigan University; Ruth Kershner, West Virginia University; Jim Kirby, Fresno City College; Cheryl Kirstein, University of Florida; Marvin Krank, Okanagan University College; Jerry Lundgren, Flathead Valley Community College; Don Matlosz, California State University—Fresno; Rustem Medora, University of Montana; Bill Meil, Indiana University of Pennsylvania; Kelly Mosel-Talavera, Texas State University; Rob Mowrer, Angelo State University; Michelle L. Pilati, Rio Hondo College; and Joseph Vlah, Flagler College.

We also want to thank other special people who helped us in completing the sixth edition. Stephen Maisto would like to thank his wife Mary Jean Byrne-Maisto for her unwavering love, support, and encouragement through his completion of this project. Stephen also thanks his two outstanding graduate students, Todd Bishop and Marketa Krenek, for all of their help in preparing this edition. Mark Galizio thanks his wife, Kate Bruce, and daughter, Annie. Their love and support make it all worthwhile. Mark also thanks the many students at the University of North Carolina at Wilmington who provide continuing challenges and inspiration. Gerard Connors thanks his wife, Lana Michaels Connors, and their daughter, Marissa, for their constant support and love throughout the preparation of the sixth edition. Gerard also thanks Jennifer Wray, Mark R. Duerr, and Julianne Deschenes for their tireless assistance and patience in preparing the chapters for this edition.

Stephen A. Maisto
Mark Galizio
Gerard J. Connors

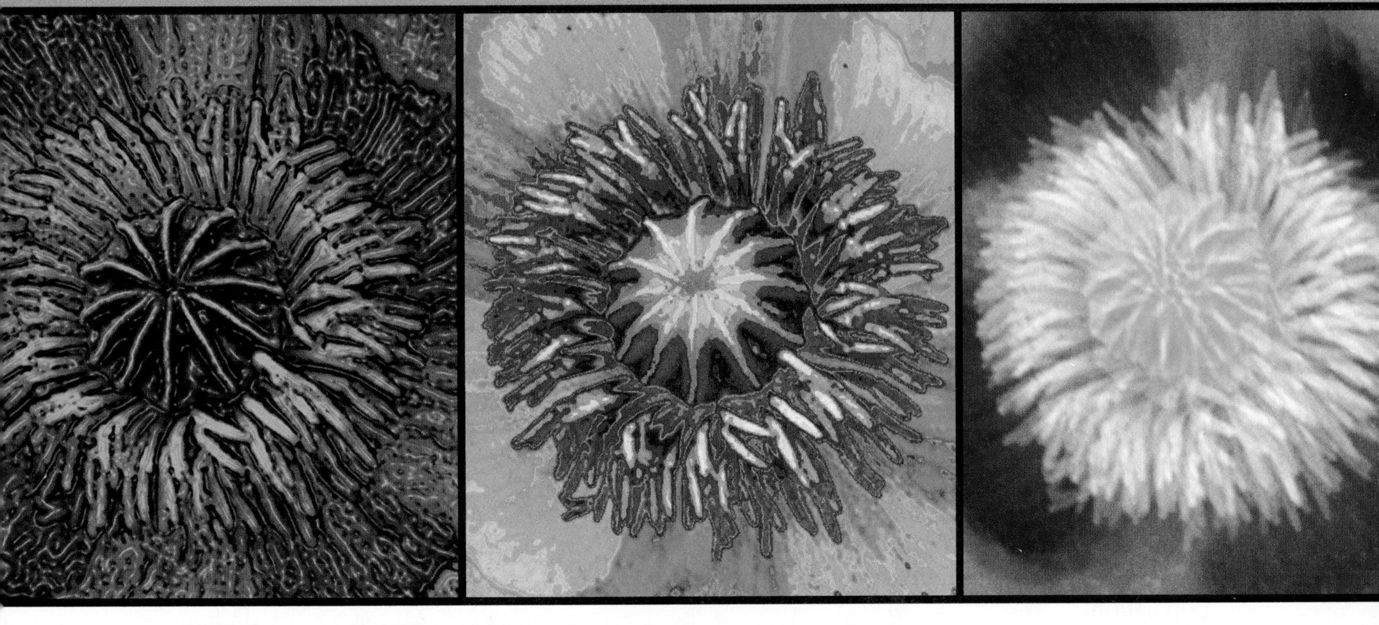

Drug Use and Abuse

What Do You Think? True or False?

Answers are given at the end of the chapter.

___ 1. Because the effects of drugs are both predictable and obvious, it is relatively easy to define drug abuse.

___ 2. A drug's street name sometimes describes the actual effect of that drug.

___ 3. A person's reaction to a drug depends mostly on the biological action of the drug in the body.

___ 4. Because drug use is complicated, it is impossible to estimate patterns of drug use for the population of a whole country.

___ 5. Within the United States, similar patterns of alcohol and other drug use are found even among different subgroups of the population.

___ 6. The highest rates of alcohol and other drug use are found among 18- to 25-year-olds.

___ 7. A person's use of more than one drug at a time is of little concern because it happens so infrequently.

___ 8. The total economic cost of alcohol and drug abuse in the United States is about a billion dollars annually.

___ 9. The use of alcohol and other drugs causes violence and crime.

___10. Modern researchers rely on definitions of alcohol and other drug use that are free of social or cultural biases.

___11. A diagnosis of drug abuse is made when a person has become either physically or psychologically dependent on a drug.

___12. Definitions of addiction emphasize overwhelming involvement with a drug.

___13. The continued use of any drug will eventually lead to tolerance of and physical dependence on that drug.

Athletic	Legal	Religious
Biological	Medical	Social/cultural
Economic	Political	
Educational	Psychological	

Q: How are these 10 systems alike?

A: They influence or are influenced by alcohol and other drug use.

This one-question quiz shows that drugs[1] may affect us in many ways, whether or not we use them. Although what we see and hear in the media often focuses on the negative consequences of drug use, drugs are popular all over the world because people perceive that they benefit from using drugs. For example, on an *individual* level, people say that drugs make them feel more relaxed, socialize more easily, feel sexier, escape boredom, and feel more confident and assertive. Drugs have also helped to ease a lot of suffering in humans and other animals when used for specific medical purposes. On a *group* or *community* level, drugs have been used for thousands of years as part of social and religious rituals. A drug used for such purposes has little to do with the drug's chemistry but rather with social or cultural factors. One society may condone the use of a drug—say, alcohol in the United States and European countries—whereas

[1]Sometimes in this book, we use the term *alcohol and drugs*; at other times we use *drugs* as the inclusive term. Because alcohol is a drug, saying "alcohol and drugs" is redundant. However, we do so on occasion, when it seems useful, to distinguish alcohol from all other drugs.

another society condemns it, such as the Islamic countries of Iran and Saudi Arabia. The array of benefits and negative consequences of drug use lies behind the image of the beautiful yet wilted poppy on the cover of this text. This complex picture of human drug use also suggests that many different factors influence drug use.

What influences drug use and how that use affects us make up the subject of drugs and human behavior and are what this text is about. Because our subject matter is so wide-ranging, this introductory chapter spans a variety of topics. We include formal definitions throughout the chapter, beginning with terms such as *pharmacology, drug,* and *drug abuse.*

Introducing a lot of terms in one chapter might be confusing at first, but there is no need to feel that you have to grasp all the terms immediately. Because the terms will be used repeatedly throughout the book, you will have time to learn them. By introducing the terms now, we give you the vocabulary to read later chapters more easily.

"Food is good. Poison is bad. Drugs may be good or bad, and whether they are seen as good or bad depends on who is looking at them."

(Weil & Rosen, 1983, p. 10)

In this chapter, we also explain the drug-classification systems used in this book and then move to a discussion of who uses drugs. The final sections of the chapter cover ways to define harmful drug use. The chapter closes with a brief overview of the rest of the text.

Pharmacology and Drugs

Humans have used drugs for several thousand years, but the scientific study of drugs is more recent. The scientific study of drugs is called **pharmacology**, which is concerned with all information about the effects of chemical substances (drugs) on living systems. Pharmacology is considered a part of biology and is allied with physiology and biochemistry (Blum, 1984). **Psychopharmacology** is an area within the field of pharmacology that focuses on the effects of drugs on behavior. Although *psychopharmacology* is a joining of the words *psychology* and *pharmacology,* it is now recognized that understanding how drugs affect human behavior requires knowledge about social and environmental factors as well. This book is about human psychopharmacology.

pharmacology
The scientific study of drugs concerned with all information about the effects of drugs on living systems.

psychopharmacology
The subarea of pharmacology that concerns the effects of drugs on behavior.

psychology
The scientific study of behavior.

drug
Broadly defined as any chemical entity or mixture of entities not required for the maintenance of health but that alters biological function or structure when administered.

Drugs are easy enough to talk about, or so it seems from the numbers and variety of people who do so. However, defining *drug* is not so simple. Although they have run into confusion along the way, experts have arrived at a workable definition. According to a World Health Organization (WHO) report published in 1981, **drug** is defined in the broadest sense as "any chemical entity or mixture of entities, other than those required for the maintenance of normal health (like food), the administration of which alters biological function and possibly structure" (p. 227). This definition remains useful today.

These fundamental definitions bring us to the question of what is drug *use* and what is drug *abuse.* We discuss this distinction in more detail later in this chapter, but it is important for you to get an idea at the outset of what is called drug use and drug abuse. Abuse has been referred to in different ways when people write about drugs, and there is no generally accepted definition. In such circumstances, one way to define a term is by a consensus of experts. A study by Rinaldi et al. (1988) achieved such a consensus definition for a number of terms used in research and clinical work on alcohol and drugs. In the Rinaldi et al. study, the experts defined **drug abuse** as "any use of drugs that causes physical, psychological, legal, or social harm to the individual or to others affected by the drug user's behavior."

drug abuse
Any use of drugs that causes physical, psychological, legal, or social harm to the individual user or to others affected by the drug user's behavior.

As you can see, the definition of abuse centers on the consequences of the drug users' behavior, both to themselves and to others in the person's social environment. Our opening quiz on the 10 systems and drug use comes into sharper relief with this definition of abuse. The definition also illustrates the difficulties in defining abuse. A major problem is that the behavior that causes consequences in one community or culture may not cause them in another, or not to the same degree. Therefore, the goal to have a standard reference for drug abuse has proved elusive. Nevertheless, in writing and other forms of communication about alcohol and other drugs, the word *abuse* is used frequently, and therefore, efforts to arrive at a more generally applicable definition should continue. For now, however, our initial definition of abuse is sufficient for understanding what we say in the first part of this chapter. Toward the end of this chapter, we discuss a "diagnostic" definition of substance (alcohol or other drugs) abuse that the American Psychiatric Association has developed.

If *abuse* is drug use with negative consequences, then drug *use* may be viewed as the larger category, with drug abuse as a subset. Drug consumption that does not meet the criteria for drug abuse is referred to as drug use.

Drug Classification

As the WHO panel of experts understood, their definition of *drug* is very broad. To make the definition useful for research and practical purposes, it is necessary to order the substances that fit the definition of drug into smaller categories. Pharmacologists have done this with their many systems for classifying drugs. These classification systems have been based on the primary properties of drugs to communicate a drug's nature and the ways it can be used. Following are some of the major ways of classifying drugs:

1. By origin. An example is drugs that come from plants, such as the opiates, which are derived from the opium poppy. The "pure" (nonsynthetic) opiates include compounds such as morphine and codeine. Heroin, which is a semisynthetic compound, is often called an opiate drug. Because this classification distinguishes only the source of the drug, a given drug class may include many drugs that have different chemical actions.
2. By therapeutic use, or according to similarity in how a drug is used to treat or modify something in the body. For example, with this system, amphetamines are called appetite-suppressant drugs. Note that the reasons some drugs are used can be much different from their therapeutic effects. Amphetamines are often used nonmedically because of their stimulant effects. Similarly, morphine may be used medically as a powerful painkiller, but street users take morphine for its euphoric effects.
3. By site of drug action, which pertains to where in the body the drug is causing physical changes. For example, alcohol is often called a depressant drug because of its depressant action on the central nervous system (CNS). Conversely, because of its CNS stimulant properties, cocaine is often called a stimulant drug. The utility of this system is limited when a drug affects several different body sites. One example is the CNS stimulant cocaine, which also has local anesthetic (pain-reducing) effects. Furthermore, drugs that differ widely in chemical structure or mechanisms of action may affect the same body site.
4. By chemical structure. For example, the barbiturates (such as phenobarbital, Amytal, and Seconal) are synthetic compounds derived from the chemical structure of barbituric acid, the synthetic compound that forms the chemical base for barbiturate drugs.

5. By mechanism of action, which means how a drug produces its **drug effects**. This is a good system in principle, and ongoing research in pharmacology is directed at specifying the mechanisms of action of an increasing number of drugs.
6. By street name, which comes from drug "subcultures" and the street drug market. For example, amphetamines are called "speed," and drugs like the barbiturates or depressants such as methaqualone (Quaalude) are called "downers." As these examples show, street names sometimes reflect actual drug effects. (Brands, Sproule, & Marshman, 1998, pp. 11–13)

drug effects
The action of a drug on the body. Drug effects are measured in different ways.

The topics of this text's drug chapters (Chapters 6 through 14) were determined according to several different ways of classifying drugs. One of the ways to classify drugs, by their effects, applies to virtually all of the drugs covered in this text. We are most interested in what are called **psychoactive** drugs—those that affect moods, thinking, and behavior. Some substances have been designated formally as psychoactive, such as alcohol, whereas others have not, such as aspirin. Psychoactive drugs are most important in this text because they are the ones that people are most likely to use, often in ways that create serious problems for them. This text mainly concerns the nonmedical use of psychoactive drugs, but we also discuss medical uses.

psychoactive
Pertaining to effects on mood, thinking, and behavior.

The Drug Experience

As we said earlier, people like many of the experiences they have when they take drugs. This raises an important question: What causes the "drug experience"? The drug's chemical action is part of the answer, but how much? Not too long ago, the chemical actions of drugs were viewed as the primary reason people experienced certain changes when they took different drugs. However, research from different disciplines, such as pharmacology, psychology, and sociology, has shown that the drug experience is a product of more factors than just the drug's pharmacological action.

Generally, we can look at three sets of factors, one pharmacological and two nonpharmacological. The first set includes *pharmacological factors,* and three of them stand out. First are the chemical properties and action on the body of the drug used. Another is **drug dosage** (or dose), which is the measure of how much of the drug is consumed. The third pharmacological factor is the **route of drug administration**, or the way the drug enters the body. This is important because the route affects how much of a dosage reaches its site(s) of action and how quickly it gets there. Chapter 4 discusses in detail major routes of drug administration and their effects on the drug experience.

drug dosage
Measure of the quantity of drug consumed.

route of drug administration
The way that drugs enter the body.

The second set of factors is nonpharmacological and consists of the *characteristics of the drug user*. Included are such factors as the person's genetic makeup (biologically inherited differences among people govern their bodies' reaction to the ingestion of different drugs), gender, age, drug tolerance, and personality. An important part of personality is the person's **psychological set** about a drug, which refers to knowledge, attitudes, expectations, and thoughts about a drug. For example, sometimes the strong belief that a drug will produce a certain effect will be enough to produce the effect, even though the person has ingested a chemically inactive substance (**placebo**).

psychological set
An individual's knowledge, attitudes, expectations, and other thoughts about an object or event, such as a drug.

placebo
In pharmacology, a chemically inactive substance.

The third and last set of factors, also a nonpharmacological one, is the *setting in which a drug is used*. The factors in this group span a wide range and include laws pertaining to drug use in the community where the drug is taken, the immediate physical environment where the drug is used, and whether other people are present at the time of drug use.

Together, these three sets of factors influence what people experience when they take a drug. You may have guessed that the path to a drug experience is not always easy to chart. However, many people are trying to do just that—to understand how drugs affect people. The accumulated knowledge from these efforts is the foundation of this book.

Alcohol and Drug Use in the United States

The way the popular media tell it, it may seem as if virtually everyone has positive experiences using drugs because everyone seems to be using them. However, scientists learned long ago that our impressions or feelings about a subject often are inaccurate, and to find out what is really going on, it is best to study the subject systematically. This means using the scientific method, which is the major way we have learned as much as we do know about drugs. One of the best ways to answer questions about the uses of alcohol and drugs in a community or larger region is to do a survey study. When we want to learn about a whole country, we do what is called a national survey study.

"I could have easily gotten stoned [before coming to this interview]; it wouldn't have bothered me. It depends on the situation. I wouldn't like to smoke in the middle of the day if I have things to do. Or I wouldn't smoke in the middle of a class. Things like that."

Research participant (Zinberg, 1984, p. 140)

In the United States, national survey studies of alcohol and drug use have involved interviewing a sample of individuals (in this case, age 12 or older) across the country. Such studies generally ensure that those interviewed are as similar as possible to the U.S. population as a whole regarding, for example, factors such as gender, age, race, region of the country, and rural-versus-urban living environment. The national survey data give us the best estimate we have of what the findings would be if we studied every person in the population that was sampled for the survey. In this case, that means the U.S. population of around 225 million people.

The federal government goes to great trouble and expense to support these national surveys of drug use because the knowledge gained from them is extremely valuable in making legal, tax, educational, and health policy decisions. More narrowly, we are interested in the information from national surveys for this text because many

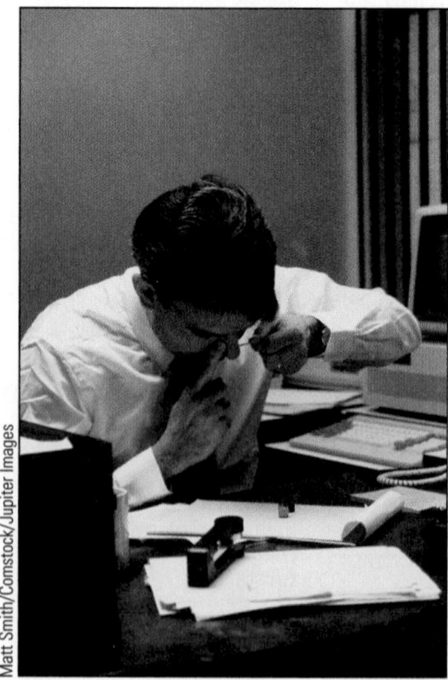

Matt Smith/Comstock/Jupiter Images

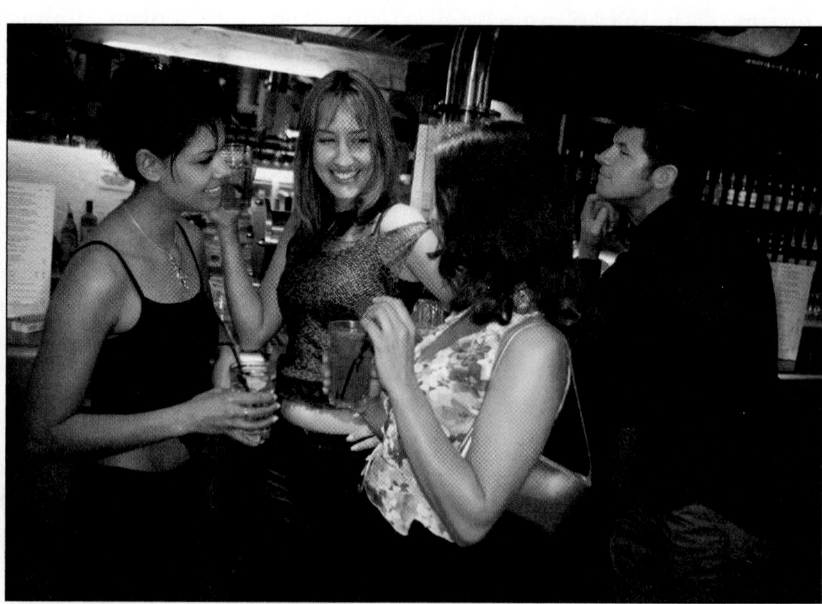

Corbis

People use drugs in a variety of situations and experience different reactions to them.

CONTEMPORARY ISSUE BOX 1.1

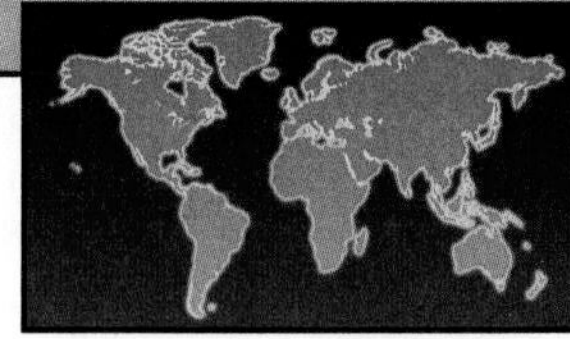

U.S. Society and Drug Use

Learning about alcohol and drug use in the United States is important. One reason is the sheer number of people in the United States who use alcohol or other drugs. Another reason is the negative consequences associated with alcohol and drug use, which are discussed later in more detail. A third reason is the amount of controversy that drugs, especially illicit drugs, create. Despite the prevalence of drug use among its citizens, popular opinion in the United States has been to eradicate illicit drug use, at times ranking such use among the nation's top problems. Indeed, a 2007 survey conducted by the University of Michigan involved collection of data on adults' perceptions of the main problems threatening children's and adolescents' well-being, and "drug abuse" was number 2 in the top 10. (Interestingly, smoking tobacco and alcohol abuse were numbers 1 and 4, respectively.) Think of some of the major headline events that have occurred and the controversies they have generated in the last few years. Some of them touch upon the basic constitutional rights of Americans:

- The right of the federal government and other public and private employers to conduct urine screens (tests for drug taking) of employees as a way to control drug abuse in the workplace
- The question of whether intravenous drug users should be supplied with clean syringes free of charge as a way of preventing the spread of human immunodeficiency virus (HIV) infection
- The continuing debate on whether marijuana should be available as a prescription drug
- Some proposed legal penalties related to selling or using drugs—the requirement of life sentences for drug dealers who are convicted twice of selling drugs to teenagers and the imposition of the death penalty for dealers when a murder occurs during a drug deal
- The argument that drugs like marijuana and cocaine should be available legally to adults because the "war on drugs" has been lost

Many Americans use alcohol or other drugs. However, the country's attitudes toward such use, especially regarding illicit drugs, are far from permissive. Society's proposed and actual solutions to drug use in the United States have far-reaching legal, social, and financial implications. Which stand out to you?

people do not know the typical patterns of drug use among Americans. For example, the popular media expose us primarily to extreme cases of use and problems associated with it. The national survey data on alcohol and drug use give us a more balanced reference for understanding any one person's or group's use. In the same way, our brief review of national survey data in this chapter will help you understand drug use patterns and related problems that we write about in later chapters of this book.

National Household Survey

To provide you with an overview of current alcohol and drug use, we used a national survey that is conducted annually by the Office of Applied Studies within the Substance Abuse and Mental Health Services Administration (SAMHSA). The National Survey on Drug Use and Health (NSDUH) includes households in all 50 U.S. states and the District of Columbia. In this section, we refer to findings from the 2007 survey (SAMHSA, 2008).

This survey included individuals 12 years of age or older. Personal and self-administered interviews were completed with 67,870 respondents. As it was a household survey, people such as military personnel in military installations, individuals in long-term hospitals, and prisoners were excluded from the sample. As a result, the data cannot be viewed as completely representative of everyone in the 50 states. Nevertheless, the NSDUH provides the best single description of frequency and quantity of drug use among a broad age range of people in U.S. society.

prevalence
The general occurrence of an event, usually expressed in terms of percentage of some population. Another common statistic in survey studies is *incidence,* or the number of first-time occurrences of an event during some time period.

In the 2007 NSDUH, a variety of data about drug use in the United States were collected. We first discuss data on the overall **prevalence** of use in the last year and the last month respectively for different drugs, including alcohol and tobacco cigarettes. In this case, "use" means the person used the drug in question at least once during the time in question; "past month" and "past year" are from the time the respondents give information about their drug use. We also offer counterpart prevalence data from the 2006 survey to allow for comparison with the 2007 data. Table 1.1 presents this first set of percentages. Several findings stand out in Table 1.1. First, alcohol leads the use list, followed by cigarettes in a distant second place. Marijuana heads the list of illicit drug use (drug use not in accord with legal restrictions). These relationships hold up for use both in the past year and in the past month.

Table 1.1 gives you an overall picture of drug use, but as we noted before, drug use differs with characteristics of people. Table 1.2 and Table 1.3 give you an initial look at some of the characteristics that are highly associated with drug use differences. Table 1.2 centers on age differences in drug use in the past year and month, as reported in the 2007 national survey. As you can see in Table 1.2, individuals in the age range 18 to 25 have the most prevalent substance use. Over three of every four of these respondents said they used alcohol in the last year, and about one of every three of them reported at least one occasion of illicit drug use in the past year. In Table 1.3, we provide 2007 substance use data for the past month according to ethnic or racial group and gender. The most striking findings in Table 1.3 are the gender differences. Men were about one and three-quarters times as likely as women to report any illicit

CONTEMPORARY ISSUE BOX 1.2

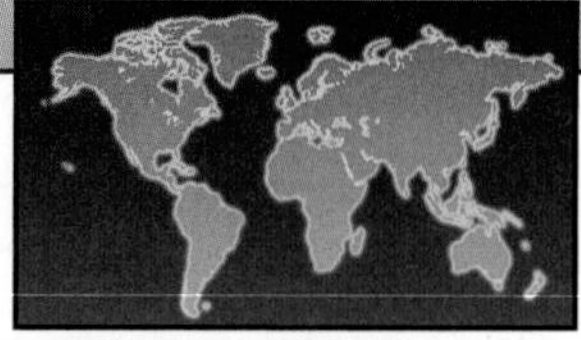

Survey Data on Drug Use: Are They Accurate?

There are compelling reasons for conducting national survey studies of drug use and its consequences. Such information can help a society formulate effective legal and social policies on the use of specific drugs. National survey data also may help to identify groups within a population that are at the greatest risk for experiencing health or other problems related to drug use, which could help in creating more effective prevention programs.

These and other benefits of national survey data on drug use are significant, but a big question is whether the information that is obtained reflects a society's *actual* drug use. That is, are the data accurate?

There are several reasons for asking this question. For example, even the largest surveys rarely collect data from every person in a target population, so it is possible that the sample of people chosen to participate in the survey is biased in some way. This means that the sample might not reflect the population's characteristics on sex of the respondent, race, religion, or education, all of which could be associated with the main behavior of interest (here, drug use). In addition, because many of the drugs asked about are illegal for nonmedical use, or for any use at all, people may be reluctant to admit to a researcher that they have used a particular drug or have used it in particular amounts or frequency. Furthermore, as surveys typically ask about past behavior, memory limits may interfere with the collection of accurate information, regardless of the respondent's intention to tell the truth.

These and other problems are real and must be addressed if national survey data on drug use are to have the utility that they are intended to have. Fortunately, the challenge to collect accurate survey information has been an active research area over the years, and methods of representative sampling and data collection to assure confidentiality or anonymity of responses have led to better survey design and procedures. These advances have resulted in data that meet high standards of reliability and accuracy. This is not to say that national survey data provide a literal picture of drug use in a population, but that the picture is getting clearer and more detailed as survey research methods continue to improve.

If you were designing a survey to study some behavior, such as drug use, in a given population, what potential sources of bias in the data would you consider? How would you handle them?

TABLE 1.1 Percentages of Individuals Aged 12 and Older Who Reported Use of Drugs for the Past Year and Past Month, 2006 and 2007

	Past Year		Past Month	
Drug	**2006**	**2007**	**2006**	**2007**
Marijuana	10.3	10.1	6.0	5.8
Cocaine	2.5	2.3	1.0	0.8
Inhalants	0.9	0.8	0.3	0.2
Hallucinogens	1.6	1.5	0.4	0.4
Heroin	0.2	0.1	0.1	0.1
Nonmedical use of any psychotherapeutic	6.7	6.6	2.9	2.8
Alcohol	66.0	65.7	50.9	51.1
Cigarettes	29.1	28.5	25.0	24.2

Note: Psychotherapeutic drugs include any prescription-type stimulant, sedative, tranquilizer, or analgesic. They do not include over-the-counter drugs. "Use" means used at least one time.

Source: SAMHSA (2008).

TABLE 1.2 Percentages of Individuals in Different Age Groups Who Reported Use of Drugs for the Past Year and Past Month, 2007

	Past Year			Past Month		
Drug	**12–17**	**18–25**	**≥26**	**12–17**	**18–25**	**≥26**
Any illicit drug	18.7	33.2	10.6	9.5	19.7	5.8
Alcohol	31.8	77.9	67.1	15.9	61.2	54.1
Cigarettes	15.7	45.1	27.3	9.8	36.2	24.1

Note: Any illicit drug use includes the nonmedical use of marijuana, cocaine, inhalants, hallucinogens, heroin, or psychotherapeutic drugs at least one time.

Source: SAMHSA (2008).

drug use in the past month, and almost 25% more likely than women to report any alcohol use. For ethnic or racial differences, whites showed the highest rate of alcohol use in the last month, followed by Hispanics and then blacks. For use of any illicit drug in the last month, blacks showed the highest prevalence, followed by whites and Hispanics.

Summary of Survey Data

The NSDUH data suggest that people in the United States use a variety of drugs, and that some drugs are used far more commonly than others. For example, alcohol and nicotine use are considerably more prevalent than is use of any illicit drug. Furthermore, characteristics of the respondents can make a considerable difference in the prevalence of substance use, as we saw for age, gender, and ethnic or racial groups in the 2007 data.

TABLE 1.3 Percentages of Individuals Aged 12 and Older of Different Ethnic and Gender Groups Who Reported Any Illicit Drug or Alcohol Use in the Past Month, 2007

	Any Illicit Drug	Alcohol
Ethnic/Racial Group		
White	8.2	56.1
Black	9.5	39.3
Hispanic	6.6	42.1
Gender		
Male	10.4	56.6
Female	5.8	46.0

Note: Any illicit drug use includes the nonmedical use of marijuana, cocaine, inhalants, hallucinogens, heroin, or psychotherapeutic drugs at least one time.

Source: SAMHSA (2008).

Multiple Drug Use

polydrug use
The same person's regular use of more than one drug.

The person who is counted in the percentage of, say, marijuana users in a survey sample may be the same person who increases the percentage of alcohol users. Such multiple drug use (also called **polydrug use**) is extremely important because of the effects that drug combinations have on the body. We explore those effects in detail in Chapter 4. For now, it is important for you to know that polydrug use is a critical health and social problem.

"I think I did every drug known to mankind, smoked crack, boozed, dropped acid, you name it."
Kid Rock

Using multiple substances on one occasion is not uncommon. According to the 2006 and 2007 NSDUH data, 5.6% of past-month alcohol users used illicit drugs on an occasion within two hours of their alcohol use. As you might expect, the illicit drug used most often with alcohol was marijuana; this pattern was most prevalent among 12- to 17-year-olds and 18- to 25-year-olds compared to older age groups. The respondents who reported "binge" drinking (5 or more drinks) on their last occasion of

CONTEMPORARY ISSUE BOX 1.3

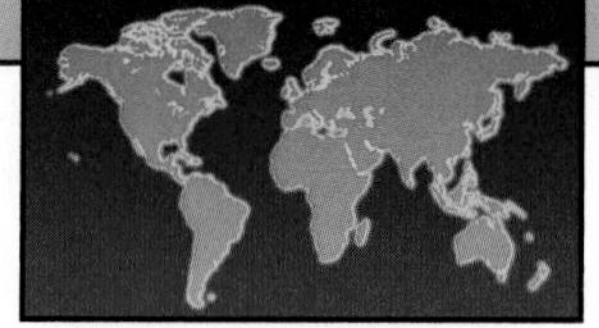

Nonmedical Use of Prescribed Drugs

You may have noticed in Table 1.1 that the illicit drug with the second highest prevalence, after marijuana, is "nonmedical use of any psychotherapeutic." These data reflect the alarm in the last few years among drug enforcement officials in the United States because of what seems to be a sharp increase in the nonmedical use of prescribed drugs. Painkillers such as OxyContin that became available relatively recently have been identified as a major source of the increased abuse rates, but many other drugs meant to be used as medical treatments to alleviate physical or psychological suffering are abused too. Another example especially prevalent on college campuses is the nonmedical use of prescription stimulant medications.

Two factors that may contribute to the increased abuse of medications are "doctor shopping" to get multiple prescriptions to treat a single physical or psychological ailment and the advertisement of prescription drugs over the Internet. Sales of drugs over the Internet are difficult for officials to track.

The abuse of prescription drugs is associated with the same kinds of physical, psychological, and social problems that come with the abuse of any other drug. Therefore, it is important to find ways to prevent or reduce such abuse. One way is for the federal government to provide resources to the individual states to develop computerized drug-prescription monitoring systems (which monitor who writes the prescriptions and who gets them). Such systems may help to address the doctor-shopping problem. Can you think of other solutions to the abuse of prescription drugs?

alcohol use were far more likely (13.9%) to report concurrent alcohol–illicit drug use than were the respondents who did not binge drink (had fewer than 5 drinks).

In its extreme, multiple drug use can include taking drugs with different or opposite physical effects in sequence on the same occasion. In such cases, the motive for use seems to be change, positive or otherwise, from one drug experience to another. An instance of extreme polydrug use, excerpted from Goldman (1971) and cited in Mendelson and Mello (1985, pp. 200–201), illustrates how people may use one type of drug after another, without apparent rhyme or reason. The example involves the famous comedian Lenny Bruce, who died in 1966, at age 40, and an associate of his:

> The night before, they ended a very successful three-week run in Chicago by traveling to the Cloisters (in New York City) and visiting the home of a show-biz druggist—a house so closely associated with drugs that show people call it the "shooting gallery." Terry smoked a couple of joints, dropped two blue tabs of mescaline, and skin-popped some Dilaudid; at the airport bar he also downed two double Scotches. Lenny did his usual number: 12, 1/16-**grain** Dilaudid pills counted out of a big brown bottle, dissolved in a 1-cubic centimeter (cc) ampoule of Methedrine, and heated in a blackened old spoon. The resulting soup was drawn into a disposable needle and then whammed into mainline (intravenously) until you feel like you're living inside an igloo. Lenny also was into mescaline that evening: Not just Terry's two little old-maidish tabs, but a whole fistful, chewed up in his mouth and then washed down with a chocolate Yoo-Hoo.

grain
As a measure, a unit of weight equal to 0.0648 gram.

International Comparisons of Drug Use

The national surveys on drug use that the United States conducts provide extremely useful information. It would be valuable if similar data were available from other countries so that comparisons would be possible. Unfortunately, this has not been

DRUGS AND CULTURE BOX 1.4

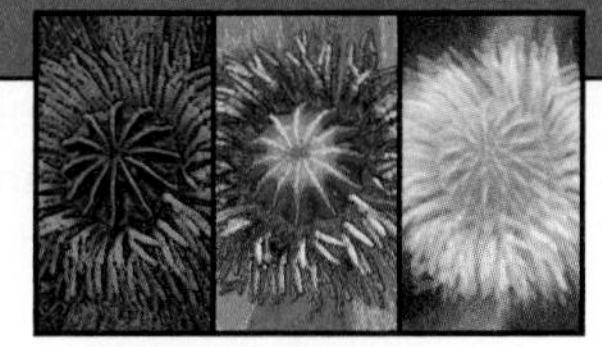

The National Survey of Drug Use and Health and Subgroup Differences

You know from our discussion that the National Survey of Drug Use and Health data give us a great description of drug use among people living in the United States. At the same time, national surveys do not actually tell us as much as they seem to. We must take into account the differences in use patterns according to characteristics—such as age, gender, and race—of the user and the user's environment—such as area of residence and local laws and policies regarding alcohol and drug use.

Demographic group differences in drug use reflect differences in complex historical or current factors common to certain groups of people or regions. Therefore, drug use differences could reflect biological, psychological, or social/environmental factors that distinguish one group from other groups or from the population as a whole. These factors are so complex that certain groups have been designated "special populations." This label emphasizes that, to understand a particular group's drug use, we need to understand its unique history and current circumstances. Groups that today are considered special populations by experts who study drug use include women (because traditionally women have received far less attention from alcohol and other drug researchers than have men), Native Americans, African Americans, the homeless, and Hispanics. A recent review suggests that adults and adolescents who identify their sexual orientation as lesbian, gay, or bisexual should also be considered a special population regarding their alcohol and drug use (Marshal et al., 2008). The drug chapters in this text incorporate cultural and regional differences with features such as a historical account of the drug or drug class in question, and with attention to special cultural differences in use of the drug.

Given the importance of subgroup differences within a total survey sample, how might you adjust the sampling in a national survey to get a more accurate look at a subgroup that is of particular interest to you?

possible with the exception of alcohol use in some cases. In this regard, population surveys of both alcohol and other drug use that different countries, including the United States, have done have not been designed with consideration of how other countries have designed their surveys, so comparisons of findings across countries have been difficult. However, it is fortunate that recent epidemiological data on lifetime drug use in specific countries in North America, South America, and Europe provide an opportunity for cross-national comparisons of general population use of alcohol and selected other drugs.

The study we focus on here involved surveys similarly constructed and administered at seven sites to over 27,000 individuals aged between 14 and 54 years (Vega et al., 2002). The emphasis of this report was lifetime use of alcohol, defined as used at least 12 times, and lifetime use of other drugs, defined as used at least five times. Surveys were conducted in the following cities/countries: Fresno County, California, United States; Mexico City, Mexico; Ontario, Canada; the Netherlands; Sao Paulo, Brazil; and Munich, Germany.

The results showed interesting similarities and differences across the countries in alcohol and other drug use. It was true in all of the countries that lifetime use of alcohol or other drugs occurred at a higher rate for men than for women. Regarding alcohol use, the Netherlands was the highest, as about 94% of the men and 78% of the women reported lifetime use. Canada was second highest (84% of the men, 60% of the women), and the United States was third (80% of the men and 63% of the women). The lowest rates were reported in Mexico City, with 73% of the men but only 21% of the women reporting lifetime alcohol use.

Other drugs showed not only some similarities across countries but also wide variability in lifetime use. Cannabis use was the second most prevalent behind alcohol for all countries. The level of cannabis use, however, varied considerably across countries. For example, the highest prevalence was in the United States, with 33% of the men and 24% of the women reporting lifetime use. Similarly, 29% of the male Canadians and 16% of the women in Canada reported cannabis use. These figures contrast with the lowest rates, recorded in Mexico: 3% of the men and 0.6% of the women. After cannabis, the rates of lifetime use of other drugs or drug classes (cocaine or other stimulants, anxiolytics, opioids, hallucinogens, inhalants) were highly variable but generally at a low level, with the exception of cocaine or other stimulants and anxiolytics in the United States. As you might guess, overall lifetime drug use, excluding alcohol and cannabis, was highest in the United States (19%) and lowest in Mexico (2%).

Although the Vega et al. (2002) data on lifetime use of alcohol and other drugs are limited, they do provide a first look at how different countries, at least those in the western part of the world, compare. Cross-national data can be a valuable vehicle to understanding how cultural, legal, psychological, and biological factors affect alcohol and other drug use. We hope the material we present in the rest of this book begins to help you to do that as well.

"No animal ever invented anything as bad as drunkenness or as good as drink."

Lord Chesterton

Negative Consequences of Alcohol and Drug Use

Describing alcohol and drug use returns us to the question of the consequences of such use. We saw that people experience positive consequences from their use of drugs. They may also experience negative effects, which definitions of drug abuse try to capture. One way to look at the negative consequences of alcohol and drug use for society is to conduct "cost-of-illness" studies. The purpose of these studies is to quantify in dollars what society "pays" for its members incurring specific illnesses. It is important to add that focusing on economic factors does not mean no psychological costs are associated with illness. However, psychological consequences are not easily quantified and thus are much more difficult to analyze.

Two major "illness" distinctions that have been studied in detail are alcohol abuse and other drug abuse. In such research, "drug abuse" concerns the use of illegal drugs and the nonprescription use of drugs typically used for therapeutic purposes. Nicotine use has not been included. (This is not to understate the costs of nicotine use to U.S. society. The costs are devastating and are reviewed in Chapter 7.)

A report by the Schneider Institute for Health Policy (2001) included estimates of the economic costs of alcohol abuse and other drug abuse to U.S. society. The study yielded the estimate that, in 1995, alcohol abuse cost the United States about $166.5 billion and drug abuse cost $109.9 billion. The total: more than $276 billion. Most people cannot even conceptualize what $1 billion is, never mind hundreds of billions of dollars. To help you understand how much money we are talking about, here is one illustration: A wealthy woman gives her sister $1 million to put in a drawer, telling her she can spend $1,000 a day and to call when the money is spent. Three years later, the sister calls. If the original sum had been $1 billion, the sister would not have called for 3,000 years. In any case, our difficulty in picturing billions of dollars does not make the cost of alcohol and drug abuse any less real.

The costs of both alcohol and drug abuse come from a wide range of sources, although the costs are not distributed in the same proportions for the two types of illnesses. The sources include illness, death, medical expenses, and crime. Crime-related costs are especially significant for drug abuse (58% of the total).

Cost-of-illness studies give us a good, well-rounded estimate of what society pays for its members' involvement with alcohol and other drugs. The multibillion-dollar cost estimates are staggering but ironically understate the impact. Some of the consequences of alcohol and drug use become clear when we think about what events make up the cost computations. For example, lifetimes of individuals will not be lived fully because the individuals were born with fetal alcohol syndrome (see Chapter 9). Or hospital emergency room resources are used for overdoses of cocaine, heroin, and MDMA (see Chapters 6, 10, and 12, respectively). Then there is the suffering of a family who lost one of its young members because he was shot and killed in a robbery to obtain drugs. Maybe you have experienced what it is like to lose a friend or family member in one of the thousands of fatal alcohol-related traffic accidents that occur every year in the United States. It is important to step away from the statistics to look at these and other realities that make up the true costs of alcohol and drugs to society.

"Unlike others, he (a heroin addict) could not find a vocation, a career, a meaningful, sustained activity around which he could wrap his life. Instead he relied on the addiction to provide a vocation around which he could build a reasonably full life and establish an identity."

Psychologist Isidor Chein (Quoted in Krogh, 1991, p. 133)

Defining Harmful Drug Use

Discussing cost-of-illness research brings our focus back to what might be called harmful drug use, or use that is associated with detrimental consequences to the drug user or to others. Indeed, to reflect on harmful use, cost-of-illness studies have used terms like *alcohol abuse* and *drug abuse*. Yet, in the beginning of this chapter, we mentioned the widely different meanings of these terms. This is a problem because it hampers communication about drug use. The lack of standard definitions also tends to slow the advance of knowledge. If there is disagreement about what it is we are trying to gain knowledge about, you can see why scientific advances might be impeded.

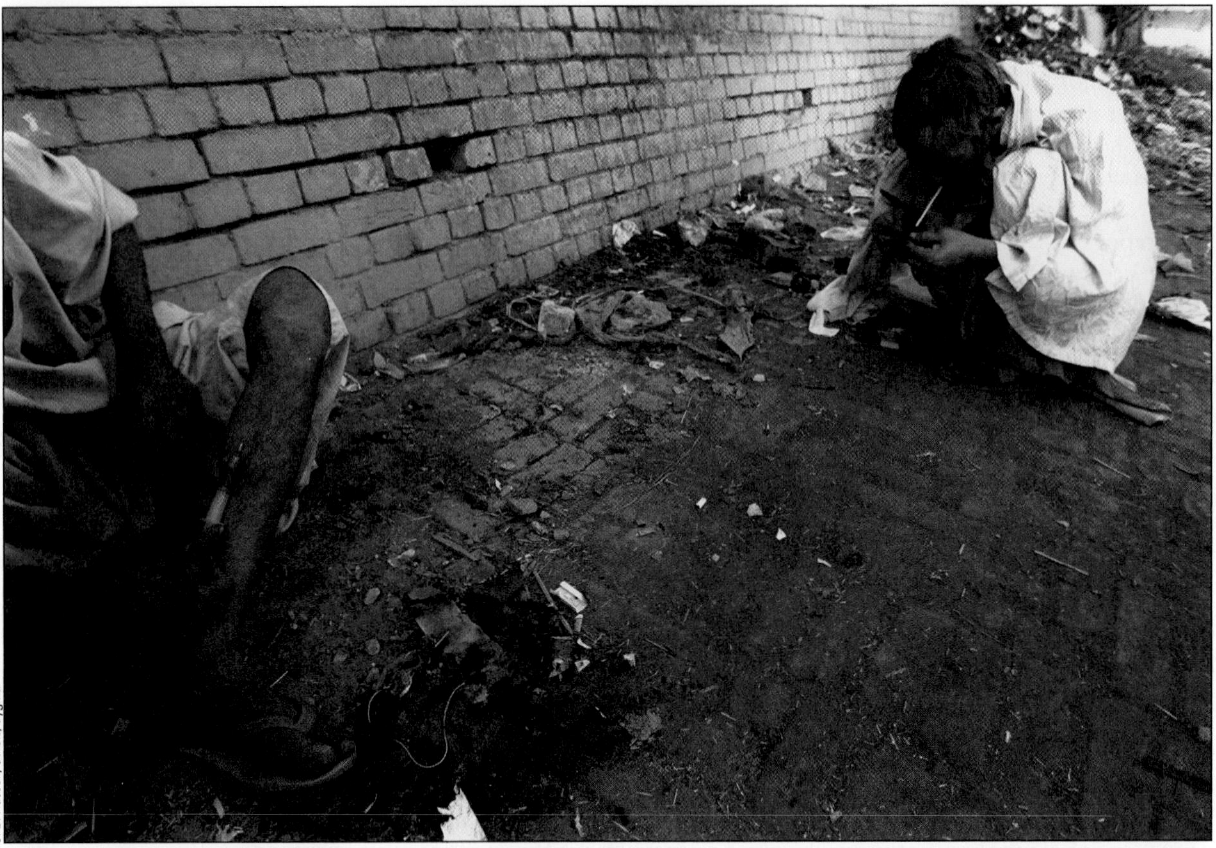

J. B. Russell/Corbis/Sygma

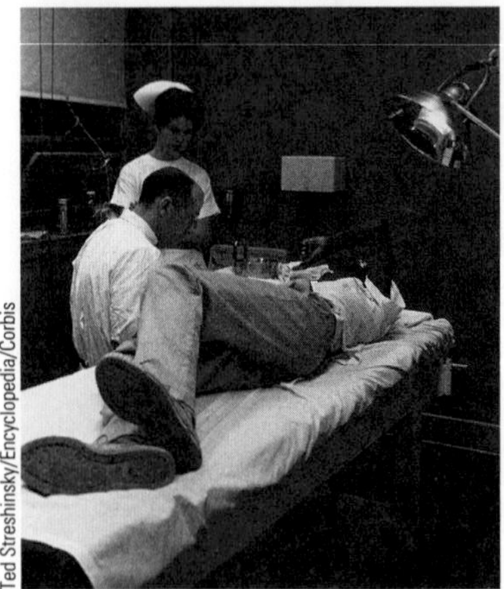

Ted Streshinsky/Encyclopedia/Corbis

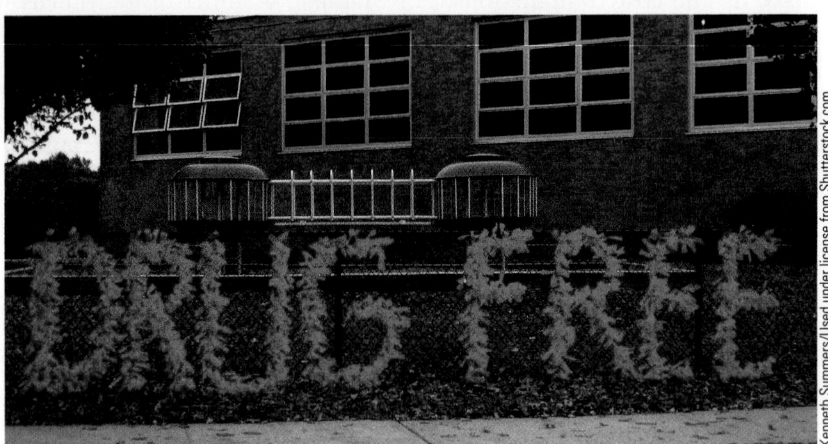

Kenneth Summers/Used under license from Shutterstock.com

The sometimes tragic consequences of drug use have drawn national attention and response.

Use of the DSM-IV

In the United States and other countries, providers of care for physical and mental illness have handled problems of definition by developing systems of definitions of illnesses, or *diagnostic systems.* A diagnosis typically is based on a cluster of symptoms that is given a name (the diagnosis). The advantage is that, say, if two physicians are communicating about pneumonia in a patient and they are following the same diagnostic system, then each knows exactly what the referent of the other is when the term

CONTEMPORARY ISSUE BOX 1.5

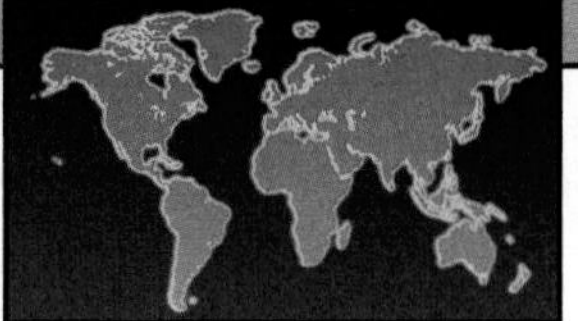

Drugs, Criminal Activity, and Aggression

We have noted how costs associated with criminal behavior are especially significant for drug abuse. The association of alcohol, drugs, and crime is one we seem to see and hear about continually in the popular media.

The problem of drugs, alcohol, and crime is an old, much-studied one. It should be clear that we are dealing with associations, or correlations, and not causes. For example, the pharmacological effects of cocaine are not known to *cause* a person to commit murder. Yet the high positive correlation between drugs and crime remains a fact: As drug use in a community increases, so does the occurrence of certain kinds of crimes, depending on the drug.

Much of the research on drugs and crime has concerned heroin. Most crimes committed by heroin addicts are either violations of the drug laws or ways to get money to buy more heroin. Therefore, the addict's most commonly committed crimes are burglary, larceny, assault, and other street crimes. These crimes are indeed serious and sometimes result in injury or death to the victims. The direct intent of the crime is not to harm the victim, however, but to get money. This same motive probably applies to much of the violence related to cocaine, and to conflicts over money among cocaine dealers and their customers.

Surprisingly, the use of some drugs has no relationship to criminal activity; there may even be a negative association between use of the drug and crime. Use of hallucinogens, for example, is not associated with crime, and marijuana seems to fall in the same category. The evidence is mixed for barbiturates and tranquilizers: Some studies show no relationship, but others suggest that the relationship between use and crime is the same for barbiturates and alcohol.

Alcohol intoxication has a high correlation with criminal activity. Because alcohol is legal and very available, little violence is connected with violating drug laws or stealing to obtain alcohol. Most of the crimes associated with alcohol intoxication are assaultive; that is, they are committed with the intent to harm the victim. Alcohol is correlated with other types of crime as well, such as aggravated assault, homicides, property offenses, sexual offenses, and check fraud.

So one point is clear: Some types of drug use are associated with criminal activity. But what is the explanation? Pharmacology figures complexly in the answer but seems to be only one of many factors. Others include the person's expectations about the drug's effects, the setting where the drug is being used, and personality characteristics of the user.

The drug–crime problem is a good example of how a society and its individual members are affected by drug use. It also illustrates that drug use and its effects on the user are influenced by many factors working together.

pneumonia is used. That is, a specific cluster of symptoms is being referred to. It also is possible to create diagnostic systems of mental illnesses. In the United States, the primary organization responsible for doing that has been the American Psychiatric Association (APA). Since the early 1950s, the APA has published formal diagnostic systems of different mental illnesses or disorders in its *Diagnostic and Statistical Manual* (DSM). The most recent version (systems are revised because of ongoing research that provides new information about different disorders) appeared in May 1994 and is called DSM-IV. The DSM-IV has a section called "substance-related" (alcohol- or other drug-related) disorders, which includes definitions of two "substance-use disorders": "substance dependence" and "substance abuse." (We should note here that the APA published DSM-IV-TR in 2000, because of changes in the coding system and some of the diagnostic categories. However, the substance-use disorders categories were not changed.)

Table 1.4 lists the criteria for defining substance dependence and abuse according to DSM-IV (American Psychiatric Association, 1994). It is important to make a few comments about the criteria. Most generally, the same criteria are applied in defining dependence and abuse for all drugs and drug classes that people tend to use for nonmedical reasons. That includes all the drugs we discuss in this text. Another general point is that dependence and abuse are considered separate diagnoses. A person could

TABLE 1.4 DSM-IV Diagnostic Criteria for Substance Dependence and Abuse

Substance Dependence

A maladaptive pattern of substance use leading to clinically significant impairment or distress, as manifested by three or more of the following occurring at any time in the same 12-month period:

1. Tolerance, as defined by either of the following:
   (a) Need for markedly increased amounts of the substance to achieve intoxication or desired effect
   (b) Markedly diminished effect with continued use of the same amount of the substance
2. Withdrawal, as manifested by either of the following:
   (a) The characteristic withdrawal syndrome for the substance
   (b) The same (closely related) substance is taken to relieve or avoid withdrawal symptoms
3. The substance is often taken in larger amounts or over a longer period than was intended
4. A persistent desire or unsuccessful efforts to cut down or control substance use
5. A great deal of time is spent in activities necessary to obtain the substance (e.g., visiting multiple doctors or driving long distances), to use the substance (e.g., chain-smoking), or to recover from its effects
6. Important social, occupational, or recreational activities given up or reduced because of substance use
7. Continued substance use despite knowledge of having had a persistent or recurrent physical or psychological problem that is likely to be caused by or exacerbated by the substance (e.g., current cocaine use despite recognition of cocaine-induced depression, or continued drinking despite recognition that an ulcer was made worse by alcohol consumption)

Specify if:
With physiological dependence: Evidence of tolerance or withdrawal (that is, either item [1] or [2] is present).

Substance Abuse

A maladaptive pattern of substance use leading to clinically significant impairment or distress, as manifested by one or more of the following:

1. Recurrent substance use resulting in a failure to fulfill major role obligations at work, school, or home (e.g., repeated absences or poor work performance related to substance use; substance-related absences, suspensions, or expulsions from school; neglect of children or household)
2. Recurrent substance use in situations in which it is physically hazardous (e.g., driving an automobile or operating a machine when impaired by substance use)
3. Recurrent substance-related legal problems (e.g., arrests for substance-related disorderly conduct)
4. Continued substance use despite having persistent or recurrent social or interpersonal problems caused or exacerbated by the effects of the substance (e.g., arguments with spouse about consequences of intoxication, physical fights)

Does not meet the criteria for substance dependence for this substance?

Source: Reprinted with permission from the *Diagnostic and Statistical Manual of Mental Disorders*, Fourth Edition. Copyright 1994. American Psychiatric Association.

addiction
In reference to drugs, overwhelming involvement with using a drug, getting an adequate supply of it, and having a strong tendency to resume use of it after stopping for a period.

not be diagnosed with both dependence and abuse of a given substance, although it is possible to meet the criteria for dependence on one substance and for abuse of another.

Regarding dependence, criteria 3 through 6 focus on what traditionally has been called "compulsive drug use," or drug **addiction**. In essence, the individual's life centers on drug use and its procurement to the point of reduced attention to or outright neglect of other aspects of life. Similarly, drug use persists despite the risk of incurring serious consequences by doing so. Individuals with addictions also have an inability to stop or to reduce drug use for any length of time, if that is the intention. This phenomenon has been called "loss of control."

The first two criteria for dependence introduce two terms: *tolerance* and *withdrawal*. We have more to say about them later in this chapter and in other chapters in this text. In DSM-IV, a distinction is made between a diagnosis of dependence without meeting criteria for either tolerance or withdrawal, and a dependence diagnosis that does meet either of those two criteria. At least three of the seven criteria listed for dependence must be met for the diagnosis to be made.

While we are discussing the DSM-IV definition of dependence, we would like to define a term that you probably have heard or read because it is so commonly used: **psychological dependence**. Like many terms used in communicating about drugs and their use, *psychological dependence* has had different meanings. So the Rinaldi et al. (1988) consensus definition is useful again. In the Rinaldi study, psychological dependence was defined as "the emotional state of **craving** a drug either for its positive effect or to avoid negative effects associated with its abuse" (p. 557). As you can see, psychological dependence is far more narrowly but less precisely defined than is dependence in DSM-IV, and it focuses on the strong desire to use a drug to alter a psychological state or to escape or avoid some unpleasant experience.

psychological dependence
The emotional state of craving a drug either for its positive effect or to avoid negative effects associated with its abuse.

craving
A term that has been variously defined in reference to drug use; typically a strong or intense desire to use a drug.

The criteria for substance abuse center on consequences in different areas of life (family, social, or job) that may reasonably be connected to substance use. Four criteria are listed for abuse, and a person has to meet at least one of them to receive the diagnosis.

We would like to say a few more words about the DSM-IV definitions before concluding our discussion of them. The DSM-IV criteria, which are based on the most current knowledge about substance-use disorders that comes from research and clinical practice, ease problems in communication because they are clearly written, descriptive criteria. This does not mean that the criteria are perfect; indeed the expectation is that the criteria will continue to evolve as new knowledge accrues. In this regard, having a generally accepted definition of a phenomenon makes it far more likely that we will acquire new knowledge about substance use and eventually have a good understanding of it. Another point you may have noticed is that the DSM-IV offers definitions of dependence on and abuse of drugs but provides no definition of drug use. In DSM-IV terms, *drug use* would be any consumption of alcohol or other drugs and related events that does not meet the criteria for dependence or abuse.

Although we may never get away entirely from the influence of societal values on definitions of substance-use disorders, the creators of DSM-IV have considerably advanced our ability to communicate about harmful drug use. Because of this, DSM-IV is ubiquitous in alcohol and other drug treatment and research settings in the United States. Accordingly, we follow the DSM-IV definitions where relevant in the remaining chapters of this text.

Drug Tolerance, Withdrawal, and Drug-Taking Behavior

The DSM-IV criteria for dependence include the term ***drug tolerance***, which was defined in parts (a) and (b) of criterion 1 in Table 1.4. Another new term is ***withdrawal symptoms***. Withdrawal is a definable illness that occurs with a cessation or decrease in drug use after the body has adjusted to the presence of a drug to such a degree that it cannot function without the drug. Not all drugs are associated with an identifiable withdrawal **syndrome** (also called *abstinence syndrome*). For any drug associated with withdrawal symptoms, the severity of those symptoms may change with the characteristics of the users and their history of use of that drug. Furthermore, psychological symptoms, such as anxiety, depression, and craving for drugs, are often

tolerance
Generally, increased amounts of a drug needed to achieve intoxication, or a diminished drug effect with continued use of the same amount of a drug.

withdrawal
A definable illness that occurs with a cessation or decrease in use of a drug.

syndrome
In medicine, a number of symptoms that occur together and characterize a specific illness or disease.

part of withdrawal syndromes. These psychological symptoms strongly influence whether the individual can stop using drugs for any length of time.

We draw your attention to drug tolerance and withdrawal in this introductory chapter because they are central topics in psychopharmacology. Tolerance and withdrawal are addressed as part of any evaluation or study of a drug. As a result, we discuss these concepts in far more detail in later chapters. It is critical to mention now, however, that tolerance and withdrawal affect drug-use patterns. For example, if tolerance to a drug develops, the individual must consume increasing amounts of it to achieve a desired drug effect. Such a trend in use may affect how much time the person devotes each day to acquiring the drug and to using it. Furthermore, with greater quantities and frequencies of drug use, the person becomes more susceptible to experiencing various negative physical, social, or legal consequences.

Drug withdrawal also makes a person more likely to continue or resume the use of a drug after a period of abstaining. Many studies have shown that relief from withdrawal is a powerful motivator of drug use. In this regard, drug withdrawal may begin when the level of drug in the blood drops. If the user takes more of the drug at this point, the withdrawal symptoms are relieved. Here the motivating force is the "turning off" of unpleasant withdrawal symptoms, which works to perpetuate a powerful cycle of drug use–drug withdrawal–drug use. Withdrawal is also associated with a higher likelihood of resuming drug use following a period of abstinence because of learned reactions to cues in the environment. We describe how this might happen in Chapter 5.

We want to emphasize here that the influences of tolerance and withdrawal are at the heart of psychopharmacology—the incentives or motivators that drive human (and other animal) drug use. Chapter 5, on the principles and methods of psychopharmacology, addresses this topic in detail.

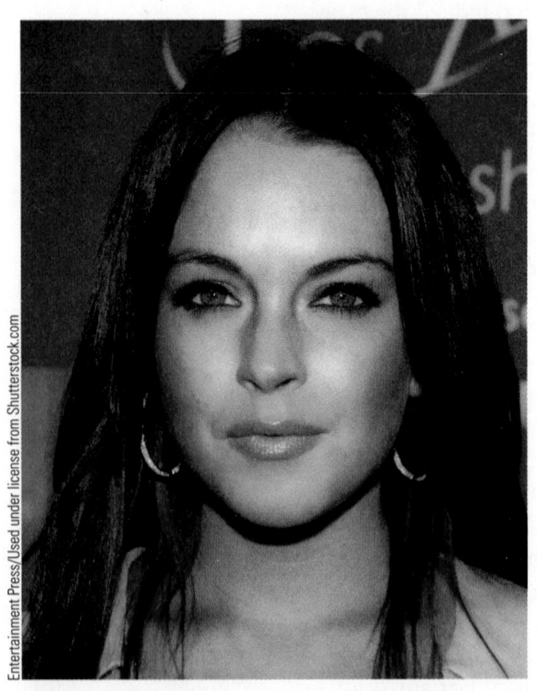

Actress and recording artist Lindsay Lohan's life illustrates a main feature of drug addiction—the neglect of professional responsibilities and personal relationships for the sake of obtaining and using drugs.

You may have observed from this discussion of drug tolerance, withdrawal, and drug-taking behavior that they may be instrumental in the development of what we defined earlier as drug addiction. Another factor that may be critical to the development of addictive drug-use patterns is "sensitization" (Robinson & Berridge, 2003). The sensitization hypothesis is that one result of repeated use of a drug in interaction with environmental factors is changes in the brain neural pathways (Chapter 3) that may heighten (sensitize) the reward value of that drug. This means that the drug's effects become more appealing to an individual, and therefore procurement of the drug may assume increasing control over the individual's behavior. Critically, the brain changes resulting from repeated drug use may be permanent, which is one reason why drug addiction may be such an intractable problem for many people, as we show later in this book.

This discussion shows that using a drug for a long time alters the patterns of use for that drug. Long-term use also relates to the DSM-IV criteria. Tolerance, withdrawal, and sensitization may result not only in changes in drug use and preoccupation but also in the likelihood that the person's life and the lives of those around that person are affected by the drug in a snowballing effect, with one consequence building on another. The outcome can reflect some of the criteria included in the DSM-IV definition of substance-use disorder.

Of course, discussion of the effects of tolerance and dependence on motivations for drug use addresses only a small minority of the different reasons that people use drugs, which takes us back to the 10 systems that influence or are influenced by drug use that we discussed at the beginning of this chapter. In this regard, people give numerous reasons for "why" they use different drugs, and different drugs may be most strongly associated with different reasons. At the same time, multiple drugs may be used for the same reasons. The same drug may be used for different reasons in different times and places. This suggests that reasons for use are not limited to a drug's pharmacological effects but by a variety of other variables as well. For example, Boys, Marsden, and Strang (2001) conducted an interview study of 364 men and women ages 16 to 22 in the United Kingdom who had used two or more substances in the last 90 days. The study showed that use of substances such as alcohol, marijuana, cocaine, ecstasy, and LSD was associated with multiple "purposes" or functions, which referred to what the participants expected to gain by using the drugs. Each substance was associated with eight to nine different functions (such as feeling better when depressed, getting intoxicated, enhancing sex, helping to relax, helping to sleep, and enhancing another activity, such as listening to music), and there was considerable overlap in the functions cited for each drug, despite their considerable differences in pharmacology. The upshot of findings such as these is that they highlight the complexity in motivations for drug use among humans, and we will spend considerable space elaborating upon this basic point in subsequent chapters of this text. The complexity of human alcohol and drug use is also represented in the models of the causes of the substance-use disorders that are summarized in Chapter 15.

"If drinking is interfering with your work, you're probably a heavy drinker. If your work is interfering with your drinking, you're probably an alcoholic."

Anonymous

"I will lift mine eyes unto the pills. Almost everyone takes them, from the humble aspirin to the multi-colored, king-sized three-deckers, which put you to sleep, wake you up, stimulate and soothe you all in one. It is an age of pills."

Malcolm Muggeridge, 1962

"In the 1960s, people took acid to make the world weird. Now the world is weird, and people take Prozac to make it normal."

Author unknown.

Overview of the Text

You now are ready for a brief overview of the rest of this text, which is divided into three main sections. The first section, which includes Chapters 1 through 5, gives you fundamental information on psychopharmacology and the history of laws and policy regarding drug use in the United States and other countries. You saw that this first chapter introduced you to important definitions of concepts and the epidemiology of drug use. Chapter 2 places human drug use in a historical context by giving you a better appreciation of today's use patterns and the social and political contexts in which they occur. Chapter 3 is a basic discussion of the nervous system and how drugs affect it. This knowledge is essential to understanding drug effects because, no matter what drug effect or experience you consider, some change in the nervous system is inevitable. Chapter 4 concerns pharmacology, as we review the methods scientists use to study drugs and their effects. Chapter 5 focuses on principles and methods of psychopharmacology, which is the central topic of this text. Chapters 4 and 5 will help you to understand how we have learned much of what we know about drugs.

Chapters 6 through 14 constitute the second section of the text and concern individual drugs and drug classes. Our drug topics include cocaine and the amphetamines, nicotine, caffeine, alcohol, opiates, marijuana, hallucinogens, psychiatric medications, and other prescription or **over-the-counter drugs**. These chapters follow a broad outline of historical overview and epidemiology; mechanisms of drug action; medical and psychotherapeutic uses; and physiological, psychological, and

over-the-counter drugs
Drugs that can be obtained legally without a medical prescription.

social or environmental effects. Your study of each of the drug chapters will give you a good understanding of that drug (or drug class) and its use.

The last section of the text consists of two chapters on topics geared to the general public that are often discussed in media. Chapter 15 is a review of the treatment of the substance-use disorders, and Chapter 16 covers the prevention of substance-use disorders before they occur. Prevention is a fitting topic on which to end this text because that is what all the research, politics, and discussion are about—reaching the goal of living in a society free of substance-use disorders.

Evaluating Websites

We will close this chapter with discussion of a topic that is relevant to your research on drugs and therefore central to this text: evaluating World Wide Web pages. College students often view "doing research" as synonymous with "searching the Web."

TABLE 1.5 Five Criteria to Help You Evaluate World Wide Web Pages

1. Accuracy of web documents
   - Who wrote the page, and can you contact him or her?
   - What is the purpose of the document, and why was it produced? Is the person qualified to write this document?
   - Make sure the author provides an e-mail or a contact address and/or phone number.
   - Know the distinction between author and web master.
2. Authority of web documents
   - What credentials are listed for the author(s)?
   - Who published the document, and is the publisher separate from the web master?
   - Check the domain of the document: What institution publishes this document?
   - Does the publisher list its qualifications?
3. Objectivity of web documents
   - What goals and objectives does this page meet?
   - How detailed is the information?
   - What opinions (if any) are expressed by the author?
   - Determine whether the page is a mask for advertising; if so, information might be biased.
   - View any web page as you would an infomercial on television. Ask why was this written, and for whom.
4. Currency of web documents
   - When was it produced?
   - When was it updated?
   - How up to date are the links (if any)?
   - How many dead links are on the page?
   - Are the links current or updated regularly?
   - Is the information on the page outdated?
5. Coverage of web documents
   - Are the links (if any) evaluated, and do they complement the document's theme?
   - Is the site all images or a balance of text and images?
   - Is the presented information cited correctly?
   - If special software is required to view the information, how much are you missing if you do not have the software?
   - Is it free, or is there a fee to obtain the information?
   - Is there an option for text only, or frames, or a suggested browser for better viewing?

Source: J. Kapoun (1998). Teaching undergrads web evaluation: A guide for library instruction. *College and Research Library News, 59,* 522–523. Reprinted with permission from the American Library Association.

There are good reasons for that. Although the World Wide Web should not be seen as eradicating the need for books, articles, and other print materials in doing research, it is a phenomenal complement to them. Indeed, we have listed several of what we judge to be good websites for each chapter of this text on the Companion Website at www.cengage.com/psychology/maisto, so you can search them if you want more information on any topic we cover.

As you know, information on the web is wide-ranging in scope and usually instantly accessed. Information on drugs is a good example. Go to Google, type in the search word *drugs,* click, and you have access to 160,000,000 (as of June 2009) potentially useful web pages! *Potential* is a key word here because web pages are not monitored for accuracy or currency or even for whether they or links related to them still exist. Therefore, in seeking nonfictional information, the web user must determine whether the data under review meet standards that would stand up in the research community.

Fortunately, a number of educators have thought a lot about evaluating web pages. Kapoun (1998) has provided a checklist of five criteria to help you to evaluate a web page: accuracy, authority, objectivity, currency, and coverage. They are summarized for you in Table 1.5. We encourage you to learn these criteria until they are second nature to you, if you have not done so already. The effort will be valuable to you in this course and in any other context that requires you to have accurate and current information.

Summary

- Psychopharmacology—the scientific study of the effects of drugs on behavior—is the subject of this text.
- Drugs may be classified in different ways; six of the major ones are reviewed in this chapter.
- The experience that humans have from taking drugs is influenced by three sets of factors: pharmacological factors, characteristics of the drug user, and the setting in which the drug is used.
- National survey data show that people in the United States use a variety of drugs. Alcohol, tobacco cigarettes, and marijuana or hashish consistently have appeared as the most commonly tried and currently used psychoactive drugs.
- Getting an accurate picture of drug use is possible only by looking at the characteristics of the users. For example, the heaviest and most frequent illicit drug use is among young adults (ages 18 to 25). Also, men are more likely than women to report alcohol and drug use in the past month.
- Some individuals use more than one drug regularly and may use different drugs together on the same occasion.
- In 1995, the estimated economic cost of alcohol and illicit drug abuse to the United States totaled more than $276 billion.
- The formal definition of substance-use disorders in the United States is given in the fourth edition of the American Psychiatric Association's *Diagnostic and Statistical Manual.*
- The DSM-IV definition includes drug tolerance and withdrawal, which may powerfully affect drug-use patterns.
- This book covers basic psychopharmacology concepts, details on major drugs and drug classes and those who use them, and discussions of prevention and treatment for a better understanding of drugs and human behavior.

Answers to "What Do You Think?"

1. Because the effects of drugs are both predictable and obvious, it is relatively easy to define drug abuse.
   F *Drugs have a variety of effects on people, and the way drugs are perceived may vary in different cultures and subcultures. As a result, it has proved difficult to create a definition of drug abuse that is generally agreeable.*
2. A drug's street name sometimes describes the actual effects of that drug.
   T *Street names, which come from drug subcultures and the street drug market, sometimes do reflect actual drug effects.*
3. A person's reaction to a drug depends mostly on the biological action of the drug in the body.
   F *Biology is important, but psychological and social or environmental factors must also be included to explain the effects of psychoactive drugs on humans.*
4. Because drug use is complicated, it is impossible to estimate patterns of drug use for the population of a whole country.
   F *Drug use is complicated, but sophisticated sampling methods and computers have made it possible to select large numbers of people and survey them to derive precise estimates of drug use in a given population.*
5. Within the United States, similar patterns of alcohol and other drug use are found even among different subgroups of the population.
   F *Drug use has been found to vary with characteristics of the person and of the environment.*
6. The highest rates of alcohol and other drug use are found among 18- to 25-year-olds.
   T *People in this age group, called "young adults," have the highest rates of alcohol and other drug use in the United States.*
7. A person's use of more than one drug at a time is of little concern because it happens so infrequently.
   F *Although multiple drug use is not as frequent as use of a single substance, it is hardly rare, especially among young people. It is of great concern because combining drugs sometimes has unpredictable effects that may be life-threatening.*
8. The total economic cost of alcohol and drug abuse in the United States is about a billion dollars annually.
   F *The most recent estimates suggest it is more than 276 times that amount.*
9. The use of alcohol and other drugs causes violence and crime.
   F *The use of alcohol and other, but not all other drugs, is associated with violence and crime but does not directly cause such behavior.*
10. Modern researchers rely on definitions of alcohol and other drug use that are free of social or cultural biases.
    F *We are improving our ability to rid our definitions of biases, but due to the influence of social and cultural factors on alcohol and other drug use and the perception of such use, it is unlikely that we will ever arrive at bias-free definitions.*
11. A diagnosis of drug abuse is made when a person has become either physically or psychologically dependent on a drug.
    F *Dependence and abuse are considered separate diagnoses. A person could not be diagnosed with both dependence on and abuse of a single drug.*
12. Definitions of addiction center on overwhelming involvement with a drug.
    T *Addiction is identified when a person has overwhelming involvement with using a drug. The person's life centers on getting an adequate supply of the drug, which takes priority over most or all other parts of life, such as school, job, family, and friends.*
13. The continued use of any drug will eventually lead to tolerance of and physical dependence on that drug.
    F *The continued use of many, but not all, drugs may lead to tolerance of and physical dependence on that drug.*

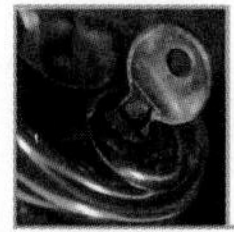

Key Terms

addiction
craving
drug
drug abuse
drug dosage
drug effects
grain
over-the-counter drugs
pharmacology
placebo
polydrug use
prevalence
psychoactive
psychological dependence
psychological set
psychology
psychopharmacology
route of drug administration
syndrome
tolerance
withdrawal

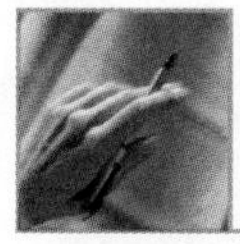

Essays/Thought Questions

1. This chapter argues that drug use has positive as well as negative consequences for humans. Considering the advantages and disadvantages of using different drugs, would you allow the use of a drug that currently is illegal for the most part, such as cocaine, marijuana, or heroin? Why or why not?
2. What are some of the advantages and disadvantages of having a formal, standard way to define a construct like "substance-use disorder," such as DSM-IV does? Should cultural differences in substance use and definitions of *abuse* matter in defining substance-use disorder? Why or why not? If you believe that cultural factors should be incorporated in definitions of substance-use disorder, how would you do it?

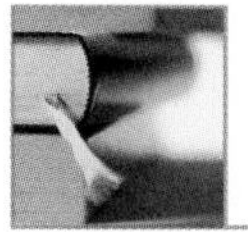

Suggested Readings

Kapoun, J. (1998). Teaching undergrads web evaluation: A guide for library instruction. *College and Research Library News, 59*, 522–523.

Weil, A., & Rosen, W. (1983). *From chocolate to morphine*. Boston: Houghton Mifflin Co.

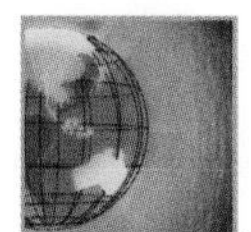

Web Resources

Visit the Book Companion Website at www.cengage.com/psychology/maisto to access study tools including a glossary, flashcards, and web quizzing. You will also find links to the following resources:

- National Institute on Alcohol Abuse and Alcoholism (NIAAA)
- National Institute on Drug Abuse (NIDA)
- Centers for Disease Control and Prevention (CDC)

The websites for Chapter 1 are meant to be resources that provide links to a broad array of valuable information on drug use and on drug abuse and its prevention and treatment. Indeed, the three sites may be used to locate specific information associated with any chapter in this book.

CHAPTER 2

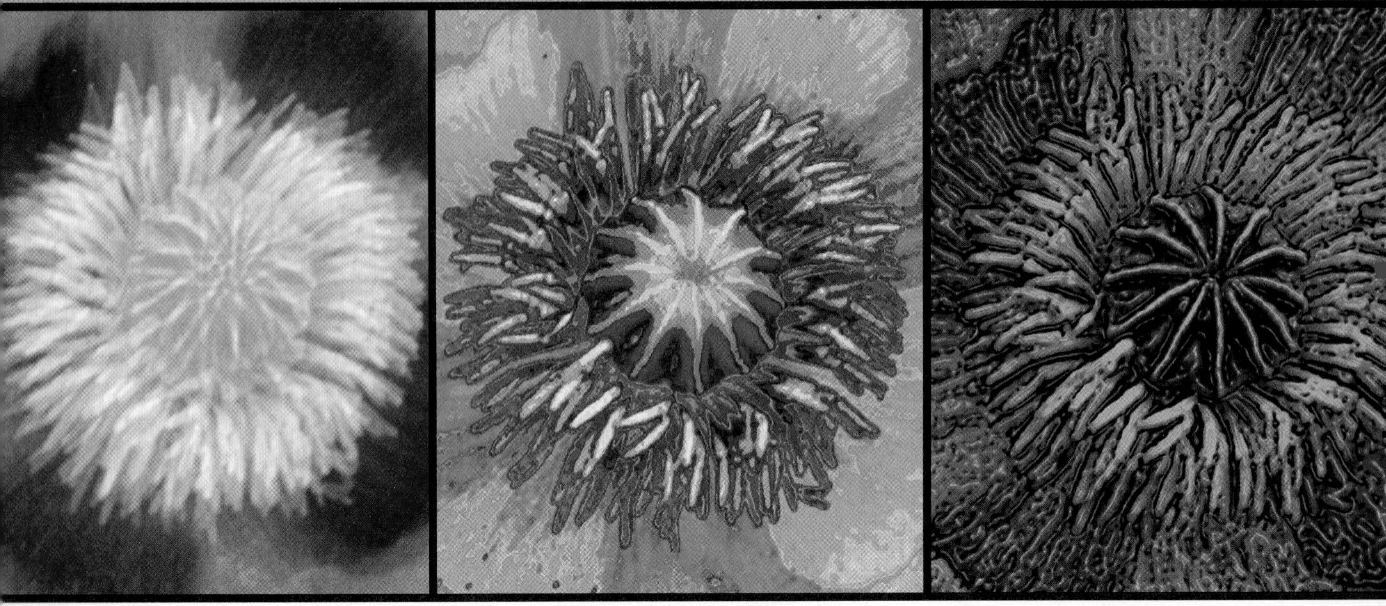

Drug Use
Yesterday and Today

What Do You Think? True or False?

Answers are given at the end of the chapter.

___ 1. The first recorded use of cannabis was in the early 1800s.

___ 2. Grape wine was the first alcoholic beverage to be used.

___ 3. The Opium Wars between China and Great Britain in the mid-1800s occurred in large part because Britain was unwilling to curtail its trade of opium into China.

___ 4. Columbus and his crew were responsible for introducing tobacco to the New World.

___ 5. Many of the drugs that are now illegal in the United States were widely used in the 1800s and early 1900s to treat a broad spectrum of maladies.

___ 6. The first notable drug law in the United States—the 1875 San Francisco ordinance—banned the smoking of opium.

___ 7. The Pure Food and Drug Act of 1906 had little impact on individuals who were addicted to drugs.

___ 8. The Harrison Narcotics Tax Act of 1914 sharply curtailed the prevalence of heroin use in the United States.

___ 9. The Eighteenth Amendment, which prohibited the production, sale, transportation, and importing of alcohol, failed because it did not have a substantial effect on drinking in the United States.

___10. Federal antidrug legislation between 1940 and 1970 failed to have a sustained influence on drug use or dependence.

___11. The most successful aspect of the war on drugs has been the interception of drugs.

___12. Urine testing is a reliable method for detecting drug use.

The use of drugs dates back thousands of years. Drugs have been used for a variety of reasons in different cultures: for religious purposes, for recreation, for altering states of consciousness, and for obtaining relief from pain or distress. In this chapter, we have three objectives. One is to provide you with a historical overview of drug use, from prehistory to recent times. This is a general overview only. More detailed histories of specific psychoactive substances appear in their respective chapters. Nevertheless, a general overview is useful as a picture of the evolution of drug use and as a background for considering the patterns of today's drug use described in Chapter 1. You will notice in some cases that history has repeated itself, and we hope an understanding of such a pattern will help us learn from past experiences. A second goal of this chapter is to discuss some parallels between developments in medicine and the nonmedical use of drugs. Finally, we review the restrictions that have been placed on drug use and summarize current drug laws.

Historical Overview

Indications of psychoactive substance use date back to the beginnings of recorded history and revolve around the use of alcohol and plants with psychoactive properties. Investigations by archeologists suggest that beer and huckleberry wine were used as early as 6400 B.C. (Mellaart, 1967). Alcohol probably was discovered following accidental **fermentation**. (Grape wine, incidentally, did not appear until 300 B.C. to 400 B.C.) Also, various plants were used for the physical and psychological changes they produced, usually in religious or medicinal contexts. As an example, what probably

fermentation
A combustive process in which yeasts interact with the sugars in plants such as grapes, grains, and fruits to produce an enzyme that converts the sugar into alcohol.

opium poppy A plant cultivated for centuries, primarily in Eurasia, for opium—a narcotic that acts as a central nervous system depressant.

Cannabis sativa The Indian hemp plant popularly known as marijuana; its resin, flowering tops, leaves, and stem contain the plant's psychoactive substances.

hashish A drug produced from the resin that covers the flowers of the cannabis hemp plant. The resin generally contains a greater concentration of the drug's psychoactive properties.

was the **opium poppy** was used in Asia Minor about 5000 B.C. as a "joy plant" (Blum, 1984; O'Brien & Cohen, 1984). The use of ***Cannabis sativa*** (brewed as a tea) dates to around 2700 B.C. in China. Emperor Shen Nung recommended it to his citizens for the treatment of gout and absentmindedness, among a host of other ailments. People in the Stone Age are thought to have been familiar with opium, **hashish**, and cocaine, and to have used these drugs to produce altered states of consciousness (typically in a religious context) or to prepare themselves for battle (Government Printing Office [GPO], 1972). Chewing coca leaves (one way to ingest cocaine) is recorded among Indian burial sites in Central and South America as far back as 2500 B.C. Something to keep in mind is that the use of a drug in one culture does not necessarily mean people in another culture were at the same time exposed to or using that substance. Instead, cultures (now as well as then) are characterized by both diversity and similarity in their patterns of drug use.

Throughout history, contact between distant cultures has often been forced by trade agreements or by wars or other hostilities. For example, the Crusades and the expeditions of Marco Polo exposed Europeans to the drugs, particularly opium and hashish, that were popular in Asian cultures. Other contacts were opened later through the travels of European explorers (particularly from England, France, Portugal, and Spain) to the Americas. The predominant psychoactive substances brought to Europe from the Americas were cocaine (from South America), various hallucinogens (from Central America), and tobacco (from North America). And according to O'Brien and Cohen (1984), the exchange was not one-sided. The trees that produced the caffeine-containing coffee bean were native to Ethiopia. The coffee beverage derived from this bean was brought to Europe in the 1600s, and European seagoers were responsible for the eventual spread of coffee bean cultivation to the current world-leading supplier of coffee, South America. In addition, Europe introduced distilled alcoholic beverages to the Americas and cannabis to Chile in 1545 (O'Brien & Cohen, 1984).

There were relatively few restrictions on drug availability or drug use prior to the beginning of the 20th century (an exception is Islamic law's edicts on alcohol consumption). Occasional efforts were made to decrease or eliminate certain substances, but these efforts tended to be short-lived or ineffective. For example, initial introductions of tobacco, coffee, and tea to Europe all met some resistance. Rodrigo de Jerez, a colleague of Columbus and the first European thought to smoke tobacco, was jailed in Spain because the authorities felt the devil had overtaken him (Whitaker, 1987). Also, at different times, efforts were made to ban the use of coffee and tea.

Cases are also known in which governments acted not to make drugs unavailable but rather to keep the drug trade open and flourishing. The best example was armed conflicts between China and Great Britain in the mid-19th century. These conflicts, because they dealt with British traders bringing opium into China, are known now as the Opium Wars. By the mid-1800s, millions of Chinese men had become addicted to opium. In fact, China appears to have had the highest national use of opium at that time. Most of the opium used in China was cultivated in India and brought to China by British traders. Chinese officials passed a variety of laws to control or eliminate opium imports, but none (including **prohibition**) had the desired effect of reducing opium use or the prevalence of addiction. Furthermore, the British were unwilling to curtail the trade of opium into China, in part for financial reasons and in part because they did not witness such a degree of addiction among users in England (where opium was widely used in medicine). Relations reached a crisis in 1839, when the Chinese government destroyed large shipments of opium being brought into China by British and American traders. Thus began the first Opium War between China and England. The British won the conflict and, as part of the 1842 Treaty of

prohibition The legislative forbidding of the sale of a substance, as in the alcohol Prohibition era in the United States, 1920–1933.

Nanking, received rights to the port of Hong Kong (rights that ended in 1997) as well as reimbursement for the shippers who lost their opium cargo. The opium trade continued until 1856, when the second Opium War commenced. The war ended in 1858, and the Treaty of Tientsin mandated that China would continue to import opium but could impose heavy taxes. Not until the beginning of the 20th century was this trade reduced and eventually terminated, dovetailing with a growing international recognition of **narcotic** drug abuse.

narcotic
A central nervous system depressant that contains sedative and pain-relieving compounds.

In the 20th century, few differences existed between Europe and North America in the types of drugs being used. What is of interest is that a large number of new or "re-discovered" drugs were first popularized in the United States and later became popular in other countries, making the United States something of a trendsetter in drug use.

Drug Use in the United States

The use of psychoactive substances in the United States has a history as old as the country itself. Upon their arrival in the New World, Columbus and his crew were amazed when they saw Indians smoking tobacco. Indeed, they described to their countrymen that these natives ate fire and belched out smoke like a dragon! The Indians who inhabited this land also introduced Columbus and the later explorers and settlers to a wide variety of psychoactive plants, including **peyote**. The Europeans, in turn, introduced distilled spirits, a major staple on the long and arduous voyage across the Atlantic. The Pilgrims, for example, brought with them large stores of alcoholic beverages.

peyote (pā-'ō-tē)
A cactus plant, the top of which (a "button") is dried and ingested for its hallucinogenic properties.

morphine
A derivative of opium best known as a potent pain-relieving medication.

One of the most interesting times in this country in terms of drug use was the 19th century. Into the mid-1800s, few restrictions were placed on drugs. Drugs such as opium, **morphine**, marijuana, heroin (at the end of the century), and cocaine were easy to obtain without prescription, often at grocery stores or through mail order.

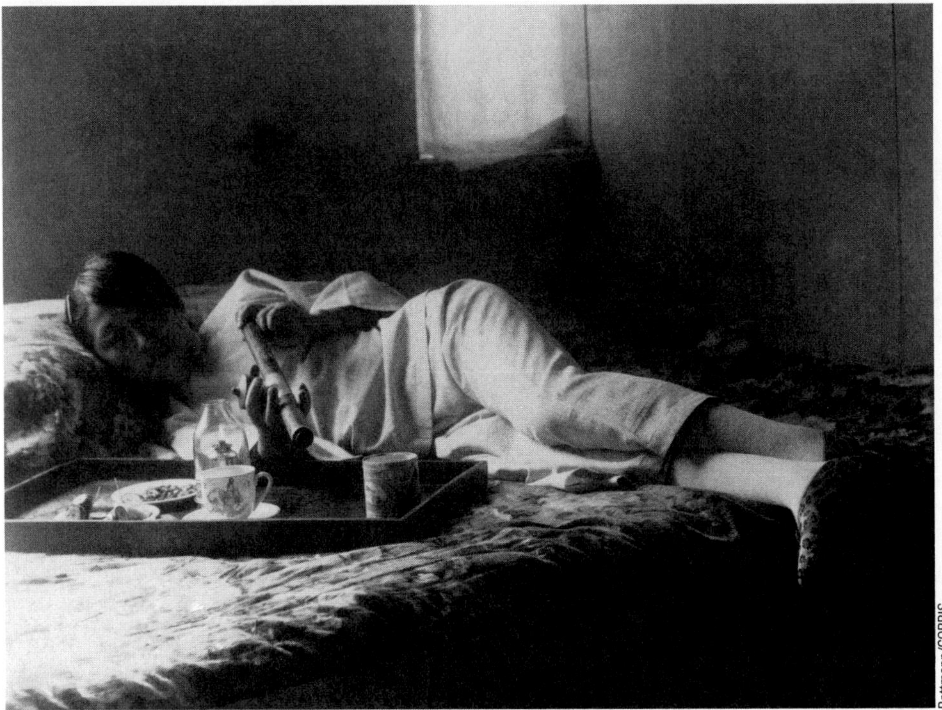
Bettmann/CORBIS

Several million Chinese men and women were addicted to opium by the mid-1800s. This photograph depicts a woman smoking opium around 1900 in China.

Opium, for example, was sold legally and at low prices; some opium poppies were grown in the United States (opium cultivation was not outlawed nationally until 1942). Morphine was commonly used, especially during and after the Civil War, and opium, morphine, and cocaine could be obtained in a variety of **patent medicines** readily available in stores. Examples were Godfrey's Cordial, Swaim's Panacea, Ayer's Sarsaparilla, and Mrs. Wilson's Soothing Syrup. Opium was frequently taken in liquid form in mixtures such as laudanum (which contained 1 grain of opium to 25 drops of alcohol), and one of its common uses was in calming and quieting crying babies!

patent medicines Products that were sold, most often in the 19th century, as medicines that would cure a host of illnesses and diseases.

Most narcotic use throughout this period was legal—whether through over-the-counter "tonics" or prescription. Physicians recommended these substances widely and referred to opium and morphine as "God's own medicine," or "G.O.M." (Morgan, 1981). Indeed these were effective calming agents. Opium was recommended for a nearly endless list of ailments. A short list includes dysentery, pain, swelling, delirium tremens (associated with withdrawal from alcohol), headache, and mental illness in certain cases. Morphine, the active agent in the opium poppy, was isolated in 1806. It was named after Morpheus, the god of sleep and dreams, and was used widely during and after the Civil War, its administration greatly facilitated by the introduction of the hypodermic needle in the late 1840s. In fact, the widespread use of morphine during the Civil War is generally considered responsible for large numbers of soldiers developing the "soldier's disease"—morphine addiction. The smoking of opium was introduced in the United States by Chinese laborers and was a widespread practice in the mid-1800s, especially on the West Coast. However, increased recognition by medical experts and others of the addictive nature of the opium poppy products—opium, morphine, and heroin—triggered efforts to control their use and availability. We discuss some of these efforts later in this chapter.

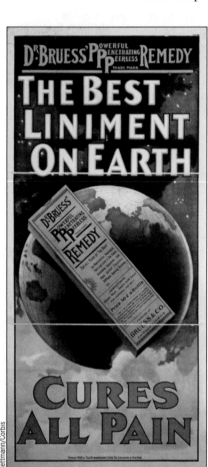

Bettmann/Corbis

Patent medicines, such as Dr. Bruess's Remedy, were widely marketed in the 1800s as cures for a variety of ailments and illnesses.

Marijuana is another substance with a long history of use. In the 1800s, physicians used a liquid extract of the *Cannabis sativa* plant as a general all-purpose medication (Nahas, 1973). Its nonmedical use was much wider in the 1920s, probably in part a reaction to alcohol prohibition (Brecher, 1972). The use of marijuana was fairly constant in the 1930s through the 1950s, but was generally limited to urban areas and to the rural areas in which the marijuana was grown and harvested. In the 1960s, its popularity soared, and that popularity has remained strong. Coinciding with this popularity have been efforts to decriminalize or legitimize marijuana sale and use. Organizations active in this effort include the National Organization for the Reform of Marijuana Laws, or NORML, and the Drug Policy Alliance. Some advocacy groups have focused their efforts on legalizing marijuana for medical uses. Via Proposition 215 in 1996, California was the first state to legalize medical marijuana. By 2009, medical marijuana use was legal in 13 states, although this number fluctuates as a function of ballot initiatives and changes in state laws. One advocacy organization supporting medical marijuana, the Drug Policy Alliance, has 45 staff members in 7 offices throughout the United States.

A drug whose popularity has fluctuated among drug users in this country is cocaine. Cocaine was widely used in various "tonics" and patent medicines in the late 1800s and early 1900s, despite concerns over negative effects associated with its extended use; not until 1914 was cocaine brought under strict legal controls and penalties. Its use was apparently limited in the United States until the 1960s. In the late 1960s and up to now, it has been in much wider use in various forms. For example, crack cocaine (a free-based form of cocaine made by cooking cocaine powder, water, and baking soda until it forms a solid) first appeared in large cities in the mid-1980s. Some experts believe that cocaine (along with heroin and methamphetamine) will be a drug of choice for many drug users in upcoming years.

Other psychoactive substances have had their distinct periods of popularity during this century. **Amphetamines**, for example, were widely used in the 1930s to treat depression. In addition, they were given to soldiers during World War II in the belief that the drug would enhance alertness (O'Brien & Cohen, 1984). Obtaining amphetamines through medical outlets such as physician prescriptions was not particularly difficult. As concern arose about the dangers inherent in the continued use of these drugs, restrictions on their availability became much tighter. At this juncture, the stage was set for a much greater production and distribution of amphetamines through illicit channels. Later, in the 1960s and 1970s, amphetamines went through another period of heavy use when they were overprescribed for weight control. Amphetamines also became widely available on the street during this time. The abuse of amphetamines remains a significant problem today, particularly when these drugs are taken intravenously.

amphetamines
Central nervous system stimulants that act like naturally occurring adrenaline.

The 1950s were the era for two central substances. Use of the minor tranquilizers became popular, and that trend continues today. As we discuss in Chapter 13, minor tranquilizers are among the most commonly prescribed psychiatric drugs in this country. The 1950s are also associated with the contemporary appearance of **solvent** inhaling. The first report of such abuse was in 1951, by Clinger and Johnson, who described the intentional inhalation of gasoline by two boys. Solvent abuse tended to be more common with other substances, however, such as model cements, lighter fluids, lacquer thinner, cleaning solvents, and more recently the propellant gases of aerosol products (Hofmann, 1975). The problem was marked in the early 1960s, with solvent inhaling causing deaths and leading hobby glue producers to remove the two most toxic solvents—benzene and carbon tetrachloride—from their products (Blum, 1984). A more recent example has been the sniffing of correction fluids that contain the solvent trichloroethane. Manufacturers of correction fluid have replaced trichloroethane with other solvents or added unpleasant substances to the fluid, such as mustard oil. Solvent inhalant abuse (such as the current "huffing" of propane and spray paint fumes) is still a serious problem, especially among boys in their teens. Indeed, there have been recent reports of teenagers using aerosol products and then diving into a swimming pool because they had heard that the underwater pressure would increase the rush. Instead, doing so has sometimes resulted in "sudden sniffing death syndrome," whereby users have a heart attack and drown.

solvent
A substance, usually a liquid or gas, that contains one or more intoxicating components; examples are glue, gasoline, and nonstick–frying pan sprays.

A historical view of psychoactive substance use might show the 1960s as the era of lysergic acid diethylamide-25, commonly known as LSD. The drug had been used in various tests during the 1950s (for example, as an adjunct to psychotherapy) but did not reach the height of its popularity until the mid-1960s, when Dr. Timothy Leary, a Harvard psychologist, began to expound on what he found to be its mind-altering advantages. LSD was banned in 1967, and its use waned considerably until a recent resurgence in its popularity, particularly in the context of the "rave" culture. A more recent psychedelic substance to appear on the scene is methylenedioxymethamphetamine, better known as MDMA or "Ecstasy." MDMA or

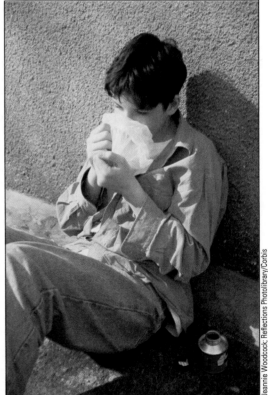
Jeannie Woodcock; Reflections Photolibrary/Corbis

Solvent sniffing remains a serious problem, particularly among teenage boys.

Ecstasy is one of a cluster of drugs collectively referred to as "club drugs" (others include methamphetamine, GHB, LSD, and ketamine; they are discussed in greater detail in Contemporary Issue Box 2.1).

Heroin is another drug with a long history of use in the United States. Heroin was first synthesized in the late 1890s, and it has been available for use since the early

CONTEMPORARY ISSUE BOX 2.1

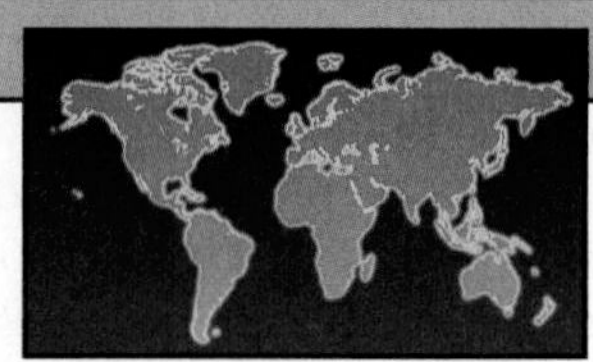

The Rise of "Club Drugs"

Throughout the 1990s and into the 2000s, the popularity of a group of substances collectively referred to as "club drugs" has been sustained. This term describes drugs being used by young adults at all-night dance parties such as "raves" and "trances" and at dance clubs and bars. All indications are that club drugs can cause serious health problems and even death in some cases. Some of these drugs are stimulants, some are depressants, and some are hallucinogens. When used in combination with alcohol, these drugs can be even more dangerous. Because some club drugs are colorless, tasteless, and odorless, individuals who want to intoxicate or sedate others (often to commit sexual assaults) can unobtrusively add them to beverages. Following is some information on the leading club drugs. More details on these substances are provided in later chapters of this text:

Methylenedioxymethamphetamine (MDMA) (street names: Ecstasy, XTC, X, Adam, clarity, lover's speed). MDMA is chemically similar to the stimulant amphetamine and the hallucinogen mescaline. MDMA can produce both stimulant and psychedelic effects and can be extremely dangerous when taken in large doses.

Gamma hydroxybutyrate (GHB) (street names: grievous bodily harm, G, liquid Ecstasy, Georgia homeboy). GHB can be produced in clear liquid, white powder, tablet, and capsule forms, and it is often used in combination with alcohol, making it even more dangerous. GHB has been increasingly involved in poisonings, overdoses, rapes, and fatalities. GHB is often manufactured in homes with recipes and ingredients found and purchased on the Internet. It is usually abused either for its intoxicating, sedative, or euphoriant properties or for its growth hormone–releasing effects, which can build muscle. When taken in smaller doses, GHB can relieve anxiety and produce relaxation; however, as the dose increases, the sedative effects may result in sleep and eventual coma or death.

Ketamine (street names: special K, K, vitamin K, cat valiums). Ketamine is an injectable anesthetic that has been approved for both human and animal use in medical settings since 1970. Ketamine is produced in liquid form or as a white powder that is often snorted or smoked with marijuana or tobacco products. Taken in larger doses, ketamine can cause delirium, amnesia, impaired motor function, high blood pressure, depression, and potentially fatal respiratory problems. Low-dose intoxication from ketamine results in impaired attention, learning ability, and memory.

Rohypnol (street names: roofies, rophies, roche, forget-me pill). Rohypnol (flunitrazepam) belongs to the class of drugs known as benzodiazepines. It is not approved for prescription use in the United States, although it is approved in Europe and is used in more than 60 countries as a treatment for insomnia, as a sedative, and as a presurgery anesthetic. Rohypnol is tasteless and odorless, and it dissolves easily in carbonated beverages. The drug can cause profound "anterograde amnesia"; that is, individuals may not remember events they experienced while under the effects of the drug.

Methamphetamine (street names: speed, ice, chalk, meth, crystal, crank, fire, glass). Methamphetamine is a toxic, addictive stimulant that affects many areas of the central nervous system. The drug is often made in clandestine laboratories from relatively inexpensive over-the-counter ingredients. Available in many forms, methamphetamine can be smoked, snorted, injected, or orally ingested. Its use is associated with serious health consequences including memory loss, aggression, violence, psychotic behavior, and potential cardiac and neurological damage. Methamphetamine abusers typically display agitation, excited speech, decreased appetite, and increased physical activity levels.

Lysergic acid diethylamide (LSD) (street names: acid, boomers, purple haze, yellow sunshines). LSD is a hallucinogen; it induces abnormalities in sensory perceptions. The effects of LSD are unpredictable, depending on the amount taken; on the surroundings in which the drug is used; and on the user's personality, mood, and expectations. Two long-term disorders sometimes associated with LSD are persistent psychosis and hallucinogen persisting perception disorder (which used to be called "flashbacks").

Source: Adapted from *Community Alert Bulletin on Club Drugs* (National Institute on Drug Abuse [NIDA], 2004). Updated 2009.

CONTEMPORARY ISSUE BOX 2.2

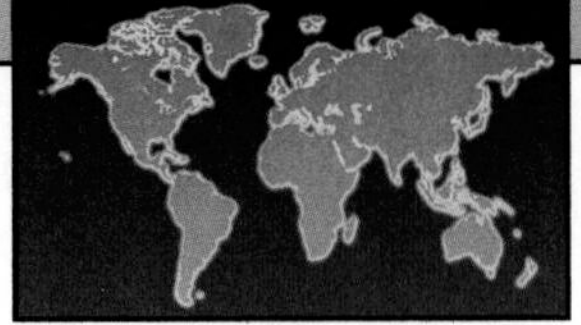

Methcathinone: Unleashing the "Cat"

One of the latest additions to the growing category of "designer drugs" is methcathinone, known most widely as "cat" and also as "goob," "jeff," "bathtub speed," "Cadillac express," "kitty," and "gagers." Methcathinone is a potent synthetic form of cathinone, a naturally occurring stimulant found in a Somali plant called khat (pronounced "kaht").

Methcathinone is a powder that most often is inhaled or smoked. It has also been injected by needle and ingested orally (mixed with a beverage such as soda). Methcathinone reportedly produces an energetic and euphoric feeling that can last for several days. Its short-term effects are similar to those following the use of methylenedioxymethamphetamine (more commonly known as MDMA or Ecstasy). These effects include increases in heart rate and respiration, heightened alertness, and pupil dilation. Higher doses can produce anxiety, insomnia, disorientation, tremors, aggression, paranoia, headaches, hallucinations (visual as well as auditory), and delusions. Withdrawal typically is accompanied by severe depression. Methcathinone is highly addictive, and methcathinone addicts have been known to suffer permanent brain damage, symptoms similar to those associated with Parkinson's disease, paranoid psychosis, and abnormal liver functioning.

Although illicitly used in Russia since the early 1980s, methcathinone was not used in the United States and most other countries until the late 1980s. In 1989, a pharmaceutical worker in Michigan obtained several vials of the drug from work and started using it with some friends. Information on methcathinone production became more widely known. With relatively easy-to-obtain ingredients, homemade methcathinone could be produced. The number of home laboratories began to increase throughout the Midwestern United States and as far away as Florida and California. Although methcathinone has been available on the streets of large cities, its use to date has mostly been in nonurban areas, such as towns and rural areas. Nevertheless, the United States Drug Enforcement Administration views methcathinone as one of its biggest challenges in upcoming years.

There have been productive legislative as well as prevention-oriented responses to concerns over the manufacture, sale, distribution, and use of methcathinone and more broadly to methamphetamines. Legislative responses have included the revision of federal and state laws to provide more severe penalties for the manufacture and distribution of methcathinone and to better control the availability of the ingredients needed to produce the drug. Many of these legislative responses were consolidated under the Comprehensive Methamphetamine Control Act of 1996. Prevention responses have also been implemented, and largely have entailed the highlighting of negative effects of methamphetamine use. Interestingly, the telling messages, at least among teenagers and young adults, have keyed on cosmetic effects, such as "meth mouth" (the rotting away of teeth associated with heavy amphetamine use). As a result of these and other responses, methamphetamine use in recent years has been in decline (Johnston et al., 2009b).

1900s. The extent of use traditionally has been greater among two populations: lower and higher socioeconomic groups (O'Brien & Cohen, 1984). During the Vietnam War, the high incidence of heroin use among U.S. soldiers in Vietnam was a significant concern, but soldiers who used the drug overseas did not tend to continue its use following their return to the States. In recent years, heroin has been showing a renewed popularity. The same factors that contributed to the spread of crack—low price and easy availability—appear to be behind this increase in heroin use. However, there are some new wrinkles and concerns. First, the level of purity of the currently available heroin is higher than in the past. In the 1980s, the purity of heroin sold on the street was less than 10%; it is now estimated at more than 60% and can be as high as 80%. Second, fewer users are injecting the drug. Instead, users have been snorting or smoking it, or mixing heroin and crack and smoking the combination. Third, heroin was a drug historically used by adults. However, early use and experimentation with heroin by U.S. teenagers have been an ongoing concern. Among those using heroin for the first time, approximately 25% are under the age of 18.

"The universal, immediate reaction is that the amphetamine high is like nothing else. You fix up a shot. You dissolve it in water. You draw it up into the dropper. You put a belt or a tie around your arm. In the meantime, you're very excited, your heart's beating fast. 'Cause you know you're going to get happy in a couple minutes. Then you give yourself a shot."

An amphetamine addict (Goode, 1972)

This overview provides only a sample of the major drugs that have been used over the years for their psychoactive properties. It is important to recognize that patterns of drug use and abuse are not static. The drugs more frequently used next year might include a drug used in the past that develops a renewed popularity or a newly synthesized substance, such as one of the so-called designer drugs. The only thing that can be said with confidence is that drugs will continue to be used and that some drug abuse will be associated with any given psychoactive substance.

Medical Science and Drug Use

Before leaving our historical perspective section, we should note the interesting long-term parallel between the development and use of psychoactive substances in medicinal forms (discussed in more detail in Chapter 5) and the nonmedicinal use or misuse of these drugs. Many of the drugs described in this text were used for medicinal purposes at one time or another. Medical science only gradually became the well-respected institution that we know today. Even in the 20th century, folk cures, potions, and so-called patent medicines were freely available and widely used.

"LSD did unlock something for me, and pot definitely did something for the old ears. Suddenly I could hear more subtle things."

Musician and former Beatle George Harrison (*Musician*, May 1992)

Perhaps the best examples of this are the opiates opium and morphine that, throughout most of the 1800s, were used to treat a variety of complaints, including rheumatism, pain, fever, delirium tremens, and colds. The opiates were also used as an anesthetic for some surgeries and for setting broken bones. As we noted earlier, physicians used and prescribed the opiates despite a lack of understanding of how they acted in the body. All that was known was that opium and morphine seemed to help alleviate pain and symptoms that simply were not understood (Morgan, 1981). Unfortunately, such widespread use contributed to a considerable number of people becoming physically addicted to these substances. Not until the 1870s did a clearer picture of the addictive properties of these drugs emerge.

Numerous other examples can be cited. Chloroform and ether were developed as anesthetics, but each also went through a period in the 1850s when its nonmedical use was quite fashionable. At one time, cocaine was used to treat complaints such as depressed mood and pain. In fact, one of its uses was as a treatment for opiate addiction. In the latter half of the 19th century, physicians recognized an array of uses for cannabis, including treatment of insomnia and nervousness, although its prescribed use was not nearly as extensive as with the opiates. The 20th century witnessed the development of the synthetic stimulant amphetamines, some of which initially were available without prescription.

"It's not good for the body; it's not good for the mind. It's the real immature adolescent in everybody that finds romance in that."

Branford Marsalis on using drugs to enhance creativity (*Musician*, May 1992)

We could provide additional examples, but the important point is that medicinal uses of psychoactive substances (whether folk medicine or more contemporary medicine), medical science, and nonmedical drug use and abuse will always be closely intertwined. In the past, folk or cultural use of a substance often became incorporated into the practice of medicine. More common today is the incorporation of a substance developed for the practice of medicine into the array of drugs that can be used in nonmedicinal ways. The reverse can still occur, however, as shown by the attention being given to the medical uses of marijuana. In any event, keeping the medical and nonmedical uses of drugs separate is impossible.

Development of Drug Laws

Legislation is the main way society establishes formal guidelines for drug use. Furthermore, such legislation essentially reflects a society's beliefs about drugs. Laws generally establish restrictions or prohibit the manufacture, importation, sale, or possession of the substance under evaluation. It is noteworthy that actual drug use in the United

States, and in other countries as well, is not a crime under federal law, nor is it a crime to be a drug addict or an alcoholic.

Drug laws for the most part have had limited effectiveness in reducing overall illicit drug availability and use (Australian Drug Law Reform Foundation, 1996; Jung, 2001; Nadelmann, 1989). In fact, the more restrictive the laws, the less effective they have tended to be in the long run (Brecher, 1972; 1986). The only time these laws seem to be more effective is when drug use or abuse is particularly unpopular (Brecher, 1986; Hofmann, 1975). However, the duration of these periods and the time between them are variable. Nevertheless, legislation remains society's central means for addressing its concerns about drugs.

Describing the history of drug laws in the United States will provide an example of one society's response to drug use and abuse. Interestingly, the implementation of drug laws in the United States did not really begin until the turn of the 20th century. This made the United States one of the last industrialized nations to formally implement drug legislation. Various efforts were mounted to regulate opiates in the second half of the 19th century, but these were largely halfhearted and ineffective. That is not to say that sanctions on drug abuse did not exist, but rather there were no legal penalties to speak of. At different times and in different locations, varying degrees of social sanctions existed, such as the ostracism of citizens who displayed certain forms of drunkenness in Colonial times.

The San Francisco Ordinance

The only notable law regarding drug use in the 19th century that had any effect was a city ordinance passed in San Francisco in 1875. Chinese men had entered this country throughout the mid-1800s, to meet demands for labor in the rapidly expanding West. Most of these immigrants worked on the building of the railways. When this construction was finished, many of the laborers made their way back to San Francisco, where they frequented "opium dens"—places where people could smoke opium. Although this drug use had little negative effect on the San Francisco community per se, some thought the practice was sinister. Rumors began to circulate that the opium den houses were evil and that unsuspecting members of the community—young women were used frequently as examples—were at risk for unknowingly heading down dangerous paths toward disrepute and drug addiction. This concern led to the 1875 ordinance. Only opium dens were banned, however, not the smoking of opium. Conviction for operating or frequenting an opium den carried a fine of $50 to $500 and/or a jail sentence of 10 days to 6 months. The actual impact of the ordinance was not great; the larger and more obvious opium dens closed, and the number of smaller dens increased. The effect was greater in the sense of setting the stage for drug regulation in other parts of the country, as a number of other cities and states passed similar ordinances in later years. Not until 1909 did Congress pass a law banning the importation of opium for smoking.

Pure Food and Drug Act

The first federal legislation of note was the Pure Food and Drug Act passed in 1906 (see Figure 2.1). This act, which was designed to control opiate addiction, legislated that producers of medicines must indicate on the packaging the amount of drug contained in their products. The law focused particularly on the opiates opium, morphine, and heroin, but also mandated the accurate labeling of products that contain alcohol, marijuana, and cocaine. The overall effect of the act was mixed: It did not ban opiates in patent medicines and thus had little impact on the addicts at the time, but the legislation may have served to decrease the number of new addicts, given the subsequent

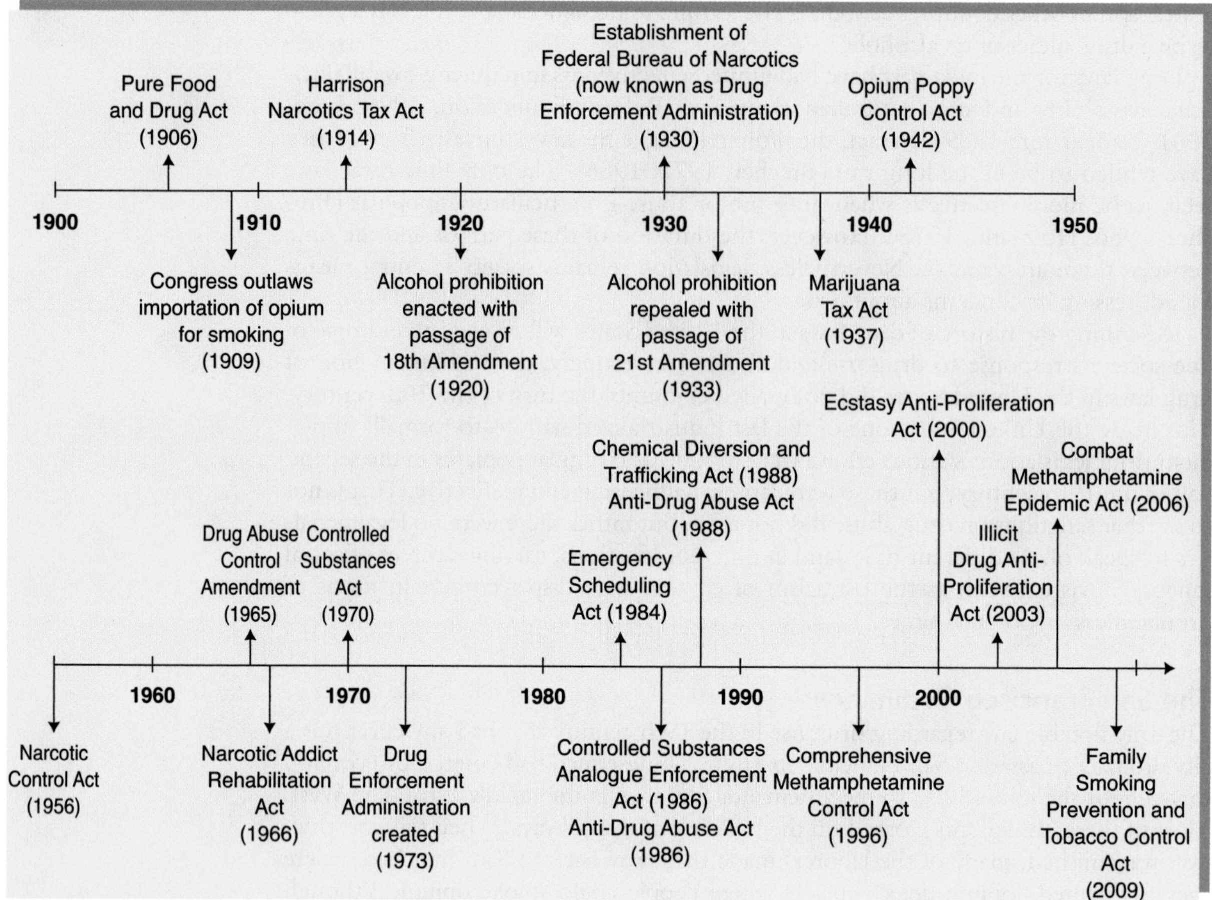

FIGURE 2.1
Major U.S. drug legislation

political and educational efforts to describe the addictive potential of patent medicines containing opiates (Brecher, 1972).

Harrison Narcotics Tax Act

Another major piece of federal legislation, the Harrison Narcotics Tax Act, was passed in 1914. Curiously, this law was passed not in response to domestic demand but rather as a consequence of the United States signing the Hague Convention of 1912, an international agreement that directed signing nations to regulate opium traffic within their respective countries (Brecher, 1986). The Harrison Narcotics Tax Act strictly regulated, but did not prohibit, the legal supply of certain drugs, particularly the opiates. The law stated that marketing and prescribing these drugs required licensing. The physician was directed to prescribe narcotics only "in the course of his professional practice." This phrase is certainly general and open to interpretation, and controversy between law enforcement agencies and physicians ensued. The central debate was whether the prescribing of an opiate for an addict was part of a treatment plan or merely served to maintain the addict's dependence on the drug. Although this confusion of the act's intent led to more restrictions on prescribing and supplying opiates, the act had little effect on opiate abuse (even when subsequent amendments mandated more severe penalties for possession). In fact, Brecher (1986) argued that the act was actually counterproductive. Brecher maintained that, in the years since its passage, the law actually has served to shift opium and morphine addicts to heroin (which became easier to obtain on the black market) and overall to double the number of addicts in the United States. This occurred despite more than 50 modifications to the act during the 50 years following its passage, each change designed to toughen the law (Brecher, 1972).

Three other facets of the Harrison Narcotics Tax Act should be mentioned. First, the act did not restrict manufacturers of patent medicines, with the exception that their preparations could "not contain more than two grains of opium, or more than one fourth of a grain of morphine, or more than one eighth of a grain of heroin . . . in one **avoirdupois** ounce" (U.S. Pure Food and Drug Act of 1906, cited in Brecher, 1972). A second interesting aspect of this narcotic control act was its inaccurate inclusion of cocaine as a narcotic. Finally, one treatment-related result of the Harrison Narcotics Tax Act was that treatment centers for addicts began to open in some of the larger cities (Morgan, 1981). Most of these centers, however, were open for only a few years and thus had limited opportunity to help alleviate opiate addiction.

avoirdupois
Something sold or measured by weight based on 1 pound equaling 16 ounces.

Alcohol Prohibition

Alcohol prohibition was enacted several years later when, in 1920, Congress passed the Eighteenth Amendment to the Constitution. The legislation was a victory for the forces that viewed alcohol as evil and destructive, notably the Anti-Saloon League and the Women's Christian Temperance Union. The amendment was not vague about its intent: It prohibited the production, sale, transportation, and importing of alcohol in any part of the United States. The only exception was that alcoholic beverages kept in the home, such as naturally fermented hard cider, could be consumed but not offered for sale (Lender & Martin, 1982).

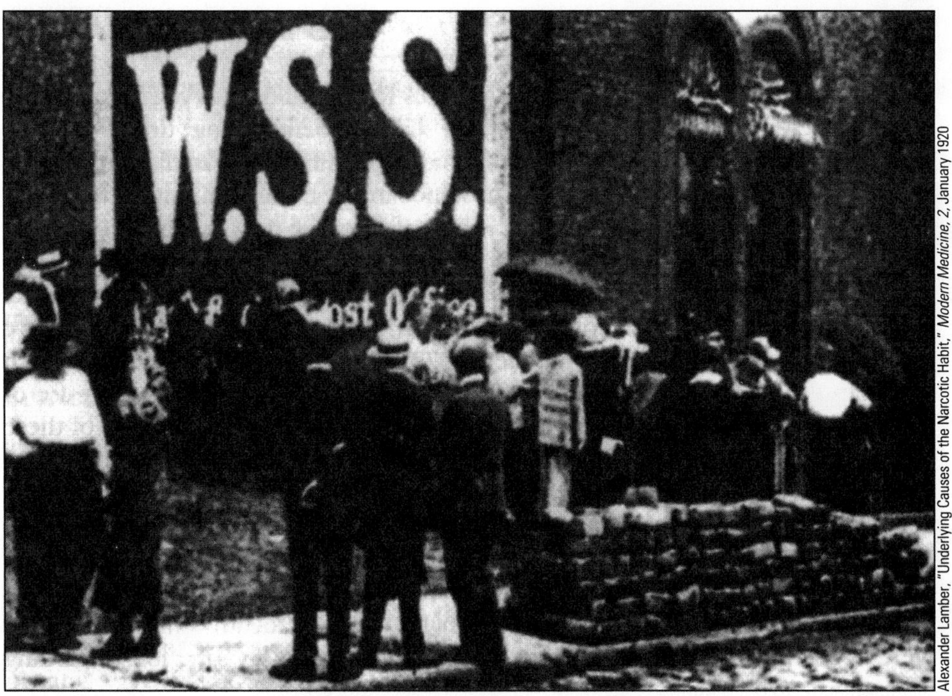

Alexander Lamber, "Underlying Causes of the Narcotic Habit," *Modern Medicine*, 2, January 1920

Addicts gathered outside a New York City drug clinic in 1920.

"Our country has deliberately undertaken a great social and economic experiment, noble in motive and far-reaching in purpose. It must be worked out constructively."

President-elect Herbert Hoover (1928, on Prohibition)

The National Prohibition Act subsequently was passed to provide the means to investigate and punish violators of the Eighteenth Amendment. The legislation, which was passed over the veto of President Woodrow Wilson, is better known as the Volstead Act because it was introduced by Minnesota Representative Andrew Volstead. Scheduled to take effect in 1920, the act defined an "intoxicating beverage" as one containing more than 0.5% alcohol.

As you may be aware, and as discussed further in Chapter 9, Prohibition was an experiment in drug control that did not succeed, and the Eighteenth Amendment was repealed 13 years later by the Twenty-first Amendment. Although Prohibition is commonly cited as a drug use control measure that failed overall, it nevertheless did have a substantial effect on drinking in the United States. For example, the rate of drinking was reduced markedly (reasonable estimates range from one-third to one-half); other decreases were in the death rates attributable to liver cirrhosis, admission rates to state hospitals for treatment of alcoholism, and arrest rates for alcohol-related offenses (Aaron & Musto, 1981). The greatest decrease in alcohol consumption was among the working population, and this made the legislation vulnerable to widespread criticism that it was a biased law. Unfortunately, a variety of other undesired consequences were associated with Prohibition, including more extensive use of marijuana, a shift in drinking habits away from beer to distilled spirits, the advent of the **speakeasy**, and the takeover of alcohol distribution by criminal groups. (Coffee intake, according to Brecher [1972], also soared during this period.) Thus, although Prohibition was successful in achieving some of its intended effects, these outcomes were tempered by other undesired results. Ultimately, Prohibition was repealed because it lacked sufficient public support to maintain it.

speakeasy
A slang expression used to describe a saloon operating without a license; popularly used during Prohibition.

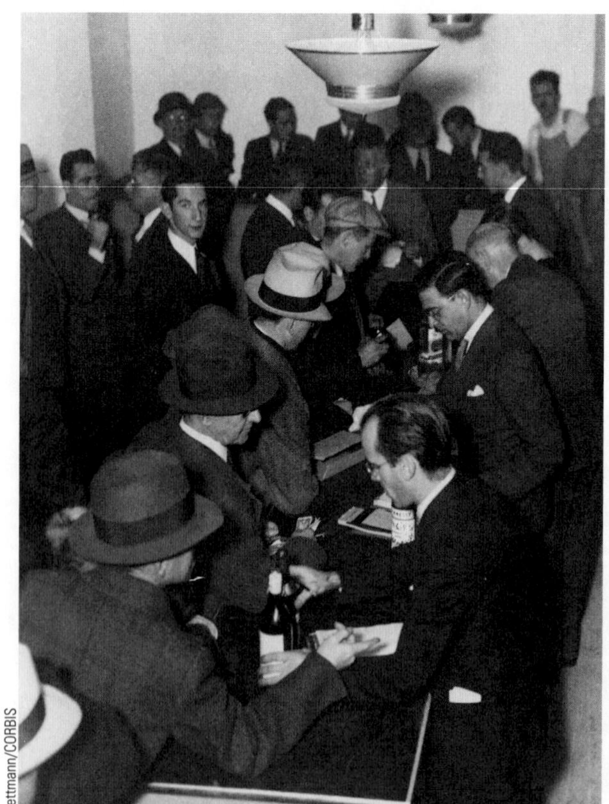

Bettmann/CORBIS

Customers turned to speakeasy establishments to drink during Prohibition.

Post-Prohibition Legislation

Following the repeal of Prohibition, the 1930s were characterized by stricter guidelines and penalties for the possession and sale of drugs, particularly marijuana. Legislative action taken in 1930 provided independent status for narcotic control agents through the establishment of the Federal Bureau of Narcotics (later to be called the Bureau of Narcotics and Dangerous Drugs and now the Drug Enforcement Administration). A major thrust of the Federal Bureau of Narcotics, spearheaded by Commissioner Harry J. Anslinger, was the eradication of marijuana use. Anslinger's crusade resulted in the Marijuana Tax Act of 1937. Like the Harrison Narcotics Tax Act, this measure did not ban marijuana but instead required authorized producers, manufacturers, importers, and dispensers of the drug to register and pay an annual license fee. Only the nonmedical possession or sale of marijuana was outlawed (Brecher, 1972). Some medical uses for marijuana were still recognized. Legislative actions regarding marijuana use gradually grew more restrictive and provided for greater penalties until the decriminalization movement began in the latter part of the 1970s.

Additional federal legislation was passed between 1940 and 1970. However, like previous legislation, these actions failed to have a sustained influence on the prevalence of drug use or dependence, despite the increased severity of the penalties for drug law infractions. Two trends are worth noting. The first is increased attention to nonnarcotic drug use, whereby stimulants, depressants, and hallucinogenic substances became regulated under legislation such as the Drug Abuse Control Amendment of 1965. The second notable change in federal legislation was a shifting of at least some attention to the treatment of drug abuse through such measures as the Community Mental Health Centers Act of 1963 and the Narcotic Addicts Rehabilitation Act of 1966.

A landmark legislative act, the Comprehensive Drug Abuse Prevention and Control Act, was passed in 1970. More commonly known as the Controlled Substances Act, this legislation is the basis for drug regulation in the United States today. We discuss this act, along with some other more recent legislation, in the following section.

Current Drug Laws

Drug classifications for law enforcement purposes are rooted in the 1970 Controlled Substances Act. Under this measure, drugs are not classified according to their pharmacological action but according to their medical use, their potential for abuse, and their likelihood for producing dependence. Almost all psychoactive substances (alcohol and nicotine are two notable exceptions) have been placed in one of the five categories, or schedules, generated by the act. A description of each of the five schedules is shown in Table 2.1, and Table 2.2 lists examples of the drugs in each classification. Several substances that have little or no potential for abuse or dependence are not classified. These include the major tranquilizers, such as chlorpromazine (trade name Thorazine), thioridazine (Mellaril), and haloperidol (Haldol); and the antidepressants, such

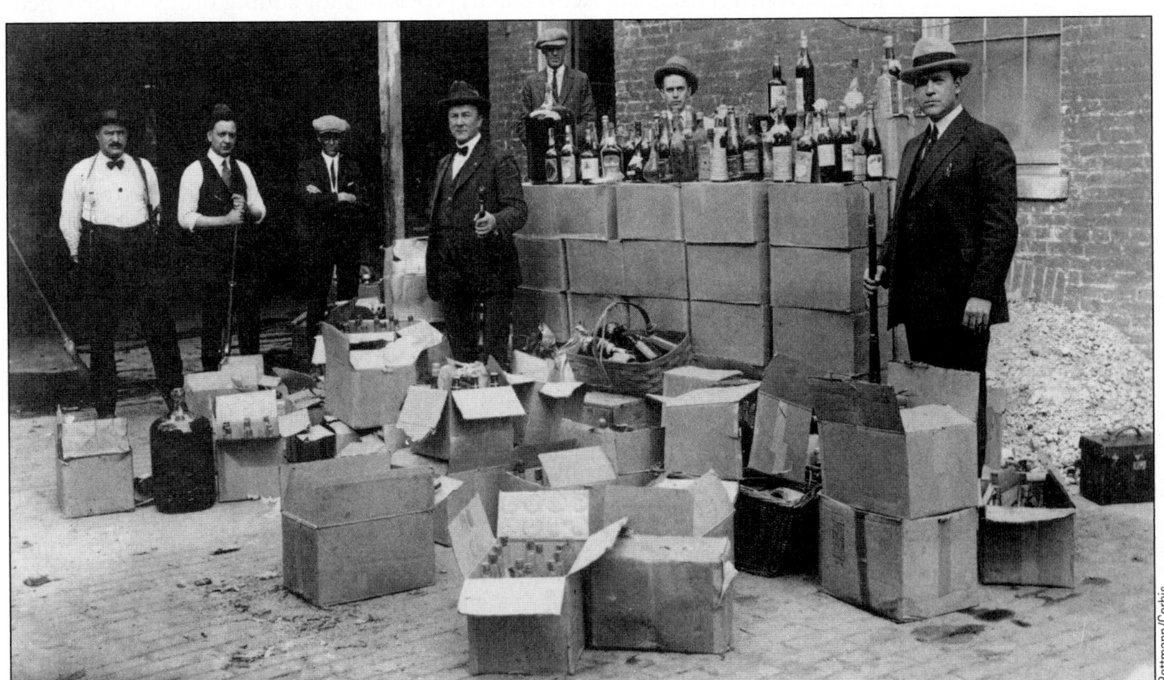

Bettmann/Corbis

Prohibition was enacted to terminate the production, sale, and distribution of alcohol. These federal agents have just completed a raid on a Washington, DC, speakeasy in 1923.

TABLE 2.1 Schedules of Controlled Substances

Schedule I: The drug or other substance has a high potential for abuse. It has no currently accepted medical use in treatment in the United States. There is a lack of accepted safety for use of the drug or other substance under medical supervision.

Schedule II: The drug or other substance has a high potential for abuse. It has a currently accepted medical use in treatment in the United States or a currently accepted medical use with severe restrictions. Abuse of the drug or other substances may lead to severe psychological or physical dependence.

Schedule III: The drug or other substance has a potential for abuse less than the drugs or other substances in Schedules I and II. It has a currently accepted medical use in treatment in the United States. Abuse of the drug or other substance may lead to moderate or low physical dependence or high psychological dependence.

Schedule IV: The drug or other substance has a low potential for abuse relative to the drugs or other substances in Schedule III. It has a currently accepted medical use in treatment in the United States. Abuse of the drug or other substance may lead to limited physical dependence or psychological dependence relative to the drugs or other substances in Schedule III.

Schedule V: The drug or other substance has a low potential for abuse relative to the drugs or other substances in Schedule IV. It has a currently accepted medical use in treatment in the United States. Abuse of the drug or other substance may lead to limited physical dependence or psychological dependence relative to the drugs or other substances in Schedule IV.

Source: From *The United States Controlled Substances Act.*

as imipramine (Tofranil) and amitriptyline (Elavil). We discuss these drugs in greater detail in Chapter 13.

The Controlled Substances Act contains provisions for adding drugs to the schedules and for rescheduling drugs. For example, diazepam (Valium) and other benzodiazepines were unscheduled when the act was passed but were classified as Schedule IV drugs in 1975. Similarly, phencyclidine (PCP, or "angel dust") was initially unscheduled but then classified as a Schedule II substance in 1978 when it began to be abused. A variety of Schedule III substances were reclassified into Schedule II during the early 1970s, including amphetamine (Benzedrine), methylphenidate (Ritalin), and secobarbital (Seconal). Methcathinone was classified as a Schedule I drug in 1992.

Consistent with its intended comprehensive character, the Controlled Substances Act also establishes the penalties for criminal manufacture or distribution of the scheduled drugs. Many of these penalties, particularly those for drug trafficking, were increased during the 1980s and 1990s, through legislation such as the 1988 Anti-Drug Abuse Act. The penalties are greatest for trafficking Schedule I and II drugs (excluding marijuana, hashish, and hashish oil, for which the penalties are only slightly less severe), and the penalties increase with the quantity involved and the number of previous offenses. For example, a first conviction for trafficking 100 to 999 grams of heroin mixture or 500 to 4,999 milligrams of cocaine mixture carries a sentence of not less than 5 years (up to 40 years) and a fine of up to $2 million. If a death or serious injury is associated with the drug trafficking, the sentence is not less than 20 years imprisonment. Larger quantities carry greater penalties, as do subsequent offenses. Penalties for trafficking any amounts of Schedule III through V substances are lower but still substantial. A first conviction for trafficking any amount of a Schedule III substance is up to 5 years and a $250,000 fine. A subsequent conviction can result in up to 10 years imprisonment and a $500,000 fine.

"Will we be able to teach the dangers of drugs to later generations who have little or no experience with them?"

David F. Musto, Yale School of Medicine Professor of Psychiatry and History, asked to ponder life in the year 2053 (*U.S. News & World Report,* October 25, 1993)

TABLE 2.2 Examples of Scheduled Drugs and Drug Products

Schedule I	
Heroin	Methylenedioxymethamphetamine (MDMA, ecstasy)
Peyote	Methaqualone
Mescaline	Tilidine
Psilocybin	Marijuana
Hash	Lysergic acid diethylamide-25 (LSD)
Hash oil	Dimethyltryptamine (DMT)
Gamma hydroxybutyric acid (GHB)	Quaalude
Nicocodeine	Methcathinone
Schedule II	
Opium	Methamphetamine
Morphine	Phencyclidine (PCP)
Codeine	Cocaine
Percodan	Benzedrine
Ritalin	Dexedrine
Seconal	Dilaudid
Oxycodone (Percodan, Percocet, OxyContin)	Demerol
	Methadone
Schedule III	
Empirin with codeine	Nodular
Tylenol with codeine	Ketamine
Paregoric	Flunitrazepam (Rohypnol)
Marinol	Butisol
Vicodan	Fiorinal
Doriden	Anabolic steroids
Schedule IV	
Luminal	Ativan
Darvon	Halcion
Valium	Restoril
Librium	Serax
Chloral hydrate	Dalmane
Placidyl	Tranxene
Darvocet	Miltown
Ambien	Xanax
Valmid	Equanil
Schedule V	
Cheracol with codeine	Phenergan
Robitussin A-C	Cosadein
Lomotil	

Source: Adapted from S. Cohen, *The Substance Abuse Problems*. The Haworth Press, 1981. Updated 2009.

Penalties for the possession of lesser amounts of a drug without intent to distribute are less severe, though still substantial. As part of the "zero-tolerance" feature of the "war on drugs" implemented in the late 1980s, law enforcement agencies may seize the assets of people who possess or sell drugs (see Contemporary Issue Box 2.3). For example, individuals caught with drugs in their cars or boats have had their vehicles seized and sold by government agencies, such as Customs, or local authorities.

"The solution to our drug problem is not in incarceration."

Barry McCaffrey, retired general and former U.S. drug czar (1996)

Each state has the opportunity to modify current drug laws according to its own needs and preferences. Most states have adopted guidelines, but many have changed certain components. For example, marijuana is classified as a Schedule I substance, but the penalties for possession in many states are less severe than those applied to other Schedule I substances. In fact, at least 11 states at some time have passed legislation to decriminalize marijuana possession.

It is important to recognize that new legislation is always on the horizon, whether in response to the latest trends in drug use and abuse or reflecting emergent political mandates. During the 1980s, law enforcement agencies were having difficulties controlling the production of the so-called designer drugs—drugs that were structurally similar but not identical to illegal substances. Each time a slight modification in the chemical structure of the drug was made, enforcement officials were forced to go through a time-consuming process of documenting the drug and having it certified as a controlled substance. In response, in 1986, Congress passed the Controlled Substances Analogue Enforcement Act, which allowed for the immediate classification of a substance as a controlled substance. In this way, drug enforcement officials were in a position to address a new drug as soon as it appeared in circulation. Similarly, legislation has been put in place to allow the Drug Enforcement Administration to monitor and regulate the distribution of chemical substances and other equipment needed for the preparation of illegal drugs. Titled the Chemical Diversion and Trafficking Act of 1988, this legislation controls the distribution of particular chemicals, tabulating machines, and encapsulating machines that are used in the manufacture of illicit substances. In 1996, the Comprehensive Methamphetamine Control Act was enacted to curb the spread of methamphetamine. The act's provisions restrict access to chemicals used to make methamphetamine, monitor

CONTEMPORARY ISSUE BOX 2.3

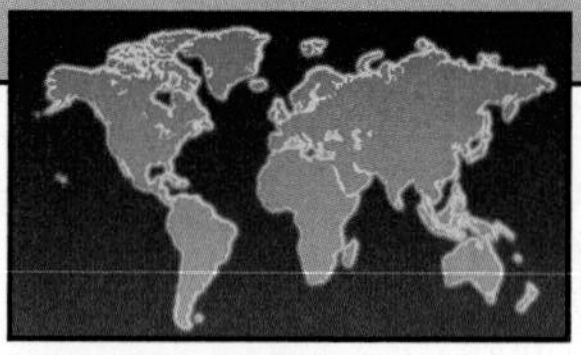

The War on Drugs

One of the foremost efforts of recent presidential administrations in the United States has been the "war on drugs," implemented in the 1980s, and continuing unabated since. Hallmark features of this "war" are efforts to catch drug smugglers and sellers (in this country and overseas) and the implementation of a "zero-tolerance" approach to drug users, including casual users of drugs. The U.S. government has been spending approximately a billion dollars a year on antidrug operations overseas alone, most of it used to catch drug smugglers.

All of these efforts appear to have had no significant impact on drug use. Most experts conclude that efforts to intercept drugs have been a failure. Hundreds of millions of dollars have been spent on these efforts, yet the flow of drugs into the United States has not been significantly altered. So what is the best strategy for combating the drug problem? Some organizations, such as the Physician Leadership on National Drug Policy, have been pushing for a greater focus on reducing the demand for drugs through prevention efforts and treatment (including the use of treatment services as an alternative to incarceration). This emphasis on demand reduction appears to reflect the attitudes of most individuals as well. An ABC News poll found that almost 70% of Americans favored treatment over jail for first- and second-time drug offenders.

It is unlikely that the war on drugs will cease anytime soon. Instead, changes in the "battle plan" will reflect shifts in focus, such as paying more attention to policing drug supply routes than to drug demand, or vice versa. Overall efforts continue to be coordinated by the head of the White House Office of National Drug Control Policy, better known as the "drug czar." The most recently appointed "drug czar," Gil Kerlikowske, appointed in 2009 by President Barack Obama, has professed a desire to abolish the use of the "war on drugs" phraseology and to shift greater emphasis on treatment relative to imprisonment.

It is noteworthy that the two drugs most associated with deaths in this country—tobacco and alcohol—are not a focus of attention in any of these efforts.

purchases of these preparation chemicals, increase penalties for the possession of chemicals or equipment used in the production of methamphetamine, and increase penalties for trafficking and manufacturing methamphetamine. In 1999, chemicals used as "date rape" drugs were added to the schedule of controlled substances. A likely candidate for upcoming legislation is ***salvia divinorum***, a hallucinogenic member of the sage family. Known as "magic mint" or "Sally-D," salvia has been used historically by Mazatec Indians in Mexico for ailments such as diarrhea, headaches, and rheumatism and for interacting with the supernatural world. Although salvia is legal to buy, sell, and smoke in most states, concerns over its use, growing popularity, and effects have led a rapidly growing number of states and also other countries to restrict or criminalize the sale and possession of salvia. The Drug Enforcement Administration is considering classifying salvia as a controlled substance, and such an action appears likely in the near future.

Finally, special note should be made of the 2009 Family Smoking Prevention and Tobacco Control Act, which authorized the Food and Drug Administration (FDA) to regulate the manufacture, marketing, and sale of tobacco products. The legislation provided the FDA with broad control over how tobacco (a product with no medical use) in its various forms is marketed and sold, and over claims made about tobacco products, although it does not provide the authority to impose an outright ban on tobacco products. A number of FDA actions were mandated in the legislation. These include the banning of candy-flavored cigarettes (within 3 months of the passage of the law), the banning of the marketing of cigarettes as "light," "mild," or "low-tar" (within 12 months), implementing stronger warnings on smokeless tobacco products that will cover 30% of the front and back package panels (within 12 months), and graphic warnings on cigarette packages covering 50% of the top front and top back of the packages (within 39 months). The mandated restrictions on marketing also included limiting advertisements and promotions to a black-and-white text-only format in stores that children can enter. The bill overall contains a strong focus on deterring young people from smoking. Because an estimated 9 out of 10 smokers begin smoking before age 18, the bill may have the effect of hindering tobacco companies' access to youth and thus dramatically reduce the number of smokers in the longer term.

We have focused on drug laws in the United States. Drug laws and their implementation in other countries reflect considerable diversity. For example, European drug policy derives largely from the framework provided by the United Nations Single Convention on Narcotic Drugs in 1961. The 12 participating European countries pledged to fight drug abuse and international trafficking through national legislation. Each country would implement a strategy of response best suited to its needs. In 1972, the Single Convention document was amended to encourage efforts to prevent substance abuse and to provide treatment services for substance abusers. Nearly two decades later, in 1990, came the Frankfurt Resolution, which involved representation from the cities of Amsterdam, Frankfurt, Hamburg, and Zurich. This resolution asserted that attempts to eliminate drugs and drug use cannot succeed. It encouraged legislation to decriminalize the purchase, possession, and consumption of cannabis. As such, many jurisdictions began to focus more on reducing the negative effects of drug use and misuse on individuals and society, a philosophy referred to as "harm reduction" or "harm minimization." Nevertheless, drug laws throughout Europe, and indeed throughout the world, continue to differ in many ways, and many do not distinguish between so-called hard drugs and soft drugs (e.g., marijuana). In addition, countries differ in the extent to which they actually enforce existing drug laws.

"We've spent a trillion dollars prosecuting the war on drugs. What do we have to show for it? Drugs are more readily available, at lower prices and higher levels of potency. It's a dismal failure."

Norm Stamper, former police chief of Seattle (*New York Times*, June 14, 2009)

CONTEMPORARY ISSUE BOX 2.4

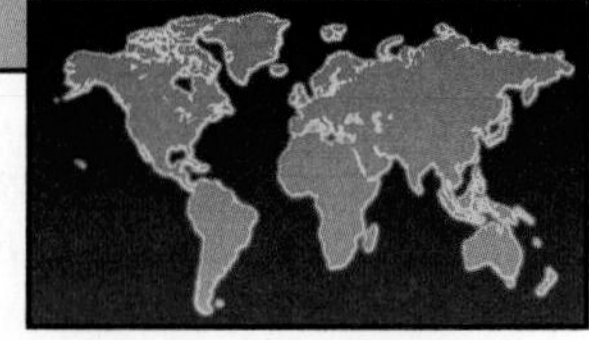

Drug Testing in the Workplace, at School, and at Home!

One result of the concern over drug use and misuse has been efforts by corporations to have their workers submit to mandatory drug tests. Employers argue the tests are needed to identify those workers who, because of their drug use, may be at risk for subpar or even dangerous work performance. Employers also believe random drug tests serve as a deterrent to drug use. More than one-third of the largest U.S. corporations currently use drug screening as part of their hiring process.

The argument put forth by employers may appear relatively straightforward: If drugs can impair work performance, then checking for drugs is a legitimate practice. However, drug testing remains controversial for several reasons. Consider three aspects of the controversy.

First is the possible infringement on constitutional rights of privacy when tests are administered randomly (that is, without warning and independent of "probable cause"). This concern has led some to suggest that tests should be used only if a demonstrable "reasonable cause" exists to believe a person is under the influence of a drug.

A second issue is the relationship between a positive test result and actual job performance. For example, traces of marijuana can be detected in a person's system for several weeks and sometimes much longer after it was smoked, even though no associated impairment in the person's functioning can be proven. Is drug use a legitimate reason for termination or other disciplinary action if no obvious effect of that drug use on the worker's job performance can be demonstrated?

A third issue is very basic yet crucial—the accuracy of the drug tests themselves. Urinalysis test results are often unreliable. In some cases, the presence of a drug is missed, and in other cases, a legitimate drug (such as a prescribed medication) is identified by the test as an illicit substance. However, the biggest factor contributing to poor test reliability is human error and carelessness on the part of the people doing the urinalysis at the laboratory. More stringent guidelines and efforts at quality control have been implemented in recent years, and progress is being reported.

Most of the problems with false readings have been associated with the use of immunoassay or thin-layer chromatography tests. These urine tests are best viewed as screening tests; they test not for the presence of the drug in the urine but rather for the metabolic products of drugs. Positive readings from immunoassay procedures should be followed by mass spectrometer procedures that identify chemical compounds associated with specific drugs. A more recent advance has been the use of radioimmunoassay procedures to test for the presence of particular drugs (such as heroin, cocaine, and marijuana) in strands of hair. However, the current scientific consensus is that the hair-testing process is not sufficiently reliable for widespread use.

Although the issues surrounding drug testing continue to be debated, similar issues are arising on a pair of new fronts—drug testing of children at school and at home by their parents. A 2008 survey by researchers at the University of New Hampshire found that around 12% of school districts nationwide now conduct drug tests with students, either on a random basis or with students in particular extracurricular activities (such as sports or serving on a school committee). The constitutionality of random testing has been upheld by several Supreme Court decisions. Testing has typically occurred through urine testing. Meanwhile, numerous companies are now offering home drug-testing products. Most such products entail testing of urine samples; others evaluate either hair samples or saliva. Yet another approach, less obtrusive in nature, involved the parent wiping a special moist pad across a child's clothing, books, or furniture. The pad is then sent to the manufacturer, which analyzes it for traces of drugs. This approach has its own set of drawbacks, as the moist pad does not necessarily prove the child has used a particular drug. Drug traces could have been left by another person or picked up through incidental contact with another person using drugs.

Summary

- Drugs have been used for a variety of reasons in different cultures for thousands of years; the earliest drug use involved ingestion of alcohol and of plants with psychoactive properties.
- Prior to the 20th century, few restrictions were placed on drug availability or drug use.
- During the 19th century, drugs such as opium, morphine, marijuana, heroin, and

cocaine could be obtained easily without prescription.

- Marijuana was used by physicians during the 1800s as a general all-purpose medication; its nonmedical use increased during the Prohibition era of the 1920s.
- Different drugs have enjoyed periods of popularity in the United States. Cocaine was widely used in medicines and tonics during the late 1800s and early 1900s. Cocaine use again became popular in the 1960s, and its popularity continues today. Amphetamines were used relatively widely during the 1930s, minor tranquilizers and inhalants during the 1950s, and LSD during the 1960s. Heroin has been showing signs of increased use in recent years. A current trend is the emergence of a group of substances collectively known as "club drugs."
- A parallel exists between the development and use of psychoactive substances in medicinal forms and the nonmedical use or abuse of these drugs.
- The main mechanism through which society establishes formal guidelines regarding drugs and drug use is legislation. However, the history of drug laws in the United States does not really begin until the turn of the 20th century.
- The first major federal legislation regarding drugs was the 1906 Pure Food and Drug Act, which mandated a listing of the types and amounts of drugs contained in medicines.
- Other major legislation of note included the 1914 Harrison Narcotics Tax Act, which regulated the legal supply of certain drugs, and alcohol Prohibition, which spanned the years between 1920 and 1933.
- Drug classifications for law enforcement today are based on the 1970 Controlled Substances Act, which classifies drugs according to their legitimate medical uses and their potential for abuse and dependence.
- Other legislation has been enacted in the years since to respond to changes in drug-use patterns. Notable recent legislation includes the 2009 Family Smoking Prevention and Tobacco Control Act.

Answers to "*What Do You Think?*"

1. The first recorded use of cannabis was in the early 1800s.
   F *The use of Cannabis sativa dates back to around 2700 B.C. in China, where it was recommended by Emperor Shen Nung for the treatment of various ailments.*
2. Grape wine was the first alcoholic beverage to be used.
   F *Beer and huckleberry wine were used as early as 6400 B.C. Grape wine did not appear until between 300 B.C. and 400 B.C.*
3. The Opium Wars between China and Great Britain in the mid-1800s occurred in large part because Britain was unwilling to curtail its trade of opium into China.
   T *Most of the opium used in China at the time was cultivated in India and brought to China by British traders. Although opiate addiction was a major problem for China, the British were unwilling to curtail this trade in part because of financial reasons and in part because the same degree of addiction was not experienced by users in England.*
4. Columbus and his crew were responsible for introducing tobacco to the New World.
   F *The Indians whom Columbus encountered introduced him and later explorers to tobacco and other psychoactive plants. The Europeans, in turn, introduced alcohol to the New World.*
5. Many of the drugs that are now illegal in the United States were widely used in the 1800s and early 1900s to treat a broad spectrum of maladies.
   T *Opiates, marijuana, cocaine, and amphetamines were all used at one time or another to treat various ailments. Use of these drugs was restricted when their addictive natures were recognized.*
6. The first notable drug law in the United States—the 1875 San Francisco ordinance—banned the smoking of opium.
   F *The San Francisco Ordinance banned opium dens but not the actual smoking of opium.*

7. The Pure Food and Drug Act of 1906 had little impact on individuals who were addicted to drugs.
   T *This act was designed to control opiate addiction and legislated that producers of medicines indicate on their packaging the amount of drugs contained in the products. The act had little impact on addicts at the time but may have served to decrease the number of new addicts.*
8. The Harrison Narcotics Tax Act of 1914 sharply curtailed the prevalence of heroin use in the United States.
   F *This act strictly regulated the legal supply of certain drugs but actually served to shift opium and morphine addicts to heroin (which became easier to obtain on the black market).*
9. The Eighteenth Amendment, which prohibited the production, sale, transportation, and importing of alcohol, failed because it did not have a substantial effect on drinking in the United States.
   F *Prohibition did have an effect on drinking. In fact, the rate of drinking decreased markedly. In addition, death rates attributable to liver cirrhosis decreased, and there was a decline in both admission rates to state hospitals for alcoholism and arrest rates for alcohol-related offenses.*
10. Federal antidrug legislation between 1940 and 1970 failed to have a sustained influence on drug use or dependence.
    T *This is true despite the increased severity of penalties for drug law infractions. However, increased attention was paid to nonnarcotic drug use and to drug abuse treatment during this period.*
11. The most successful aspect of the war on drugs has been the interception of drugs.
    F *Most experts conclude that this effort has been a failure, even though hundreds of millions of dollars were spent on it. The flow of drugs into the United States has not been significantly altered.*
12. Urine testing is a reliable method for detecting drug use.
    F *Many urinalysis tests continue to be unreliable, although progress is gradually being made. Technological deficiencies and human error make test results questionable.*

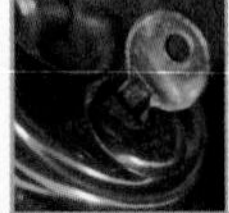

Key Terms

amphetamines
avoirdupois
Cannabis sativa
fermentation
hashish
morphine
narcotic
opium poppy
patent medicines
peyote (pā-'ō-tē)
prohibition
solvent
speakeasy

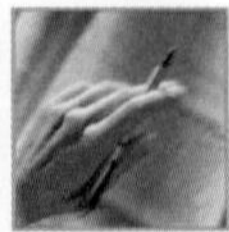

Essays/Thought Questions

1. What efforts might be taken to reduce or eliminate the availability and use of "club drugs"?
2. What are the potential benefits of reducing the availability of illegal drugs versus reducing the demand for such substances?
3. Should efforts be supported to decriminalize or even legalize the use of certain drugs, such as marijuana?
4. Describe the 2009 Family Smoking Prevention and Tobacco Control Act. Discuss whether the mandated elements of this act will impact on smoking among children and young adults.

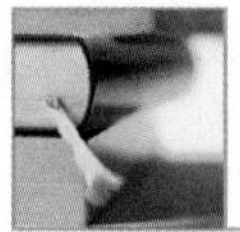

Suggested Readings

Aaron, P., & Musto, D. (1981). Temperance and prohibition in America: A historical overview. In M. H. Moore & D. R. Gersten (Eds.), *Alcohol and public policy* (pp. 127–181). Washington, DC: Academy Press.

Burnham, J. C. (1993). *Bad habits: Drinking, smoking, taking drugs, gambling, sexual misbehavior, and swearing in American history*. New York: New York University Press.

Jonnes, J. (1999). *Hep-cats, narcs, and pipe dreams: A history of America's romance with illegal drugs*. Baltimore, MD: Johns Hopkins University Press.

Lender, M. E., & Martin, J. K. (1982). *Drinking in America*. New York: The Free Press.

McKenna, T. (1992). *Food of the gods: The search for the original tree of knowledge*. New York: Bantam Books.

Morgan, H. W. (1981). *Drugs in America: A social history, 1800–1980*. Syracuse, NY: Syracuse University Press.

Rudgley, R. (1993). *Essential substances: A cultural history of intoxicants in society*. New York: Kodansha International.

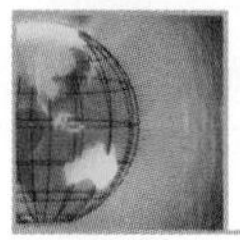

Web Resources

Visit the Book Companion Website at www.cengage.com/psychology/maisto to access study tools including a glossary, flashcards, and web quizzing. You will also find links to the following resources:

- National Institute on Drug Abuse
- Information on club drugs
- Partnership for a Drug-Free America
- U.S. Department of Justice, Drug Enforcement Administration
- National Organization for the Reform of Marijuana Laws
- The History of the Non-Medical Use of Drugs in the United States
- U.S. Department of Justice, Drug Enforcement Administration (schedules of controlled substances)
- Information on street drugs

CHAPTER 3

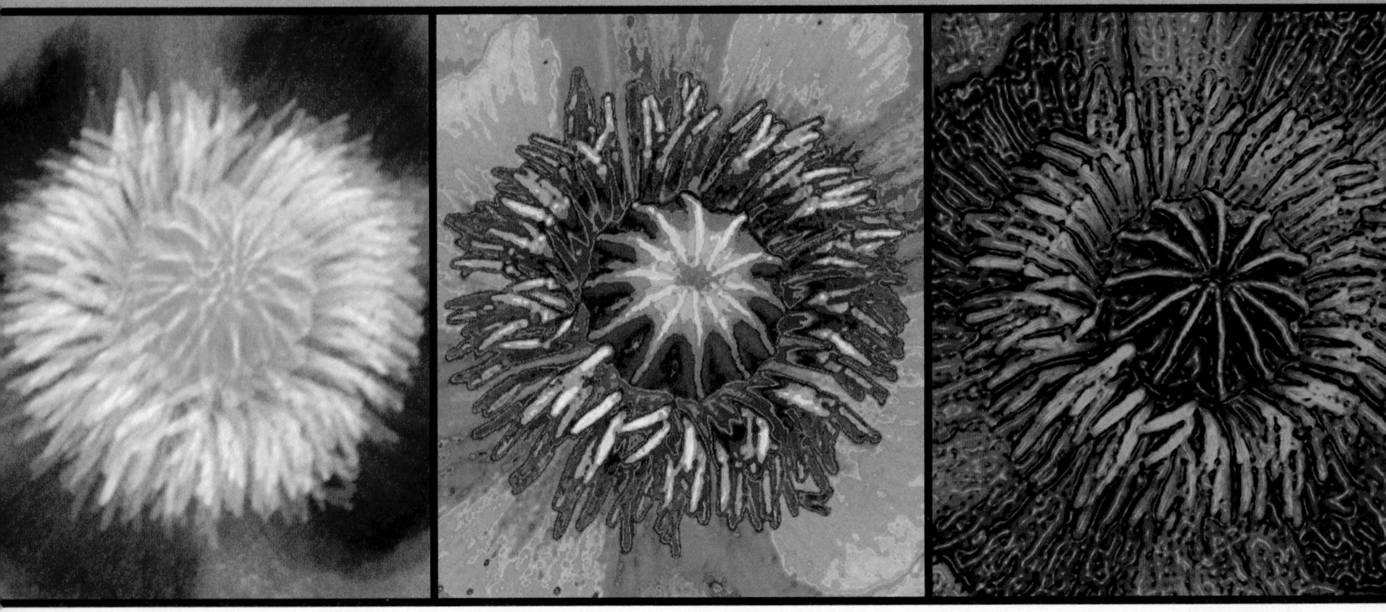

Drugs and the Nervous System

What Do You Think? True or False?

Answers are given at the end of the chapter.

___ 1. Certain cells in the nervous system have the unique ability to "talk" with each other.

___ 2. The effects of drugs always involve naturally occurring physiological processes.

___ 3. Some drugs may act by mimicking a neurotransmitter.

___ 4. All drugs have the same basic effect on a cellular level; that is, they all block neural firing.

___ 5. The brain is shielded from many toxic substances by a protective barrier.

___ 6. The two main branches of the nervous system are the peripheral nervous system (PNS) and the autonomic nervous system (ANS).

___ 7. The brain and the spinal cord make up the peripheral nervous system.

___ 8. The brain is firmly attached to the inside of the skull by tough membranes known as the meninges.

___ 9. The autonomic nervous system is responsible for regulating food and water intake.

___10. Animals will work for the electrical stimulation of certain parts of the brain.

Every feeling or emotion you have—in fact, all psychological experience—is based on brain activity. The fact that this physical entity, the brain, is the basis of conscious experience is the key to understanding how the chemical agents we call drugs alter psychological processes.

One feature all psychoactive drugs have in common is that they produce their effects by acting in some way on nervous system tissue; this chapter is concerned with these physiological actions of drugs. Most of these actions occur at the level of the brain. As recent discoveries in neuroscience have led to a greater understanding of how the brain works, parallel advances have taken place in our understanding of drug actions. These developments have led to some radically new ways of thinking about drug effects and drug problems such as addiction. Before we discuss how drugs act on the brain, however, we must first cover some of the fundamentals of just how the brain works.

The Neuron

The basic building blocks of the nervous system are cells called **neurons**. Neurons are similar to other cells in the human body, such as blood cells or muscle cells, but they have the unique feature of being able to communicate with one another. The structural properties of neurons provide us with some clues to the nature of the neural transmission process.

Notice that the neuron depicted in Figure 3.1 has a cell body similar to those of any other cell. The cell body includes a nucleus that contains the genetic material for the neuron and other processes that control the metabolic activities of the cell. Extending from the cell body of the neuron are a number of small spine- or branchlike structures called **dendrites** and one long cylindrical structure called the **axon**. These structures are unique to the neuron and are responsible for some of its remarkable properties.

Axons vary in length but are usually much longer than shown in the illustration—sometimes thousands of times longer than the diameter of the cell body. The axon

neurons ('nü-'rän)
Individual nerve cells that are basic building blocks of the nervous system.

dendrites ('den-'drīt)
Spiny branchlike structures that extend from the cell body of a neuron, typically contain numerous receptor sites, and are thus important in neural transmission.

axon ('ak-'sän)
A long cylindrical extension of the cell body of the neuron; conducts an electrical charge from the cell body to the axon terminals.

FIGURE 3.1
Diagram of a Neuron

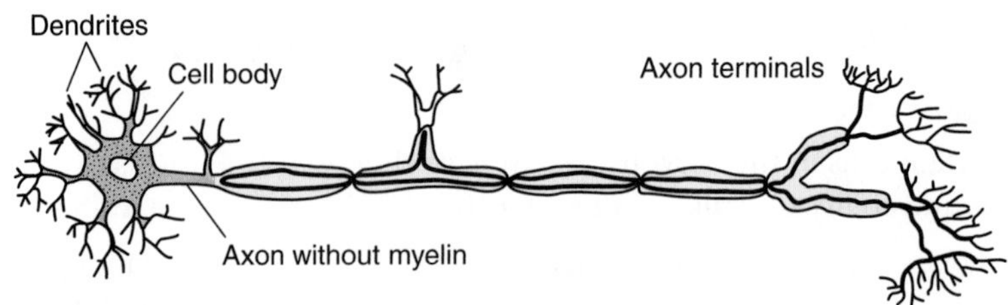

myelin ('mī-ə-lən) A fatty white substance that covers the axons of some neurons.

action potential The electrical impulse along the axon that occurs when a neuron fires.

depicted in Figure 3.1 is enclosed within a sheath of a white, fatty substance called **myelin** (not all axons are covered by myelin sheaths; "unmyelinated" axons are gray). Myelin provides insulation for the axon, similar to insulation for a wire. The comparison is fitting because the principal function of the axon is to conduct electrical current. The axon transmits information by conducting an electrical signal from one end of the neuron to the other. Generally, information is gathered by dendrites and the cell body and transmitted along the axon in the form of an electrical signal called the **action potential**.

The action potential does not work in precisely the way that electricity travels along a wire. Rather it is produced by the flow of charged particles called ions through channels in the membrane that covers the axon. When the neuron is at rest, the concentration of positively charged sodium ions is greater outside the axon membrane, whereas negatively charged protein and chloride ions are concentrated within the axon. When the neuron is stimulated, certain ion channels open, permitting positive ions into the axon, and some depolarization of the axon will occur. If the level of stimulation becomes high enough, a threshold of excitation is reached, and a massive depolarization of the axon membrane occurs as positively charged sodium ions rush into the axon. This rapid depolarization that produces a change of about 110 millivolts is also termed the *action potential.* The action potential travels rapidly along the axon like a wave and is said to be "all or none," in that the axon is either "firing" with the full voltage charge or at rest. Once the neuron has fired, sodium ions are pumped out of the axon, channels close, and the neuron returns to its resting potential.

Neural Transmission

axon terminals (or terminal buttons) Enlarged buttonlike structures at the ends of axon branches.

synapse ('si-'naps) The junction between neurons.

neurotransmitters Chemical substances stored in the axon terminals that are released into the synapse when the neuron fires. Neurotransmitters then influence activity in postsynaptic neurons.

The branches at the end of the axon shown in Figure 3.1 terminate in small buttonlike structures known as **axon terminals** or **terminal buttons**. These axon terminals hold the key to an important puzzle: how the electrical message actually gets from one neuron to another. When advances in microscopy made possible the viewing of neurons as they are seen here, a surprising finding was that most axon terminals of one neuron do not come into direct contact with the dendrites of the neighboring neuron as had been supposed; instead, the junction between two neurons, the **synapse**, is generally separated by a gap called the synaptic cleft (see Figure 3.2). The question is: How does one neuron communicate with another without direct contact between them? It is now known that, when an action potential reaches the axon terminal, chemical substances stored in the terminal button are released into the synapse, and these chemical substances, called **neurotransmitters**, actually trigger activity in the adjacent neuron.

Thus, neural transmission may be thought of as an electrochemical event—electrical along the axon and chemical at the synapse. This is of some importance for our purposes;

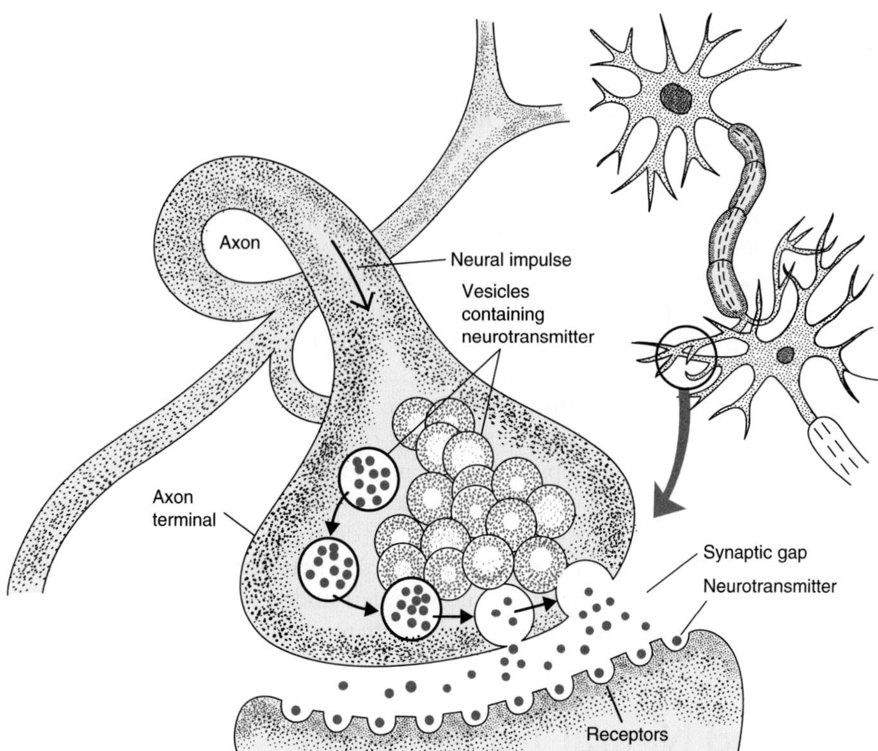

FIGURE 3.2
Diagram of a synapse showing an enlarged axon terminal with vesicles containing neurotransmitter molecules

it suggests that drugs may interact with the nervous system at the synapse because that is where chemical transmission takes place. In fact, we now know that most psychoactive drugs produce their important effects by action at the synapse (see Valenstein, 2005, for an account of the discovery of neurotransmitters and synaptic transmission). Therefore, more detailed analysis of the chemical processes that occur at the synapse is required.

A lock–key analogy is useful for depicting the neural transmission process. Scattered along the dendrites and cell body are special structures known as **receptor sites**, or receptors. These structures may be viewed as locks that must be opened before the neuron fires. To fire, the receptors must be "unlocked," which is accomplished by the neurotransmitter substances released at the terminal button. The neurotransmitter molecules may be thought of as keys. The idea is illustrated in Figure 3.2. Receptor sites are depicted as circular holes in the dendrite and neurotransmitters as circles being released from the axon terminal. The notion is simple: The key must fit the lock to trigger an event such as neural firing.

receptor sites
Specialized structures located on dendrites and cell bodies for neurons that are activated by neurotransmitters.

In fact, neurotransmitter molecules and receptors have chemical structures that are considerably more complex than is illustrated, and the lock–key analogy does not completely explain the process. Transmitters and their receptors are said to have an affinity for one another; that is, the transmitter is attracted to the receptor site, and when a transmitter key occupies a receptor lock, they briefly become attached in a process called binding. When a neurotransmitter molecule binds to a receptor, changes occur in the neuron that may make the neuron more or less likely to fire. The two major mechanisms for these changes are ionotropic and metabotropic.

Ionotropic receptors are directly coupled to the ion channels that regulate the number of charged molecules inside and outside the neuron. When the transmitter binds to such a receptor, it causes the channel to open and allows charged particles to enter or leave the cell. If the receptor opens a channel that allows more positively charged ions

ionotropic receptors
Receptors that are coupled to ion channels and affect the neuron by causing those channels to open.

into the neuron, then the neuron will be more likely to fire. If enough of these channels are opened, the neuron will generate an action potential, and such receptors are referred to as *excitatory*. At other synapses, when the neurotransmitter binds to a receptor, it may open ion channels that result in more negative ions entering the neuron, and this will hyperpolarize the neuron and make it *less* likely to fire. Because activating such a receptor actually makes it more difficult to produce an action potential, this is referred to as *inhibitory* neurotransmission. Ionotropic receptors are sometimes termed "*fast*" *receptors* because the entire process is completed in just a few milliseconds.

metabotropic receptors Receptors that act through a second messenger system.

In contrast, another class of receptors, **metabotropic receptors**, are said to be "*slow*" *receptors* because they produce changes in the neuron that are slightly delayed (by a few hundred milliseconds) and that can be relatively long lasting. Metabotropic receptors are not directly coupled with ion channels but rather cause the release or activation of specialized molecules (e.g., G proteins) that are referred to as "second messengers." Second-messenger molecules can have a number of effects within the neuron, but generally they act much like ionotropic receptors and open ion channels somewhere in the neuron. Also like ionotropic receptors, some metabotropic receptors increase the likelihood of neural firing (excitatory) and others may decrease firing (inhibitory). An important point is that there are many different types of neurotransmitter keys and many corresponding receptor site locks. We now understand that the brain is chemically coded with different pathways that respond to different neurotransmitter chemicals.

Drugs and Neural Transmission

Several ways that drugs can interfere with synaptic transmission may have already occurred to you. For example, suppose the chemical structure of some drug is similar to the structure of a naturally occurring (endogenous) neurotransmitter. If the similarity is close enough, the drug molecules might bind to the receptor sites, thus duping the receptor into reacting as if the natural transmitter is present and stimulating the neuron. Just such a process, called *mimicry*, actually does occur with some drugs. For example, morphine and heroin are now thought to act by mimicking natural neurotransmitters called endorphins.

Mimicry is an obvious mechanism of drug action, but drugs can influence neural transmission in numerous other ways as well. A sampling of these mechanisms is listed in Table 3.1. Neurotransmitters must be manufactured from simpler building blocks, or precursor molecules. Transmitters are usually manufactured in a cell body or axon terminal, but if the substance is manufactured in the cell body, it must still be transported to the terminal before it is functional. Some drugs interfere with transmitter production or transport. Neurotransmitter molecules are stored in small packages called **vesicles** located in the terminal buttons. Some drugs affect the ability of the vesicles to store neurotransmitter substances. For example, the drug reserpine, once used to treat high blood pressure, causes certain vesicles to become leaky and then the transmitters involved are not effectively released into the synapse. Alternatively, other drugs can enhance the release of neurotransmitter substances into the synapse; this is one of the ways stimulants such as amphetamines are thought to act.

vesicles ('ve-si-kəl) Tiny sacs in axon terminals that store neurotransmitters.

enzyme breakdown One process by which neurotransmitters are inactivated. Chemicals called enzymes interact with the transmitter molecule and change its structure so that it no longer is capable of occupying receptor sites.

reuptake One process by which neurotransmitters are inactivated. Neurotransmitter molecules are taken back up into the axon terminal that released them.

Another important rule of neural transmission is that neurotransmitters, once released, must be deactivated to terminate cell activity. Neurotransmitters are deactivated in two ways: **enzyme breakdown** and **reuptake**. Certain chemicals called enzymes act both to build the complex molecules of neurotransmitters and to break down neurotransmitters to inactive form. These processes are complex and reveal one reason that identifying and isolating the functions of neurotransmitters in the brain are difficult. The brain contains

TABLE 3.1 Neurochemical Mechanisms of Drug Action

Drug effects can be produced by altering the following neurochemical systems:

1. *Neurotransmitter synthesis.* A drug may increase or decrease the synthesis of neurotransmitters.
2. *Neurotransmitter transport.* A drug may interfere with the transport of neurotransmitter molecules to the axon terminals.
3. *Neurotransmitter storage.* A drug may interfere with the storage of neurotransmitters in the vesicles of the axon terminal.
4. *Neurotransmitter release.* A drug may cause the axon terminals to release neurotransmitter molecules into the synapse prematurely.
5. *Neurotransmitter degradation.* A drug may influence the breakdown of neurotransmitters by enzymes.
6. *Neurotransmitter reuptake.* A drug may block the reuptake of neurotransmitters into the axon terminals.
7. *Receptor activation.* A drug may activate a receptor site by mimicking a neurotransmitter.
8. *Receptor blocking.* A drug may cause a receptor to become inactive by blocking it.

many different chemicals, and they are constantly changing form. Consider the processes involved in the production and destruction of **acetylcholine**, one of the better-known neurotransmitters. The precursor molecule choline is acted on by an enzyme (choline acetyltransferase) to make acetylcholine. Acetylcholine itself is broken down by a different enzyme—acetylcholinesterase—to yield two metabolites: choline and acetate. By the way, enzymes are named by the stem of the chemical that they influence and always have an "-ase" ending. A drug can alter neural transmission by affecting enzyme activity. For example, some antidepressant drugs alter brain levels of the neurotransmitters norepinephrine, dopamine, and serotonin by inhibiting the activity of monoamine oxidase, the enzyme that breaks down these compounds.

acetylcholine (ə-'se-t° l-'kō-lēn)
A neurotransmitter linked with cognitive processes and memory that is found both in the brain and in the parasympathetic branch of the autonomic nervous system.

A second mechanism for removing neurotransmitters from the synapse is called reuptake. Neurotransmitters are taken back up into the terminal button after they have been released—hence the term *reuptake.* This is an economical mechanism of deactivating transmitters because the neurotransmitter molecule is preserved intact and can be used again without the expense of energy involved in the manufacture of new transmitters. Some drugs (notably cocaine) exert some of their action by blocking the reuptake process.

As noted, an important site of drug action is directly at the receptor. Some drugs directly affect the receptor by mimicking the activity of natural neurotransmitters—similar to a duplicate key that fits into and opens a lock. Other drugs seem to act as if they fit into the lock but then they jam the lock and prevent the neuron from firing. Such a drug is called a *blocking agent.* In general, any chemical—natural or otherwise—that fits a receptor lock and activates it is said to be an **agonist** of that receptor. Any compound that occupies a receptor and does not activate it, but rather prevents other compounds from activating the receptor, is said to be an **antagonist** (see Table 3.2). For example, naloxone is an antagonist of the receptors on which opiate drugs (such as heroin) work. If naloxone is promptly administered to a patient who has just taken a potentially lethal dose of heroin, the patient will survive and will rapidly be brought to a state in which it appears as if the heroin had never been taken. In fact, all effects of heroin and other opiates are blocked completely or reversed by naloxone. Thus, naloxone is called an opiate antagonist. The terms *agonist* and *antagonist* may also be used more generally to refer to drugs that enhance (agonist) or inhibit (antagonist) the activity of a particular neurotransmitter system.

agonist ('a-gə-nist)
A substance that occupies a neural receptor and causes some change in the conductance of the neuron.

antagonist
A substance that occupies a neural receptor and blocks normal synaptic transmission.

TABLE 3.2 Major Neurotransmitters with Representative Agonists and Antagonists

Neurotransmitter	Agonist	Antagonist
Acetylcholine	Nicotine	Atropine
Dopamine/norepinephrine	Cocaine/amphetamines	Chlorpromazine
Serotonin	LSD	Chlorpromazine
Endorphins	Morphine	Naloxone
GABA	Barbiturates	Bicuculline
Glutamate	Aspartic acid	Ketamine

Up to now, we have considered only the acute effects of drugs on neural transmission, that is, effects that occur during a single use of the drug. When drugs are used more regularly, long-lasting changes in neurotransmission can occur that are important in the development of drug tolerance and dependence. For example, chronic use of some drugs can result in a long-term reduction of the amount of neurotransmitter produced and released in affected neurons. Alternatively, the number of available receptor sites can be reduced. Such changes result in the affected pathway becoming less sensitive to the drug and thus illustrate neural mechanisms of tolerance development. Depending upon the functions of the affected pathway, these changes may alter responsiveness to nondrug environmental stimuli as well. If the user stops taking the drug, the loss of stimulation in these pathways may result in withdrawal symptoms (see Nestler, 2009).

We have seen a number of ways that drugs can act to influence neural transmission (see Iversen et al., 2009, for a more detailed review). A point to remember, however, is that although drugs can interact with the brain in many different ways, the effects of the drugs always involve naturally occurring processes. That is, some systems in the brain or body with defined natural functions are made more or less active by the drug. The different effects of various drugs are coming to be understood in terms of which transmitter systems they influence and exactly how they influence them. Therefore, we next take a brief look at the neurotransmitter systems of the human brain and note some of their known functions.

Major Neurotransmitter Systems

Acetylcholine

One of the first neurotransmitters to be discovered was acetylcholine, probably because it is found in the more easily studied neurons located outside the brain. Acetylcholine resides in the axon terminals of neurons that activate the skeletal muscles. At sites where nerves meet muscles, there is a space similar to the synapse called the **neuromuscular junction**. When the neurons that synapse with muscle fibers fire, they release acetylcholine into the neuromuscular junction, and the muscle contracts. Some muscle disorders are related to problems with this process. For example, myasthenia gravis, a disease characterized by severe muscle weakness and fatigue, is caused by a blockage of acetylcholine at the neuromuscular junction. A related similar process is the basis for one of the deadliest toxins known: botulinum. One gram of botulinum toxin (about the weight of a dollar bill) is enough to fatally poison more than 3 million people (Meyer & Quenzer, 2005). Botulinum toxin is produced by a bacterium that grows in oxygen-free environments such as improperly prepared canned goods, and as you might well imagine, is a major concern with respect to biological warfare and terrorism. The basis for botulinum toxicity is that it

neuromuscular junction Junction between neuron and muscle fibers where release of acetylcholine by neurons causes muscles to contract.

blocks the release of acetylcholine at the neuromuscular junction, resulting in muscle paralysis and, in sufficient doses, death by asphyxiation. Interestingly, a carefully prepared form of botulinum toxin is now being marketed and used cosmetically under the brand name Botox. When Botox is injected into one of the facial muscles, it causes that muscle to become partially paralyzed; this can produce a temporary smoothing of certain types of facial wrinkles and lines.

As a point of terminology, if the name of a neurotransmitter is to be used as an adjective, simply take the stem of the name (e.g., *choline*) and add the suffix "-ergic." Thus, neurons that contain acetylcholine are *cholinergic* neurons, and drugs that block acetylcholine, such as atropine, are *anticholinergic* drugs. Nicotine is an example of a cholinergic drug because it is an agonist at acetylcholine receptors.

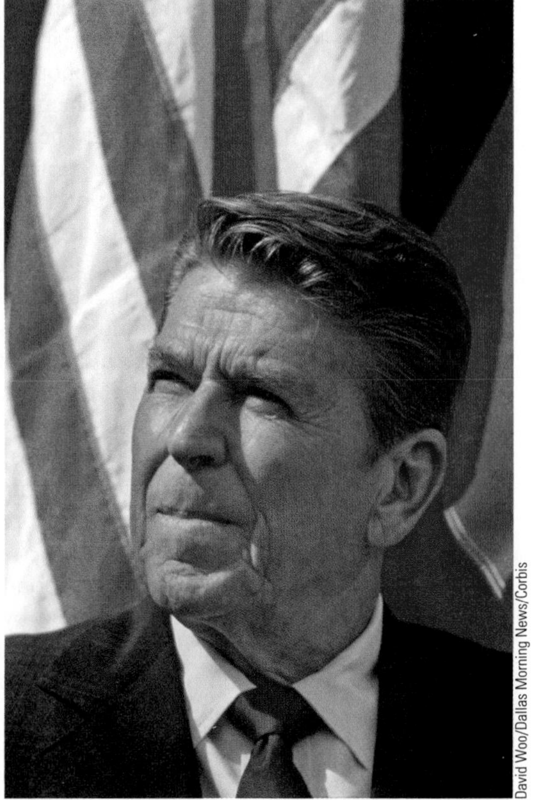

David Woo/Dallas Morning News/Corbis

Late President Ronald Reagan retreated from public life after it was revealed that he suffered from Alzheimer's disease.

Acetylcholine is also important in the brain, but like most neurotransmitters, its function in the brain is not thoroughly understood. Acetylcholine is thought to be important in sensory processing, attention, and memory. In fact, there is substantial evidence that **Alzheimer's disease**, a progressive loss of memory function that occurs in the elderly, is related to the loss of neural function in some of the brain's cholinergic pathways. Much current research on Alzheimer's disease is attempting to determine just what might be going wrong in these pathways and to develop ways of correcting or preventing the problem. Drugs such as Aricept (donepezil) and Exelon (rivastigmine) reduce the symptoms of Alzheimer's disease by elevating levels of acetylcholine in the brain through inhibition of the enzyme acetylcholinesterase. The problem of Alzheimer's disease underscores an important point: When neurotransmitter systems malfunction, disease states are a likely consequence, and drugs that target the affected system may provide effective treatments. These ideas have been critical to contemporary theories of the biological basis of mental illness, which are considered in the next section.

Alzheimer's disease ('älts-'hī-mərz-)
One of the most common forms of senility among the elderly; involves a progressive loss of memory and other cognitive functions.

norepinephrine ('no·r-'e-pə-'ne-frən)
A neurotransmitter in the brain that is involved in activity of the sympathetic branch of the autonomic nervous system.

dopamine ('dō-pə-'mēn)
A neurotransmitter in the brain that is involved with movement and reward.

serotonin ('sir-ə-tō-nən)
A neurotransmitter in the brain that is involved with sleep and mood.

monoamines ('mä-nō-ə-'mən)
A class of chemicals characterized by a single amine group; includes the neurotransmitters norepinephrine, dopamine, and serotonin.

Monoamines

Three important neurotransmitters—**norepinephrine** (noradrenaline), **dopamine**, and **serotonin**—are collectively known as the **monoamines** because the chemical structure of each contains a single amine group. Like acetylcholine, norepinephrine was discovered early because it is found outside the brain. It serves as a key chemical to mediate the physical changes that accompany emotional arousal. Norepinephrine is also found in the brain as a neurotransmitter, where it seems to be important in the regulation of hunger, alertness, and arousal. Serotonin is found throughout the brain and has been shown to be important in the regulation of sleep. Dopamine is a key neurotransmitter in the pathways that regulate coordinated motor movements. This discovery led to the hypothesis that dopamine insufficiency may be the basis of **Parkinson's disease**, a disorder characterized by progressive loss of fine motor movements, muscle rigidity, and tremor primarily afflicting elderly people.

The dopamine deficiency hypothesis of Parkinson's disease led to new treatment approaches involving the administration of **L-dopa**, a precursor of dopamine. L-dopa was administered to patients in hopes of correcting the dopamine deficiency and proved to

Parkinson's disease
A disease that primarily afflicts the elderly and involves a progressive deterioration of motor control.

L-dopa ('el-'dō-pə)
A chemical precursor of dopamine used in the treatment of Parkinson's disease.

blood-brain barrier
The system that "filters" the blood before it can enter the brain.

be dramatically effective in relieving the symptoms of this disease. Dopamine itself is not effective because it does not enter the brain from the bloodstream. The brain is protected from toxic compounds that might enter the bloodstream by a **blood-brain barrier** that screens many chemicals, including dopamine. But L-dopa does penetrate the barrier, and once it reaches the brain, it is converted to dopamine (Deutsch & Roth, 2009). Using L-dopa in the treatment of Parkinson's disease is a dramatic example of the value of new knowledge about neurotransmitters for the treatment of disease. Although L-dopa does not cure the disease process (dopaminergic neurons continue to be lost and eventually even L-dopa cannot correct the loss), it has brought years of productive living to many whose lives would otherwise have been prematurely ended by Parkinson's disease.

In addition to these functions, the monoamine neurotransmitters norepinephrine, dopamine, and serotonin have been closely linked to mood states and emotional disorders. In fact, drugs that influence the monoamine systems have revolutionized modern psychiatry. For example, considerable evidence shows that severe clinical depression may have a biological basis. Current theories propose that clinical depression is associated with dysregulation of monoamines, particularly norepinephrine and serotonin. This monoamine theory of depression originated with the finding that certain drugs that depleted monoamines seemed to produce depression. Reserpine, once used to treat high blood pressure, makes monoaminergic vesicles leaky (as we noted earlier) and the transmitters are then destroyed by enzymes, resulting in a depletion of norepinephrine, serotonin, and dopamine. This process often causes depression in people whose mood states were normal before treatment (as you may have guessed, it also produces Parkinson's symptoms due to dopamine depletion, and this side effect led to the use of L-dopa previously mentioned). Evidence of abnormal monoamine activity in clients who suffer from depression has been reported; for example, numerous studies have linked deficient serotonin activity to suicidal behavior (Arango & Mann, 2009). Finally, the drugs that are useful in the treatment of depression (e.g., Prozac) generally influence either norepinephrine or serotonin transmission or both, which further supports this monoamine-dysregulation hypothesis. Increased knowledge of neurochemical processes linked to depression is suggesting new and promising approaches to the understanding and treatment of depressive disorders (Berman et al., 2009—see Contemporary Issue Box 3.1).

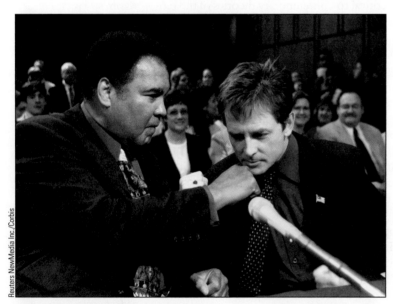

Reuters NewMedia Inc./Corbis

Boxing legend Muhammad Ali pretends to punch actor Michael J. Fox. Both suffer from Parkinson's disease.

Monoamines, particularly dopamine and serotonin, appear to be important as the biochemical basis of another important mental illness: schizophrenia. Schizophrenia involves a major loss of contact with reality, characterized by false beliefs or delusions, hallucinations, social withdrawal, and distortions of emotionality. Strong evidence ties these symptoms to high levels of monoamine activity. First, all the drugs that are effective in the treatment of schizophrenia also block monoamine transmission. In fact, it has long been known that a close correlation exists between the clinical potency of the various drugs used and their ability to block dopamine receptors (Snyder, Burt, & Creese, 1976). Another interesting piece of evidence is that stimulant drugs such as cocaine and amphetamines increase monoamine activity

CONTEMPORARY ISSUE BOX 3.1

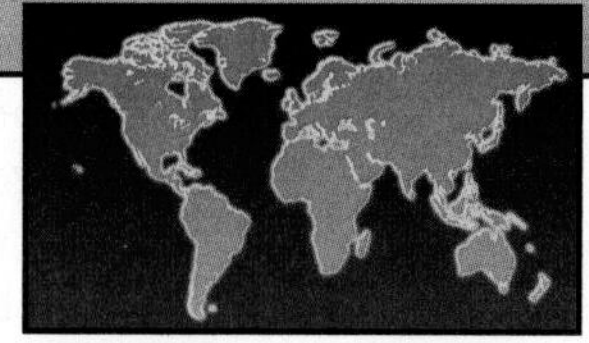

You Are Never Too Old to Make New Neurons: Adult Neurogenesis and Depression

Until very recently, it was almost universally accepted that the birth of new neurons—neurogenesis—ended very early in development. Young adults were considered to possess all the neurons they would ever have. It was believed that cells lost due to stroke, injury, or drug abuse could never be replaced. However, in the 1990s, it was discovered that new neurons were born in certain brain regions in adult rats (Gould et al., 1999). These findings were subsequently confirmed in adult humans, and it is now believed that neurogenesis may occur in the hippocampus and certain other brain areas throughout adulthood. As yet, little is known about the functions of adult neurogenesis, but the possibilities for treatments of neurological disease are enormous if the process can be harnessed. The role of neurogenesis in mental health has become a major research emphasis. One of the most exciting early developments in this research is the possible linkage between neurogenesis and depression. A number of studies have shown that various types of stress can suppress production of new neurons (Duman, 2009). Stress is also linked to depression, and there is evidence of reduced hippocampus size in depressed patients, which may indicate less neurogenesis (Jacobs, 2004). We noted earlier that antidepressant medication generally elevates levels of the neurotransmitter serotonin, and several studies now indicate that elevated serotonin levels increase neurogenesis. Importantly, it requires several weeks for new neurons to become integrated into functional neural pathways, and this corresponds well with the time course of antidepressant action. These drugs generally increase serotonin levels fairly rapidly, but it takes several weeks for the depression to lift, which suggests that it may be the increased birth of new neurons, rather than the elevation of serotonin per se, that is responsible for antidepressant action. If this new neurogenesis theory of depression is correct, it could lead to new and more effective treatments for this serious disorder (see Duman, 2009, for a review).

in the brain. Although low or moderate doses of these stimulants enhance mood, overdoses often lead to paranoid delusions and a loss of reality contact that strongly resembles some symptoms of schizophrenia. When the drug wears off and monoamine activity returns to normal, these symptoms generally dissipate—a finding that further supports the link between abnormal monoamine activity and schizophrenia (see Sawa & Snyder, 2002). Although complex disorders such as schizophrenia and depression cannot be understood completely without considering a host of psychological and social factors, the biological approaches just noted have certainly improved our understanding and treatment of them. We consider the use of drugs to treat these and other disorders in more detail in Chapter 13.

Endorphins

During the late 1970s, compounds were discovered in mammalian brain tissue that were functionally similar to opiate drugs such as morphine and heroin. Unlike acetylcholine and the monoamines, these compounds were large molecules in the peptide family. Because they appeared to be, in effect, a naturally occurring morphine, they were named **endorphins**—a contraction of *endogenous morphine*. We now understand that the effects of opiate drugs are mediated through endorphinergic activity. The natural functions of the endorphins themselves are still far from clear but they certainly modulate pain relief. The endorphins are explained in more detail in Chapter 10.

endorphins (en-'do•r-fənz) Neurotransmitters in the brain that are mimicked by opiate drugs.

GABA Short for gamma-aminobutyric acid; the most abundant inhibitory neurotransmitter in the brain.

glutamate An excitatory amino acid neurotransmitter.

Amino Acid Neurotransmitters

Two additional neurotransmitters are the amino acids gamma-aminobutyric acid, commonly referred to as **GABA**, and **glutamate**. GABA is among the most abundant of the known neurotransmitters in brain tissue, and it is the most significant inhibitory transmitter of the brain. That is, GABA opens negatively charged chloride ion channels that do not cause the neuron to fire but rather hyperpolarize the membrane and impede neural firing. If a neuron has a GABAergic receptor site that is activated, a larger quantity of the excitatory transmitter is required for the neuron to fire. A number of drugs are now thought to act on the GABA system; as you might guess, they are the classic depressant drugs: barbiturates, tranquilizers such as Valium (diazepam) and Xanax (alprazolam), and alcohol. Glutamate is among the most abundant of the excitatory neurotransmitters and is known to be important in learning and memory processes. Some hallucinogenic drugs (PCP and ketamine) act on glutamate receptors in some parts of the brain (see Chapter 12).

Other Transmitters

The development of more sophisticated research techniques has led to the recognition that many more neurotransmitters await discovery. A thorough discussion of recent advances in neuropharmacology is beyond the scope of this text, but some developments have already had a substantial impact on our understanding of psychoactive drug actions. Indeed, many neurotransmitters have been discovered beyond those previously mentioned, and no doubt many more remain to be found. We have much to learn about the brain's chemical code. Often the discovery of a new neurotransmitter increases our understanding of drug action. For example, one of the most recently discovered neurotransmitters is a lipid called **anandamide**. It is of considerable interest because the active chemical in marijuana appears to act by mimicking anandamide.

anandamide
A lipid neurotransmitter mimicked by marijuana.

The Nervous System

central nervous system (CNS)
The brain and the spinal cord.

peripheral nervous system (PNS)
Sensory nerves, motor nerves, and the automatic nervous system.

autonomic nervous system (ANS)
Part of the PNS; has two branches: sympathetic and parasympathetic.

sympathetic branch
Branch of the ANS that is activated during emotional arousal and is responsible for such physiological changes as increased heart and respiratory rate, increased blood pressure, and pupil dilation.

sympathomimetic
Drugs such as cocaine and amphetamines that produce the physiological effects of sympathetic activity.

beta-blockers
Drugs that block beta-adrenergic receptors of the sympathetic system and thus act to relieve high blood pressure.

We have been focusing on a microscopic view of the nervous system as we considered how drugs might act at the level of the single neuron. We now turn to the larger picture and consider a macroscopic view of the nervous system. The structure of the nervous system is outlined in Figure 3.3. The major distinction is between the **central nervous system (CNS)** and the **peripheral nervous system (PNS)**. The CNS includes the brain and spinal cord. All nervous tissue outside (or peripheral to) the CNS is part of the PNS. The PNS includes nerves (nerves are simply bundles of axons) that send input from the senses to the brain (sensory nerves) and nerves that send output from the brain to muscles (motor nerves).

The PNS also includes an important regulatory system known as the **autonomic nervous system (ANS)**. The ANS regulates various nonconscious or automatic functions and is divided into two parts. The **sympathetic branch** of the autonomic nervous system is activated during emotional arousal by a release of epinephrine and norepinephrine from the adrenal glands. This branch is responsible for the physiological changes that characterize the "fight-or-flight" reaction. During sympathetic arousal, heart rate increases, blood pressure increases, respiratory rate increases, sweating increases, pupils dilate, the mouth becomes dry, and changes occur in blood flow as blood is shunted away from the internal organs and to the brain and large muscle groups. These physiological effects are important to keep in mind because some psychoactive drugs mimic sympathetic arousal. Such drugs are said to be **sympathomimetic**; they include cocaine, amphetamines, and some hallucinogens such as LSD. Another group of drugs blocks a type of norepinephrine receptor in the sympathetic nervous system called "beta-noradrenergic" receptors. These beta receptors regulate blood pressure, and the so-called **beta-blockers** (drugs such as propranolol) are widely used in the treatment of hypertension.

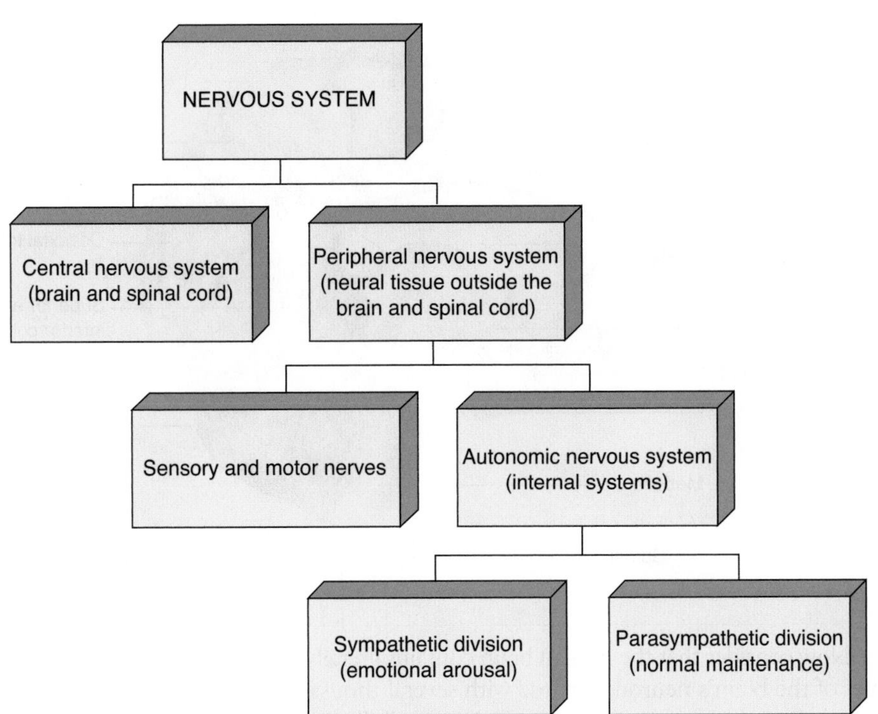

FIGURE 3.3
Organizational structure of the nervous system

The other branch of the autonomic nervous system is the **parasympathetic branch**, which in general balances the actions of the sympathetic branch by exerting opposite effects. Parasympathetic activity reduces heart rate, blood pressure, and so on. In contrast to sympathetic neurons, parasympathetic synapses are primarily cholinergic.

parasympathetic branch
Branch of the ANS that is responsible for lowering heart rate and blood pressure.

The Brain

The key organ of the nervous system is the brain (see Figure 3.4). Covered with tough membranes called the *meninges*, the brain floats within the skull in a liquid known as cerebrospinal fluid. Although weighing just a few pounds, the human brain is an extremely complex structure. We have just examined the processes involved when a single neuron

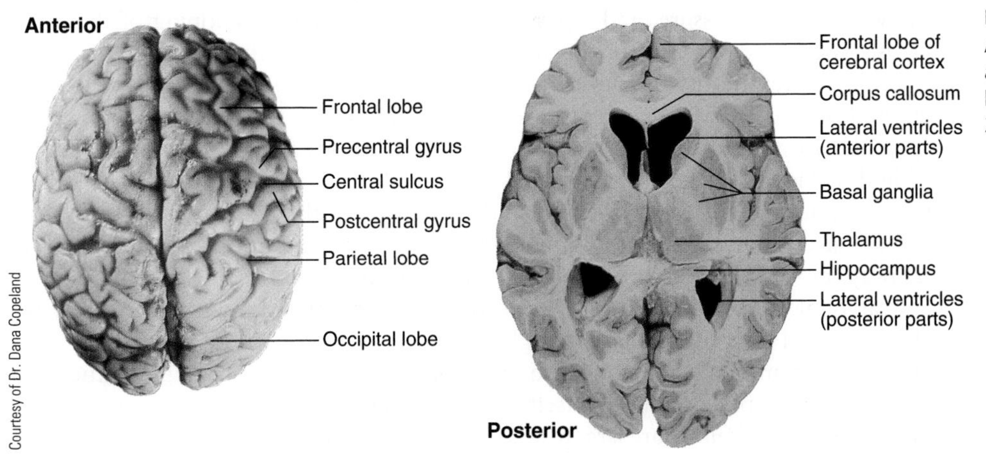

FIGURE 3.4
A dorsal view (from above) and a cross-section of the human brain (from Kalat, 2009)

FIGURE 3.5
A sagittal (inside) view of the human brain (from Kalat, 2009)

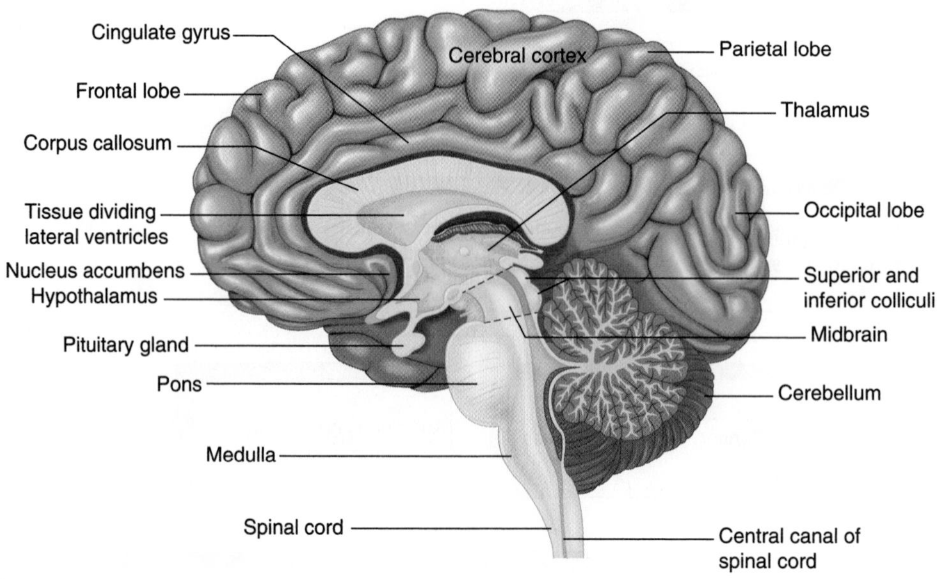

fires. Now consider that the human brain contains literally billions and billions of neurons. Many of the brain's neurons synapse with several thousand other neurons because of an elaborate branching of axons. The complexity of billions of neurons and more billions of synapses is absolutely staggering and almost beyond comprehension. Despite the enormity of the task, great strides have been made in understanding how this most complex of organs works. One fruitful approach is to consider the different parts of the brain separately in an attempt to determine their individual functions.

The major divisions of the human brain are the **hindbrain**, **midbrain**, and **forebrain**. Figure 3.5 shows the relative locations of these three divisions. If a voyage through the brain began at the spinal cord and moved up, the first part of the brain encountered would be the hindbrain.

hindbrain
The lower part of the brain, including the medulla, pons, and cerebellum.

midbrain
Part of the brain that includes the inferior and superior colliculi and the substantia nigra.

forebrain
The largest part of the human brain; includes the cerebral cortex, thalamus, hypothalamus, and limbic system.

medulla oblongata (mᵊ-'də-lə-'ä-bl-oŋ-gä-tə)
The lowest hindbrain structure of the brain; important in the regulation of breathing, heart rate, and other basic life functions.

cerebellum ('ser-ᵊ-'be-ləm)
Hindbrain structure important in motor control and coordination.

pons ('pänz)
Hindbrain structure important in the control of sleep and wakefulness.

reticular activating system
Pathway running through the medulla and pons that regulates alertness and arousal.

The Hindbrain

The hindbrain consists of three main components: the **medulla oblongata**, the **cerebellum**, and the **pons** (see Figure 3.5). The medulla is located just above (and is really a slight enlargement of) the spinal cord. A highly significant structure for the regulation of basic life functions, the medulla controls breathing, heart rate, vomiting, swallowing, blood pressure, and digestive processes. Normal functioning of the medulla is critical, and when drugs begin to affect the medulla, the person is often in danger due to respiratory or cardiovascular failure. When toxic chemicals reach high levels in this area, the vomit center is often triggered to purge the body, which may be why drinking large quantities of alcohol often causes nausea and vomiting. Farther up the hindbrain is an enlarged section called the pons. In addition to providing the pathways for input up and output down from the spinal cord, the pons plays a role in the control of sleep and wakefulness. Running along the pons and through the medulla is a pathway (not visible in Figure 3.5) known as the **reticular activating system**, which is critical for alertness and arousal. Drugs that lower arousal and induce sleep (such as barbiturates and tranquilizers) are thought to act in this region of the brain.

The cerebellum, the last major organ of the hindbrain, is a highly complex structure containing several billion neurons itself. The cerebellum is critical for motor control. Activities of the cerebellum are largely unconscious but do involve balance, coordinated movement of all kinds, and speech. The loss of motor control and balance produced by drugs such as alcohol may be caused by their action on the cerebellum.

The Midbrain

The midbrain consists of a number of structures, including the **inferior colliculi**, the **superior colliculi**, and the **substantia nigra**. The inferior colliculi form part of the auditory system. The superior colliculi function in localization of visual stimuli. These structures are specifically involved with localization of stimuli and mediation of reflexes. The actual recognition and interpretation of visual and auditory stimuli take place elsewhere in the brain (see the section on the cerebral cortex).

inferior colliculi (ko-'lik-yü-lī) Midbrain structures that control sound localization.

superior colliculi Midbrain structures that control visual localization.

substantia nigra (səb-'stan(t)-shē-ə-'nī-grə) Literally "black substance," this basal ganglia structure is darkly pigmented; produces dopamine. Damage to this area produces Parkinson's disease.

Parkinson's disease involves damage to the substantia nigra and the nigrostriatal motor pathway. Specifically, Parkinson's disease develops when nerve cells in this brain region begin to degenerate. The substantia nigra produces dopamine, which is transported through this motor pathway, and as the substantia nigra deteriorates, less and less dopamine is available for neurotransmission. Parkinson's symptoms do not appear until about 80% of the substantia nigra is destroyed. Although the causes of Parkinson's disease are not completely understood, some toxins, including some "designer drugs," appear to be capable of killing neurons in the substantia nigra and triggering the disorder (see Chapter 10).

The Forebrain

The Thalamus and Hypothalamus

The most important brain regions from the perspective of interpreting complex human behavior are in the forebrain, particularly the cortex, but also including the **thalamus** and **hypothalamus** (see Figure 3.5). The thalamus is often referred to as a relay station because it receives incoming sensory stimuli and then "relays" that information to relevant centers throughout the brain. The hypothalamus is a critical structure in the motivation of behavior. It contains areas that appear to be involved in the regulation of eating and drinking, and the control of body temperature, aggression, and sexual behavior. Worth noting is that information about the particular function of a given brain region has not been easily determined and remains somewhat controversial. Historically, the methods for analyzing brain structures were primarily lesions and stimulation. Lesioning a structure involves performing surgery on an animal subject and causing localized damage to the structure in question. When the animal has recovered from surgery, changes in behavior are then attributed to the damaged structure. For example, lesions in one part of the hypothalamus result in greatly reduced food intake, whereas if another part is damaged, overeating and obesity occur. Thus, the hypothalamus contains at least two sites that appear to be important in the regulation of food intake. One area seems to inhibit eating (because its loss results in overeating) and the other seems to excite hunger (because its loss results in less eating). The effects of electrical stimulation of a brain region generally are the opposite of the effects of lesioning or removing that region.

thalamus ('tha-lə-məs) Forebrain structure that organizes sensory input.

hypothalamus ('hī-pō-tha-lə-məs) Forebrain structure that regulates eating, drinking, and other basic biological drives.

A note of caution accompanies these findings. When cells in the brain are lesioned or stimulated, the effects extend beyond those specific cells, and indeed entire pathways may become damaged or stimulated. Thus, rather than speaking of the hunger or satiety *centers*, a more appropriate term is hunger or satiety *pathways*. However, even this may be an oversimplification because some researchers have noted that the role of these pathways may not be as specific to hunger as we first thought. That is, these pathways could affect motor movements, the sensation of taste, or more general motivational variables, and much current research is devoted to these effects. However, there is general agreement that the hypothalamus is an important structure in the regulation of hunger, thirst, and other basic biological motives (Carlson, 2008).

The Neural Basis of Reward

Despite the difficulties of such research, electrical stimulation of brain regions led to one of the most significant discoveries in the quest to understand the relationship of brain, behavior, and drugs. During the 1950s, the psychologist James Olds was trying to map the effects of stimulation on the rat brain by implanting electrodes into various regions. The rat seemed to enjoy the electrical stimulation in some areas of the brain. Here is how Olds describes his serendipitous discovery:

> I applied a brief train of 60-cycle sine wave electrical current whenever the animal entered one corner of the enclosure. The animal did not stay away from the corner, but rather came back quickly after a brief sortie which followed the first stimulation and came back even more quickly after a briefer sortie which followed the second stimulation. By the time the third electrical stimulus had been applied the animal seemed indubitably to be "coming back for more." (Carlson, 2001, p. 457)

mesolimbic dopaminergic pathway Pathway that is rewarding when stimulated.

Following up on this finding, Olds and Milner (1954) discovered that when electrodes are implanted in some brain areas, particularly in a region called the **mesolimbic dopaminergic pathway**, rats could actually be trained to press a lever to electrically stimulate themselves. The mesolimbic dopaminergic pathway includes a small subcortical area called the nucleus accumbens and travels through the ventral tegmental area all the way to the frontal cortex. When rats have been trained to self-stimulate this area, they often respond with great vigor (more than 1,000 responses per hour), and the potency of the reinforcement related to this center led Olds and others to refer to it as the "pleasure center." The notion is that the region may represent the final common pathway for pleasurable stimulation and reward. It has been argued too that this brain region is of significance in understanding the rewarding properties of drugs. The nucleus accumbens is rich in dopamine, and some investigators have suggested that dopamine is a critical chemical in producing the rewarding properties of drugs (Koob & Le Moal, 2006; Nestler, 2009). Indeed, some have viewed this region of the brain as critical to drug addiction: "There is now a wealth of evidence that [the mesolimbic dopaminergic pathway] is a crucial substrate for the acute rewarding effects of virtually all drugs of abuse and for the derangements in reward mechanisms that contribute to drug addiction" (Nestler, 2009, p. 777). As Dackis and Gold (1985) once put it, addicts can be seen as individuals who have "tampered chemically with endogenous systems of reward and lost control of this shortcut to pleasure" (p. 476).

It is true that many pleasurable events result in the release of dopamine in this pathway—good-tasting food (especially chocolate), sex, and indeed many drugs such as cocaine, heroin, and nicotine (Goldstein, 2001). However, the idea that dopamine release in this pathway always translates into the psychological experience of pleasure appears to be an oversimplification. For example, events that are surprising or arousing but not especially pleasurable (like an electrical shock) seem to release dopamine in the nucleus accumbens, so perhaps activity in this pathway reflects events that have motivational significance or are "attention-getters" (Baron & Galizio, 2005; Berridge & Robinson, 1998; Martin-Soelch et al., 2001).

limbic system Forebrain structures including the amygdala and hippocampus.

basal ganglia ('bā-səl-'gaŋ-glē-ə) Forebrain structures important for motor control; include the caudate nucleus, the putamen, and the globus pallidus.

cortex The outermost and largest part of the human brain.

The Limbic System, Basal Ganglia, and Cerebral Cortex

The forebrain also includes three complex systems: the **limbic system**, the **basal ganglia**, and the **cortex**. The aspects of behavior that are most uniquely human, such as complex reasoning, memory, logic, speech, and planning, are largely derived from these structures.

The limbic system includes several structures in the interior of the forebrain. One limbic structure, the amygdala, seems to be important in mediating certain types of aggression, fear, and other emotional experiences. Another important limbic structure is the **hippocampus**, which appears to be critical in memory storage. People with damage to the hippocampus can remember things that occurred in their lives prior to the damage but, for the most part, are unable to store new memories. In other words, their long-term memories are intact, but they have difficulty in forming new permanent memories. The basal ganglia include the caudate nucleus, the putamen, and the globus pallidus. These structures are critical for motor movements.

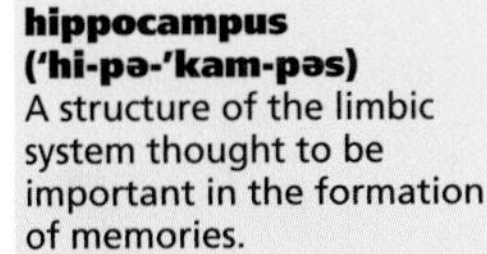

hippocampus ('hi-pə-'kam-pəs) A structure of the limbic system thought to be important in the formation of memories.

One feature that distinguishes the human brain from those of most other animals is the greatly enlarged cerebral cortex. Indeed, many of the complex psychological functions that are characteristically human are thought to involve the cortex. Figure 3.4 shows the lobes of the cerebral cortex. The occipital lobe is at the back of the brain and is often referred to as the visual projection area. Stimulation of the eye is eventually perceived as a visual stimulus when the signal reaches the occipital cortex. The temporal lobe is similarly specialized for auditory stimulation and also appears to be important in language. Damage to the left temporal lobe results in severe impairment of language abilities (at least for most right-handed individuals). Right temporal lobe damage often results in dysregulation of emotions. This relationship between right and left temporal lobe mediation of language and emotions is reversed in some cases (e.g., left-handed individuals). The frontal lobe is important in the initiation of movement and is involved with emotionality, intelligence, and personality. Tactile stimuli are registered in the parietal lobe.

Because most nonhuman species do not share the enlarged cortex of humans, using animal models to study the functions of the cortex is more difficult. Much of what we know about the cerebral cortex then has come from unfortunate accidents and diseases such as strokes and tumors, which in effect produce lesions in the patient's brain that may result in some loss of psychological function. Upon autopsy, the nature of the psychological impairment can be matched to the site of the damage. For example, consider the tragic but instructive example of Phineas Gage. Gage was a 25-year-old railroad worker in 1848, when an accidental explosion drove an iron rod through his head. Remarkably, Gage not only survived but after a recovery period was able to walk, talk, and remember as well as he had before the accident. It was clear, however, that Gage's personality had changed. His friends said that he was no longer himself. Before the accident, he was regarded as a mild-mannered, well-adjusted, friendly man, but his brain damage left him impulsive, ill-tempered, and unreliable. He was apparently unable to execute or stick to even the simplest plans. His skull was preserved, and nearly a century and a half later, a reconstruction of the trajectory of the rod showed that the likely area of damage was the frontal lobe, which is now recognized to be important in the ability to plan, to control impulses, and generally to consider the long-term consequences of behavior (Damasio, 1994). Some researchers have suggested that frontal lobe abnormalities may be caused by exposure to some drugs of abuse such as cocaine (e.g., Kalivas & Volkow, 2005).

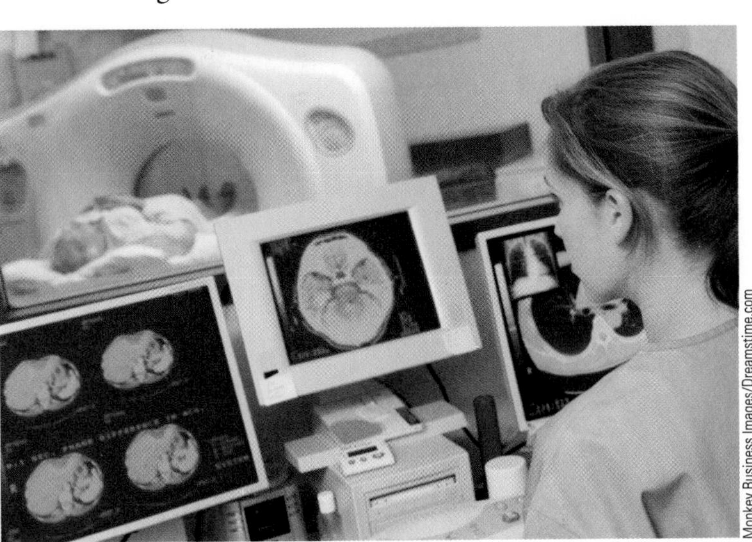

A technician monitors a patient during a CAT scan.

Monkey Business Images/Dreamstime.com

Imaging the Human Brain

Although much of what we know about the brain comes from a combination of research with animals and autopsy data from humans, new imaging technologies in recent years have opened new windows on the human brain. These technologies are teaching us much about the functional neuroanatomy of the normal brain. They also provide us with more sophisticated answers to questions that come up whenever chronic effects of drugs are discussed: the issue of drug-induced brain damage. We discuss this problem throughout the text as we consider individual drugs, but now, after this lengthy discussion of the brain, a few general comments are warranted. Detecting brain damage caused by drugs is often very difficult. Rarely do psychoactive drugs produce such dramatic long-term effects as those seen with Phineas Gage, for example, so we must rely on specialized methods to determine whether damage has occurred. Various neuropsychological tests are available that can be used to detect impairment in memory, perceptual motor skills, language, and other functions that may be influenced by chronic drug use. More direct analysis of brain tissue may be accomplished through **electroencephalography (EEG)**. This technique involves measuring the brain's electrical activity through the scalp. These brain waves change in predictable ways with sleep or various kinds of arousal, and abnormalities in EEG patterns can reveal gross brain damage.

electroencephalography (EEG) Technique used to measure electrical activity in the brain.

computerized axial tomography (CT) Technique that produces a three-dimensional X-ray image of the brain.

positron emission transaxial tomography (PET) Technique used to measure activity in selected brain regions.

magnetic resonance imaging (MRI) Technique that creates a high-resolution, three-dimensional image of the brain.

A more recently developed and more sensitive measure of brain impairment is **computerized axial tomography,** better known as the CT or CAT scan. The CT scan involves passing X-rays through the head in a circular pattern to get a three-dimensional image of the brain. The focus can be changed to different depths of the brain to detect internal tumors, enlarged spaces or ventricles, and other internal abnormalities.

CT scans provide a picture of the brain but reveal nothing about its functioning. However, a technique called the PET scan may greatly increase our ability to detect brain activity. **Positron emission transaxial tomography (PET)** involves injecting weak radioisotopes into the brain. Radioactive glucose or oxygen or even radioactive neurochemicals are then measured by sensitive detectors that can determine where the isotopes are absorbed, their rate of absorption, and so on. Then changes in activity in various brain regions can be assessed, including changes induced by drugs. Techniques like the PET scan and the closely related SPECT (single photon emission computed tomography) scan promise to greatly increase our ability to determine where in the brain damaging drugs produce their effects.

Another sophisticated and sensitive technique used to image the brain is **magnetic resonance imaging (MRI)**. With this technique, a strong magnetic field is passed through a person's head. Radio waves are then generated, which cause the molecules of the brain to emit energy of different frequencies, depending on their properties. This technique creates a localized and detailed brain image and eventually may greatly improve our ability to detect and understand brain dysfunction (Uttal, 2001). A modification of MRI technology called functional MRI (fMRI) has been developed; fMRI permits very rapid imaging and enables us to measure oxygen levels in blood vessels of the brain. Oxygen levels are correlated with the metabolism

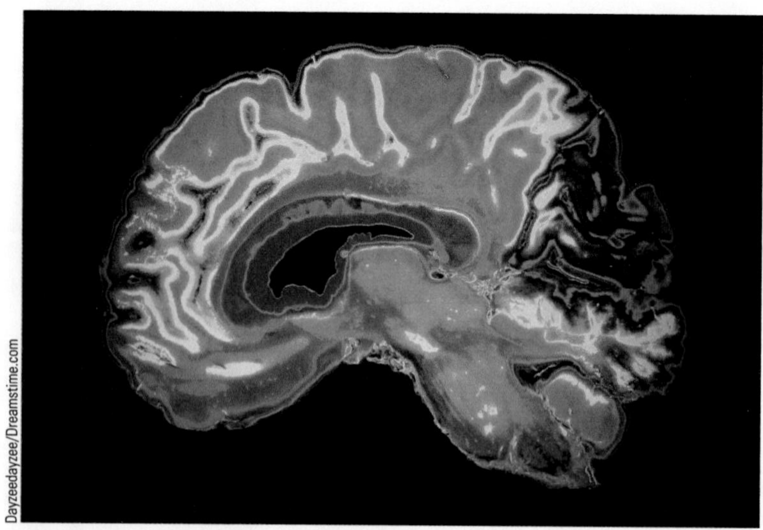

Dayzeedayzee/Dreamstime.com

An MRI image of the brain

CONTEMPORARY ISSUE BOX 3.2

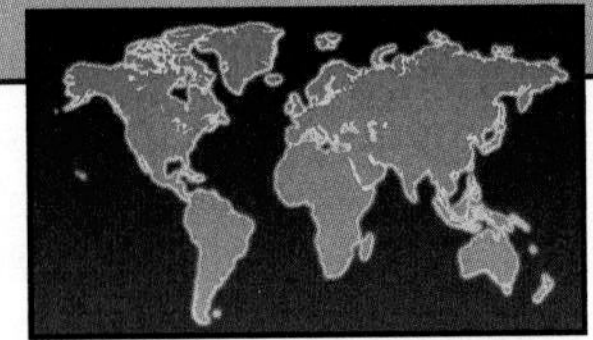

Drug Craving and the Brain

Drug abusers often report experiencing strong reactions when they are exposed to environmental stimuli associated with drug use. For example, being in a place where they have frequently used drugs or with friends who use them can evoke drug craving, excitement, and even physical symptoms such as elevated heart rate. Using some of the sophisticated brain-imaging tools described in the text, researchers are now able to characterize how the brain reacts to drug-related stimuli. In one study, Childress et al. (1999) used the PET scan to compare the reactions of cocaine users (not using at the time of the study) with those of control subjects who had never tried cocaine. Subjects in both groups watched two videos in the laboratory while measurements were taken. One video showed an individual purchasing, preparing, and smoking crack cocaine; the other video was a nature film unrelated to drugs. The cocaine users, but not the control subjects, reported strong craving after watching the crack video. The PET scans revealed increased activity in the limbic region of the brain, particularly the amygdala and a limbic structure called the anterior cingulate, that correlated with cocaine craving. That is, the cocaine users exhibited limbic activity while watching the crack video but not the nature video.

The nonusers did not show limbic activation during either video. Subsequent studies have replicated these findings with fMRI technology (Wexler et al., 2001) and shown similar patterns of brain activity when alcoholics and cigarette smokers experience craving as well (Lim et al., 2005; Myrick et al., 2004). Brain-imaging techniques have the potential to identify the brain regions involved with the psychological experiences, such as craving, that are thought to be important aspects of drug dependence.

of a particular brain region and are taken as an index of brain activity in that region. Thus, fMRI images obtained while a subject is engaged in some psychological activity (e.g., doing mental arithmetic) can be used to make inferences about the brain regions that were most active during the activity. These various imaging techniques are increasingly being used to learn about the neural mechanisms of drug action and dependence (see Contemporary Issue Box 3.2), as well as to evaluate changes in the brain after long-term exposure to drugs.

Summary

- All psychoactive drugs produce their effects by action on the nervous system—primarily by altering normal brain function.
- The brain is composed of specialized cells called neurons. Neurons transmit information by conducting electrical currents along their axons and releasing chemical substances called neurotransmitters into the synapse. Most drugs act by altering this chemical phase of neural transmission.
- Neurotransmitters work through a lock–key mechanism. The transmitter substance is like a key, and specialized areas on the neuron, called receptor sites, are like locks. Neurotransmitter chemicals must occupy the receptor sites for the neuron to fire.
- Drugs alter neural transmission in several ways. For example, a drug may mimic a natural or endogenous neurotransmitter by activating receptor sites. Alternatively, a drug may block a receptor site. Drugs can also affect the deactivation or release of neurotransmitters.
- Dozens of different chemicals have been proposed to act as neurotransmitters in the human brain; several are known to be related to drug effects. These include acetylcholine, anandamide, dopamine, endorphins, GABA, glutamate, norepinephrine, and serotonin.
- The nervous system is divided into two main sections. The central nervous system includes the brain and spinal cord. The peripheral nervous

system includes the sensory nerves, motor nerves, and the autonomic nervous system.

- The autonomic nervous system is divided into two branches. The sympathetic branch produces the physiological effects that accompany emotional arousal, and the parasympathetic branch controls the body when at rest.
- For convenience of description, the brain is divided into three divisions: the hindbrain, the midbrain, and the forebrain.
- The evolutionarily primitive hindbrain includes the medulla, the pons, and the cerebellum.
- The midbrain includes the superior and inferior colliculi and the substantia nigra.
- The forebrain includes the cerebral cortex, the thalamus, the hypothalamus, the basal ganglia, and the limbic system.

Answers to *"What Do You Think?"*

1. Certain cells in the nervous system have the unique ability to "talk" with each other.
   T *Neurons are able to communicate with each other through an electrochemical process known as neural transmission.*
2. The effects of drugs always involve naturally occurring physiological processes.
   T *Drugs act by making defined natural functions of the brain or body either more or less active.*
3. Some drugs may act by mimicking a neurotransmitter.
   T *Some drugs bind to receptor sites just as natural transmitters do.*
4. All drugs have the same basic effect on a cellular level; that is, they all block neural firing.
   F *Although some drugs, called antagonists, do block receptor sites and prevent activation of the receptor, other drugs, called agonists, activate the receptor.*
5. The brain is shielded from many toxic substances by a protective barrier.
   T *The brain is protected from toxic compounds that might enter the bloodstream by a blood-brain barrier that screens many, but not all, chemicals.*
6. The two main branches of the nervous system are the peripheral nervous system (PNS) and the autonomic nervous system (ANS).
   F *The two main branches of the nervous system are the central nervous system (CNS) and the peripheral nervous system (PNS).*
7. The brain and the spinal cord make up the peripheral nervous system.
   F *The brain and the spinal cord make up the central nervous system.*
8. The brain is firmly attached to the inside of the skull by tough membranes known as the meninges.
   F *The brain floats within the skull in a liquid known as cerebrospinal fluid.*
9. The autonomic nervous system is responsible for regulating food and water intake.
   F *Food and water intake appears to be regulated by the hypothalamus, a structure found in the brain.*
10. Animals will work for the electrical stimulation of certain parts of the brain.
    T *The mesolimbic dopaminergic pathway is sometimes called the pleasure center of the brain.*

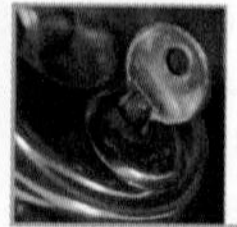

Key Terms

acetylcholine (ə-'se-tᵊl-'kō-lēn)
action potential
agonist ('a-gə-nist)
Alzheimer's disease ('älts-'hī-mərz-)
anandamide
antagonist
autonomic nervous system
axon ('ak-'sän)
axon terminals (or terminal buttons)
basal ganglia ('bā-səl-'gaŋ-glē-ə)
beta-blockers

blood-brain barrier
central nervous system (CNS)
cerebellum ('ser-ə-'be-ləm)
computerized axial tomography (CT)
cortex
dendrites ('den-'drīt)
dopamine ('dō-pə-'mēn)
electroencephalography (EEG)
endorphins (en-'do·r-fənz)
enzyme breakdown
forebrain
GABA
glutamate
hindbrain
hippocampus ('hi-pə-'kam-pəs)
hypothalamus ('hī-pō-tha-lə-məs)
inferior colliculi (ko-'lik-yū-lī)
ionotropic receptors
L-dopa ('el-'dō-pə)
limbic system
magnetic resonance imaging (MRI)
medulla oblongata (mə-'də-lə-'ä-bl·oŋ -gä-tə)
mesolimbic dopaminergic pathway
metabotropic receptors
midbrain
monoamines ('mä-nō-ə-'mēn)
myelin ('mī-ə-lən)
neuromuscular junction
neurons ('nü-'rän)
neurotransmitters
norepinephrine ('no·r-'e-pə-'ne-frən)
parasympathetic branch
Parkinson's disease
peripheral nervous system (PNS)
pons ('pänz)
positron emission transaxial tomography (PET)
receptor sites
reticular activating system
reuptake
serotonin ('sir-ə-tō-nən)
substantia nigra (səb-'stan(t)-shē-ə-'nī-grə)
superior colliculi
sympathetic branch
sympathomimetic synapse ('si-'naps)
thalamus ('tha-lə-məs)
vesicles ('ve-si-kəl)

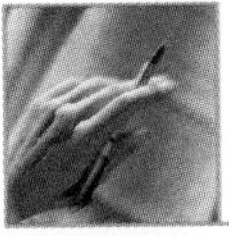

Essays/Thought Questions

1. Drugs produce psychological effects by chemical action on neurons. What implications does this mechanism have for the traditional distinction between mind and body?
2. Should addiction be viewed as a brain disease? Consider the implications of drug actions on the mesolimbic dopaminergic pathway.

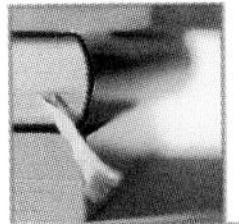

Suggested Readings

Iversen, L. L., Iversen, S. D., Bloom, F. E., and Roth, R. H. (2009). *Introduction to neuropsychopharmacology.* New York: Oxford University Press.

Charney, D. S., & Nestler, E. J. (Eds.) (2008). *Neurobiology of mental illness* (3rd ed.). New York: Oxford University Press.

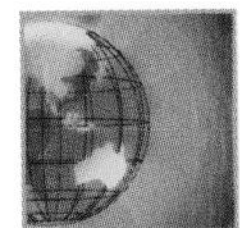

Web Resources

Visit the Book Companion Website at www.cengage.com/psychology/maisto to access study tools including a glossary, flashcards, and web quizzing. You will also find links to the following resources:

- Society for Neuroscience: The major international organization dedicated to brain research
- Neuroscience on the Internet: Presents various topics in neuroscience
- Whole Brain Atlas: Covers neuroanatomy and related materials
- Brain Science Podcast Archive: Podcasts of interviews with leading neuroscientists on various topics

CHAPTER 4

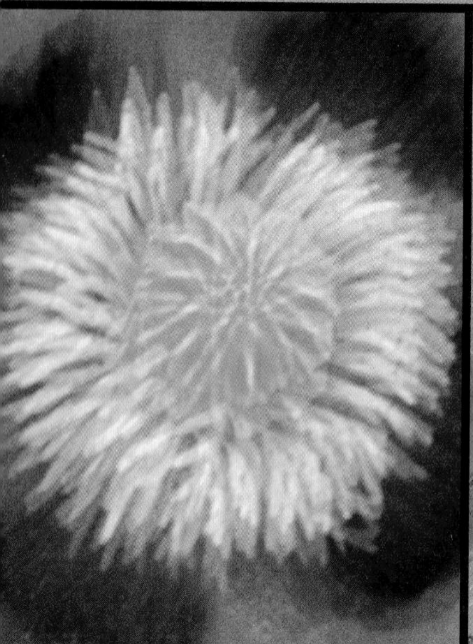
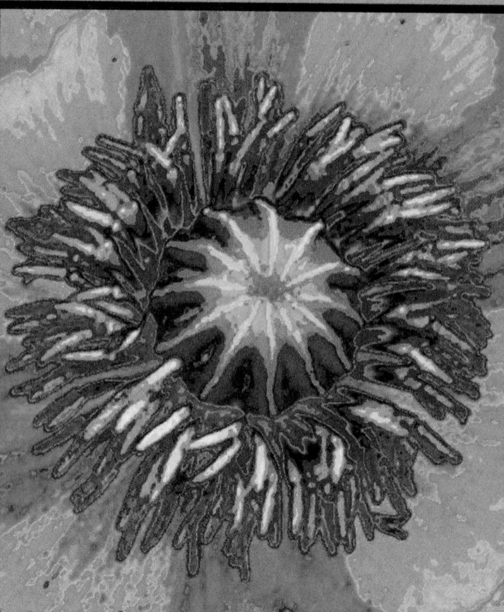
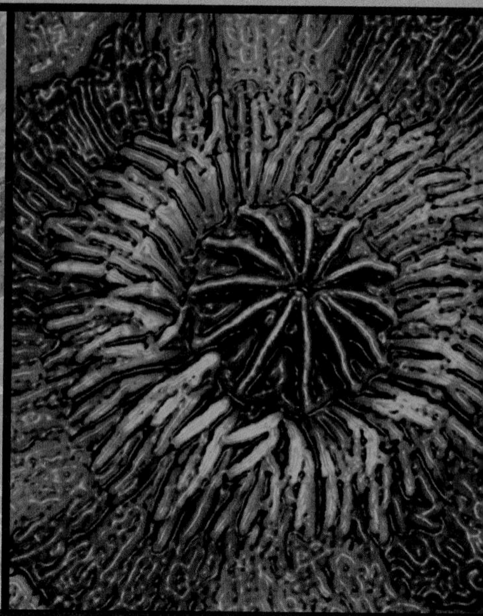

Pharmacology

What Do You Think? True or False?

Answers are given at the end of the chapter.

___ 1. A given amount of a drug has similar biological effects on different people.

___ 2. Despite the large number of known drugs, there are only three ways that drugs are commonly administered or taken.

___ 3. The safest way to take a drug is orally, but that is the slowest way of getting the drug into the blood.

___ 4. Taking a drug intravenously is a highly efficient, safe way to get a drug into the blood.

___ 5. Smoking is a relatively slow way of getting a drug into the blood.

___ 6. Some drugs can enter the body through the skin.

___ 7. The body protects the brain from toxic substances.

___ 8. The kidneys play the major role in drug metabolism.

___ 9. Scientific study of the effects of drugs is difficult because there is no way to represent such effects quantitatively.

___10. When more than one drug is taken at a time, the effects of one can enhance or diminish the effects of the other(s).

___11. Caffeine and alcohol have antagonistic effects.

___12. It is important to know about drug interactions because of the increasing prevalence of using more than one drug at a time among people who present themselves for drug treatment.

The aim of this chapter is to cover the basic principles and methods of pharmacology that apply to the description and evaluation of all drugs. We will elaborate on an idea we first mentioned in Chapter 1—the drug experience, or a person's perception of the effects of a drug. A series of interrelated factors contributes to a given drug effect. The importance of any one factor, or set of factors, for a given drug-taking occasion depends on the importance of the other factors. This idea sounds complicated, and it is even more complicated to analyze in practice. To evaluate the importance or contribution of any one factor to a drug effect or experience, researchers must comprehend or at least somehow **control** the effects of other relevant factors.

We will try to walk down the path of the drug experience from beginning to end as if it were a logical and linear route. That analogy is flawed, however, because not only are the contributory factors of a drug effect interdependent, but **feedback** relationships may also occur among those factors. For example, a large quantity of some drug may be taken and **absorbed** into the blood. Then the drug is carried to its site of action (distributed). In some cases, a large quantity of a drug may cause the body to slow absorption or quicken **metabolism** of the drug to defend itself against a toxic drug effect. In this event, the **distribution** of the drug is information that the body "feeds back" to its regulators of absorption and metabolism to, in effect, reduce the drug quantity.

Still, including all the possible feedback loops would strangle this discussion, so we review the drug experience and the factors that influence it as if everything proceeds linearly. We chart the path in Table 4.1. For each of the "steps" in the table, there may be two or more factors to consider. By the end of this chapter, you will begin to understand the great complexity of what humans experience when they take drugs.

To the pharmacologist, the drug experience involves two branches of that science: pharmacokinetics and pharmacodynamics. **Pharmacokinetics** concerns "the absorption, distribution, biotransformation, and excretion of drugs" (Benet, Mitchell, & Sheiner, 1990a, p. 1). Drug absorption and distribution are essential for determining

control
In research, to be able to account for variables that may affect the results of a study.

feedback
In this context, in a series of events, what happens in a later event alters events that preceded it.

absorbed
When drugs have entered the bloodstream.

metabolism
The process by which the body breaks down matter into more simple components and waste.

distribution
The transport of drugs by the blood to their site(s) of action in the body.

pharmacokinetics
The branch of pharmacology that concerns the absorption, distribution, biotransformation, and excretion of drugs.

TABLE 4.1 "Steps" in the Drug Experience

1. A drug of a specified chemical structure is present.
2. A certain quantity of this drug is measured.
3. This quantity of the drug is administered in one of a number of possible ways.
4. The drug is absorbed into the blood and distributed to site(s) of action.
5. Some pharmacological effect is produced.
6. In humans, a drug's pharmacological effects may be modified depending on characteristics of the person, such as genetic constitution, gender, age, personality, and drug tolerance.
7. The setting or context of drug use may also modify a drug's pharmacological effects.

how much drug reaches its sites of action and therefore its effects. Absorption and distribution are key factors in the drug experience (see Step 4 in Table 4.1).

Once in the body, drugs do not stay forever. The basics of how the body eliminates drugs and how that is studied are also covered in this chapter. Knowing about drug excretion or elimination is required for learning the effect a drug will have after it enters the body.

pharmacodynamics The branch of pharmacology that concerns the biochemical and physiological effects of drugs and their mechanisms of action.

Pharmacokinetics might be viewed as the vehicle for **pharmacodynamics**, which is the study of the "biochemical and physiological effects of drugs and their mechanisms of action" (Benet et al., 1990a, p. 1). The neural mechanisms of drugs were discussed in Chapter 3. In this chapter, we introduce some of the language that pharmacologists use to describe drug effects and some ways that have been developed to depict them. In later chapters on individual drugs and drug classes, pharmacodynamics enters into our description of a drug's biological mechanism of action. Pharmacodynamics is relevant to the drug experience because this branch of pharmacology concerns the biological bases of observed drug effects. It will be valuable for you to know what standards are followed in describing and representing these effects.

The emphasis of this chapter is on the characteristics of drugs and the role the body plays in producing drug effects. Unique characteristics of people (see Step 6 in Table 4.1) and setting factors that affect the drug experience (see Step 7) are the subject of Chapter 5.

Pharmacokinetics

We begin our overview of pharmacokinetics by describing how to specify and measure a given amount of a drug and how the drug gets into the body. The combination of drug and body chemistry determines the drug experience.

Drug Dose

You know from Chapter 1 that the effect of a drug depends most fundamentally on how much of the drug is taken (see Steps 1 and 2 in Table 4.1). A science about drugs relies on a standard way to determine drug quantities. How do pharmacologists compute drug dose? How is that quantity communicated? A drug's dose is computed according to a person's body weight, because heavier people have a greater volume of body fluid than lighter people do. Therefore, a given amount of a drug is less concentrated in the body of a heavier person, and similarly at the site of drug action, than it is in the body of a lighter person (White, 1991). As you will see later in this chapter, in general, the greater the drug concentration at a site, the greater the drug effect. Therefore, the amount of a drug that is administered has to be adjusted according to body weight to assure that the drug is given in equivalent strength (dose) to people who have different weights.

The first step is to determine the desired dose, expressed in milligrams of the drug per kilogram (mg/kg) of body weight. The next step is to weigh the person and record the weight in kilograms. With these two quantities, the amount of drug required for the desired dose is easily determined. For example, if the desired dose is 0.08 mg/kg and the person weighs 80 kg, the necessary amount is 0.08 x 80 = 6.4 mg of the drug (Leavitt, 1982).

Routes of Administration

In pharmacology, the "route of drug administration" may refer to either the site where a drug is taken or how a drug is taken.[1] The route of drug administration can strongly influence the effects that a drug has (see Step 3 in Table 4.1). In this section, we discuss eight administration routes. The five most common are oral, by injection (includes three ways—subcutaneous, intramuscular, and intravenous), and by inhalation. Three other important routes are intranasal (sniffing), sublingual (under the tongue), and transdermal (through the skin).

Oral

Oral administration, or swallowing, is the route with which you probably are most familiar. Drugs taken orally are usually in the form of pills, capsules, powders, or liquids. Examples are the variety of headache medicines, cough syrups, and cold remedies available at any drugstore. Such accessible medications are virtually always prepared for oral administration because it usually is the safest, most convenient, and most economical way to administer a drug.

When drugs are swallowed, they pass through the stomach and are absorbed primarily through the small intestine. This travel course affects both how fast a drug can register its effect physically and how much effect is registered. A major factor in determining the effect is how much food is in the digestive tract when the drug is taken. The presence of food delays the stomach from emptying and may dilute the concentration of a drug. The result: delayed absorption and a decrease in the maximum drug level achieved. People may notice this result when they compare drinking alcohol after eating a full meal to drinking on an empty stomach. Another point about oral administration is that food may encapsulate the drug so that it is passed out of the body in the feces. Finally, oral administration, even without the complications of food in the stomach, causes the drug to be absorbed into the blood more slowly than with other routes.

So, the pluses of oral administration—relative safety, convenience, and economy—must be balanced against considerations of time to absorption and the maximum drug effect that can be reached with a particular drug dose. With some drugs, such as heroin, the stomach acids used in digestion actually break down the drug to some degree before it is absorbed into the blood. Once in the blood, the chemically altered drug is passed through the liver before it reaches the brain. Because the liver is the major site of the metabolization of most drugs, only a fraction of the drug dose actually reaches the brain. The outcome is a diminished drug effect.

Injection

Three of the most common routes of drug administration involve injecting drugs into the body using a needle and syringe. When drugs are taken this way, they typically are

[1]Our discussion of routes of drug administration draws heavily from Benet, Mitchell, and Sheiner (1990a; 1990b); Brands et al. (1998); Jacobs and Fehr (1987); and Julien, Advokat, and Comaty (2008).

dissolved
When a drug changes from solid to liquid by mixing it with a liquid.

suspended
When a drug's particles are dispersed in solution but not dissolved in it.

dissolved or **suspended** in some solution ("vehicle") before injection. The routes for administration when injecting drugs are subcutaneous, intramuscular, and intravenous.

Subcutaneous

This route involves injecting the drug under the layers of the skin. It is the easiest of the injection routes to use because the target site of the needle is just below the skin surface. Many beginning drug abusers take their drugs subcutaneously. This route may also be preferred medically for drugs that are not irritating to body tissue because of the route's relatively slow (but faster than oral) and constant absorption rate. In fact, the solution in which the drug is administered may be selected to adjust the drug's absorption rate. A drug should not be taken subcutaneously when the drug irritates body tissue and when large volumes of solution must be taken to introduce enough of the drug to achieve the desired effect.

Intramuscular

The name of this route means "within the muscle." Intramuscular injection requires a deeper penetration than the subcutaneous method but is associated with a faster absorption rate when the drug is prepared in a water solution and there is a good rate of blood flow at the site of administration. Absorption rates may differ depending on the rate of blood flow to the muscle group the drug is injected into; in practice, the most common muscle sites are the deltoid, thigh, and buttocks. The absorption rate can also be modulated by the solution that the drug is prepared in for administration.

One disadvantage is that intramuscular injection can result in localized pain (at the site of injection). Furthermore, when a person who is not formally trained administers drugs intramuscularly, the risk of infection from irritating drugs and tissue damage is high.

Intravenous

Intravenous means "into the veins," and therefore most absorption problems are avoided. A common street term for the route is "mainlining." The drug is injected in solution directly into the veins. The effects can be immediate. As a result, intravenous administration is valuable in emergency medical situations, and doses can be precisely adjusted according to the person's response. In addition, irritating drugs as well as irritating vehicles can be taken intravenously (as opposed to, say, subcutaneously or intramuscularly) because blood vessel walls are relatively insensitive and the drug is further diluted by blood.

The apparent advantages of intravenous administration raise the question of why this is not the preferred route for prescribed medications. A major reason is that the intravenous route is the one most highly associated with complications because large quantities of the drug quickly reach the site of action. This feature contrasts with oral administration, which is considered safe because drugs reach their sites of action relatively slowly. Another point to consider is that if a drug is repeatedly administered intravenously, then a healthy vein must be maintained. In general, intravenous injection is associated with such risk that administration must be done slowly and with careful monitoring of a person's response. Obviously, this care is much more likely in a controlled medical environment than in other settings where drugs are taken.

> *"I had not taken a bath in a year nor changed my clothes or removed them except to stick a needle every hour in the fibrous wooden flesh of heroin addiction. I did absolutely nothing."*
>
> William S. Burroughs

Those who regularly take drugs like heroin, cocaine, or heroin and cocaine together (called "speedball") intravenously are called "hard-core addicts." These users take drugs intravenously because they want immediate and powerful drug effects. However, the risks of taking a drug intravenously, coupled with the assault that such drug taking has on the body, usually take a toll on a person. Drug-induced deaths, intentional or not, are an ever-present danger among addicts and other nonmedical drug users who take their drugs intravenously.

CONTEMPORARY ISSUE BOX 4.1

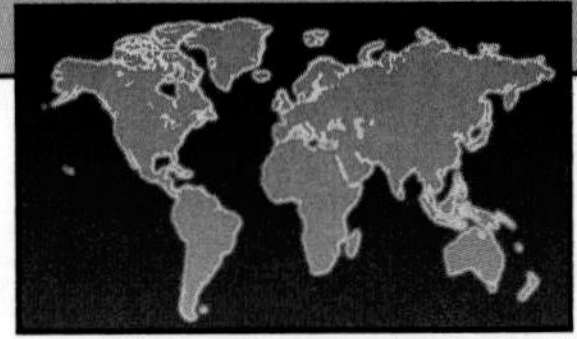

Needle Sharing and AIDS

Intravenous (IV) drug use remains a risk factor for AIDS. The reason the risk for AIDS is high among IV drug users is that they often share needles while taking drugs. The risk for becoming HIV positive increases when one or more of the needle sharers are HIV positive and the needle is not sterilized before being passed from person to person.

IV drug users share needles for several reasons. It may be a simple matter of syringe availability. If few needles are around, then sharing becomes more likely. In this regard, the addicts' first priority is to get the drug into their body. However, a more entrenched and difficult-to-modify reason for needle sharing is that it may be part of local drug-taking social norms. In addition, needle sharing is often part of socialization into the drug-taking subculture and has been viewed as a way that addicts can feel a sense of group belonging and friendship.

Several approaches have been taken to combat the problem of HIV risk and needle sharing. One is education. In the last 10 years or so, it would be difficult not to have heard or read about one or more campaigns directed at addicts, alerting them to avoid needle sharing or, if the practice is followed, to clean the needle before reusing it. A related approach has been to directly supply addicts with clean syringes. So-called needle exchange programs, in which addicts trade their used syringes for clean ones, seem promising. Reviews of such programs in the United States, Canada, and Europe show that addicts in exchange programs do less needle sharing and more often clean their syringes with bleach. In addition, needle exchange programs have not increased IV drug use where they have been implemented (Center for AIDS Prevention Studies, 1998; Rich et al., 2004).

Despite research evidence that needle exchange programs can make inroads into the risk of HIV or IV drug use problem, such programs still are controversial in many parts of the United States and in other countries, such as Sweden. The controversy is rooted in the fear that free exchange of syringes without a physician's prescription will accelerate the spread of IV drug use. If you were a local official, what would you consider the pros and cons of needle exchange programs in your city?

Another critical point to consider when drugs are taken by injection is that, to prevent diseases such as AIDS, hepatitis, and tetanus, drugs must be injected using sterile needles and solutions (see Contemporary Issue Box 4.1). When any of the three injecting routes are used, the body's natural protections against microorganisms, such as skin and mucous membranes, are bypassed. Therefore, dirty needles or nonsterile solutions may carry illness-inducing microorganisms that the body cannot "screen out." This is why, for instance, street drug abusers who share their needles are at high risk for contracting AIDS.

"Your veins get hard. They died out. You killed them and they're gone, and then you can no longer have any more veins. Then you have to skin pop it (intramuscular injection)."

Research participant in a study of long-term injection drug users reported by Anderson and Levy (2003)

Inhalation

Some drugs may be inhaled and then absorbed through the lung's membranes. For such drugs, inhalation results in a fast and effective absorption. A drug has to be in one of a few states to be inhaled. Drugs that can be changed into gaseous states may be inhaled. For example, the vapors of one class of substances may be inhaled. Three examples of these substances, which typically are ingredients of commercial products and are aptly called *inhalants* when used for their psychoactive properties, are benzene, toluene, and naphtha. We have more to say about this important group of substances in Chapter 10. Drugs that can be administered in the form of fine liquid drops also may be inhaled. Furthermore, drugs in small particles of matter that are suspended in a gas may be inhaled (Jacobs & Fehr, 1987). For example, tobacco smoke contains tiny drops of nicotine. Similarly, the smoke from **freebase** cocaine (crack) contains droplets of cocaine.

freebase
When a substance is separated, or "freed," from its salt base. The separated form of the substance is thus called "freebase."

As we noted, inhaling a drug results in rapid and effective absorption. However, it is possible to absorb only a small amount of a drug by inhalation in one administration.

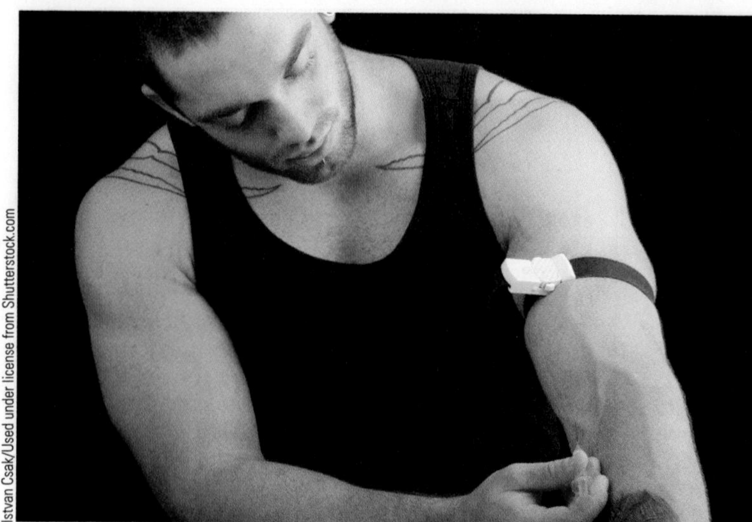
Istvan Csak/Used under license from Shutterstock.com

Intravenous drug injection is associated with rapid drug effects, making it the preferred route of some drug abusers. Intravenous injection of drugs is considered dangerous because large quantities can reach the site(s) of action so quickly.

Intranasal

In this route, a drug in powdered form is taken through the nose. The drug is then absorbed through the mucous membranes of the nose and the sinus cavities. Other terms for intranasal administration that you may have heard are *snorting* and *sniffing*. Examples of drugs commonly absorbed this way are cocaine, heroin, and powdered tobacco snuff. When a drug is fat soluble, sniffing is a rapid and effective way to absorb it. If a sniffed drug is irritating and disrupts blood flow, however, it can cause damage. An example that has been cited often is the damage that cocaine sniffing causes to the nasal septum and lining of the nose.

Sublingual

With this route, a drug tablet is placed under the tongue and dissolves in saliva. The drug is absorbed through the mouth's mucous membranes. Nitroglycerin, which is taken for treatment of angina pectoris (heart pain), is usually taken sublingually. Nicotine may be taken in the form of chewing tobacco or "dipping" snuff by the sublingual route.

The sublingual route results in faster and more efficient drug absorption than oral administration. It also is preferred to oral administration for drugs that irritate the stomach and cause vomiting. Almost any drug with the right chemical properties may be taken in pill form sublingually. However, this route is used less frequently than might be expected because of the unpleasant taste of many of the drugs that may be taken sublingually.

Transdermal

Some drugs may be taken transdermally, or "through the skin" (Wester & Maibach, 1983). One common medical use of the transdermal route is to provide an alternative to oral administration when a drug may cause unwanted gastrointestinal effects. The transdermal route actually is not an effective one for many drugs because the skin acts as a barrier to some chemicals and thus is relatively nonpermeable. For those drugs that more readily penetrate intact skin, absorption is better because the drug is applied to a wider area.

Drugs that penetrate the skin are absorbed better at sites that have a higher rate of cutaneous blood flow. In addition, a drug dose may be modified by mixing it with other substances, such as an oily preparation, to improve penetration at the site of administration. In Chapter 7, we discuss a patch containing a preparation of nicotine and other substances that is applied to the skin so that nicotine can enter the body. This is one type of pharmacological treatment of nicotine dependence. Nitroglycerine may be administered by patch, which avoids the problem of metabolizing the drug before it reaches its site of action when it is taken orally (see the earlier discussion of the oral route and the discussion of "first-pass effects" later in this chapter). Finally, patches may be used to place a drug at a site of the skin that is advantageous for its increased blood flow.

Routes of drug administration should be thought of as ways to get drugs into the body, and they can have a considerable influence on the drug experience. No route is inherently better than any other. Rather, determining the preferred route depends on the drug administered, the goals of administration, and the advantages and disadvantages of using a particular route with a particular drug under particular circumstances.

Table 4.2 is a summary of general considerations in using the eight routes of drug administration that we have discussed. Table 4.3 is a summary of the routes typically used with drugs taken for medical and nonmedical reasons.

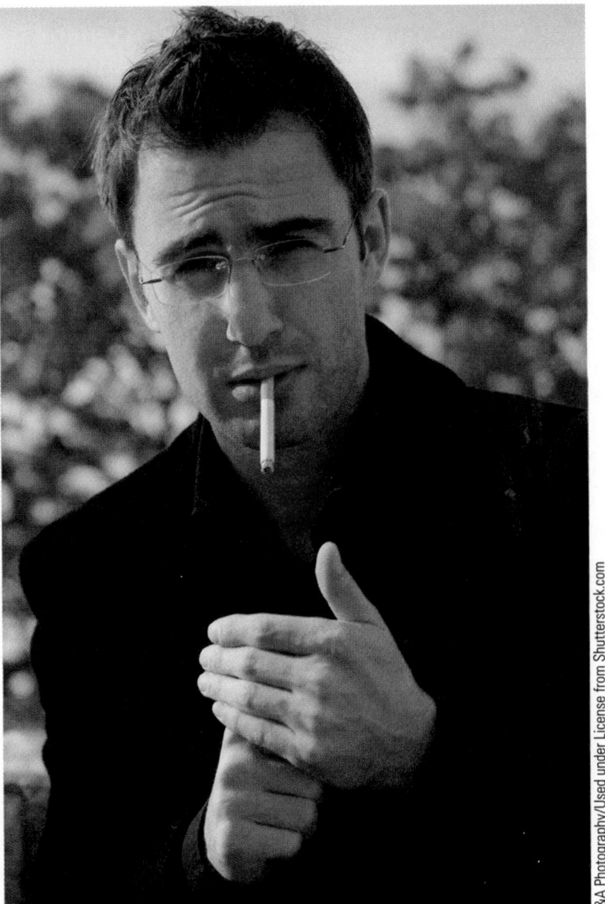

Probably the best-known way of ingesting a drug by inhalation is taking nicotine by smoking cigarettes.

Drug Absorption

Absorption (of a drug into the bloodstream) also may be defined as the rate and extent to which a drug leaves its site of administration, and it plays a major role in the drug experience. Absorption and the factors that affect it are extremely important because they influence **bioavailability**. Bioavailability is the portion of the original drug dose that reaches its site of action or that reaches a fluid in the body that gives the drug access to its site of action (Benet et al., 1990b). As such, the bioavailability of a drug tells us about its effects.

We have explained in detail how the route of administering a drug affects its absorption. Actually, differences among the routes in absorption rates are related to the factors that influence absorption in general. We cite a few major examples here (Benet et al., 1990b; White, 1991). For all routes besides intravenous, the drug must pass through at least one body membrane before it can reach the circulatory system. Because membranes consist largely of lipids (fats), drugs that are more soluble in lipids are much more readily absorbed. Alcohol is an example of a drug that dissolves in lipids. Another factor is the form in which the drug is administered: Drugs taken in water solution are absorbed more rapidly than are drugs taken in suspension, in oily solution, or in solid form because they are dissolved more readily at the site of absorption. When a drug is taken in solid form, as aspirin is, for example, its solubility depends on conditions at the site of absorption. For instance, aspirin is fairly insoluble in the acidic environment of the stomach, and this places a limit on its absorbability. This point relates to the importance of the environment in the gastrointestinal system and its influence on the absorption of drugs that are taken orally, as we have discussed. Circulation at the site of absorption also influences it, as more blood flow speeds absorption. Finally, the size of the absorbing surface makes a difference. Drugs are absorbed more rapidly from larger surface areas.

bioavailability
The portion of the original drug dose that reaches its site of action or that reaches a fluid in the body that gives it access to its site of action.

Because each of these and other factors may singly or in combination affect absorption, you can see why it is so difficult to specify a drug effect for a person under specific conditions at a given time. This discussion also reaffirms why intravenous injection is the most efficient way to get a drug to its sites of action. Intravenous injection bypasses many factors that may retard absorption because it puts the drug in direct contact with the blood—the vehicle of drug distribution.

Drug Distribution

The biochemical properties of both the body and the drug have a lot to do with a drug's distribution to its sites of action. Because the blood transports a drug, it follows

TABLE 4.2 General Considerations for the Eight Major Routes of Drug Administration

Route	Considerations
Oral	• Among the safest, most convenient, and most economical routes of administration • Food in the stomach retards absorption or may diminish the amount of drug absorbed • Stomach acids may break down some drugs, resulting in reduced drug effect
Subcutaneous	• Easiest of the three injection routes to use • Associated with absorption rates faster than oral administration but slower than intramuscular and intravenous routes • Preferred for medical use of drugs that are not irritating to body tissue because of its relatively slow but constant absorption rate with sustained drug effects • Should not be used when a drug irritates body tissue or when large volumes of solution must be used for taking the drug
Intramuscular	• Requires deeper penetration of injection than subcutaneous but results in a faster absorption rate with proper preparation of solution and an injection site with good blood flow • May be painful at the injection site • Use by untrained people is associated with a high risk of infection from irritating drugs and tissue damage
Intravenous	• Considered one of the fastest absorption rates • Valuable for emergency medical needs because the resulting drug effects can be immediate • Doses can be adjusted precisely according to the person's response because of immediacy of drug effects • Better than subcutaneous or intramuscular routes for irritating drugs because blood vessel walls are relatively insensitive and the blood further dilutes the drug • Danger in the potential for a large quantity of a drug to reach its site of action • Repeated use requires maintenance of a healthy vein • Drug dose must be administered gradually and the person's response monitored carefully to prevent serious complications
Inhalation	• When feasible, absorption is effective and the most rapid for some drugs • Only a small amount of drug can be absorbed in any one administration
Intranasal	• For a fat-soluble drug, absorption is rapid and effective • Can cause damage when the drug is irritating or disrupts blood flow
Sublingual	• May be used for many drugs in pill form • Results in faster and more efficient absorption than oral administration • Preferable to oral administration for drugs that irritate the stomach and cause vomiting • Not used as often as it might be because of the unpleasant taste of many drugs
Transdermal	• An alternative to the oral route when a drug may cause unwanted gastrointestinal effects • Not used for many drugs because the skin is a relatively impenetrable barrier to many chemicals • Resulting absorption is enhanced at sites that have greater cutaneous blood flow, and mixing a drug with another substance may improve penetration of the skin

TABLE 4.3 Drugs Used for Medical and Nonmedical Reasons and Their Routes of Administration

Drug	Route
Alcohol	Oral
Amphetamines	Oral; intravenous (preferred by the chronic high-dose abuser); sniffed by occasional or new users
Barbiturates	Oral; rectal (through the mucous membrane of the rectum); subcutaneous; intramuscular; intravenous
Benzodiazepines	Most commonly oral; some intravenous or intramuscular
Caffeine	Most commonly oral; medically, occasionally by injection for mild stimulant properties; intravenous injection by abusers
Cannabis	Almost all routes; most commonly smoking (inhalation); injection not efficient because THC is not water-soluble
Cocaine	Cocaine hydrochloride is taken through nasal or other mucous membranes, such as those of the mouth, vagina, and rectum; also intravenous. Cocaine freebase (crack) is volatile and therefore most often vaporized in a freebase pipe and inhaled into the lungs
Heroin	Most commonly is dissolved in water and injected subcutaneously, intramuscularly, or intravenously; may be inhaled by smoking or sniffed
Nicotine	Inhaled by smoking (cigarettes); nicotine in cigar or pipe smoke mainly absorbed across membranes of the mouth and upper respiratory tract; may be absorbed through membranes of the mouth (chewing tobacco) and nose (snuff) and through the skin
LSD (lysergic acid diethylamide-25)	Oral; inhalation; the three injection routes; through the skin
MDA (methylenedioxy-amphetamine)	Most commonly oral
PCP (phencyclidine)	Oral; sniffed; inhalation by smoking (sprinkled on marijuana, parsley, tobacco, or other substance that can be smoked); intravenous injection

that regions of the body that receive the most blood get the most drug. Indeed the heart, brain, kidney, liver, and other systems that receive a lot of blood get major portions of the drug shortly after absorption. Other parts of the body that receive less blood flow, such as muscle, viscera, and fat, may take considerably longer to receive the drug. Besides blood flow, the **diffusibility** of membranes and tissues affects distribution: The more diffusible tissues receive the drug more rapidly.

diffusibility
A more diffusible substance is more easily entered into or "receptive" of another.

solubility
The ease with which a compound can be dissolved or entered into a solution.

Drug properties may influence distribution considerably. One such property is fat **solubility**. Drugs that are more soluble in lipids penetrate body membranes and therefore reach sites of action more easily than do less lipid-soluble drugs. The fat solubility of a drug also plays a role in how much of it can reach the brain. This is important to us because we concentrate on drugs that affect the CNS in this text. Although the blood flow to the brain makes it a natural repository for drugs (and other chemicals) that enter the body, substances must cross the blood-brain barrier before they can reach the brain. As we noted in Chapter 3, the blood-brain barrier filters out toxins from the blood before they reach the brain. Pores of the capillary walls in the brain are small and close together, so they restrict the passage of substances through them. In addition, a thick wall of glial cells encloses the capillaries to form another line of defense. A drug that is highly fat-soluble, like the benzodiazepine diazepam (Valium), can easily pass through the capillary and glial cell membranes, but passage of less fat-soluble drugs is impeded (Johanson, 1992).

Another feature of a drug's chemistry that affects its distribution is whether it selectively binds to elements of the body. Some drugs, such as the barbiturates, may bind chemically to certain proteins in the plasma. The more "tightly" bound a drug is, the slower its distribution to sites of action (Benet et al., 1990b; Leavitt, 1982; White, 1991). Similarly, some drugs have an affinity for fatty tissue in the body. In this case, the drug may be released, but it can take a relatively long time. With such longer-term unbinding, the drug may remain in the blood for some time, yet the drug's release from fat tissues is slow enough that the psychoactive effects are negligible (White, 1991). A notorious example of a drug that has an affinity for fat is marijuana. Its distribution is uneven throughout the body because of selective binding, and the effects achieved by taking the drug are attenuated. Part of the dose does not immediately reach its sites of action.

In summary, the processes of drug absorption and distribution illustrate that a drug is a chemical that, when introduced into the body, disrupts its steady biochemical state. Absorption and distribution are the complex fundamentals of bioavailability, or how much drug reaches its sites of action. Bioavailability tells us most about drug effects. To understand the effects of a drug over time, it is essential to track its excretion or elimination from the body.

Drug Elimination

Drugs may be excreted from the body directly or first metabolized into pharmacologically inert, water-soluble by-products that are less likely to be reabsorbed. The metabolic by-products are then excreted. Enzymes in the liver play the major part in drug metabolism. These enzymes also are present in other organs such as the kidneys and gastrointestinal (GI) tract. As a result, a drug administered orally is subject to a "first-pass effect," which means that enzymes in the GI tract break down a drug to some degree. Therefore, less drug than was administered is eventually distributed to its sites of action. In Chapter 9, we discuss a study of differences between men and women in first-pass effects with alcohol.

side effects
Effects of a drug other than those of central interest; used most often in reference to the other-than-therapeutic effects of medications, such as the side effect of drowsiness for antihistamines. Note that what are considered a drug's side effects depend on what specifically the drug is being used for.

One question that may have occurred to you is whether the drug metabolic by-products themselves have pharmacologic action. If they do, then it is difficult to see how a drug state could ever become deactivated. In fact, some drug metabolites are pharmacologically active and are responsible for unwanted **side effects** of different medications, for example. The metabolites of other drugs have desired psychoactive effects. Two examples are the metabolites of diazepam (Valium) and of chlordiazepoxide (Librium). In fact, one of Valium's metabolites is eliminated from the body more slowly than is Valium (Jacobs & Fehr, 1987). When metabolites are active, the action ends with further metabolism of the by-products or by their direct excretion in the urine (Benet et al., 1990b).

"There are three side effects of acid: enhanced long-term memory, decreased short-term memory, and I forget the third."

Timothy Leary.

The kidney is by far the most important organ for excretion of both drugs and their metabolites, but excretion may occur in other ways as well. For example, drugs that are taken orally may be excreted directly in the feces. Drug metabolites may be excreted in liver bile. Drugs are excreted in mother's milk, which is not critical so much because of the proportion of drug that leaves the body this way but because of the dangers posed to the nursing infant. Drugs also may be excreted through the lungs, which is why you can smell alcohol on a person's breath after he or she drinks it. Finally, drugs may be excreted in perspiration.

Pharmacologists have discovered that the rate of elimination of drugs from the body obeys two general laws: zero-order kinetics and first-order kinetics (Clark,

Brater, & Johnson, 1988). On one hand, zero-order kinetics means that the rate at which a drug is metabolized is independent of its concentration in the blood; a well-known example is alcohol (Julien, 1996). First-order kinetics, on the other hand, means that the amount of drug that is metabolized in a unit of time depends on how much drug is in the blood. Most drugs obey the law of first-order kinetics. Knowledge of these laws is a great help to people who do research on drugs and to physicians when they prescribe medications.

A term relevant to drug elimination that you may come across is **half-life**, which is the time that must pass for the amount of drug in the body to be cut by half. *Drug half-life* actually is a term that has been given more importance than is warranted. It has been discovered to be a result of other statistics that reflect the body's ability to clear a drug. These other statistics are directly linked to the kinetics law that the drug is obeying. In any case, you will see the term *half-life* again in this text and likely in other sources, so it is useful to know it.

half-life
The amount of time that must pass for the amount of drug in the body to be reduced by half.

Drug Testing

Discussing drug-elimination processes raises the topic of procedures that are used in drug testing. *Drug testing* is a term applied to various methods of determining drug use, most commonly by analyzing urine or blood samples. In recent years, drug testing by analysis of sweat, saliva, and hair samples has also been applied with increasing frequency as the technology for such application improves (Dolan, Rouen, & Kimber, 2004). Analysis of urine samples (urinalysis) remains the most commonly used method, in part because its technology is the best developed among the main methods, and its cost is relatively low. In addition, urinalysis is a sensitive method if samples are not adulterated, because a drug's metabolites may be detected in urine. If a drug is detected in the blood directly, it is an indication of recent use (Miller, 1991).

The validity of drug testing depends on factors such as the dose last taken of the drug, the testing method used, and the laboratory quality control procedures used in testing. The detectability of drug use is determined by the drug's clearance rates from the body and the clearance rates of the drug's metabolites. Table 4.4 is a list of common drugs of abuse, their range of elimination times, and their range of detectability in days by testing of urine samples. The range of elimination times pertains to elimination of the drug itself (shorter time) and to elimination of the drug's metabolites (longer time) from the body. Alcohol has no range because its metabolites are used too efficiently in the body to be measured reliably (Miller, 1991).

The right-hand column of Table 4.4 gives the ranges of detection times under the best testing conditions. Detection times are substantially longer if the drug's metabolites can be measured by the testing method. Note that the detection time ranges are generally much shorter than the elimination time ranges of drugs and their metabolites. This is because the testing method is not sensitive enough to pick up the metabolite(s) at some point. Where that point is depends on the metabolite and the testing method. Therefore, a positive drug test does not necessarily provide precise information about when the drug actually was used. The exception, as we noted, is that if the drug is detected in blood, we then know that use was recent. A final point about Table 4.4 is that an acute dose of marijuana can be detected for up to eight days after use. In chronic users, the drug can be detected for longer than a month after the last dose was taken.

Drug testing is highly accurate if a two-step drug-testing process is used (screening of the urine sample followed by a confirmatory test if the sample shows positive for some drug) and high-quality specimen collection procedures and laboratory protocols are followed (Bina, 1998). Nevertheless, many methods have been tried to undermine the validity of drug tests. Most often these methods are designed to result in a false-negative

TABLE 4.4 Common Drugs of Abuse and Their Ranges of Elimination and Detection Times

Drug	Range of Elimination Times	Range of Detection Times (Days)
Alcohol	Hours	Up to 1
Cocaine	Hours to days	0.2–4.0
Marijuana	Weeks to months	2–8 (acute), 14–42 (chronic)
Benzodiazepines	Weeks to months	7–9
Opiates	Days to weeks	1–2
Barbiturates	Weeks to months	3–14

Note: Shorter time in the elimination range refers to the drug itself and longer time to the drug's metabolites.
Source: Adapted with permission from N. S. Miller, *The Pharmacology of Alcohol and Drugs of Abuse/Addiction.* Copyright © 1991 Springer-Verlag.

finding—that is, for the test to show a negative result for a given illicit drug when in fact the individual has used the drug. The main goal is to trick the screening test into giving the false-negative finding, which virtually always stops the drug-testing process. Typically only positive results are confirmed because of cost considerations. To give you an idea, the screening procedure costs only pennies to complete, but the most current and accurate confirmatory test costs about $200. The confirmatory test (of positive screens) is essential to the drug-testing process because the screening methods that are used are wrong 25% to 35% of the time.

"Put 30 drug-testing workers in a room together for a few hours and it isn't long before they start trading strange—and somewhat indelicate—tales of urine collection. Stories of specimens doctored to the most vivid hues of blue, green, and purple, and others spiked with bleach or diluted with chewing tobacco. Talk of . . . synthetic urine formulated in separate his and hers versions. And accounts of mystery concoctions ingested or added to try to ensure that urine does not betray the drug use of the provider."

San Jose Mercury News, March 29, 2004

Three major methods have been used to get a false-negative finding on a drug screen: substitution, adulteration, and dilution. Substitution is the simplest method and is the exchange of a "dirty" urine sample (one that shows evidence of use of a banned substance) for a clean one. Urine samples may also be adulterated with compounds that interfere with the mechanism that the screening test uses to detect the presence of a given drug or its metabolites. Dilution refers to drinking large quantities of liquids before the drug screen so that the urine is diluted and the drug metabolite concentration falls below the level that the test can detect. Each of these methods of deception, if done correctly and without detection, can fool the drug screen. However, after years of experience in managing deception, drug-testing laboratories have developed procedures for determining that a urine sample has been somehow altered or substituted. You also should be aware that some products, especially aids to sample dilution, purport to be effective but are not.

A false-positive screen also might be a concern to an individual. Some legal drugs or compounds show positive for an illicit substance on both the screen and the confirmatory tests. In fact, some people who use illegal drugs try to get a prescription for a fitting legal substance before a drug test so that a positive finding may be attributed to the prescribed substance. Other legal substances yield a positive screen, but the confirmatory tests negate such a result (Connecticut Clearing House, 2001). For example, poppy seeds eaten in sufficient quantities (about the amount on a hundred bagels) give a positive screen for opiates (see Chapter 10), and over-the-counter decongestants give a positive screen for amphetamines (see Chapter 14).

In summary, drug testing is a major social concern in the United States and other countries because of the consequences to individuals in the workplace and other environments of confirmed illicit drug use. From the technical side of this issue, if current laboratory technology and protocol are followed, then drug testing may be seen as performing its task well. And it is important to note that research is ongoing to improve the technology of drug testing by using biological samples. For example, as we noted earlier, there is a developing technology in the use of hair samples, which offers the potential

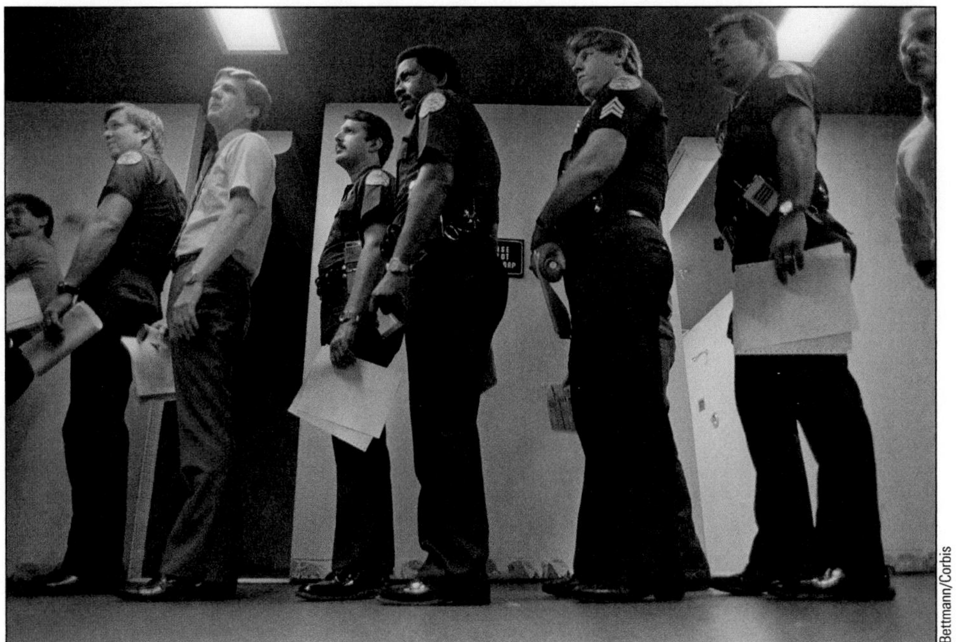

Bettmann/Corbis

Drug testing is becoming a more frequent requirement for obtaining and keeping employment.

major advantage of enabling detection of drug use from longer periods before the sample is taken than is possible with any of the other drug-testing methods. In general, it is important to remember that the different methods of drug testing have different advantages and disadvantages, and the one chosen depends on the purpose of administering the test and the context in which it is administered (Dolan et al., 2004).

"I'm in favor of it as long as it's multiple choice."

Kurt Rambis, on drug testing

Summary

Our discussion of drug elimination concludes our review of the first four steps of the drug experience and of pharmacokinetics. Figure 4.1 is a summary of what we have covered in this chapter so far. A given quantity of a drug (dose) may be administered by one of several methods (routes of administration). The drug then leaves its site of administration (absorption) to be distributed to the sites of drug action. The route of administration and biochemical factors influence the speed and amount of drug absorption. Biochemical factors also affect the amount of drug that is distributed. The latter refers to bioavailability, which determines what portion of the original dose reaches sites of drug action. Bioavailability is the pharmacological basis of the drug experience. Once they reach their sites of action, drugs are eliminated from the body either by direct excretion or by metabolism into by-products that are excreted. The course of elimination of a drug is one influence of a drug effect over time.

It is important to point out that a drug's exit from the body may not be the end of the drug experience. In later chapters on specific drugs, you will see that elimination of a drug from the body often is associated with physical and psychological changes that are the opposite of those that were caused by the drug. For example, the feelings of euphoria and tranquility that heroin causes switch to irritability and intense, extremely unpleasant physiological changes when the drug leaves the addict's body. The euphoria and high energy that cocaine and amphetamines typically induce turn to lethargy and depression as the drugs end their course of action. Such opposite (sometimes

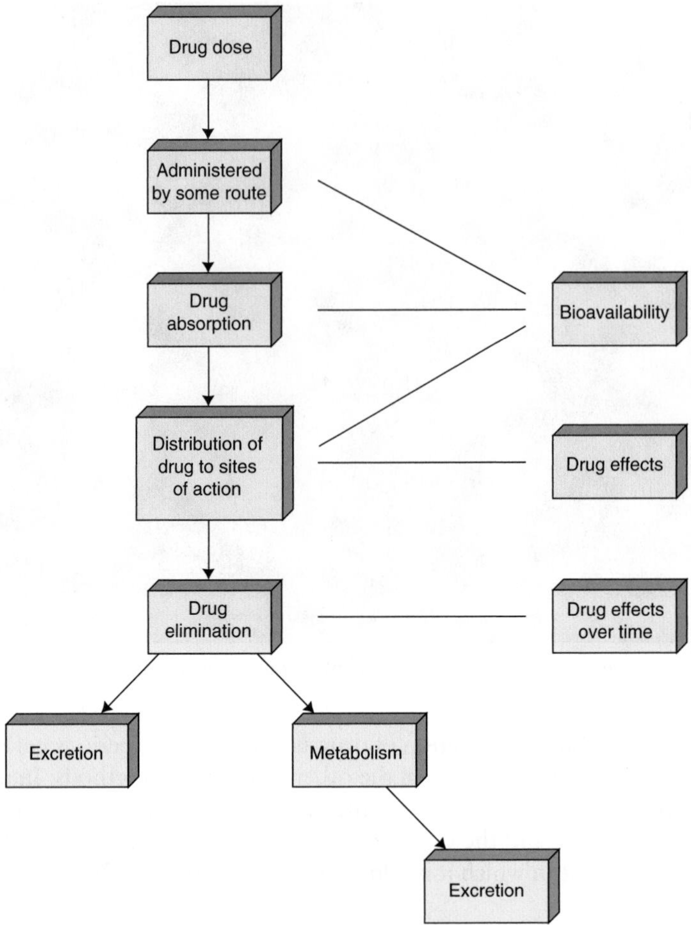

FIGURE 4.1
A summary of the first four steps of the drug experience and pharmacokinetics

called "rebound") effects are important to us because of their influence on drug use patterns. The rebound effect of depression that follows cocaine use is sometimes so unpleasant, for example, that users feel a strong need to take more cocaine to stop the bad feelings. Avoiding the effects of heroin abstinence is a powerful force in addicts' continued use of the drug. When coming down from a dose of alcohol, people often feel sleepy and somewhat depressive, so they may start drinking again to try to recapture the more euphoric mood associated with just starting to drink.

Pharmacodynamics

Our overview of pharmacokinetics prepares you for the description and explanation of drug effects—the subject of pharmacodynamics. In the remainder of this chapter, we present terms that pharmacologists use to describe drug effects and graphic representations of such effects. This standard language of drug effects is essential to your understanding of not only information in this text but also much other information that is available on drugs and human behavior.

The Dose-Effect Curve

Knowing the size or magnitude of an effect for a range of drug doses is important. Earlier we saw that drug effects differ according to drug doses. Because representing the different effects a drug can have over a number of doses can become complicated quickly, a tool that represents such information as clearly and efficiently as possible would be useful. In pharmacology, this tool is the dose-effect curve (formerly commonly called the dose-response curve), a standard way of representing drug effects that result from taking different drug doses. This curve is a representation of some effect according to a dose of the drug. For example, several groups of people may drink different doses of alcohol and be asked to report their degree of relaxation at a given point. If the average reports of relaxation for each group were then plotted, we would have a dose-effect curve.

"Tout est poison, rien n'est poison, tout est une question de dose." ("Everything is poisonous, nothing is poisonous, it is all a matter of dose.")

Claude Bernard, experimental pathologist

Figure 4.2 is a prototype dose-effect curve. The vertical axis of the graph, labeled "Effect size," represents the change we are interested in recording. The changes that we emphasize in this text are reported in some generally accepted measurement of mood, behavior, or nervous system function. Examples might include memory task performance, ratings of mood, or some measure of physiological arousal such as heart rate. On the vertical axis, the effect is generally depicted as going from smaller to larger. The graph's horizontal axis represents the range of doses under investigation, from smaller to larger doses. (Often the logarithm of the drug dose is represented on the horizontal axis.) Typically, a minimum of three doses is studied. Creating the curve is then simply a matter of plotting the effect, however measured, for the individuals who have received a given dose of the drug under evaluation. Usually, different groups of subjects each receive a given dose, or the same subjects receive all the doses studied in an experiment lasting a number of days. In either case, the average effect of each dose is plotted. When the effect is plotted for each dose investigated, the resultant graph represents effect **as a function of** drug dose.

as a function of
A term expressing correlation. In graphs of functional relationships between two variables, changes in one variable (for example, drug effect) associated with changes in another (drug dose) are represented.

Figure 4.2 shows that the effects of this hypothetical drug are not constant across different doses. Rather, the S shape (sigmoid) of the curve reflects that an accurate description of this drug's effects requires the specification of a dose. The hypothetical drug in Figure 4.2 produces a larger effect as the dose increases. However, a limit

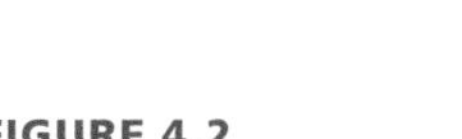

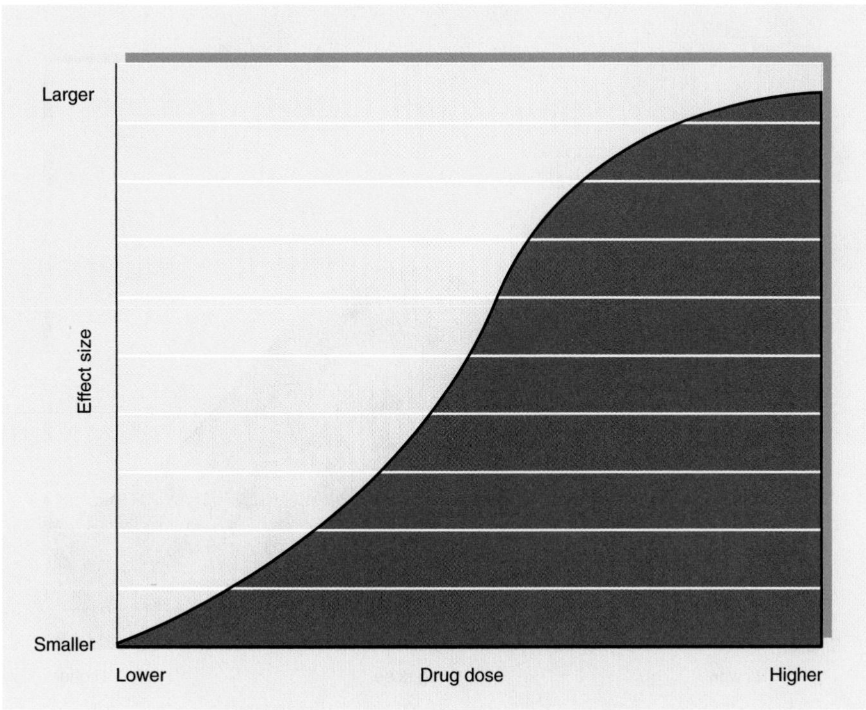

FIGURE 4.2
A typical dose-effect curve

exists; the graph plateaus for the highest doses. This means that increasing the dose beyond a given level does not increase the drug's effects. One illustration of this is the effect of alcohol on simple reaction time, which is formally measured by timing a person's "yes–no" response to the presence or absence of some stimulus, such as a light. For the "average" drinker (see Chapter 9), having two 12-ounce beers in an hour has little effect on simple reaction time. After about four beers, however, reaction time is significantly increased (the person's response is slower). After five beers, reaction time is slowed even further. A person who drinks about nine beers in an hour might find it hard to stay conscious, so measuring any further deterioration in reaction time with additional drinking would yield little new information. At that point, if the person is having a hard time maintaining consciousness, then the possibility of—and the utility of—measuring further slowing of reaction time with a higher dose of alcohol would hover around zero. The plateau of the dose-effect curve in this instance would be reached at the alcohol dose equivalent of about nine beers. The example of alcohol and simple reaction time shows that the question is not what effects drug X has but rather what the effect of drug X is at a specified dose.

Variations of the Dose-Effect Curve

Not all drug effects look like Figure 4.2 when plotted over a range of doses. One variant is a *biphasic* drug effect. This means that the effect of a drug may go in one direction—say, increase as the dose goes up—but then the effect changes direction (decreases) as the dose continues to go up. A biphasic drug effect is represented in Figure 4.3.

As illustrated, the drug effect gets larger as the drug dose increases to the moderate range. As the dose continues to increase, however, the curve changes direction to represent the decrease in drug effect with higher drug doses. In this example, the size of the effect essentially returns almost to the level at the lowest drug doses. Heart rate is an effect that has been reported to be biphasic for both alcohol and marijuana (Blum, 1984).

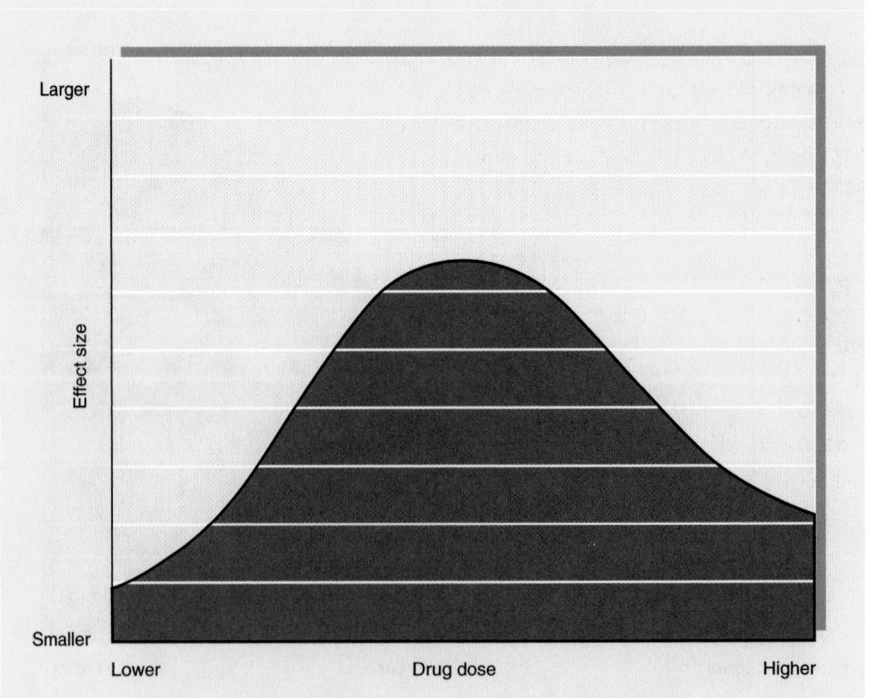

FIGURE 4.3
Dose-effect curve for a biphasic drug effect

Any drug may cause many different effects that can be measured, and for each of these effects, a dose-effect curve can be plotted. Many of the curves look alike and they usually are similar to the curve in Figure 4.2. Some dose-effect curves for a given drug could look quite different, however, depending on what effects are being measured. This brings out a major point: The dose-effect curve for a drug depends on the effect being measured. Figure 4.4 shows how college women in laboratory studies perceive their sexual arousal (one effect) and a physiological measure (such as vaginal blood flow) of their sexual arousal (a second effect) at lower to moderate doses of alcohol. Figure 4.4 looks different from the other dose-effect curves we have shown because we have changed how effect is represented (vertical axis) to accommodate a negative drug effect. As the figure shows, the college women perceived that their sexual arousal increased with increasing doses of alcohol, at least up to moderate doses (very high doses have not been studied). However, physiological measures of the women's sexual arousal show decreases as the dose increased (Abel, 1985).

Slope, Efficacy, and Potency

Pharmacologists use a few terms to more specifically describe a drug's action. These terms are illustrated in Figure 4.5, which shows the dose-effect curves for two hypothetical drugs, A and B. The first feature of the curves is the *slope*, or steepness. The slope of the curve reflects how much the drug dose changes before the effect gets larger. Slope can have very practical implications in prescribing drugs therapeutically or in considering potentially life-endangering effects of drugs taken nonmedically. Examples of the latter are the sedating effect of barbiturates and the effects of taking a benzodiazepine drug and alcohol together. In Figure 4.5, curve A has a steeper slope than curve B, so as the curves rise to a plateau, a given dose of A yields a larger effect.

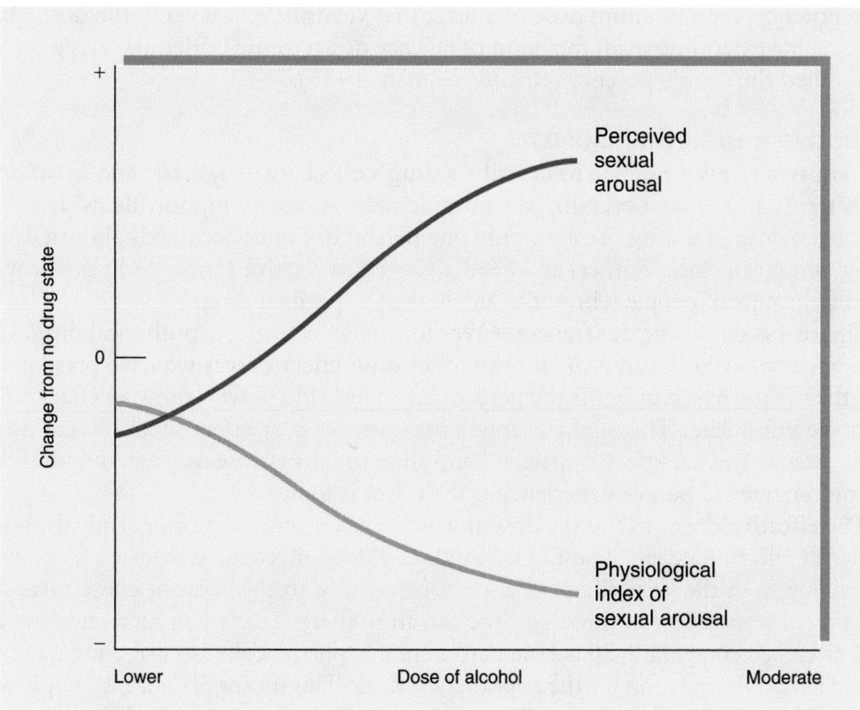

FIGURE 4.4
Dose-effect curves for perceived sexual arousal and a physiological measure of sexual arousal in college women after drinking low to moderate doses of alcohol

FIGURE 4.5
The dose-effect curves for two hypothetical drugs, A and B—the terms slope, efficacy, and potency are illustrated on the curves

Source: Adapted from *The Pharmacological Basis of Therapeutics*, 7/e, by E. M. Rose and A. G. Gilman. © 1985 McGraw-Hill.

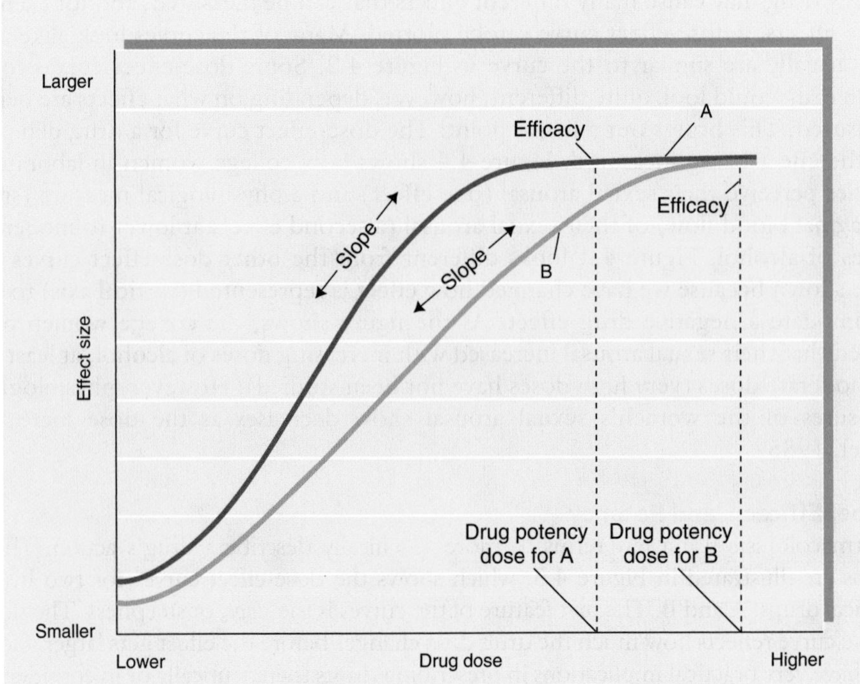

efficacy
The most intense, or peak, level of a drug effect.

drug potency
The minimum effective dose of a drug.

Two other terms illustrated in Figure 4.5 are a drug's **efficacy** and **drug potency**. Efficacy is defined as the peak of the dose-effect curve for a given effect. In Figure 4.5, that peak is where each curve reaches a plateau. Curves A and B are drawn to show two drugs with the same efficacy. The last concept we have included in Figure 4.5 is drug potency: the minimum dose of a drug that yields its efficacy. On the dose-effect curve, a line extending from the point of efficacy down to the horizontal axis gives the dose called the drug's potency (Ross & Gilman, 1985).

Effective and Lethal Doses

The last two terms we define to describe a drug's effect are its *effective* and *lethal doses*. Both terms arise from observing the considerable variability in individuals' reactions to a given dose of a drug. Testing only one person does not accurately show a drug's effect at a given dose. Rather, an effect is viewed in relative terms, or in the proportions of groups of people who show an effect at a specified dose.

Figure 4.6 shows the dose-effect curves for two effects of a hypothetical drug. One difference between Figure 4.6 and the other dose-effect curves we have presented is that the vertical axis represents the percentage of individuals who show an effect rather than the effect size. This slight change enables us to plot effective and lethal doses. With these terms, an effect is specified and then the drug dose associated with different percentages of people experiencing the effect is found.

effective dose
The dose at which a given percentage of individuals show a particular effect of a drug.

The **effective dose** (ED) is the dose at which a given percentage of individuals show a particular effect of a drug. The ED is found on a dose-effect curve by extending a horizontal line from the vertical axis at a given percentage to the relevant effect curve and dropping a vertical line to the drug dose axis from there. That point represents the ED for a given percentage. ED 50 is a standard term that pharmacologists use, and Figure 4.6 shows *ED* 50 for sedation for the hypothetical drug. This means 50% of the people who receive that amount of the drug will experience sedation. Of course, the ED for any percentage can be found in the same way. Two other EDs are also shown in Figure 4.6.

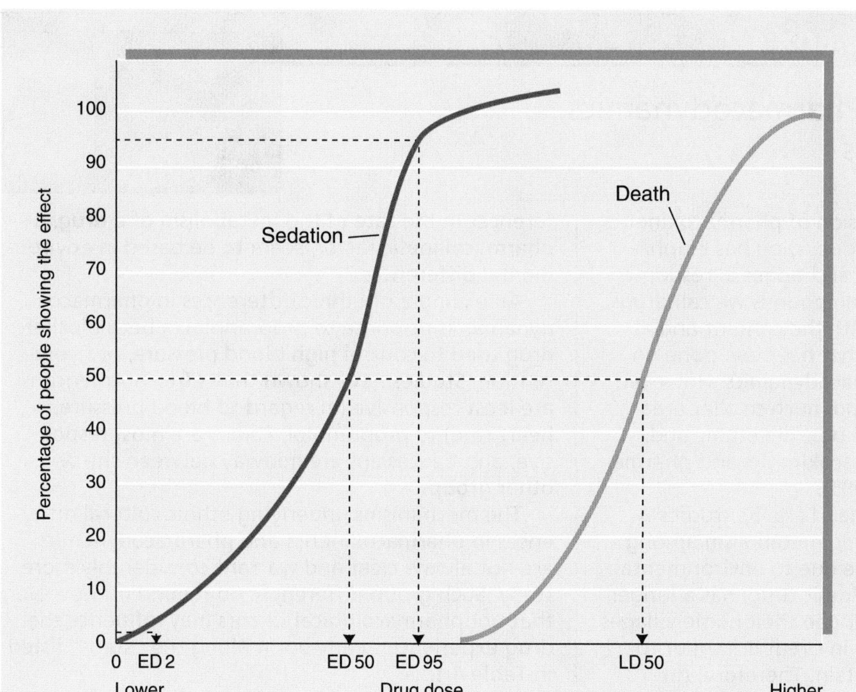

FIGURE 4.6
The dose-effect curves for two hypothetical drug's effects, sedation and death—the curves are used to compute three effective doses for sedation and the drug's LD 50

Source: Adapted from *The Pharmacological Basis of Therapeutics*, 7/e, by E. M. Rose and A. G. Gilman. © 1985 McGraw-Hill.

The **lethal dose** (LD) of a drug is a special case of the effective dose. As the name implies, in lethal dose, the effect of interest is death, and the LD is the dose at which a given percentage of nonhumans (human subjects are not used in experiments to determine the lethal doses of drugs) die within a specified time. A standard referent in pharmacology is a drug's LD 50, which is the dose at which 50% of the animals administered a given dose of a drug died within a stated time. Determining the LD 50 of a drug in humans is a matter of extrapolating the findings with animal subjects to humans. (Contemporary Issue Box 5.2 in Chapter 5 is devoted to the complex considerations involved in using animals in research for the benefit of humans.) The LD 50 of our hypothetical drug is illustrated on the curve on the right in Figure 4.6.

lethal dose
The dose of a drug at which a given percentage of individuals die within a specified time.

A drug's EDs and LDs are of more than casual interest. Of particular importance for a city's health officials, for example, is the difference between a drug's ED and LD. When the difference is small, much more danger of accidental suicide exists for a person who is using drugs for nonmedical reasons. For some drugs, such as caffeine, the ED–LD difference is large; however, other drugs pose more of a problem. Accidental deaths due to heart damage from a dose of cocaine have been described in the popular media, especially during the late 1980s. Alcohol is another example. A 160-pound man with average tolerance to alcohol typically would report feeling relaxed after drinking about two drinks in an hour on an empty stomach. However, that person would reach LD 50 for alcohol if he drank about a fifth (25.3 ounces) of whiskey in an hour. Such drinking occurs more often than you might think and has been responsible for serious injuries and deaths in fraternity hazings (initiation rites). Furthermore, when some drugs are combined, such as alcohol and the barbiturates, the resulting ED and LD are pushed even closer and the danger is greater. We discuss the effects of combining drugs in the next section of this chapter.

A final point: The ED–LD difference is also important when a physician or nurse practitioner administers a drug for medical reasons. In medicine, the goal is to find a drug that can be given in a dose that is therapeutic (that is, effective) for all patients, has no side

DRUGS AND CULTURE BOX 4.2

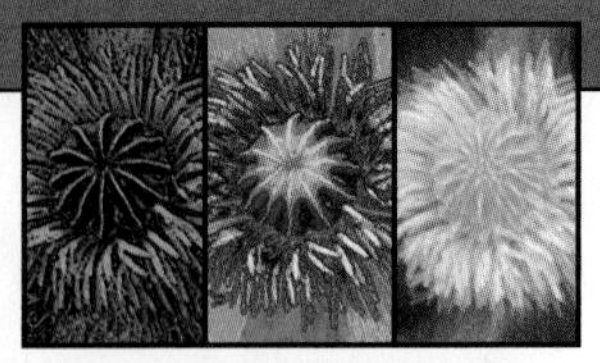

Pharmacokinetics, Pharmacodynamics, and Cultural Factors

Up to this point in our discussion of pharmacokinetics and pharmacodynamics, our discussion has emphasized the body's neurochemical changes in response to its ingestion of chemical compounds we call drugs. This emphasis is consistent with the content and long history of the research that has been done on pharmacokinetics and pharmacodynamics. However, a more recently developed and much smaller area of research is concerned with possible ethnic and cultural differences in pharmacokinetics and pharmacodynamics (Lin & Poland, 1995).

As reviewed in Lin and Poland (1995), studies have shown differences in drug metabolism among ethnic groups that seem to be due to environmental variables. Antipyrine, an analgesic drug, has a longer half-life among Sudanese living in their home villages compared to Sudanese living in Great Britain or to Caucasians living in Great Britain. Therefore, differences in the rate of the metabolism of a drug, a pharmacokinetic factor, seem to be based in environmental differences.

An example of ethnic differences in pharmacodynamics is response to propranolol, a beta-blocker drug used to control high blood pressure, or hypertension. Studies have shown that African Americans are least responsive (in regard to blood pressure, heart rate) to propranolol, Asians are most responsive, and Caucasians are midway between the two other groups.

The mechanisms underlying ethnic/cultural differences in pharmacokinetics and pharmacodynamics are not always clear and warrant considerably more study. Such group differences do remind us, however, that nonpharmacological factors may influence the drug experience at any point along the "steps" listed in Table 4.1.

therapeutic index A measure of a drug's safety in medical care; it is computed as a ratio: LD 50/ED 50.

effects, and is not lethal. Accordingly, the **therapeutic index** has been derived: the ratio LD 50/ED 50 for a given drug. Here, the ED of interest is the alleviation of the symptoms of some disease or injury. You can see that the higher a drug's therapeutic index, the more useful the drug is in medical treatment. Another point is that steeper dose-effect curves tend to have smaller therapeutic indices. The therapeutic index gives health care providers a quick idea of the benefits of prescribing a drug as part of a specific treatment.

Drug Interactions

So far we have simplified our discussion by considering only one drug at a time. The study of pharmacodynamics often involves the actions of two or more drugs, however. A person could take multiple drugs at the same time, or take one drug before another has totally cleared from the body. The extremes are seen in polydrug abuse, which we illustrated in Chapter 1.

interact When the effects of one drug are modified by the presence of another drug.

Using more than one drug at a time increases the complexity of the drug experience because two or more drugs entering the body may **interact**. Two drugs have an interaction if the effect of one modifies or alters the effect of the other. Drug interactions may be analyzed qualitatively or quantitatively; the degree of effect, or quantitative study, is by far better understood in pharmacology. The quantitative study of drug interactions considers both enhancing and diminishing effects of combining drugs.

Enhancing Combinations

synergism Any enhancing drug interaction.

Drug synergism is a confusing term because it has been used in different ways. Here we will use it to denote any enhancing drug interaction. Another word that currently is used in the same way as synergism is *potentiation*. When two drugs are synergistic, the effects of taking them together are greater than the effects of taking either drug alone. In practice, pharmacologists find it difficult to tell for sure whether synergistic effects are a simple result of adding the separate effects of the two drugs together or if somehow one of the drugs is "multiplying" the effects of the other.

In quantitative studies of combining drugs, interactions are represented by changes in the dose-effect curve. Figure 4.7 represents a synergistic relationship between drug A and drug B. You can see that the solid line is like the typical dose-effect curve for a drug that we illustrated in Figure 4.2. The effect of synergy between the two drugs, then, is to "shift" the dose-effect curve to the left, represented by the broken line in Figure 4.7. The broken line curve shows that larger effects of drug A are evident at lower doses of it when drug B is present.

Diminishing Combinations

Drug antagonism is a term that refers to the diminished or reduced effect of a drug when another drug is present. As you might guess, drug antagonism is represented by a shift to the right of a drug's dose-effect curve. For example, the amphetamines, which are CNS stimulant drugs, antagonize alcohol's CNS depressant effects. However, the amphetamines do not reduce alcohol's impairment of motor skills, like driving (Blum, 1984).

antagonism
The diminished or reduced effect of a drug when another drug is present.

The Importance of Interactions between Drugs

An awareness of interactions between drugs is important for several reasons. In medical practice, knowledge of drug interactions is vital because drugs are often used in combinations for more effective treatment of an illness. Therefore, drug interactions may be used to improve medical care. On the other hand, interactions could be a problem, for example, for a physician. Difficulties may occur if the physician is not aware of all the drugs a patient may be using at a given time. For example, the effects of one drug could cancel the therapeutic effects of another. Furthermore, prescribed medication could have detrimental or even lethal effects in the presence of other drugs. Fortunately, pharmacies now commonly have computerized profiles of the medications that a patient has been prescribed. Such information allows pharmacists to inform customers how newly prescribed medications interact with other medications they may be taking and what precautions they should follow to avoid harmful combined drug

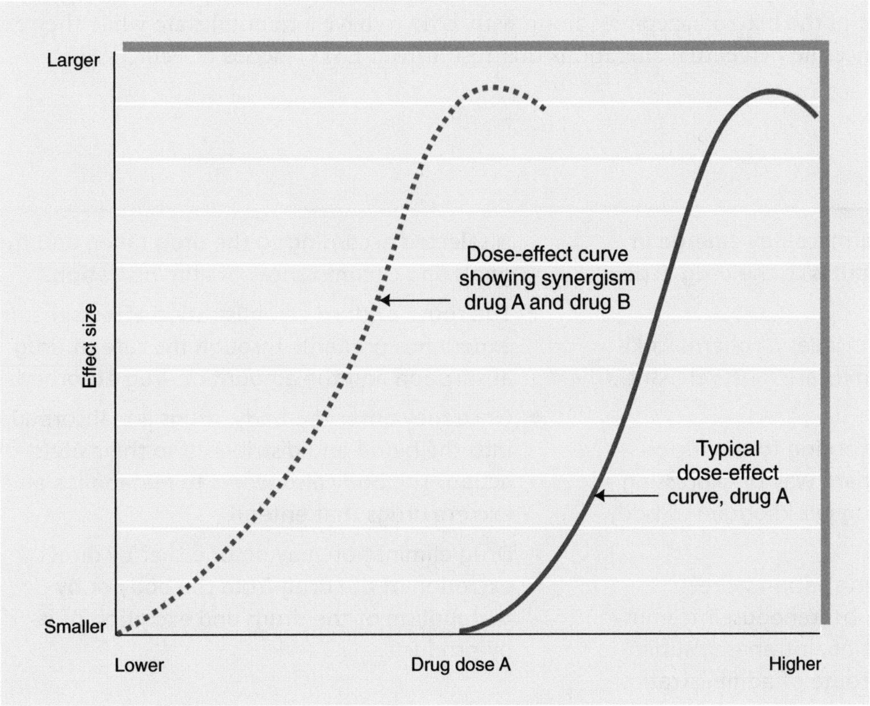

FIGURE 4.7
Representation by dose-effect curves of a synergistic relationship for drugs A and B

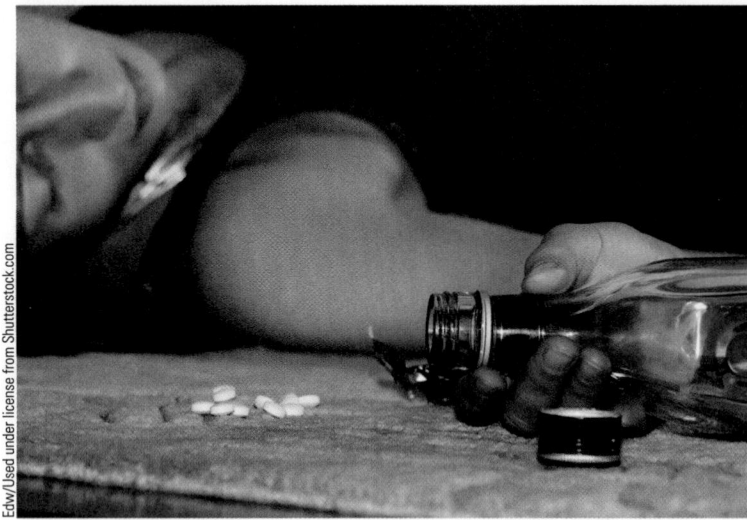

People often use more than one drug at a time, which sometimes can pose considerable risks to safety.

effects. This backup to physician advice is available to all patients but is probably of most help in treating the elderly, who often take more than one prescribed medication at a time.

Drug interactions also may cause problems with different nonprescribed drugs or combinations of prescribed and nonprescribed drugs. The most common examples are mixing drugs that depress the central nervous system. For example, as we said earlier, alcohol and the barbiturates may be lethal in enhancing the sedative effects of each. This drug combination has caused many intentional and accidental deaths.

Drug interactions also are important for their influences on the reasons for and patterns of human drug use, so they are of central concern in this text. Individuals may intentionally combine drugs that have the same or similar action to achieve a "super" high or effect. Or individuals may use drugs that have opposite effects in a deliberate effort for one drug to modify the other. An example heard commonly in treatment settings is using alcohol's depressant effects to modify the overstimulation sometimes induced by cocaine. Drinkers sometimes consume large amounts of black coffee (containing caffeine) in hopes of antagonizing alcohol's CNS depressant effects. In truth, however, caffeine seems to do little to counter alcohol's effects on the CNS. These two examples illustrate the drug user's attempt to modify the intensity (quantitative) of drug effects. However, drugs also may be combined to achieve **qualitative** interaction effects that could not be achieved by any of the drugs separately. Users might take a depressant drug, such as one of the benzodiazepines, along with LSD to have a tranquil state while they experience the perceptual alterations that result from LSD (Jacobs & Fehr, 1987).

qualitative
The kind, as opposed to quantity, of effect.

Summary

- The basic principles of pharmacology emerge in discussions of what contributes to the drug experience.
- To the pharmacologist, principles of pharmacokinetics and pharmacodynamics are most relevant to the drug experience.
- Drug dose is computed according to the recipient's body weight. A standard way of expressing dose is in milligrams of drug per kilogram of body weight (mg/kg).
- Eight routes of drug administration were discussed in detail: oral, subcutaneous, intramuscular, intravenous, inhalation, intranasal, sublingual, and transdermal. A route of administration is selected according to the drug taken and the goals and circumstances of administration.
- The route of drug administration affects the drug experience primarily through the rate of drug absorption and the amount of drug absorbed.
- Once they enter the body, drugs are absorbed into the blood and distributed to their site(s) of action. The body also works to metabolize and excrete drugs that enter it.
- Drug elimination may occur either by direct excretion of the drug from the body or by metabolism of the drugs and excretion of its by-products.

- A common term related to drug elimination is drug half-life.
- Drug absorption, distribution, and elimination are affected by different biochemical factors and accentuate the complexity of the drug experience.
- Pharmacodynamics most directly concerns actions of the drug on the body and thus drug effects. This chapter covered fundamental terms that pharmacologists use to describe drug effects and ways to depict them graphically.
- Pharmacologists use the dose-effect curve as a standard way to represent graphically the size of an effect in relation to the dose of a drug taken. The prototype dose-effect curve has an S shape, but variations depend on the effects studied.
- Three concepts derived from a dose-effect curve offer valuable information about a drug's action: slope of the curve, drug efficacy, and drug potency.
- Two other important features of a drug's actions are its effective dose and lethal dose. The relationship between these two doses is essential information for medical and nonmedical drug use.
- Pharmacodynamics often involves the consideration of more than one drug in the body at the same time. Multiple drugs interact to contribute to the drug experience. Interactions may be enhancing or diminishing.
- Drugs that enhance the effects of each other are called synergistic. Antagonism between drugs creates diminished drug effects.
- Enhanced and diminished drug effects refer to the quantitative (degree of effect) study of drug interactions. Qualitative study of drug interactions also is possible.
- It is essential to be aware of drug interactions in both medical and nonmedical drug use.

Answers to "What Do You Think?"

1. A given amount of a drug has similar biological effects on different people.
   F *The quantity of a drug is adjusted for a person's body weight to yield pharmacologically equal amounts of the drug.*
2. Despite the large number of known drugs, there are only three ways that drugs are commonly administered or taken.
   F *There are a variety of ways to take drugs; we described eight of them in this chapter.*
3. The safest way to take a drug is orally, but that is the slowest way of getting the drug into the blood.
   T *The most common and the safest way to take a drug is orally. However, the absorption of a drug when it is taken orally is slowed.*
4. Taking a drug intravenously is a highly efficient, safe way to get a drug into the blood.
   F *The intravenous route is highly efficient because it bypasses problems of absorption associated with, say, the oral route. Because the drug is injected directly into veins, however, the intravenous route is the most risky because of problems of overdosing. Great caution is required when drugs are administered intravenously.*
5. Smoking is a relatively slow way of getting a drug into the blood.
   F *For drugs that can be taken by inhalation, that route results in very rapid absorption.*
6. Some drugs can enter the body through the skin.
   T *Some drugs can be taken through the skin, or transdermally. Nicotine is among the best known of such drugs.*
7. The body protects the brain from toxic substances.
   T *The blood-brain barrier prevents many toxic substances from reaching the brain. Drugs that are less fat-soluble have a tougher time getting through the blood-brain barrier.*
8. The kidneys play the major role in drug metabolism.
   F *The liver is the organ primarily responsible for drug metabolism.*
9. Scientific study of the effects of drugs is difficult because there is no way to represent such effects quantitatively.
   F *The effects of drugs can generally be measured and can be represented with dose-effect curves.*
10. When more than one drug is taken at a time, the effects of one can enhance or diminish the effects of the other(s).

T *Drugs modify the effects of each other when taken simultaneously. Sometimes the outcome is difficult to predict.*

11. Caffeine and alcohol have antagonistic effects.

F *Although it is intuitive that caffeine and alcohol are antagonists, research shows that caffeine does little to alter alcohol's effects on the CNS.*

12. It is important to know about drug interactions because of the increasing prevalence of using more than one drug at a time among people who present themselves for drug treatment.

F *Although using more than one drug is more common among people who present themselves for treatment, knowledge of drug interactions also is important because many people are prescribed more than one medication.*

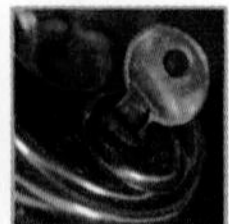

Key Terms

absorbed
antagonism
as a function of
bioavailability
control
diffusibility
dissolved
distribution
drug potency
effective dose
efficacy
feedback
freebase
half-life
interact
lethal dose
metabolism
pharmacodynamics
pharmacokinetics
qualitative
side effects
solubility
suspended
synergism
therapeutic index

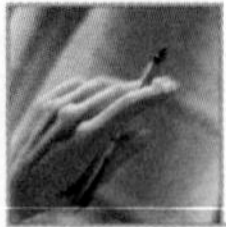

Essays/Thought Questions

1. Sketch a map marking the steps of the drug experience, from the point of a drug's entry into the body to an individual's perception of that drug's effects.
2. What factors might be considered in determining the "safety threshold" of a drug's therapeutic index?

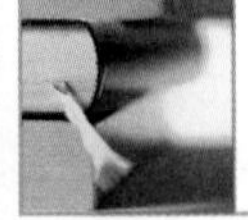

Suggested Readings

Center for AIDS Prevention Studies. (1998). Does needle exchange work? Chicago: American Medical Association.

Bina, C. (1998). Drug testing 101: Detecting tainted samples. Corrections Today, 60, 122–128.

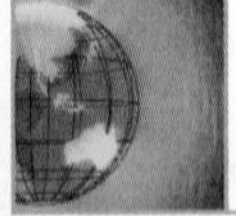

Web Resources

Visit the Book Companion Website at www.cengage.com/psychology/maisto to access study tools including a glossary, flashcards, and web quizzing. You will also find a link to the following resource:

- The Center for AIDS Prevention Studies (CAPS): Up-to-date information on HIV prevention research and related topics, including needle exchange programs

CHAPTER 5

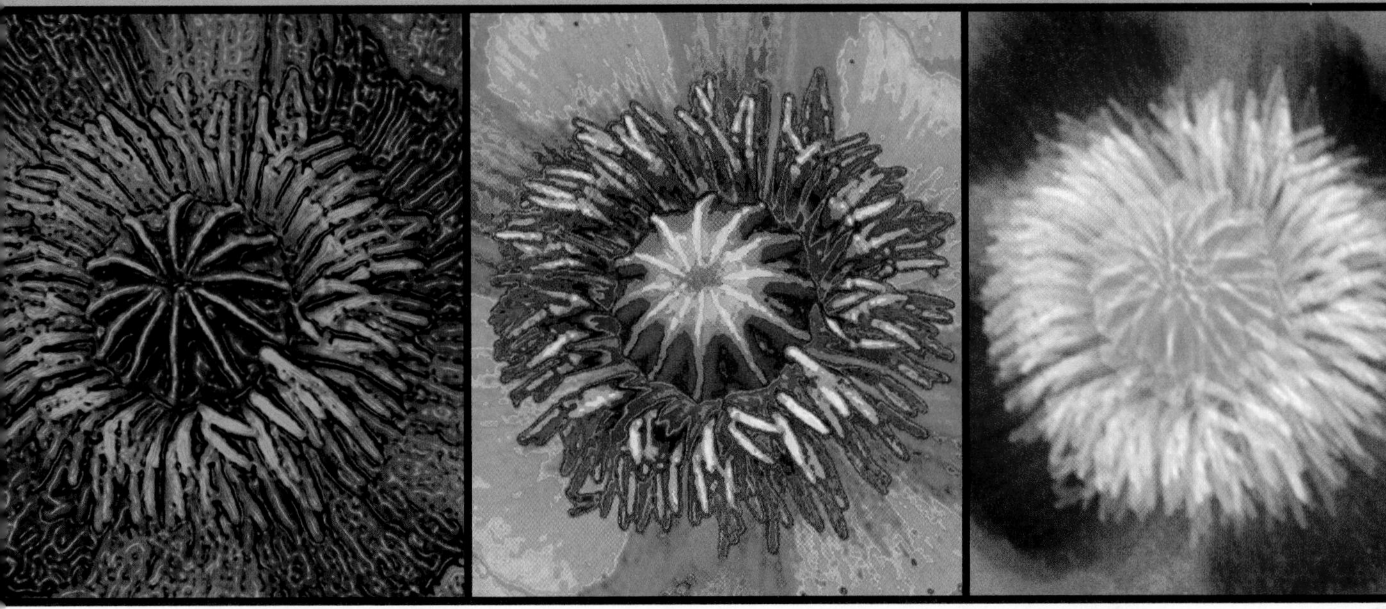

Psychopharmacology and New Drug Development

What Do You Think? True or False?

Answers are given at the end of the chapter.

___ 1. Gender differences in the effects of drugs are due primarily to body weight differences.

___ 2. Some individuals have an "addictive" personality that predisposes them to alcohol or drug-use disorders.

___ 3. Expectancies about alcohol's effects may be a more powerful determinant of its effects than is the pharmacological action of alcohol.

___ 4. Theories about the effects of drugs on humans always have taken into account social and environmental factors.

___ 5. Tolerance to a drug develops because of biological changes that occur as a result of using the drug.

___ 6. Tolerance to a drug may be evident within the same occasion of using it.

___ 7. People who have tolerance to alcohol will also demonstrate tolerance to barbiturates the first time they use them.

___ 8. There is no relationship between the drugs that animals show preference for and the drugs that humans prefer.

___ 9. The effects of a drug on animals tell us little about how that drug will affect humans.

___10. In general, drug researchers are not concerned with placebo effects when studying the actions of a drug.

___11. Because new medications are needed to treat diseases like AIDS, government regulation of the process of drug development and marketing has been greatly simplified.

___12. Folk uses of naturally occurring products are important sources for discovering new drugs.

In Table 4.1, we listed seven steps of the drug experience, but only five were discussed in Chapter 4. In this chapter, we focus on Steps 6 and 7; Step 6 concerns biological and psychological characteristics of drug users that affect the experiences humans have when they use drugs, and Step 7 concerns social and environmental factors and their influence on the drug experience. Our discussion of the steps listed in Table 4.1 raises the question of how the drug experience relates to human drug use, which leads to our consideration of research methods in the field of psychopharmacology. (Another narrower use of the term *psychopharmacology* is the study of drugs used to treat mental illness.) Psychopharmacology research, as you might guess, focuses on the reasons behind drug-use patterns and on the patterns of use themselves. Information on research basics will prepare you for understanding the process of discovering and developing new drugs, which we review in the last sections of this chapter.

Characteristics of Users

Differences among people probably account for most of the differences in how they react to a given dose of a drug. We present only the major factors in this section because any more extended discussion would preclude the presentation of anything else in this text. Roughly, we can divide user characteristics into two types: biological and psychological.

Biological Characteristics

Inherited Differences in Reactions to Drugs

Major differences in how people react to drugs are genetically based (Nies, 2001). For example, the way people are affected by their first dose of a drug is called their

initial sensitivity to a drug. Differences in sensitivity are thought to be determined genetically. More generally, a lot of money is spent on research to discover the role genetics plays in causing the various substance-use disorders. Alcohol-use disorders in particular have received much attention from scientists. It is believed that inherited differences in how alcohol is experienced (as a result of action in the brain) and metabolized may be of major importance in some individuals developing alcohol abuse or dependence (see Chapter 9).

initial sensitivity The effect of a drug on a first-time user.

Gender

A specified dose of a drug administered to a man and a woman on average will have somewhat greater effects on the woman. One major reason for this difference is the tendency for women to have a higher percentage of body fat and therefore a lower percentage of body water than men do. So, based on information you learned in Chapter 4, percentage of body fat may influence drug effects in two ways. If there is less body water because of more body fat, then a drug will be more concentrated in the body and thus have greater effect. In addition, some drugs selectively bind to fat molecules in the body, so the drug is eliminated more slowly with a higher percentage of body fat and thus remains active in the body for a longer time.

Weight

In Chapter 4, you saw that body weight is part of the formula for computing drug dose. This is because the concentration of a drug in the blood depends on how much blood and other body fluids are in the body. These fluids dilute an absorbed drug. Simply put, heavier people have more blood and other fluids, so for a given quantity of drug, they would have a smaller concentration of it than would lighter people. As we noted earlier for gender differences, this contributes to a lesser drug effect in heavier people.

Age

Age can influence drug effects if the users are very young or old. Children are more sensitive to drugs because enzyme systems that metabolize drugs may not be fully developed. As a result, the drug stays active longer. In the elderly, these same enzyme systems may be impaired, with the same result of increased duration of drug action.

Psychological Characteristics

How an individual's psychological characteristics affect the drug experience has often been studied in research on personality and drug use. It is not surprising that the relationship between personality and the drug experience is difficult to understand. *Personality* is a term used to represent a cluster of characteristics that describe the ways in which an individual thinks, perceives, feels, and acts. These characteristics are thought to be fairly constant, although variations occur in how a person acts in different situations. Nevertheless, personality characteristics are for the most part viewed as enduring.

One personality characteristic that has received a lot of attention regarding its relationship to drug use is sensation seeking. Zuckerman (1979) defined *sensation seeking* as "the need for varied, novel, and complex sensations and experiences and the willingness to take physical and social risks for the sake of such experience" (p. 10). Four different aspects of sensation seeking have been discovered: thrill and adventure seeking, experience seeking, disinhibition, and boredom susceptibility.

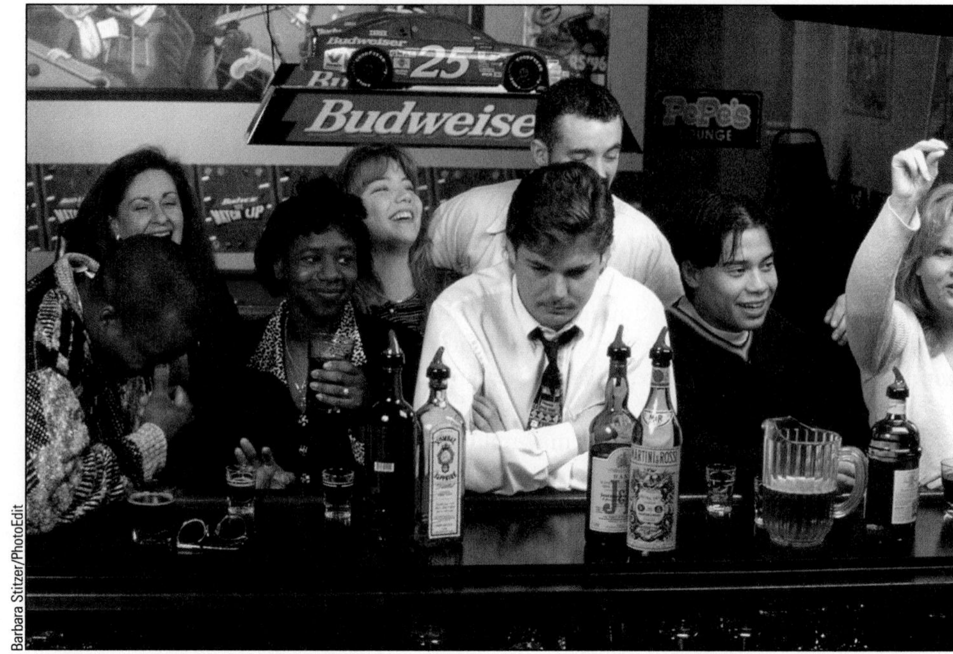

Barbara Stitzer/PhotoEdit

People differ in how they react when they use drugs in a given setting as a result of differences in biological and psychological factors.

"The great art of life is sensation, to feel that we exist, even in pain."
Lord Byron

A number of studies have shown a positive relationship between sensation seeking and frequency of drug and alcohol use and the variety of drugs that are used. The more sensation seeking a person is, the more the person tends to use alcohol and drugs and to use more kinds of drugs (Earleywine, 1994). One explanation for these findings is that sensation seeking represents the individual's higher degree of sensitivity to the pleasurable effects of drugs. That is, *sensation seeking* is a summary term for one source of the differences in how people experience drugs.

Personality factors also have been shown to influence the degree of stress reduction that people get from taking alcohol and other drugs. This is particularly important because stress reduction has long been held to be a major reason people drink and use drugs, particularly people who develop drug- or alcohol-use disorders (Greeley & Oei, 1999). For example, Sher (1987) developed the "stress response dampening" (SRD) model of alcohol and other drug use. Alcohol and drugs such as the benzodiazepines have anxiety-reducing effects. People who experience such effects therefore are more likely than others to use drugs to cope with unwanted stress. Of particular interest here is that individuals seem to vary in the SRD of alcohol they experience according to their personality characteristics. For example, Sher and Levenson (1982) showed that people characterized as aggressive, impulsive, and extroverted were more sensitive to alcohol's SRD effects. Notably, studies have shown that those individuals who developed alcohol-use disorders tended to be high on these characteristics before they began to experience problems with alcohol.

addictive personality The hypothesis of a personality structure common to all people with substance-use disorders.

A general discussion of research on personality and drug use cannot ignore the topic of the **addictive personality**. Essentially, this is the idea of a personality structure common to all individuals who have substance-use disorders. The notion of an addictive personality has generated a lot of research and discussion, and it remains a popular idea among people who treat individuals who have substance-use disorders. The addictive personality idea is important to us because the idea implies that people who have a particular personality makeup experience a unique reaction to alcohol and drugs, or that they find alcohol and drugs especially valuable in coping with life's stressors. As a result, people with an addictive personality would be more likely to develop substance-use problems than people who do not have such a personality.

Although the idea may have some appeal, the research yields little evidence for an addictive personality. Instead, it seems that people identified as having substance-use disorders have considerable personality differences. In short, people who have problems with drugs may have as many personality differences as any other group of people. However, we should note that men and women who have developed substance-use disorders may be distinguished from people who did not develop such problems by personality characteristics predating development of the disorders (Barnes, 1979; Cox, 1986; Goldstein & Sappington, 1977; USDHHS, 1993). For example, young men who later developed alcohol problems were characterized as self-centered, rebellious, impulsive, thrill seeking, talkative, gregarious, and in need of personal power. Note that these studies do not provide evidence for an addictive personality. But this research does suggest that some personality characteristics may interact with other factors, like stress, influences of peers, and quality of family life, to make it more likely that a person will develop problems with alcohol and drugs.

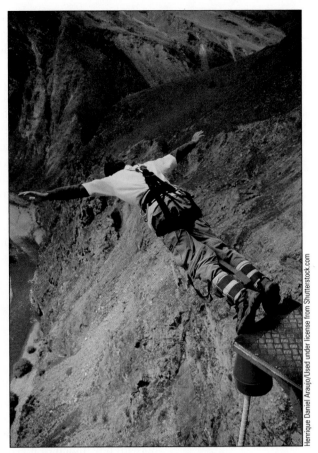

Individuals who enjoy bungee jumping probably would score high on a measure of sensation seeking.

Drug Expectancies and Beliefs

The history of experience with drugs, beliefs, knowledge, attitudes, and other thoughts about drugs that people have are part of their uniqueness and therefore personality. These nonpharmacological variables can exert powerful influences on the drug experience. One factor that is prominent in this regard is what a person expects to achieve or happen when using a drug. This anticipation is called a **drug expectancy**.

drug expectancy
A person's anticipation of or belief about what he or she will experience upon taking a drug.

A person's expectancies are based on previous experiences with a given psychoactive substance and its effects. These experiences could have been direct (that is, the person has used the substance) or indirect (the person has been exposed to the substance and its effects through instruction, friends' use, television, advertising, reading, and so on).

Most of the research on expectancy has been conducted on alcohol use, and we review some of that work in Chapter 9. In one early discussion, MacAndrew and Edgerton (1969) proposed that what people have learned and believe about alcohol is an important determinant of how they conduct themselves while drinking. Thus, what people expect to happen when they drink can be an important factor in determining their response to the alcohol consumed. In some cases, this may be more influential than alcohol's pharmacological action! Researchers have investigated alcohol-related expectancies by conducting studies in which some participants are

"Over the course of socialization, people learn about drunkenness what their society 'knows' about drunkenness; and, accepting and acting upon the understandings thus imparted to them, they become the living confirmation of their society's teachings."

MacAndrew & Edgerton (1969, p. 88)

told they are drinking alcohol but actually receive a nonalcoholic "placebo" beverage. An earlier summary of such research showed that expectancy effects are most prominent with behaviors or emotions that society proscribes from free expression, such as aggression, sexual arousal, and humor (Hull & Bond, 1986). Therefore, it would be predicted that people who believe alcohol fosters aggression or enhances sexual arousal would experience those effects, but at least partly because they expect that result, along with any specific pharmacological effect of alcohol. Expectancies may affect other kinds of behaviors, too. For example, one experiment showed that young adult men's beliefs about alcohol and skills on a motor task (for example, tracking a target moving on a rotating disk with a stylus) affected their performance on such tasks while they were under the influence of a dose of alcohol equal to about four 12-ounce beers in a 175-pound man (Fillmore & Vogel-Sprott, 1996). In this regard, as expected, alcohol did affect motor performance. However, the impairment was reduced in experienced drinkers who expected alcohol to have only mildly impairing effects on the task, even though they were told that alcohol would severely impair their performance.

Expectancies appear to have a considerable effect on the way people respond to other drugs as well (Vogel-Sprott & Fillmore, 1999). Marijuana is a good example (Orcutt, 1987). People who anticipate a relaxed, "mellow" feeling are more likely to experience that result than people who anxiously anticipate some type of drug-induced "loss of control" over their behavior. In part, this relates to the ways that smokers interpret or understand the various sensations that marijuana produces. The same sensation might be interpreted positively by one user but negatively by another, and much of that discrepancy is likely attributable to what the user expects to occur as a result of smoking. Marijuana is not the only other drug besides alcohol that seems to be affected by expectancies. Brandon, Juliano, and Copeland (1999) found that expectancies about the positive effects of smoking tobacco are associated with its use and with how much of it is used. Finally, although expectancy effects have been studied primarily in the context of using one drug on an occasion, a few studies have investigated how expectancies affect responses to the use of more than one drug. A common combination of drug use is alcohol and caffeine. Fillmore and Vogel-Sprott's (1996) study showed that behavioral impairments related to alcohol intoxication tended to increase or decrease with participants' beliefs about how combining the drugs would affect them.

Social and Environmental Factors

"I wasn't really persuaded to smoke (marijuana). I just watched everybody. I saw nobody going mad or anything; they were all laughing and having a good time. So . . . I smoked and got high. I liked the high and I smoked."

Research participant (Zinberg, 1984, p. 85)

It has not always been the case, but it now is generally accepted that the drug effects people experience are strongly influenced by social and environmental (setting) factors (Zinberg, 1984). *Environment* is an extremely broad term, and its components range from government laws about alcohol and other drug availability (see Chapter 2) to the people and places that define the immediate drug-use setting (McCarty, 1985).

Setting seems to be a particularly important influence on the effects of alcohol, marijuana, and hallucinogenic drugs. Pliner and Cappell (1974) demonstrated this point with alcohol. In their study, men and women drank moderate amounts of alcohol alone and with others. When subjects drank alone, they mostly reported experiencing physical changes, like fuzzy thinking, sleepiness, and dizziness. In contrast, subjects who drank the same amount of alcohol but with others said their mood changed to feeling friendly and more pleasant. Because subjects who drank an alcohol placebo beverage reported no changes whether drinking alone or with others, it seems that the number of people you drink with affects how you interpret the physiological changes that alcohol induces.

Another example of the influence of the setting involves reactions to marijuana. Carlin, Bakker, Halpern, and Post (1972) noted that, with lower doses of marijuana, smokers viewed others in the setting as more intoxicated than they actually were. The experimenters were able, again using lower doses of the drug, to enhance or diminish the degree of reported marijuana intoxication by having an accomplice act "up" or "down." Setting was not so influential with higher doses of marijuana. Studies such as these support Becker's (1963) ideas about the "making" of a marijuana user. Becker described this as a sociocultural process in which experienced users essentially "teach" new users what to anticipate, how to interpret the effects, what effects to enjoy, and what effects to ignore. Becker's ideas imply that what people experience when taking marijuana is influenced by their expectations about the drug's effects and by others' presence in the drug-taking setting.

Tolerance

Repeated administration of a given dose of a drug often results in reduced response to the drug (O'Brien, 2001). This phenomenon, known as tolerance, was defined and briefly introduced in Chapter 1. Here we summarize the major principles and explanations of tolerance. Our discussion of tolerance follows our overview of biological, psychological, and social/environmental characteristics of users because, as you will see, tolerance involves all three types of factors.

Types of Tolerance

It is widely agreed that there are three distinct types of tolerance involving different mechanisms. Regular use of a given drug results to some degree in **dispositional tolerance**, which is an increase in the metabolism rate of a drug so that users must consume greater quantities of the drug to maintain a certain level of it in their body.

Another type of tolerance is **functional tolerance**. Functional or pharmacodynamic tolerance means that the brain and other parts of the central nervous system become less sensitive to a drug's effects. The two types of functional tolerance are acute and protracted. **Acute tolerance** (sometimes called tachyphylaxis) is measured within the course of action of a single dose or the first few doses of a drug. When a person takes a dose of a drug, the amount of drug in the body—measured as the amount of drug in the blood, or the blood level—rises to some peak level. With some drugs, at any point when the blood level is rising to peak, users may experience greater drug effects than at that same point when the blood level is falling. For example, people show acute tolerance to alcohol. One effect of alcohol when consumed in moderate amounts is impairment of short-term memory, or memory for events that occurred, say, in the past 30 seconds. Because of acute tolerance to alcohol, we are more likely to see impairment in short-term memory when the blood level of alcohol is rising than when it is falling.

A second example of acute tolerance is with regard to stimulant drugs like cocaine. Cocaine is a short-acting drug, and when the highly pleasurable effects of an initial dose begin to wear off, users are prone to taking another dose. However, the second administration—even when the same amount is taken—generally produces much less of a pleasurable high due to rapidly developing acute tolerance.

dispositional tolerance
An increase in the rate of metabolizing a drug as a result of its regular use.

functional tolerance
Decreased behavioral effects of a drug as a result of its regular use.

acute tolerance
A type of functional tolerance that occurs within a course of action of a single drug dose.

protracted tolerance A type of functional tolerance that occurs over the course of two or more drug administrations.

Protracted tolerance pertains to the effects of a given dose of a drug when it is administered more regularly or chronically. Protracted tolerance means that the individual consumes greater amounts of a drug to achieve an effect that was once achieved with a lesser dose. So, in our example of alcohol and short-term memory, people who drink may show impairment in memory today after drinking six cans of beer, when they formerly showed the same degree of impairment after drinking only three beers.

behavioral tolerance Adjustment of behavior through experience in using a drug to compensate for its intoxicating effects.

The third type of tolerance involves a behavioral adjustment by the subject and is called **behavioral tolerance** (or learned tolerance). For example, individuals who have had considerable experience with the effects of alcohol on motor coordination may learn to compensate for their intoxication by walking slowly or with a lower center of gravity to keep from falling—even if they are quite drunk (for example, Vogel-Sprott, 1992). Other examples of learned or behavioral tolerance are discussed later.

cross-tolerance Tolerance to a drug or drugs never taken that results from protracted tolerance to another drug or drugs.

In addition to these three types of tolerance, there are other mechanisms to be introduced. For example, tolerance to one drug may extend to other closely related drugs—a phenomenon called **cross-tolerance**. People who have developed tolerance to one drug also will have tolerance to certain other drugs, even though they may never have taken those other drugs. A practical consequence of cross-tolerance commonly occurs in surgical treatment. People who are highly tolerant to drugs that depress the central nervous system, such as alcohol or the barbiturates, are a problem for anesthesiologists. Anesthetic drugs are used in surgery because of their depressant effects, so drugs like alcohol or the barbiturates show cross-tolerance to drugs used medically as anesthetics. As a result, it may be difficult to determine a safe yet therapeutically effective dose of anesthetic to administer to cross-tolerant patients.

Tolerance is an extremely complicated topic. For example, people may develop tolerance to some effects of a drug but not to others. The barbiturates present a complex case. Tolerance develops rapidly to the sleep-inducing and pleasantly intoxicating (e.g., euphoria) effects of these drugs, but tolerance does not develop as readily to their effects of impaired motor coordination and slowed reaction time. And tolerance to the anticonvulsant effect of the barbiturate phenobarbital does not seem to occur at all (Jacobs & Fehr, 1987). Another example is the amphetamine drugs. Tolerance to their appetite-suppressant and euphoric effects may develop rapidly, but the **psychosis**-like effects of amphetamines are not subject to tolerance. Similarly, one amphetamine drug, methylphenidate (Ritalin), is used to treat **attention deficit/ hyperactivity disorder** in children. Fortunately, tolerances do not develop to the **paradoxical** attention-focusing and calming effects that Ritalin has on these children. Finally, we have **reverse tolerance** (sensitization) to a drug, which is increased sensitivity to the effects of a drug with its repeated use. Reverse tolerance has been reported, for example, for marijuana and cocaine. Much less research has been done on drug sensitization than on drug tolerance.

psychosis A severe mental disorder whose symptoms include disorganized thinking and bizarre behavior.

attention deficit/ hyperactivity disorder A disorder with features such as a greater-than-normal amount of activity, restlessness, difficulty concentrating or sustaining attention, and impulsivity.

paradoxical Contrary to what is expected. A paradoxical drug effect is opposite in direction to what is expected based on the drug's chemical structure.

reverse tolerance Increased sensitivity to a drug with repeated use of it.

Explanations of Tolerance

Because tolerance is so important in psychopharmacology and is so fascinating, there has been no shortage of efforts to explain how tolerance to a drug develops. So far, no one theory has been able to account for all the nuances in tolerance that have been observed, but a few theories can account for portions of what has been discovered. These theories reflect current thinking that tolerance is multifaceted and involves both biological and learning processes.

Cell Adaptation Theory

One explanation for tolerance that has been around for more than 40 years is called the adaptation-**homeostasis** hypothesis (Cicero, 1980). This theory assumes that a drug acts on specific cells in the central nervous system (CNS). Because of the plasticity of the CNS, the cells become "adapted" to the presence of the drug with repeated exposure to it. The adaptation allows the cells to maintain normal functioning at a given drug dose. As a result, more drug is required to disrupt cell functioning. This required increase is called tolerance.

homeostasis
A state of equilibrium or balance. Systems at homeostasis are stable; when homeostasis is disrupted, the system operates to restore it.

Cell adaptation actually is a general notion that some kinds of changes occur in the cells of the CNS to account for the changes we call tolerance to drugs. The idea of cell adaptation is important because it seems that changes in a drug's effects as a result of its repeated use are due only in minor part to dispositional tolerance. Instead, protracted functional tolerance is more important, and the reduced sensitivity to a drug in the CNS seems to be caused by cellular changes there. Several hypotheses have been proposed for the specific changes that might explain tolerance at the cellular level. For example, chronic exposure to a drug that affects a particular neurotransmitter system results in a reduced synthesis of that transmitter. Because of reduced transmitter levels, more of the drug might be required to effect the same overall neurochemical actions. Alternatively, there is evidence that repeated exposure to drugs may reduce the number of receptor sites on neurons that the drug activates. This process is called *down-regulation* and could also explain the phenomenon of cellular tolerance. The specifics of those changes have not yet been determined (Kalant, 1996; Koob & Bloom, 1988).

Drug Compensatory Reactions and Learning

In the 1970s, scientists discovered that tolerance to drugs is learned, in part. To illustrate the observations that led to this conclusion, imagine that two people who are "theoretically equal in all ways" take a particular dose of a drug on 10 occasions. Person A takes the drug every time under the same conditions, whereas person B takes the drug under different conditions every time. For example, the room where B takes the drug may vary, or the color of the drug tablets may change. Then on the 11th occasion, tolerance for some effect of the drug at the specified dose is measured in A and B under the conditions in which A took the drug 10 previous times. Who would show greater tolerance? The cell adaptation hypothesis predicts equal tolerance for A and B. Yet numerous studies of humans and other animals show that A has the greater tolerance (Hinson, 1985).

To understand this idea, you have to know about compensatory reactions. When an event, like taking a drug, occurs to disrupt the body's homeostasis, then sometimes the body counteracts the disruption with a reflex-like response. In this case, the counterreaction is an effect opposite to the drug effect. So, for example, when you drink two cups of coffee, the caffeine is absorbed and acts to increase your heart rate. Simultaneously, your body begins to work to counteract this effect; that is, a compensatory reduction in heart rate begins. This mechanism of compensatory reactions means that when you take a drug, two major actions are biologically triggered: one is the drug effect, whatever it might be, and the other is homeostatic counterreaction.

One more aspect of compensatory reactions is that drugs are thought to become stronger with repeated use of a given dose of the drug. You can see that we have the makings of an explanation of tolerance here, one that two psychologists, Richard Solomon and John Corbit, made prominent in the 1970s, when they published their "opponent process" theory of motivation (Solomon & Corbit, 1974).

Learning enters into the final part of the explanation, which involves the phenomenon of classical conditioning.[1] The cues associated with drug taking, such as where it is taken, who is there, and what colors the pills are, are "conditioned stimuli" that become associated with drug actions and compensatory reactions. Over repeated pairings of drug taking and drug-taking cues, just presenting the drug-taking cues alone may elicit a drug compensatory reaction. For example, presenting drug-taking paraphernalia, such as a syringe and tourniquet, may elicit strong urges in IV heroin or cocaine users to consume their respective drugs. This urge to use is based on elicitation of biological reactions associated with drug deprivation. Therefore, drug compensatory reactions—one hypothesis of what underlies tolerance—seem to grow stronger with their repeated pairings with the same environment. They seem to be tied to the specific drug-taking context. As a result, the "sum" of the drug effect and countereffect that is observed when a person takes a drug depends on how often the same drug-taking conditions have occurred in the past. The higher the number of pairings, the larger the compensatory reaction and the smaller the observed drug effect. In our initial example, that is why person A showed more tolerance than B did: The drug-taking event never changed for A, so that conditioning or learning in that context was stronger than it was in B, who changed contexts every time.

In addition, because the stimuli paired with drugs come to elicit reactions opposite to those elicited by the drug, exposure to these stimuli in the absence of the drug may produce discomfort or craving in users. For example, people who are trying to quit cigarette smoking often report that the smell of tobacco produces cravings, and users of crack cocaine may react strongly to the sight of a crack pipe. Only when people have been exposed to these stimuli many times without the drug do these effects dissipate—a process called *extinction*.

Final Notes on Tolerance

Once tolerance to a drug effect has developed, it is not irreversible. A period of abstaining from a drug increases users' sensitivity to drug effects that they may have become highly tolerant to in the past. This, for example, has resulted in the deaths by overdose of some abusers of heroin who have resumed heroin use after a relatively long time of not using the drug. When use was resumed, the user failed to take into account the loss of tolerance that resulted from the long period of abstinence. In general, acute tolerance reverses in a short time, whereas protracted tolerance requires more extended abstinence to reverse. Learned or behavioral tolerance may not reverse at all unless special procedures such as extinction are used.

Another point about tolerance concerns its reacquisition. Often resumption of the use of a drug after a long period of abstinence from it results in the reacquisition of tolerance more quickly than it developed when first acquired (Kalant, LeBlanc, & Gibbins, 1971).

Our consideration of factors included under Steps 6 and 7 and their effects on the drug experience raises a final point: As we have mentioned before, factors from different "domains" (biological, social) may interact in affecting the drug experience. For example, the major advances in genetics that have been made in the last few decades have paved the way for increasing our understanding about genetically based differences in

[1]Classical conditioning is a type of learning in which, by repeated pairing, a second stimulus elicits a response similar to the response elicited without prior learning by another stimulus. For example, a puff of air (a type of stimulus) blown at the eye elicits an eye blink. If a buzzer, which normally does not elicit an eye blink, is repeatedly followed by an air puff directed at the eye, then at some point, presenting the buzzer alone will elicit an eye blink. We then say that classical conditioning has occurred: The buzzer now elicits a reaction that it did not before the repeated pairing with the puff of air.

CONTEMPORARY ISSUE BOX 5.1

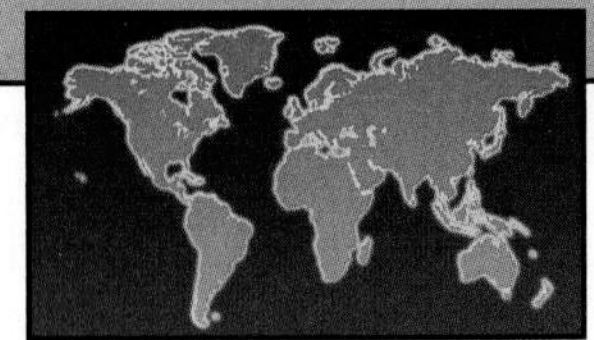

Tolerance and DUI Laws

There have been almost radical changes in the attitudes and behaviors of U.S. politicians and other citizens about the availability of alcohol and its legal and social consequences. For example, the legal drinking age in the United States is now 21 for all alcoholic beverages, compared to less than 20 years ago when many states had a legal drinking age of 18 or 19. Another major area of change is the set of laws about driving under the influence (DUI) of alcohol (and other drugs). At this writing, the blood alcohol level at which an individual is declared legally intoxicated is 0.08% in most states and the District of Columbia; one state does not specify a legal level of intoxication. Arrest and conviction for driving at this level of intoxication now bring far harsher penalties than before, especially for repeat offenders. The main reason behind this change is compelling: For years, it had been a consistent finding that about 50% of U.S. traffic fatalities are associated with alcohol use.

A blood alcohol level of 0.08% was chosen for several reasons, but a central one is that the driving skills of the average person are greatly impaired at that level. Now that you know something about tolerance to a drug and that alcohol is one of the drugs to which people develop a tolerance, what do you think of the "average driver" approach to the DUI law? Do you see any value in the argument that arrest should be based on behavioral (especially driving skills) impairment of the driver at a given blood alcohol level, whether it is above or below some specified level? What do you see as the health, social, and political consequences of this stance?

how individuals react to a given dose of a psychotherapeutic drug (Chapter 13). We referred to one genetically based difference in reactions to drugs earlier when we discussed initial sensitivity to a drug. But there also are genetically based differences that underlie differences among racial and ethnic subgroups around the world in reactions to a dose of a given psychotherapeutic medication. A major reason for these differences is inherited variations (mutations) of the genes responsible for the enzymes that metabolize drugs, and they occur both within subgroups of individuals and between racial and ethnic subgroups (Keh-Ming, Smith, & Ortiz, 2001). Genetically based differences such as these combine with other culturally based beliefs, attitudes, and expectancies about psychotherapeutic drugs, which of course overlap to a degree with racial and ethnic differences, to affect how individuals react to a given dose of psychotherapeutic medication. This same process may occur for other types of drugs as well.

The information presented so far in this chapter and in Chapter 4 completes our overview of the drug experience and the factors that affect it. We have shown that the drug experience in humans is complex because biological, psychological, and social/environmental factors influence it. This knowledge about the drug experience prepares us to address the fundamental topic of this text: the links between the drug experience and the behavior of drug use or, as commonly referred to by scientists, "drug-taking behavior." We now turn to some of the principles and methods of **behavioral pharmacology**, which is the specialty area of psychopharmacology that concentrates on drug use as a learned behavior.

behavioral pharmacology
The specialty area of psychopharmacology that concentrates on drug use as a learned behavior.

Behavioral Pharmacology

The premise of behavioral pharmacology is that drug use is a learned behavior governed by the same principles as any other learned behavior. We already saw in this chapter how a learning process called classical conditioning may influence some aspects of drug use, so we do not discuss that further. Instead, in this section, we emphasize drug use as an "operant" or voluntary behavior.

Reinforcement and Punishment

The basic principle of operant learning is that behavior is controlled by its consequences: reinforcement and punishment. A **reinforcer** is a consequence of a behavior that increases the likelihood that it will occur in the future. For example, if studying for an exam is followed by getting an "A" on it, then studying is more likely to occur when it is time for the next exam. If a person who has not eaten for 12 hours goes to the refrigerator and finds food, then at the next occasion of hunger, going to the refrigerator is a more likely event. In these two examples, getting an "A" and finding food are reinforcers.

reinforcer A consequence of a behavior that increases its future likelihood.

"Consider the ordinary lab-rat, once taught that pressing a lever will give him a rat-sized hit of crack. . . . This rat, I can identify with. Until recently he could, I fancy, identify with me. But Facebook is an addiction ole Ratty would look on with pity and contempt."

Sam Leith

When receipt of something, such as an "A" or food, results in an increase in the likelihood of the behavior it followed, it is called positive reinforcement. Another concept is negative reinforcement: The likelihood of a behavior increases if it results in avoidance of or escape from something. In this case, the reinforcer is avoidance of or escape from something, in contrast to receipt of something in positive reinforcement. Common examples of negative reinforcement are turning on the air conditioner to escape the heat of a summer day, slamming on the brake of your car to avoid an accident, and changing the subject of a conversation to escape an unpleasant topic.

A **punisher**, on the other hand, is a consequence of a behavior that suppresses or decreases its future likelihood. We touch a hot stove only once because of the consequence that was transmitted to our fingertips. If inviting someone out for a date is followed by insults and rejection, the likelihood of trying again will probably decline.

punisher A consequence of a behavior that suppresses or decreases its future likelihood.

You may reasonably wonder what getting an "A," changing conversation topics, and burning your fingers have to do with drug use. If drug-taking behaviors are controlled by their consequences, as behavioral pharmacologists believe, then drug users must derive either positive or negative reinforcement from their behavior and experience relatively little punishment for it. Thus, the study of drugs as reinforcers has become an important research area. Behavioral pharmacologists often study drug access as consequences for behavior in what are called **self-administration studies**. As the name implies, a drug self-administration study involves testing whether research participants will "give themselves," or self-administer, a drug. Imagine that an animal—say, a rat—has no experience whatsoever in psychopharmacology experiments. The essential question is whether the rat can be trained to perform a simple behavior, like pressing a lever, if the lever press is followed by access to or infusion of some drug. If the rat meets the challenge of learning to press the lever, then the question becomes whether it will continue to press the lever to get the drug. Based on years of research, the answer to both questions is a resounding yes. And not just rats—the yes applies to monkeys, baboons, dogs, mice, and humans as other examples. An impressive array of drugs has been tested, including alcohol, marijuana, cocaine, opioids, PCP, barbiturates, benzodiazepines, amphetamines, and nicotine (Bickel, DeGrandpre, & Higgins, 1995; Bozarth, 1987; Mello & Griffiths, 1987; Young & Herling, 1986).

self-administration study A study that involves testing whether research participants will "give themselves" a drug.

"I think maybe it is time we stopped all the . . . nonsense about social milieus and how your daddy fell off a horse . . . and just say . . . what you mean, which is 'I got loaded because I love to do it.'"

Respondent cited in Le Dain Commission Interim Report (Brecher, 1972, p. 456)

These robust findings suggest that humans and other animals, under given environmental, biological, and psychological conditions, "prefer" the drug experience. They show this preference experimentally by voluntarily working to obtain the drug. As one research group put it: "[A]bused drugs are those that serve as positive reinforcers and thereby maintain drug-seeking behavior" (Henningfield, Lukas, & Bigelow, 1986, p. 75).

In our concern about human drug use, the temptation is strong to "get behind" the preference to find out its basis, to discover why the drug state is a preferred one under some circumstances. This question has been the topic of numerous studies. For example, we did an informal review of survey questionnaire items that have been used among adults (18 years and older) in the United States. We found almost 50 reasons for using alcohol! Some examples are to expand awareness and understanding, to celebrate something important, to relax, to make sex better, to overcome shyness, to help forget worries, and to increase courage and self-confidence. The same array of mood and behavior changes has been recorded for the "drugs of abuse" other than alcohol (Barrett, 1985).

It is important to insert a note of caution here. There is a high positive correlation, or association, between pleasant or desired drug effects and their reinforcing effects in humans (Griffiths & Woodson, 1988b). The correlation is not perfect, however. Therefore, asking people why they use a drug or what they like about it is only an indirect way of studying a drug's reinforcement value. Technically, the reinforcement efficacy of a drug is measured by its ability to maintain or increase the frequency of a behavior that precedes access to a drug.

Self-administration studies also are an important source of knowledge about drug use because they show that not all drugs have reinforcement value. Again, it seems that drugs that humans tend not to abuse, such as the psychiatric drugs (see Chapter 13) chlorpromazine and imipramine, are not self-administered by other animals. Another insight about drug abuse that can be derived from reinforcement principles is that reinforcers are most effective when they are presented immediately following a behavior. When a drug like crack is smoked or heroin is injected intravenously, the drug taking is reinforced almost instantly by the "rush" or flash, and it is thus not surprising that these methods of delivery lead to addiction more frequently.

Operant Principles and Drug Dependence

Principles of operant learning and drug self-administration may help us understand changes that take place in drug use over time. For example, the initial use of most drugs is not determined by drug reinforcement; rather, it is typically in response to the instructions or advice of peers, parents, or a physician. Only when an individual has actually taken the drug will the user experience the drug effects that may reinforce behavior. Thus, in regard to drugs with powerful reinforcing properties, the observation that an "ounce of prevention is worth a pound of cure" may be quite valid.

Although social factors may instigate initial drug use, continued use is more likely determined by the positive reinforcement effects noted previously. As drug use continues and increases in frequency, however, a change in motivation may occur. Consider that with chronic use, tolerance develops to the effects of many drugs, and withdrawal symptoms may occur when the drug wears off. Thus, because of tolerance, the effects users desire are more difficult to experience, but unless users take the drug, they feel withdrawal distress. Taking the drug now relieves the unpleasant withdrawal symptoms and thus produces negative reinforcement. The general principle is that incentives for use of some drugs, especially those associated with significant physical dependence, may come to include negative as well as positive reinforcement contingencies as initial use becomes more chronic (Crowley, 1981).

Negative reinforcement may also be important in the early use of some drugs. For example, people often say that they drink alcohol to escape unpleasant feelings of anxiety or depression. Because drugs such as alcohol can elevate mood rapidly, people who are prone to negative mood states may be more vulnerable to abuse.

So far we have shown that getting a drug as a consequence of behavior can be a powerful force in maintaining drug use. But we still have not addressed the negative drug effects we reviewed in Chapter 1 that have been extremely serious for some individuals

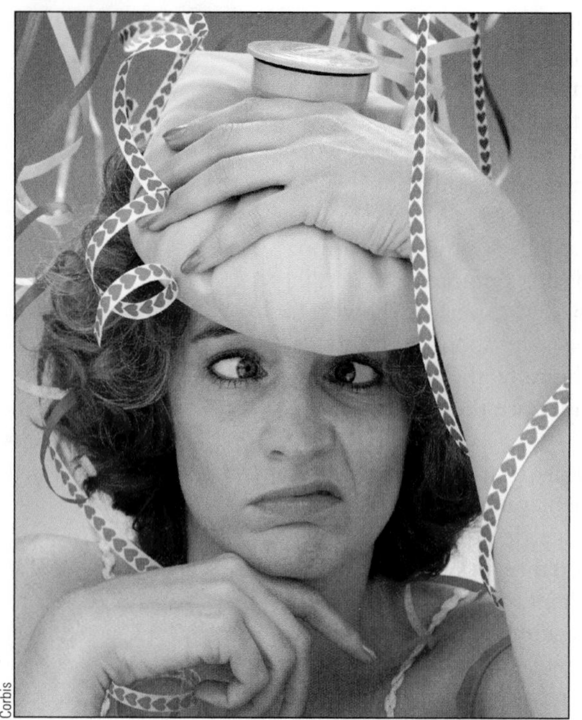
Corbis

Despite the possible consequences of a hangover from overindulgence in alcohol, its consumption remains popular.

and for society in general. Perhaps the major challenge for people who study addiction is to explain humans' continued use of drugs in the face of punishing consequences. At least part of the explanation may be that punishment, like reinforcement, is most effective when it is immediate.

In general, the impact of a consequence decreases the more removed it is from the target behavior. For example, the decision of whether to eat a piece of luscious chocolate cake is usually affected more powerfully by how the cake will taste if eaten now than by the possible weight gain or tooth decay later. Similarly, some negative consequences of drug use, like social, family, and health problems, do not tend to occur until some time, often years, after any given episode of drug use. Furthermore, such consequences are not certain. This contrasts sharply with the immediate, desirable effects of drugs of abuse. Immediate consequences have a lot more control over an individual's drug use patterns than do the distant, more negative consequences. Note that this idea of delay of reinforcement holds even if the delay is not very long. People have been known to put off considerations of a hangover tomorrow for the pleasures of drinking alcohol tonight, for example.

These behavioral principles have proved to be useful in developing treatment strategies for drug dependence. The idea is to reduce drug use by arranging punishment for drug use and reinforcement for abstinence (see Bickel & DeGrandpre, 1995; Higgins et al., 1991; Iguchi et al., 1997, for examples). We say more about these approaches to treatment in Chapter 15.

The drug self-administration procedure is perhaps the most obvious method in behavioral pharmacology through which research with animals can provide important information about human drug abuse. There are other important methods, however, and we now consider two of them: drug discrimination and the conflict paradigm.

Drug Discrimination

drug discrimination study A research procedure that primarily concerns the differentiation of drug effects.

Another research method in behavioral pharmacology is the **drug discrimination study**, which is important because it provides a way of asking nonhuman subjects about the subjective effects of drugs. Many species of animals can be trained to make a target response to achieve some reinforcer, such as food, based only on a drug state. For example, a rat may first learn to press a lever for food reinforcement. Then over multiple sessions, the rat is injected with either some drug—for example, an amphetamine—or a placebo saline solution (a solution containing salt but no drug) and placed in an experimental chamber that has two levers. Pressing one of the levers results in food when the animal has been injected with the amphetamine, and pressing the other lever is reinforced when the animal has been given the placebo. Pressing the "wrong" lever for a respective drug state (here, drug or placebo) results in no food. With only the drug state as a signal, the animal can learn what lever to press to receive food. This shows that the animal can learn to discriminate between drug and nondrug states. Naturally, this basic paradigm can be extended to test ability to discriminate among different doses of a drug and among different drugs.

Drug discrimination studies provide important knowledge about drug use because they can help us to explain the bases of perceived similarities and differences between internal changes produced by different drugs and by different doses of the same drug (part of what we have called the drug experience). Thus, an animal trained to discriminate amphetamine from saline will respond on the amphetamine lever when injected with the related stimulant cocaine but not when alcohol or other depressants are administered. Similarly, if LSD is the training drug, other hallucinogens will be "recognized." These techniques have allowed behavioral pharmacologists to classify experimental drugs according to their "subjective" effects even before they have been administered to people (Colpaert, 1987).

Conflict Paradigm

The last major research method in behavioral pharmacology that we present involves the **conflict paradigm**. The conflict paradigm is generated by creating a history of some behavior being followed by both reinforcement and punishment. So, to return to our previous example, a rat may be trained to press a lever to get food as a reinforcer. Then, after this learning occurs, the rat is also punished by pressing the lever—say, by administering electric shock if the lever is pressed during some programmed time period. You can see why this is called the conflict paradigm: The rat has a learning history of both reinforcement and punishment for the same behavior. This arrangement of consequences typically suppresses the behavior in question.

conflict paradigm
A research procedure that concerns the effects on a behavior of a drug that has a history of both reinforcement and punishment.

The conflict paradigm is important because it has been shown to be sensitive to drugs such as benzodiazepines that are in the family we call "antianxiety drugs." When an animal is injected with such drugs, the usual disruption in behavior seen by introducing the punishment component of the conflict does not occur when the animal has been given an antianxiety drug. Anticonflict effects in animals have been found for a range of drugs that have been shown to have the effect of reducing the perception of anxiety in humans (see Chapter 10).

These basics of behavioral psychopharmacology have advanced our knowledge about drug use and drug effects. A lot of what we say in the rest of this text about specific drugs or drug classes was discovered using behavioral pharmacology principles and methods. Another way those principles and methods have been extremely important is in the development of new drugs, which we review later in this chapter (Sanger, Willner, & Bergman, 2003). For example, self-administration studies with animals can tell us a lot about the abuse potential of a drug that is being developed for medical reasons, or whether prolonged use of a new drug has toxic consequences. Self-administration studies of the abuse potential of a drug also may be conducted with human participants. One excellent example is Troisi, Critchfield, and Griffiths's (1993) experiment, which helped to establish that BuSpar, an antianxiety drug, is less likely to be abused than the benzodiazepine drug lorazepam, which also is used to treat anxiety. This conclusion was based on sedative abusers' ratings of liking (or disliking) the drug as well as on the size of the dose they selected to take.

Knowledge of the principles and methods of behavioral pharmacology in animals is essential to your understanding of new drug development. Before we get to that, however, we address questions about generalizing from animal research and using human subjects in drug research.

Animal Models and Human Drug Use

Much has been learned about drug effects in humans from research on animals other than humans. Yet questions frequently arise about the relevance of findings about drugs based on nonhuman animals. A more technical way to ask this question is: How

generalizable Applicability of a research finding from one setting or group of research participants to others.

generalizable to humans are findings based on animals? The answer is that generalizability is remarkably good. In our discussion of drug self-administration studies, you saw the similarities among different animal species, including humans, in the reinforcement value of drugs. Other areas of comparable generalizability are the effects of drug dose, age, the presence of other drugs in the body, and environmental factors on drug use (Johanson & Uhlenhuth, 1978; Vuchinich & Tucker, 1988).

causal relationship A relationship between variables in which changes in a second variable are due directly to changes in a first variable.

Fortunately, what we learn about drugs in animal studies can be used to learn more about human drug use and effects. Such research has vastly increased our knowledge without unduly risking human health. Furthermore, a **causal relationship** between drugs and functioning in parts of the human body, like the brain, could never have been established with certainty without animal studies.

You should keep in mind that, in science, generalizability is always an "empirical question." We cannot safely assume that what we find in one experimental setting will automatically apply to the next. Rather, we do a second experiment, varying some essential factor about the individual or the setting, to see whether what was found in the first experiment applies to the second one also.

Human Behavioral Pharmacology

In studying the effects of a drug on human behavior, there are a number of issues to consider. Here we discuss two major issues, the ethics of conducting drug administration research with humans and the related matter of using placebo substances as part of such research.

Ethical Issues

Just as there are ethical issues in animal research, using humans as participants in drug research poses a number of ethical dilemmas. Many kinds of biomedical research hold the potential to harm subjects. Atrocities committed in the name of biomedical research in Nazi Germany led the postwar scientific community to adopt a set of ethical guidelines called the Nuremberg Code to govern scientific research. One basic principle of the code is that research with humans cannot be conducted without the subjects' responsible, voluntary, informed consent. That is, the subjects must agree to participate in the study and must give their consent without coercion after being told all the risks or potential problems related to the research.

Despite the principle of informed consent, ethical difficulties in human research remain. After all, when a new drug is developed, someone has to be the first person to take it. Even though federal law says that a drug must be tested extensively in animals before it is tried with people, some side effect not detected in the animal studies could still occur.

control group The reference or comparison group in an experiment. The control group does not receive the experimental manipulation or intervention whose effect is being tested.

placebo control A type of control originating in drug research. Placebo subjects have the same make up and are treated exactly like a group of subjects who receive a drug, except that placebo subjects receive a chemically inactive substance.

Placebo Controls

A second research, and, in some contexts, an ethical issue in human behavioral pharmacology is a methodological one: the need for placebo controls. A **control group** or control condition is a referent that scientists usually build into their experiments to tell whether the drug they are investigating is really causing an effect. In psychopharmacology, an important control condition is the **placebo control**. The idea that such a control is essential to determining the pharmacological part of a drug's effect arose long ago, when placebo effects were discovered.

Earlier in this chapter, we noted that drug effects might be influenced by subjects' histories with and beliefs and expectancies about drugs. These nonpharmacological effects of drug administration are often called *placebo effects* and may be difficult to disentangle from the pharmacological effects of drugs. When drugs are used as part of medical treatment, placebo effects seem to be most pronounced in administering drugs to treat symptoms that tend to fluctuate over time, such as pain and depression (Julien et al., 2008). Indeed, one study used brain imaging techniques to show that the administration of a placebo to subjects who expected to receive a painkiller drug may result in chemical changes in the CNS that follow those induced by actual painkillers (Zubieta et al., 2005). Therefore, in many experiments, the effects of administration of an actual chemical compound of interest can be specified only by comparing conditions in which people are told that they receive a drug, and then half actually get a chemically active substance and half do not. Sometimes all the experimental participants are told that they may or may not receive the real drug and then half really get the drug and half do not. In either case, neither the experimenter nor the subject knows whether the drug or placebo is administered to any one subject. This "double-blind" method is used so that biases from the experimenter or subject, according to their respective beliefs and expectancies about the drug or the experimental situation in general, are less likely to affect the results of the study. For example, a person who takes the drug may have specific expectancies about what effects it will have. Similarly, a person who administers the drug may have expectancies about its effects and accordingly may react to the person receiving the drug in a certain way. Both the subject's and the experimenter's expectancies may influence the effects of the drug that the subject experiences. Even professionals who are skeptical about whether a person's expectancies can affect the response to a medication agree that placebo controls are needed in drug research (Hrobjartsson & Gotzsche, 2001).

CONTEMPORARY ISSUE BOX 5.2

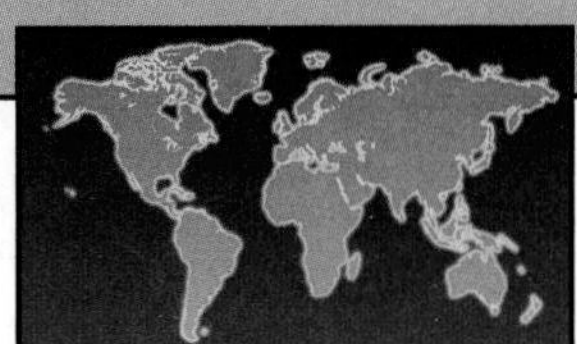

Advances in Discovering Drugs

The great success that has marked efforts to find new drugs in the 20th century has its roots in the earth. Soil and plants are sources of microbes that produce disease-fighting compounds. For example, penicillin was discovered in mold more than 60 years ago, and many painkillers have their sources in plants and soils.

Advances in technology have helped us to tap another of earth's resources—the sea—to find drugs. For example, animal and plant microbes taken from the sea in the Bahamas provide chemicals that seem to inhibit the growth of certain cancer cells. Bacteria taken from jellyfish in Florida produce compounds that kill some cancer cells and fight inflammation and swelling.

Scientists have found ways to discover drugs that do not have their source in nature, as developments in biochemistry make the synthesis of useful new drugs more promising than ever before. For instance, new knowledge of neurotransmitter and receptor chemistry has made it possible to use computers to design drugs tailored to bind to specified brain receptors, thus having highly selective biological activity.

Whether their roots are natural or synthesized, large groups of compounds traditionally have been screened to test their potential value as drugs. Advances in genetic engineering in the last few years (the human genome was mapped in its entirety in 2003) have allowed the definition of "large" (groups of compounds) to go from about 5,000 a year to billions (Fisher, 1992; Rowberg, 2001). The advance is not so much in synthesizing compounds to be screened as in the ability to generate and screen large numbers of them. The method essentially involves generating millions of peptides, which are chains of amino acids that constitute proteins. Then through successive stages of screening, it is discovered which peptides bond best with (and thus neutralize) disease-causing bacteria or viruses. Although these methods have been used only in the last few years, some drugs have been developed that are ready for human clinical trials. Examples are drug treatments for blood clots, high blood pressure, and asthma.

group design A type of experimental design in which groups (as compared to individual cases) of subjects are compared to establish experimental findings.

Using a placebo and control **group design** can get complicated, as you can imagine. And, when new drugs are being tested for their effectiveness in treating illnesses, many argue that it is unethical to have a placebo control group if there is an alternative drug that has demonstrated some effectiveness to use as a comparison. The notion here is that it is unethical to give subjects who are ill a compound that is thought to be ineffective (the placebo) if there is a compound that has some effectiveness compared to a placebo but that potentially may be less potent than an experimental drug. However, many view such a design as essential to learning how drugs affect people, and this does seem to be the case at least in the treatment of some disorders. For example, Walsh, Seidman, Sysko, and Gould (2002) reviewed all double-blind randomized clinical trials of the use of medications to treat major depression that were published in English from 1981 to 2000. They found that the average proportion of the participants in each study showing a "therapeutic response" to taking the medications in question was about 50%. However, the average for the placebo groups was about 30%. Moreover, the strength of both the drug and placebo response was greater the later in the 20-year period that a study was published. This suggests that it is indeed ethical practice to use placebo control groups in trials of drugs designed to treat depression, as one case, and reaffirms why a placebo control group is part of clinical trial research designs: It allows the experimenter to say with confidence what the chemical action of a drug has to do with the way a person reacts upon taking it. In this respect, it is reasoned that if the measured effect in the people who take the real drug is greater than the effect in the people who take the placebo, then the chemical action of the drug must be responsible for the effect.

You now have the foundation for understanding the last section of this chapter, which concerns how a new drug is developed according to guidelines established by the U.S. government. All of what we have discussed here and in Chapter 4 enters into drug development.

This text concerns mostly nonmedical drug use, yet this emphasis does not diminish the importance of drugs developed legally for medical reasons. First, many of these drugs are in fact used in a way that was not prescribed by a physician, as you saw in Chapter 1. Second, medical drug use is far more prevalent among adults than is nonmedical use. A final point is that legal drug development and distribution make up a major economic force in the United States. For these reasons, your knowledge about drugs and human behavior is not complete without understanding how legal drugs are developed.

New Drug Development

The "discovery" of new drugs generally occurs in one of three ways (Baldessarini, 1985): the rediscovery of folk usages of various naturally occurring products, the accidental observation of an unexpected drug effect, or the synthesizing of known or novel compounds. No matter how a drug's potential usefulness is discovered, however, the procedure for testing and marketing it is fairly standard. In the United States, the Food and Drug Administration (FDA) details these guidelines. The typical stages of the procedure are shown in Table 5.1.

Clinical Trials and FDA Approval

A "new" drug may be a novel molecular synthesis, a recombination of known ingredients, or a new use of an existing compound (Walters, 1992). In all these cases, the

TABLE 5.1 Stages in the Testing and Marketing of a Drug

1. Belief that a particular compound has clinical value
2. Animal studies
3. Experimental studies with healthy volunteers
4. Experimental studies with clinical patients, rigorously conducted
5. Broader clinical trials
6. Licensing and marketing approval
7. Aftermarketing evaluation of clinical use, particularly short-term and long-term effects

FDA has guidelines that must be met to make a "new drug application," which must be approved before a drug can be marketed. The extensive process of meeting the guidelines is outlined in Table 5.2.

As you can see in Table 5.2, the first step is, where relevant, synthesis and adequate chemical description of the compound and a series of preclinical or animal studies. The animal studies are done to establish the safety of the compound for use by humans. The first step in the process may take one to three years, and the animal research relies heavily on research designs such as drug self-administration and drug discrimination that we described earlier. Because of differences among animal species in their reactions to drugs, these initial studies must be done on at least two species. If the compound at this point is deemed to have therapeutic potential, then the drug developer applies to the FDA for designation of the new product as an Investigational New Drug (IND), which, if approved, allows the drug to be distributed for purposes of completing the three phases of clinical trials or studies in humans, as outlined in Table 5.2.

TABLE 5.2 Steps, According to FDA Guidelines, in the Development of a New Drug

Step	Duration
Initial synthesis and preclinical studies	1–3 years
↓	
Phase 1 clinical trials: to establish safety, up to 50 normal volunteers	
↓	
Phase 2 clinical trials: controlled studies in patients with a target disease, 50–200 patients	2–10 years
↓	
Phase 3 clinical trials: controlled and open studies of 1,000 or more patients monitored for drug effectiveness and for adverse reactions; data used for determining doses and labeling requirements	
↓	
FDA review/approval	1–2 years
↓	
Post-marketing testing	1–2 years

Source: Adapted from information in Rowberg (2001, p. 13) and Walters (1992, p. 334).

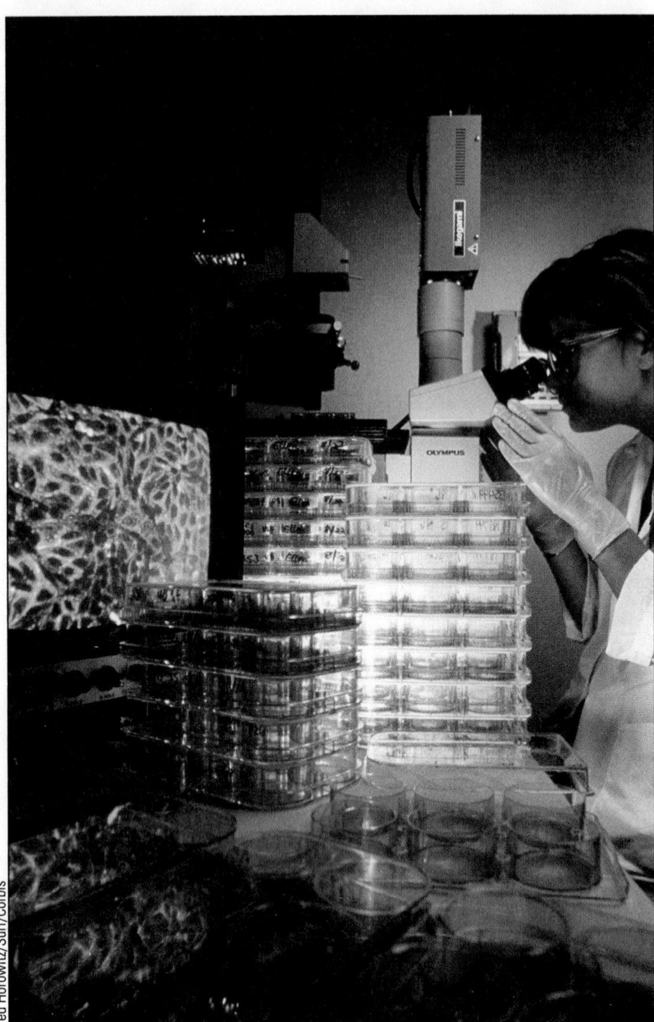
Ted Horowitz/Surf/Corbis

Methods of drug discovery have been aided substantially in recent years by advances in computer technology, biochemistry, and genetic engineering.

The three phases of clinical trials are straightforward, if not easily accomplished. Phase 1 involves normal (not ill) human volunteers and is completed to specify human reactions to the drug and to determine that it is safe for human use. In Phase 2, the efficacy of the drug in alleviating or curing a target disease is determined through controlled clinical trials in humans who are diagnosed as having the disease. Phase 3 expands Phase 2 by increasing the number of patients involved in clinical trials and also by evaluating the drug's effects in less controlled trials (Spiegel & Aebi, 1983). Throughout the Phase 1–3 trial process, drug developers are required to be in frequent contact with the FDA to monitor the development of the drug. Phases 1 through 3 may take 2 to 10 years (Nies, 2001; Tyrer, 1982a; Walters, 1992).

When Phase 1–3 clinical trials are completed, the developer files a New Drug Application with the FDA, which contains the data on the drug that have been collected so far. The FDA has up to six months to act on the application; if the drug is approved or determined to be safe and effective, then the developer may market the drug within the United States and may export the drug for sale outside the United States. Anything less than approval means more time must be spent to correct deficiencies or solve problems so that a new application for approval may be filed.

Distribution and Marketing

Monitoring is not over once the developer begins to distribute and market the new drug. Clinical researchers continue to evaluate the effectiveness of the drug and the appearance of any unforeseen side effects associated with its use. In recent years, controversy has surrounded the FDA with criticism that it does not allocate sufficient resources to identifying untoward drug side effects after a drug is approved for marketing and is used by millions of consumers (Harris, 2004; Harris, 2007).

chemical name The name given to a drug that represents its chemical structure.

brand name The commercial name given to a drug by its manufacturer.

generic name The general name given to a drug that is shorter (and easier for most people to say) than its chemical name.

Drugs are designated in different ways once they reach commercial status. First is the **chemical name** of the drug, which indicates the drug's structural formula and allows chemists to reproduce the drug's structure. The manufacturer of the drug also gives it a **brand name** or trademark. Most people would know this name because it is the commercial name for the drug that the manufacturer uses exclusively until its sole rights to market the drug expire. The brand name says nothing about the drug's chemical structure. Finally, a drug also is given a **generic name**, a general name that is shorter than its chemical name. Like its trade name, a drug's generic name tells nothing about its chemical structure.

As one example, consider the names of Valium (brand name): The generic name is diazepam, and its chemical name is 7-chloro-1, 3-dihydro-1-methyl-5-phenyl-2H-1, 4-benzodiazepin-2-one.

The U.S. pharmaceutical industry reported that, in 2003, it spent $25.3 billion on developing new drugs (Golan, 2005). You can guess part of the reason the costs of this critical research are so high from our summary of the drug development and approval process; in time alone, the sequence of steps averages about 15 years to market approval. The process also results in a lot more failure than success: For every drug that makes it to market approval, 5,000 to 10,000 drugs have been screened, 250 enter clinical testing, and 5 enter clinical trials.

Generic Drugs

No introduction to marketing and distributing new drugs is complete without mention of generic drugs. Generics have fueled heated debate. When a drug is approved, the source of its invention, usually a drug company, is granted sole rights to market the drug for 20 years after the filing date of the patent for the drug. After that, generic drug companies can sell their versions of the same compound as long as they use the generic rather than the brand name. Generic versions are not chemical copies of the respective brand name drugs, but the FDA officially designates the generics as equivalent in effect to the brand names. Generic drugs usually are sold at a price lower (an average of 50% lower) than that charged for the drug of the company that invented it. Therefore, not only can the widespread use of generic drugs considerably lower the costs of health care, but also, because generic drugs are less expensive, people are more likely to be compliant with their treatment if they can access generic drugs rather than be restricted to brand name drugs.

"Don't stop trials too early: Whatever the pressures are, keep going as long as possible. We must look to the longer term regarding benefit and harm."

Dr. Ian Weller, head of the British Concorde Research Team (*New York Times,* April 16, 1993, p. c3)

"Silence = Death"

Campaign banner to lobby the FDA to release experimental drugs to AIDS patients (1987)

Generic drug companies have made a significant impression in the drug market. For example, a July 1987 article in the *New York Times* noted that, between 1981 and 1986, generic drug sales tripled to $5.1 billion. This was 23% of the $21 billion-prescription drug market for 1986. In 2002, the National Center for Policy Analysis estimated that generic drugs accounted for 50% of the prescription drugs that are dispensed, and in 2007, they accounted for 60%. The sales of generic drugs in the United States are expected to exceed $25 billion in 2010 (Saul, 2007).

The drug companies that are awarded patents have not always appreciated the generic drug market. Their gripe is understandable, considering all the time, money, and energy they have spent in gaining new drug approval. And we did not even discuss compounds that fail to meet all the criteria for approval. Efforts put into testing such compounds are written off as losses. Brand-name drug companies did fight back by claiming that using generics may be unsafe for some patients. However, there is little evidence to support this claim, as shown in a recent review of drugs used to treat cardiovascular disease (Kesselheim et al., 2008). Such findings are not surprising, because the FDA requires that generic drugs meet the same standards of safety as innovator drugs meet. It is fair to say that the generics are probably here to stay. Consumers support their use (saving $8 billion to $10 billion each year at pharmacies by using them), as does the American Medical Association.

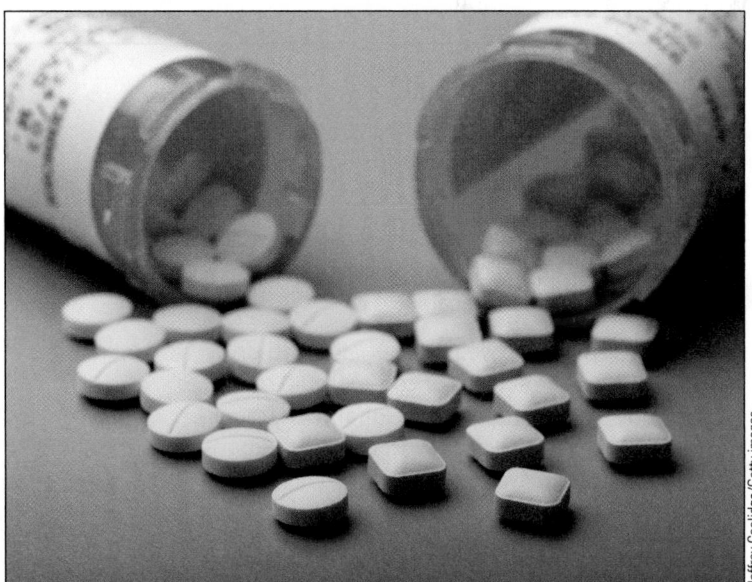

Jeffrey Coolidge/Getty images

Generic drugs have become a popular pharmacy item.

CONTEMPORARY ISSUE BOX 5.3

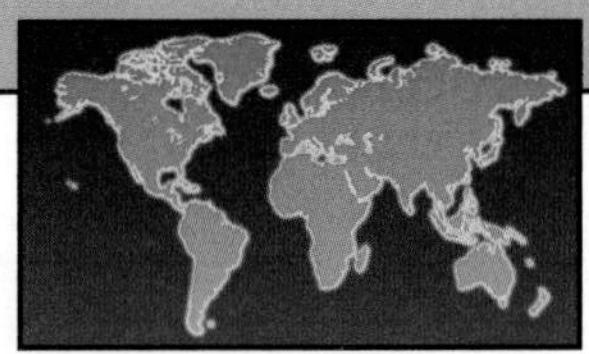

Awaiting Drug Approval

As we have seen, going from preliminary indications of a drug's usefulness to its final approval for prescription use is a long and rigorous process. The main reasons the process takes so long are to ensure the drug's effectiveness and to study possible side effects. Probably the best-known example in support of the FDA's exhaustive new drug approval process is the case of thalidomide. Its use by women in Europe as a sedative in early pregnancy in the 1960s (although banned in the United States by the FDA) resulted in damage to thousands of developing embryos. Nevertheless, the time needed to complete the FDA's approval process can seem interminable to the person who now suffers from a fatal disease that in a few years may be treatable with a new drug.

A case in point is the ongoing testing of potential drug treatments for AIDS. This syndrome, first identified in the early 1980s, grew in five years from being an isolated clinical oddity to near epidemic proportions. Moreover, there is only a short time between patients' initial medical treatment for AIDS symptoms and their death. This rapid course of AIDS created pressure on the FDA to shorten the drug approval process. In fact, in 1987, the FDA eased its regulations to expedite commercial use of the drug AZT, which then seemed to be a major and singular hope for slowing the advance of AIDS in some patients. That change has become a more general policy that allows less lengthy approval requirements for drugs that may be of help in fighting fatal diseases like AIDS.

This change was a victory for patient advocate groups, but a 1993 study conducted in England, Ireland, and France, called the Concorde study, shows the importance of scientists' concerns about the risks of shortening drug approval requirements. The Concorde study suggests that AZT may show benefits in slowing the progression of AIDS during the first several months but not in the longer term.

The results of the Concorde study suggest that the clinical trials process will continue to take a substantial period of time, although it was reduced by almost 1.5 years during the 1990s. Other parts of the drug approval process have also been reduced in recent years with little apparent harm. Legislation enacted during the late 1990s called the Prescription Drug User Fee Act and the FDA Modernization Act have reduced the average time of FDA approval to about 12.5 months in 1999. And advances in biotechnology and genomics may considerably reduce the time for the beginning part of the drug discovery/approval process, synthesis, and preclinical testing.

Decisions about drug approval requirements are extremely complex and are of interest to patients, scientists, clinicians, and drug companies. If you were a top FDA administrator, would you continue to relax drug approval requirements for quicker distribution of a drug that may help fight a fatal disease? In what part(s) of the approval process? Why?

Summary

- Step 6 of the drug experience concerns characteristics of the user, which may be classified as biological or psychological.
- The relationship between personality and drug use has been the subject of considerable research attention. Although some personality characteristics seem to be associated with the drug experience, there is no evidence for an "addictive personality."
- Step 7 of the drug experience concerns environmental factors, which range from government laws about alcohol and drug availability to the immediate drug-use setting.
- Tolerance is an extremely important concept in understanding human drug-use patterns. There are several different types of tolerance.
- Both biological and learning factors seem to be involved in the development of tolerance.
- Behavioral pharmacology provides the link between the drug experience and drug use.
- Drug use has been shown to follow the operant principles of reinforcement and punishment.
- An extremely important way to learn about drug use is self-administration studies.
- The effects of delay of consequences on behavior may be at least part of the explanation for

continued drug use by humans in the face of negative consequences.

- Two methods of learning about drug effects are drug discrimination and conflict paradigm studies.
- A lot of knowledge that we have today in psychopharmacology is the result of experiments with nonhuman animals, yet the question of what research on nonhuman animals says about the human drug experience is still debated.
- Ethical questions must be addressed carefully in the administration of both active and inactive (placebos) drugs to human research participants.
- New drugs become available through a process of drug discovery, development, marketing, and distribution.
- Once a drug is commercially available, it is given a chemical name, a brand name, and a generic name. Generic drugs have had a major impact on the prescription drug market in the United States.

Answers to "What Do You Think?"

1. Gender differences in the effects of drugs are due primarily to body weight differences.
   F *Although men tend to be heavier than women, drugs tend to have a greater effect on women than on men because men tend to have less body fat.*
2. Some individuals have an "addictive" personality that predisposes them to alcohol or drug-use disorders.
   F *The idea of an addictive personality is a popular one in some circles, but there is no scientific evidence for it.*
3. Expectancies about alcohol's effects may be a more powerful determinant of its effects than is the pharmacological action of alcohol.
   T *Alcohol expectancies, especially at lower doses of alcohol, are powerful determinants of behaviors and emotions that normally are socially proscribed.*
4. Theories about the effects of drugs on humans always have taken into account social and environmental factors.
   F *The importance of social and environmental factors in understanding the effects of drugs on humans has been generally recognized only in the last 30 years.*
5. Tolerance to a drug develops because of biological changes that occur as a result of using the drug.
   F *Important biological changes do seem to occur at the cellular level and they seem to explain tolerance in part. However, learning and environmental variables also seem related to demonstrations of tolerance.*
6. Tolerance to a drug may be evident within the same occasion of using it.
   T *For example, impairment in some behavior, like driving with a given concentration of alcohol in the blood, is greater when the blood alcohol level is rising than it is at that same concentration when the level is falling.*
7. People who have tolerance to alcohol will also demonstrate tolerance to barbiturates the first time they use them.
   T *These people are demonstrating cross-tolerance to the two drugs, which have similar action in the body.*
8. There is no relationship between the drugs that animals show preference for and the drugs that humans prefer.
   F *Self-administration studies show that the drugs that animals "take" are similar to the ones subject to human abuse. Conversely, the drugs that animals tend not to self-administer are less prone to abuse by humans.*
9. The effects of a drug on animals tell us little about how that drug will affect humans.
   F *There is remarkably good generalizability from how drugs affect animals to how they affect humans. Some examples are the effects of drug dose, age, and environmental factors on drug use.*
10. In general, drug researchers are not concerned with placebo effects when studying the actions of a drug.
    F *Subjects' expectancies and beliefs about a drug may influence what drug effects are experienced. Therefore, a "placebo control" group(s) is often included in drug experiments.*
11. Because new medications are needed to treat diseases like AIDS, government regulation of the process of drug development and marketing has been greatly simplified.
    F *Some of the regulations have been eased, resulting primarily in a potentially shorter time*

from drug discovery to distribution for public use. However, the process still is extensive and takes a considerable amount of time.

12. Folk uses of naturally occurring products are important sources for discovering new drugs.

T *Rediscovery of old folk medicines based on, for example, plants growing "wild," is an important source of creating new drugs.*

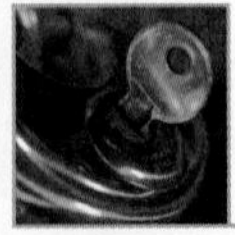

Key Terms

acute tolerance
addictive personality
attention deficit/hyperactivity disorder
behavioral pharmacology
behavioral tolerance
brand name
causal relationship
chemical name
conflict paradigm
control group
cross-tolerance
dispositional tolerance
drug discrimination study
drug expectancy
functional tolerance
generalizable
generic name
group design
homeostasis
initial sensitivity
paradoxical
placebo control
protracted tolerance
psychosis
punisher
reinforcer
reverse tolerance
self-administration study

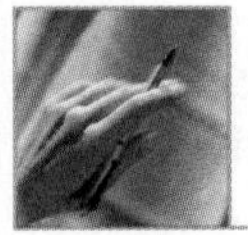

Essays/Thought Questions

1. What are some ethical factors to consider when using placebo controls in experiments? What are some of the ethical factors in the administration of experimental drugs to patients?
2. There remains considerable pressure on the FDA to shorten the drug approval process. What arguments support a speedier drug approval process? What argues against it?

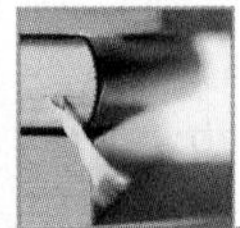

Suggested Readings

Hrobjartsson, A., & Gotzsche, P. C. (2001). Is the placebo powerless? An analysis of clinical trials comparing placebo with no treatment. *New England Journal of Medicine, 344,* 1594–1603.

MacAndrew, C., & Edgerton, R. B. (1969). *Drunken comportment.* Chicago: Aldine.

Rowberg, R. E. (2001). *Pharmaceutical research and development: A description and analysis of the process: A CRS report for Congress.* Washington, DC: Library of Congress.

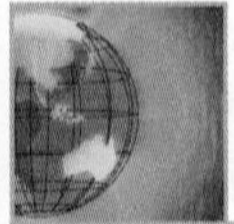

Web Resources

Visit the Book Companion Website at www.cengage.com/psychology/maisto to access study tools including a glossary, flashcards, and web quizzing. You will also find links to the following resources:

- The U.S. Department of Health and Human Services
- The U.S. Food and Drug Administration (FDA)

CHAPTER 6

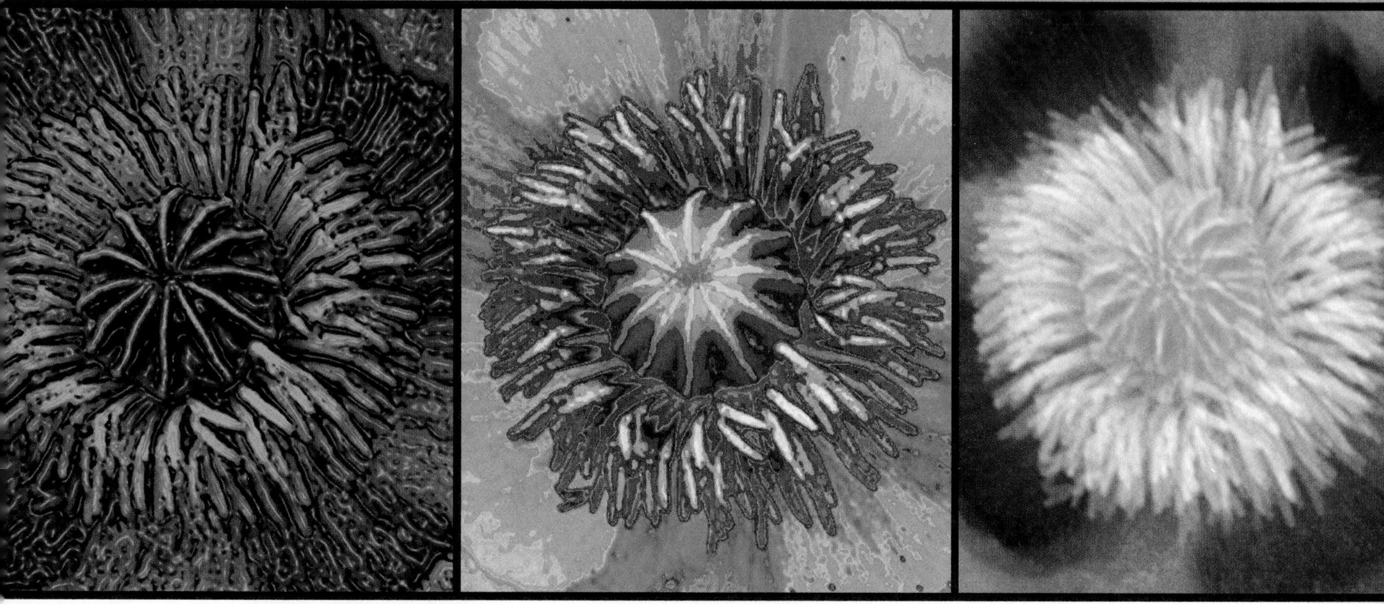

Cocaine, Amphetamines, and Related Stimulants

What Do You Think? True or False?

Answers are given at the end of the chapter.

___ 1. Cocaine is a synthetic drug developed during World War II.

___ 2. Cocaine abuse was epidemic in the United States in the 1880s.

___ 3. Stimulant drugs are often used to treat children who have attention deficit/hyperactivity disorder.

___ 4. Amphetamine effects are very similar to cocaine effects.

___ 5. Overdoses of cocaine and amphetamine may produce a psychotic state.

___ 6. Amphetamine has been used medically as a sleeping pill.

___ 7. Crack is a smokable form of amphetamine.

___ 8. The most common withdrawal symptom associated with cocaine is depression.

___ 9. Stimulant drugs enhance learning and intellectual performance.

___10. One difference between cocaine and the amphetamines is that cocaine has a longer duration of action.

___11. Severe physical withdrawal symptoms follow heavy cocaine use.

___12. Cocaine and amphetamines act by blocking the reuptake of endorphins.

Many drugs used for recreational as well as medical purposes are referred to as stimulants because they heighten mood, increase alertness, and decrease fatigue. We separate stimulants into two groups according to their legal and social status. Controlled stimulants such as cocaine, amphetamines, methylphenidate (Ritalin), and related compounds are treated in this chapter, and over-the-counter stimulants such as nicotine and caffeine are dealt with in Chapters 7 and 8, respectively. We first consider the history of stimulant use and discuss some of the effects of cocaine and the amphetamines as we review their history. Then we turn to a more detailed treatment of the pharmacology of these stimulants.

The Coca Leaf

Our story begins in the Andean regions of Bolivia, Ecuador, northern Argentina, and Peru, where a low shrub called the coca bush or coca tree (*Erythroxylum coca*) grows. From the leaves of this plant comes the powerful stimulant cocaine. The use of this drug is truly ancient. For centuries, the native inhabitants of this region of South America, including the Incas and their descendants, have engaged in the practice of chewing the coca leaf. Although no one knows when this practice began, archeological evidence suggests several thousand years ago. The coca leaf had important religious significance to the Inca people but was used for medicinal and work-related purposes as well. When the Spanish *conquistadores* encountered the Incas during the 16th century, they were at first disturbed by the religious use of coca, which was, of course, inconsistent with Catholicism (see Drugs and Culture Box 6.1). After conquering the Incas, the Spanish permitted and actually encouraged the use of coca because they believed it helped the Incas to work harder and longer. The Spanish ultimately came to control Inca access to the coca leaf by using it as a form of payment and levying taxes to be paid in coca leaves. The Spanish considered chewing coca a vice and neither used coca themselves nor encouraged other Europeans to use it (Kennedy, 1985; Streatfeild, 2001).

DRUGS AND CULTURE BOX 6.1

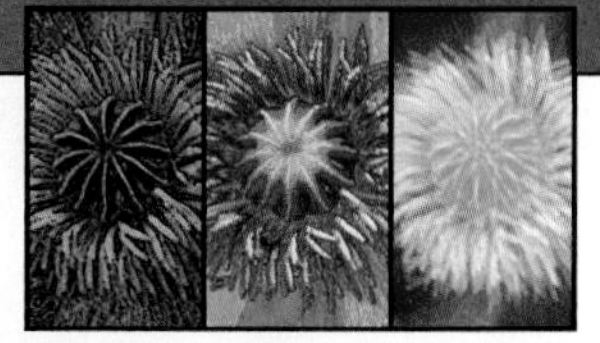

Cocaine and the Incas

The use of cocaine by humans dates back to prehistoric times. The Incas of the Andes regions of Bolivia, Ecuador, and Peru developed the practice of chewing the coca leaf more than 3,000 years ago. Archeological sites in Peru that date back to 1300 B.C. contain mummified bodies with shell vessels for coca and the powdered lime used even today to enhance absorption of cocaine from the leaf (Streatfeild, 2001). Coca was a sacred drug to the Incas. "Mama Coca" was viewed as possessing a goddesslike essence. One myth had it that coca had been a beautiful woman who was executed for adultery. From her remains, the divine coca plant grew, to be consumed only by royalty in her memory (Petersen, 1977).

Spanish *conquistadores* recounted tales of early coca use as in this quote from the journal of Pedro Cieza de Leon:

> In all parts of the Indies through which I have travelled, I have observed that the Indians take great delight in having herbs or roots in their mouths. . . . They go about with small coca leaves in their mouths, to which they apply a mixture, which they carry in a calabash, made from a certain earth-like lime. Throughout Peru the Indians carry this coca in their mouths, and from the morning until they lie down to sleep they never take it out. When I asked some of these Indians why they carried these leaves in their mouths . . . they replied that it prevents them from feeling hungry, and gives them great vigour and strength. I do believe that it does have some such effect although, perhaps, it is a custom only suited for people like these Indians. (Streatfeild, 2001, p. 39)

The Spanish missionaries took a dim view of coca because they saw it as idolatry and thus a barrier to conversion. Because of its social importance, however, the Spanish eventually took over coca production and distribution and used coca as a tool to control the conquered population.

Thus, until the 1800s, the coca plant was relatively unknown in Europe. Then European naturalists began to explore Peru and experiment with coca, and soon strange and often conflicting tales began to circulate about coca. Some, such as the German naturalist Edward Poeppig, viewed coca as deadly: "The practice of chewing the leaf is attendant with the most pernicious consequences, producing an intoxication like that of opium. As indulgence is repeated the appetite for it increases and the power of resistance diminishes until at last death relieves the miserable victim" (Kennedy, 1985, p. 55). Others, such as the Italian biologist Mantegazza who chewed coca while in Peru, were more positive: "I sneered at poor mortals condemned to live in this valley while I, carried on the wings of two coca leaves, went flying through the spaces of 77,438 worlds, each more splendid than the one before" (Mortimer, 1901, p. 137).

Neither of these quotes is a very accurate depiction of the effects of chewing the coca leaf. Of the two, however, apparently Mantegazza's was more compelling because nearly every historical reference attributes the rise of scientific interest in coca to his praise. This scientific interest led to the increased availability of the coca leaf in laboratories, and in the 1850s, European chemists were able to isolate the far more potent active agent in the leaf, which they called cocaine. The extraction of cocaine from the leaf led to a new era in the history of stimulant drug use. This is because of the greater potency of cocaine (a single coca leaf contains only a tiny amount of cocaine) and because cocaine seems to produce different and more intense effects when taken through intravenous injection or smoking methods of administration made possible only by the extraction of cocaine from the leaf. Presumably the more rapid delivery of large amounts of cocaine to the brain is responsible for the more intense actions of cocaine when it is injected.

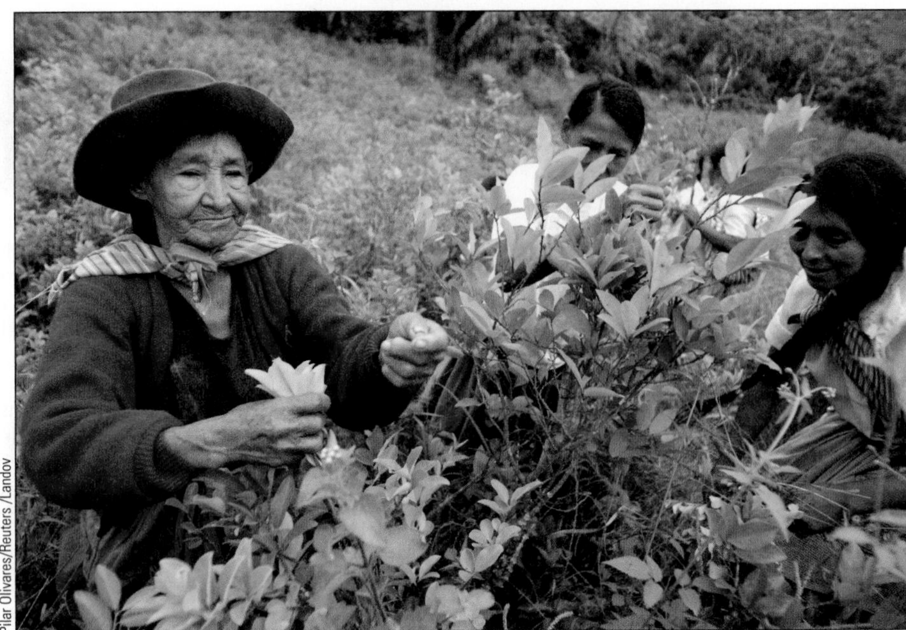
Pilar Olivares/Reuters /Landov

Andean woman harvests coca in Peru.

Early Use of Cocaine

The next chapter in the history of cocaine is fascinating because it involves an ambitious young physician working in Vienna who was looking for some medical breakthrough to make his mark. Though he is now best known for other contributions, Sigmund Freud was first recognized for his writings on cocaine. Freud obtained a sample of cocaine in 1884 and, after taking it a few times, felt he had come across a miracle drug. In his first major publication, "On Coca," he advocated cocaine as a local anesthetic and as a treatment for depression, indigestion, asthma, various neuroses, syphilis, morphine addiction, and alcoholism. Freud also thought cocaine was an aphrodisiac (Byck, 1974).

"Cocaine produces . . . exhilaration and lasting euphoria. . . ."
Freud on cocaine

Only one of these therapeutic uses has turned out to be valid, and that is the use of cocaine as a local anesthetic. When cocaine makes direct contact with peripheral neurons, it prevents neural firing, which has the effect of "numbing" the area. This action is unlike cocaine's effects on the central nervous system. Cocaine was the first local anesthetic and revolutionized surgery. Now, of course, related "-caine" drugs such as procaine and xylocaine are used more frequently, but because cocaine also constricts blood vessels, it is still used for surgery on areas such as the face, due to the fact that it reduces bleeding as well as pain.

Freud was mistaken in his early suggestions about cocaine, and he helped launch a major period of cocaine abuse. Ironically, an indication of what was to come was observed in one of Freud's friends, Ernst von Fleischl-Marxow. Fleischl-Marxow suffered from chronic pain and had become a morphine addict. Freud prescribed cocaine, and Fleischl-Marxow began to consume larger and larger doses of it. Although doing quite well at abstaining from morphine, Fleischl-Marxow eventually was consuming a gram of cocaine daily. Not only had he become the first European cocaine addict, but he also began to show bizarre symptoms that we now recognize as characteristics of cocaine overdose. These symptoms included paranoid delusions, which are often seen in paranoid schizophrenia, and a feeling of itching called the **formication syndrome**, which is described as something like insects or snakes crawling just under the skin. Today these symptoms are recognized as caused by cocaine overdose, but Fleischl-Marxow was the first reported to experience these effects.

formication syndrome Symptoms of itching and feeling as if insects were crawling under skin, caused by cocaine and amphetamine.

Surprised by the disastrous effects of cocaine on Fleischl-Marxow, Freud in his later writings on cocaine was not quite so enthusiastic, but the damage had been done. The cocaine epidemic of the '80s was on—the 1880s, that is! Not only was cocaine prescribed by physicians but it also was readily available in patent medicines that could be obtained without prescription, such as Mariani's Coca Wine, a top seller in Europe, and yes, Coca-Cola. Coca-Cola's early advertising touted it as containing the "tonic and nerve stimulant properties of the coca plant"—back when it *was* the real thing! Cocaine was popularized in music and literature as well. Author Sir Arthur Conan Doyle depicted the famous fictional detective Sherlock Holmes as using cocaine to give him energy and aid his powers of deductive reasoning. Robert Louis Stevenson apparently wrote the Jekyll and Hyde story while taking cocaine treatments for tuberculosis, and others who provided testimonials to the value of cocaine include Thomas Edison, Jules Verne, Emile Zola, Henrik Ibsen, Czar Nicholas of Russia, and President Ulysses Grant (Grinspoon & Bakalar, 1976). An advertisement from another coca product, Metcalf's Wine of Coca, again illustrates how cocaine became so popular:

> Public Speakers, Singers, and Actors have found wine of coca to be a valuable tonic to the vocal cords. Athletes, Pedestrians, and Base Ball Players have found by practical experience that a steady course of coca taken both before and after any trial of strength or endurance will impart energy to every movement, and prevent fatigue. Elderly people have found it a reliable aphrodisiac superior to any other drug. (Siegel, 1985, p. 206)

It is not hard to understand how cocaine became popular with this kind of publicity, and with so many people using cocaine, casualties began to emerge. By the end of the 19th century, many users had discovered firsthand the hazards of cocaine, and

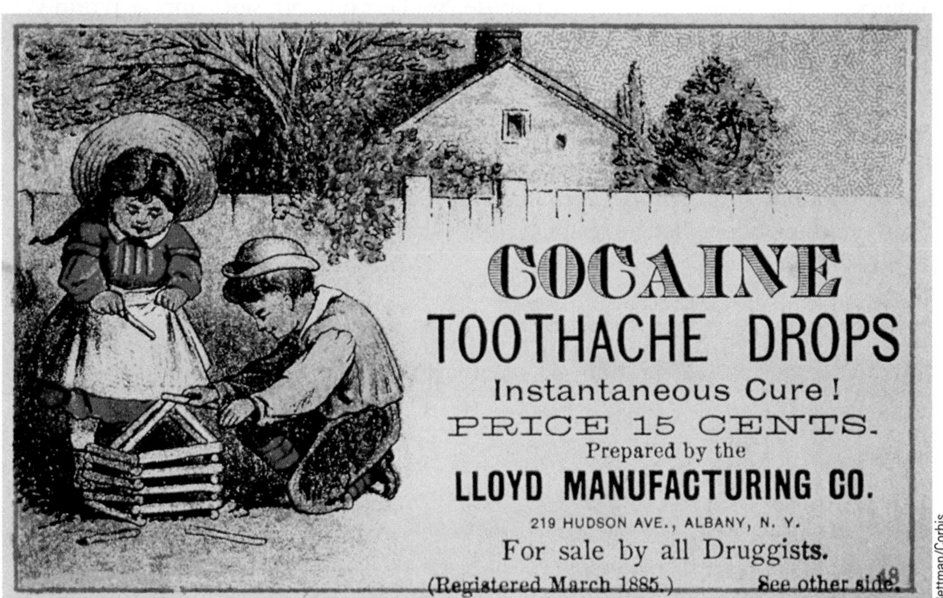

Bettman/Corbis

Cocaine was a popular ingredient in many remedies and tonics of the late 1800s, as shown in this advertisement for toothache drops.

with cocaine psychosis, overdose death, and severe dependence becoming major problems, popular sentiment turned against cocaine (Spillane, 2000).

One of the most influential works that changed ideas about cocaine was an article that described the case of Annie C. Meyers, who had been a successful businesswoman and a "well-balanced Christian woman" before becoming a "cocaine fiend." The depth of addiction to cocaine was well described by Meyers who, upon finally running out of money for cocaine, recounted: "I deliberately took a pair of shears and pried loose a tooth that was filled with gold. I then extracted the tooth, smashed it up, and the gold went to the nearest pawnshop (the blood streaming down my face and drenching my clothes) where I sold it for 80 cents" (Kennedy, 1985, p. 93).

Thus, beliefs and attitudes about cocaine continued to change. In addition to dramatic accounts of addiction to cocaine, reports of violent acts committed under the influence of the drug led to a dramatic swing of public opinion, culminating in the control of cocaine under the 1914 Harrison Narcotics Act. Although the Harrison Act was primarily designed to control opiates such as morphine and heroin, cocaine's inclusion as a dangerous drug was no accident.

The Amphetamines

Use of cocaine in the United States declined during the years following the Harrison Narcotics Act, but new stimulants soon entered the scene: the amphetamines. The amphetamines are a class of drugs first synthesized in the late 19th century that include amphetamine, dextroamphetamine, and methamphetamine (see Table 6.1). Although amphetamines had been available for research for many years, the first medical applications were developed in the 1920s. Amphetamines have been used as a treatment for cold and sinus symptoms (the original inhalers contained Benzedrine, an amphetamine), obesity, narcolepsy (a disease in which the patient uncontrollably falls asleep), and paradoxically, attention deficit/hyperactivity disorder. Amphetamines also have a high potential for abuse. Soldiers on both sides during World War II used these drugs for their stimulant properties. After the war, amphetamine abuse reached epidemic proportions in Japan, Sweden, and other parts of Europe, yet the drugs were not recognized as dangerous in the United States until the 1960s. Ironically, amphetamines became a major problem in the United States when physicians began to prescribe methamphetamine as a treatment for heroin addiction. Like Freud's cocaine treatment of morphine addiction, this treatment backfired, resulting in an explosion of amphetamine abuse, particularly on the West Coast during the early 1960s (Brecher, 1972).

TABLE 6.1 Controlled Stimulants

Generic Names	Brand Names	Slang Terms
Cocaine	—	coke, snow, freebase, base, crack
Amphetamine	Adderall, Benzedrine	bennies, white crosses
Dextroamphetamine	Dexedrine, Biphetamine	black beauties, cadillacs, dexies
Methamphetamine	Desoxyn	speed, crank, ice, crystal, Tina
Methylphenidate	Ritalin, Concerta	Vitamin R
Methcathinone	—	cat

The use of injected amphetamine resulted in a pattern of abuse reminiscent of the cocaine problems seen at the turn of the century and again today. Users experience a brief but intense "flash" or "rush" immediately after the drug is injected. The strongly pleasurable feeling produced following amphetamine or cocaine injection is often described as orgasmic in nature, but because it lasts only a few minutes, users are soon craving a return to the heights of pleasure even though the level of the drug in the body remains high. A series of injections often follows; users become more and more stimulated but have difficulty obtaining a rush as pleasurable as the first. Because both cocaine and amphetamines suppress appetite and prevent sleep, people may go for days without sleep, eating very little and administering dose after dose.

In the 1960s, people who engaged in this pattern of use came to be called "speed freaks." When speed freaks burst onto the drug scene, it became clear that amphetamine shares virtually all the effects of cocaine. For example, when dose levels of amphetamine get large enough, users develop formication symptoms (called "speed bugs" or "crank bugs" by users) and paranoid delusions. Thus, a psychosis is produced not only by cocaine; amphetamines can cause an almost identical phenomenon. Here is a description of a speed freak from the San Francisco street scene of the late 1960s:

> He is a very nice person, and extremely generous; however when he gets all jacked up and he is wired (stimulated with speed) . . . then he is in trouble. Because pretty quick he's got a shotgun . . . I've seen him out in front of . . . the freeway entrance herding the hitchhikers away because he's paranoid of them. At four o'clock in the afternoon with a full-length shotgun, he's screaming "move on, you can't stand there, move on." That's just the way he gets. (Brecher, 1972, p. 287)

So the paranoid psychosis produced by cocaine and amphetamine overdose is properly called **stimulant psychosis**. By the late 1960s, the word was out on the street—"Speed kills!" What was referred to in this slogan was not just death by overdose. Amphetamine overdose deaths did occur, but they were relatively rare. Far more common was the development of a paranoid state that often led to acts of violence. In addition, after a long binge of amphetamine abuse, users may crash (sleep for an extended period) and then awaken deeply depressed. The depression could last for days and is now recognized as a common withdrawal symptom after heavy use of either amphetamine or cocaine. The depression often leads users back to drugs to try to get "up" again, and the cycle is repeated. Eventually, users' physical and mental health deteriorates badly unless they can break out of the cycle.

stimulant psychosis
Paranoid delusions and disorientation resembling the symptoms of paranoid schizophrenia, caused by prolonged use or overdose of cocaine and/or amphetamine.

As the word spread about the hazards of amphetamine abuse, users tried to obtain other stimulants they thought might be safer. For example, a compound related to the amphetamines called phenmetrazine had a run of popularity in the 1970s, but soon it was recognized that it, too, produced all the adverse effects of the amphetamines. By the middle of that decade, a different trend was clear: A "new" stimulant drug was on the scene, an "organic" or "natural" drug—surely there could be nothing wrong with . . . cocaine?

Cocaine Epidemic II

It has been said that those who do not know history are condemned to repeat it, and that certainly seems to be true with cocaine. Why did cocaine reemerge as a stimulant of choice? One reason is that, in the early 1970s, cocaine was fairly difficult to obtain and was quite expensive. It became glamorized as the drug of movie stars and pro athletes (who were among the few who could afford to buy it), and thus acquired a reputation as the "champagne" of the stimulants. Most users during this period experimented with low doses taken intranasally and thus rarely encountered the problems associated with intravenous use. There were occasional exceptions: One of the first of many athletes to admit to a major cocaine problem was former Dallas Cowboy linebacker Hollywood Henderson, who acknowledged he had acquired a $1,000-a-day habit in 1978. But this type of cocaine casualty was relatively rare. Cocaine was believed to be a fairly innocuous drug. To give you a feeling of the times, Ashley (1975) concluded in a popular book that cocaine was "not an addictive, especially dangerous drug" (p. 186).

Unquestionably, the contemporary view is that cocaine is, in fact, a very dangerous drug. Today Ashley's comments seem naive because there have been many well-documented deaths from cocaine overdose and, through the media, we have witnessed the struggles of many famous personalities trying to recover from cocaine dependence. Several factors led to the increase in cocaine-related problems. One has been the increased availability of cheaper cocaine. This has led to changing patterns of use, as more people were able to regularly use the drug in high doses. Another critical factor was the practice of smoking freebase cocaine or crack. Although free-basing cocaine seemed to emerge in the late 1970s, **crack** burst upon the national scene in 1986.

crack
A freebase cocaine produced by mixing cocaine salt with baking soda and water. The solution is then heated, resulting in brittle sheets of cocaine that are "cracked" into small smokable chunks or "rocks."

The form in which cocaine is administered is an important determinant of abuse liability (see Table 6.2). Street cocaine, which takes the form of a white powder, is produced by combining a paste made from coca leaves with a hydrochloric acid solution to form a salt—cocaine hydrochloride. Because it is a salt, street cocaine is water-soluble and can be injected or taken intranasally (sniffed or snorted). Intranasal cocaine can produce intense effects, but because it causes constriction of blood vessels in the nose, absorption is slowed. By the way, it is this vasoconstriction that results in inflammation and tissue damage of the mucous membranes of the nose in chronic intranasal users. Overdose deaths, psychosis, and dependence are all possible consequences of intranasal cocaine but are less common than with injected cocaine. Because sniffing was the major method of administration on the street until the late 1980s, the hazards of cocaine abuse were underestimated.

Freebasing is the term used to describe the practice of smoking cocaine, but as a point of clarification, it should be noted that cocaine is not burned like tobacco but rather is heated until it vaporizes. When the vaporized cocaine is inhaled, it is absorbed rapidly and completely in lung tissue and produces an intensely pleasurable high of very short duration followed by a severe crash. However, cocaine is broken down at the high temperatures necessary to smoke it when it is in the salt form. To smoke cocaine, the hydrochloride salt must be separated from the cocaine base and this is where "freebase" and crack come in.

Freebase cocaine is made by mixing street cocaine with a highly flammable substance—ether. Many people have been badly burned by failing to handle the

TABLE 6.2 Types of Cocaine and Routes of Administration

Cocaine	Form	Method
Coca leaf	—	Oral
Coca paste (basuco)	Cocaine sulfate	Smokable
Street cocaine	Cocaine hydrochloride	Intranasal injection
Crack	Freebase cocaine	Smokable

ether properly. The late comedian Richard Pryor developed a popular routine in which he spoofed the severe burns he received in a freebase accident. Base cocaine can be produced more simply and safely by dissolving the cocaine salt in an alkaline solution (for example, baking soda). When the water in the solution is boiled off, what remains is a hard, rocklike substance called "crack" or "rock" cocaine. Crack has a low melting point and thus can be heated and the fumes inhaled while the potency of the cocaine is preserved. The name *crack* comes from the crackling sound made by the baking soda left in the compound when it is heated (Inciardi, 2002). Smoking crack results in rapid and concentrated delivery of cocaine to the brain, and the intense "rush" is so pleasurable that addicts actually prefer it to comparable doses of injected cocaine (Foltin & Fischman, 1993). The euphoria is short-lived, however, and within 10 to 20 minutes, users report a "crash" and begin to crave another hit.

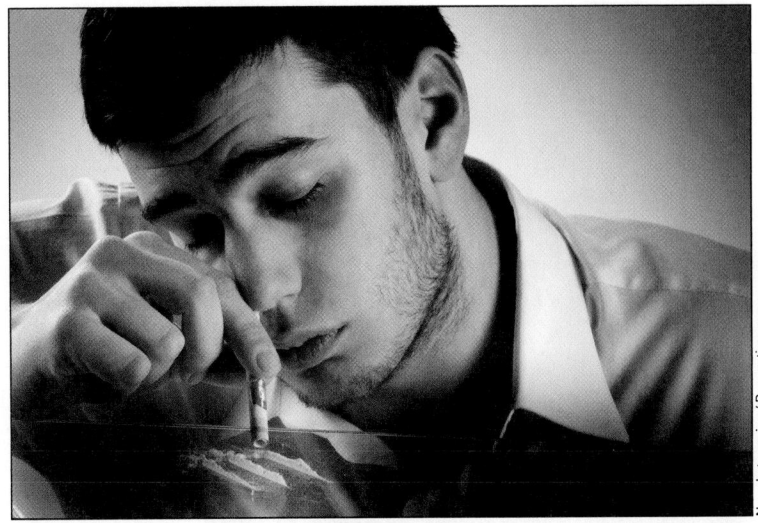

Newphotoservice / Dreamstime.com

Sniffing lines of cocaine through a rolled dollar bill.

Crack is cheaper and less dangerous to produce than other forms of freebase, so dealers became attracted to it. Also it is so potent that it can be sold in small chunks or rocks and so is relatively affordable. Because it produces such strong cravings and dependence, a large market for crack developed almost overnight. Although there is evidence of sporadic crack use in the 1970s, it came to the attention of the media in late 1985, and by early 1986, national media such as *Time, Newsweek,* and various television documentaries reported that crack use had emerged as a national crisis. By the late 1980s, millions of Americans had tried crack, and overdose deaths were increasing. Cocaine can kill, especially when smoked. Other cocaine overdose emergencies, such as paranoid reactions, also increased rapidly during this period. According to National Institute on Drug Abuse (NIDA) statistics, more than 80,000 cocaine-related emergency room visits occurred in 1990, up from 10,000 in 1985, and almost none in the early 1970s (NIDA, 1991). Dependence on cocaine, once viewed as a minor problem, came to be seen as one of the nation's major health problems with the introduction of crack. The National High School Senior Survey reported peak levels of use in 1986, when 4.1% of students reported using crack and 12.7% used powdered cocaine during the past year. By 1992, these figures had dropped to a low of 1.5% using crack and 3.1% using powdered cocaine during the year, and use has remained relatively stable since then. The 2008 survey (the most current data available at this writing) revealed 1.3% using crack and 2.6% using powdered cocaine during the past

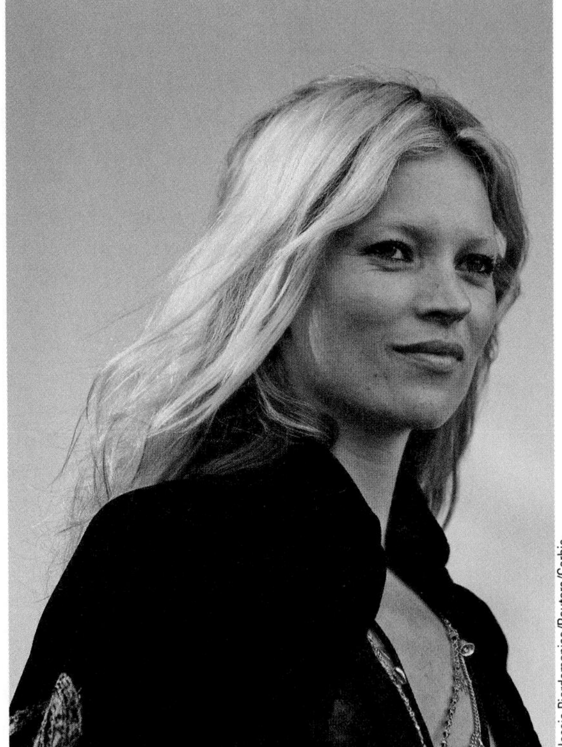

Alessia Pierdomenico/Reuters/Corbis

Supermodel Kate Moss lost many of her high-profile contracts when a video showing her snorting cocaine was released in 2005.

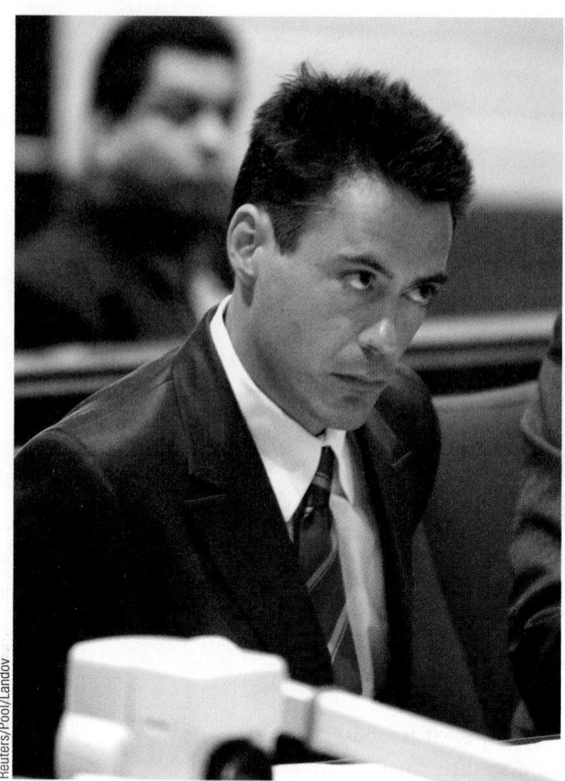
Reuters/Pool/Landov

Robert Downey Jr. has had a history of problems with cocaine. He is shown here in court on drug possession charges.

year (Johnston et al., 2009a). Contemporary use among adults is somewhat higher, with 6.4% of Americans between the ages of 18 and 25, and 3.6% of those between the ages of 26 and 34 reporting use of some cocaine during the past year in a recent national survey (SAMHSA, 2008). Medical problems associated with cocaine use continue to be quite high with over 548,608 cocaine-related emergency department visits in the most recent survey. In recent years, cocaine has accounted for more drug-related hospital emergency department visits than any other illegal drug (U.S. Department of Health and Human Services, 2006).

Despite the intense war on drugs in the United States and Latin America, it has proven difficult to prevent cocaine from reaching the United States. Although the United States has spent billions of dollars since 2000 on a plan for drug eradication in Latin America, availability of cocaine in the United States remains high, and the street price has remained relatively low (Lacey, 2009). Historically, the distribution of cocaine was controlled by large and well-organized criminal groups based in Colombia, and these Colombian cartels supplied most of the cocaine that reached the United States. As the United States and Colombian governments began to crack down on cocaine smuggling in the 1980s, the war on drugs became a literal war. For example, the city of Medellín, Colombia, was a quiet, conservative town; then the powerful Medellín Cartel emerged, and more than 2,000 murders were reported during the first six months of 1989 alone. Government officials, judges, and court employees were often targets of assassination, and the impact of this terror on the fabric of the city and perhaps the entire country has been enormous (Roldan, 1999; Streatfeild, 2001). Pablo Escobar, former head of the Medellín Cartel, was eventually killed in a gunfight with police in 1993, but the decline of the Medellín Cartel simply allowed another group, the Cali Cartel, to take control. During the early 1990s, the Cali Cartel is thought to have made billions of dollars in the cocaine trade annually and was rich enough that they once tried to lease their own satellite to avoid eavesdropping by the Central Intelligence Agency (CIA) and U.S. Drug Enforcement Administration (DEA). By the end of the decade, the Colombian National Police working with the U.S. DEA had arrested virtually all the Cali Cartel leaders. The cocaine trade did not vanish but simply became less centralized, with former Cali Cartel members moving their operations to multiple sites (Inciardi, 2002). Cooperative efforts to control cocaine production in Colombia did result in an 11% decline in production in that country, but this was offset by increased production in Peru and Bolivia (Efron, 2005). Most of the cocaine entering the United States comes through Latin America, so you might think that preventing access to U.S. borders would be straightforward. But land, air, and sea routes provide many possible entry points, and despite significant interdiction efforts, it continues to be difficult to control the amount of cocaine that reaches the United States.

"You want to know why I grow coca, right? The answer is: because I can live on it."

Colombian coca farmer (Streatfeild, 2001)

Once in the United States, cocaine distribution continues to contribute to crime and violence. Organized gangs generally control the cocaine market. These highly organized criminal elements pose a major threat to police and civilians alike. Unlike

DRUGS AND CULTURE BOX 6.2

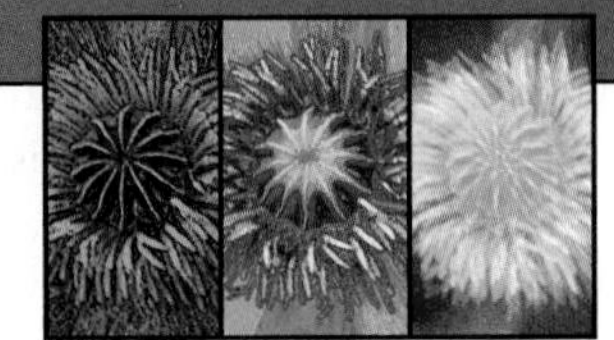

The Coca Leaf Today

The practice of chewing the coca leaf in the Andean countries of South America was never eliminated, despite the efforts of the early Spanish colonists. Use of coca remains very popular today in the mountainous regions of Argentina, Bolivia, Colombia, Ecuador, and Peru. Today, populations in these countries are all predominantly Catholic, so use of the coca leaf has lost its religious significance, but rather is primarily based on the desired stimulant effects. Chewing coca and drinking tea brewed from coca leaves are common daily activities in the region, and these practices are thought to stimulate alertness, reduce fatigue, and combat altitude sickness, among other health benefits. Despite pressure from the United States to eradicate coca production, limited cultivation of coca is legal in Bolivia, Colombia, and Peru, and coca leaves and coca teabags are sold legally at local markets throughout the region. Opposition to the U.S. coca eradication policies has become a nationalistic issue in several Latin American countries. As an example, Evo Morales was elected president of Bolivia in 2006, in part because of his pledge to decriminalize coca production. President Morales spoke to delegates at the Vienna meeting of the United Nations Commission on Narcotic Drugs in March 2009, to demand that coca be removed from the United Nation's list of prohibited drugs. He is not arguing for the legalization of cocaine powder or crack, but rather argues that the small amounts of cocaine absorbed by chewing coca are not harmful, a position that has some scientific support (Grinspoon & Bakalar, 1976). He dramatized his speech by holding up a coca leaf and chewing it after his presentation.

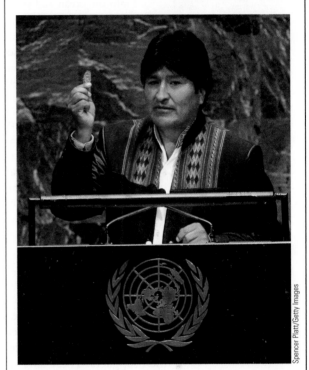

Spencer Platt/Getty Images

Bolivian President Evo Morales held up a coca leaf at a United Nations conference to dramatize his defense of the traditional use of coca in South America.

the traditional notion of the small-time drug dealer, modern drug criminals often possess high-tech weapons and sophisticated transportation systems. Many drive-by shootings and other acts of urban violence are linked to cocaine.

Cocaine, particularly crack cocaine, has also been extremely destructive to users. Because the allure of crack is so great, dependence on the drug leads many people to tragic levels of desperation and self-destruction. The "crack house"—a place where crack is sold and smoked—has become the contemporary den of iniquity, and the media are filled with stories of degradation. When addicts run out of money, sexual activities become the medium of exchange, and then the transmission of HIV is an additional risk factor. Studies of crack house activities chronicle examples of prostitution, murder, rape, child abuse, and other acts of violence (Inciardi, 2002). Publicity about the dangers of crack is impossible to avoid. So why are people still smoking crack?

Consider this seductive and sinister description from a cocaine smoker:

> Imagine you are on an island and offshore about a dozen yards is this orange-pink haze that is glowing and extremely enticing. So you walk out into that cold, dark water and you swim a ways to get near that glow and you're out on the edge of it and it feels so good and so warm, but it moves away a little. So you swim out into deeper water and this time you get even closer to the center and it is so incredibly seductive. But now it's moving a little faster out into the ocean and you swim harder trying to keep up and you're getting farther and farther away from shore. That's how with the first few tokes you feel pretty good and then with a deep toke you are near the center and it's so exhilarating but you come down and keep wanting more. Pretty soon you are way the hell out in the cold black ocean and you're faced with keeping up swimming harder toward that warm, wonderful, glowing haze just out of reach or turning back and swimming miles back to shore in that dark, cold water. (Kirsch, 1986, p. 49)

Concerns about the dangers of smoking crack cocaine led to the passage of the Anti-Drug Abuse Acts of 1986 and 1988, which specified penalties for sale (1986) and possession (1988) of crack. These laws have become highly controversial, and some discussion here is warranted. A conviction for selling large quantities (500 grams or more) of cocaine powder (the salt form) triggers a minimum sentence of five years in prison. The 1986 law created a five-year minimum sentence for selling only five grams of crack—100 times less than that needed for cocaine in the powder form. The 1988 law extended the five-year minimum penalty to those convicted only of *possession* of five grams of cocaine. Although these extreme penalties were designed to curb the very real crack problem in the United States, the laws were based in part on misunderstandings about the actual potency of crack and overstatements regarding its dangers. Today, inequities caused by these crack laws are increasingly seen as problematic. Basically, small-time crack dealers and users are often punished more severely than major, high-volume dealers of cocaine powder. Ironically, powder dealers may actually be the suppliers of cocaine for crack users, thus crack users are hit harder than their suppliers! These laws also disproportionately affect African Americans, as blacks represent more than 80% of crack prosecutions. Although these laws remain in effect at this writing, there is reason to think change is coming, as the Obama administration recently announced a Justice Department review of the policy. In the words of Attorney General Eric Holder: "This administration firmly believes that the disparity in crack- and powder-cocaine sentences is unwarranted, creates a perception of unfairness, and must be eliminated" (Cose, 2009, p. 25).

The Return of Meth

Although the United States was coming to grips with the dangers of cocaine during the 1980s, a "new" stimulant drug began to appear on the street called "ice," "crystal," "crank," or "meth." Of course, this was really nothing new. The drug is methamphetamine, and we reviewed its devastating impact on users in the 1970s earlier in this chapter. Now the "speed freak" phenomenon is back. In the early 1990s, methamphetamine (meth) reappeared on the West Coast and Hawaii, and it has steadily spread east since then. Illegal methamphetamine laboratories began to spring up with great frequency in the Midwest in the early 2000s, and by 2005, it began to reach the East Coast as well. Some describe methamphetamine use as reaching epidemic proportions across the United States, but use today is relatively stable and still remains most concentrated in the West and Midwestern regions of the country

(Owen, 2007). Figure 6.1 shows the distribution of the methamphetamine abuse problems by presenting methamphetamine treatment admissions as a percentage of total drug admissions (excluding primary alcohol admissions) in 2008 (Community Epidemiology Work Group, 2009). Clearly, meth problems are most prevalent in Hawaii and on the West Coast, but note that high percentages were also seen in parts of the Midwest and South as well—particularly in Texas, Minneapolis, and Atlanta. Percentages were uniformly low in Eastern cities. Another indication of meth activity is shown in Table 6.3, which lists the number of meth labs detected and/or seized in selected states between 2004 and 2008. Meth labs were much more common in the Western states in 2004, but the numbers declined by 2008. In contrast, meth lab activity went up dramatically in the Midwest over the four-year period. In the Eastern states, activity also went up but remains at a relatively low level (U.S. Drug Enforcement Agency, 2009).

Some other aspects of the epidemiology of meth use are of interest. In the 1980s and 1990s, meth was known as a "biker" drug, and it was associated with blue-collar white males. Today, meth is often referred to as a "club" drug, and its use has become more cosmopolitan. Methamphetamine use is now more common among women and nonwhite populations and is very prevalent among gay and bisexual men (Halkitis, 2009). However, the High School Senior Survey shows relatively low and declining levels of meth use, with a peak of 4.1% in 1999 dropping to 1.3% in the Class of 2008 (Johnston et al., 2009a).

Although overall levels of meth use have declined in recent years, the drug continues to have a significant social impact. As noted in Chapter 2, the 1996 Comprehensive Methamphetamine Control Act was passed in the early stages of the problem to increase penalties for meth manufacture and trafficking. At that time, meth trafficking appears to have been controlled by organized criminal groups primarily located in California and Mexico, and although these large-scale operations may have been

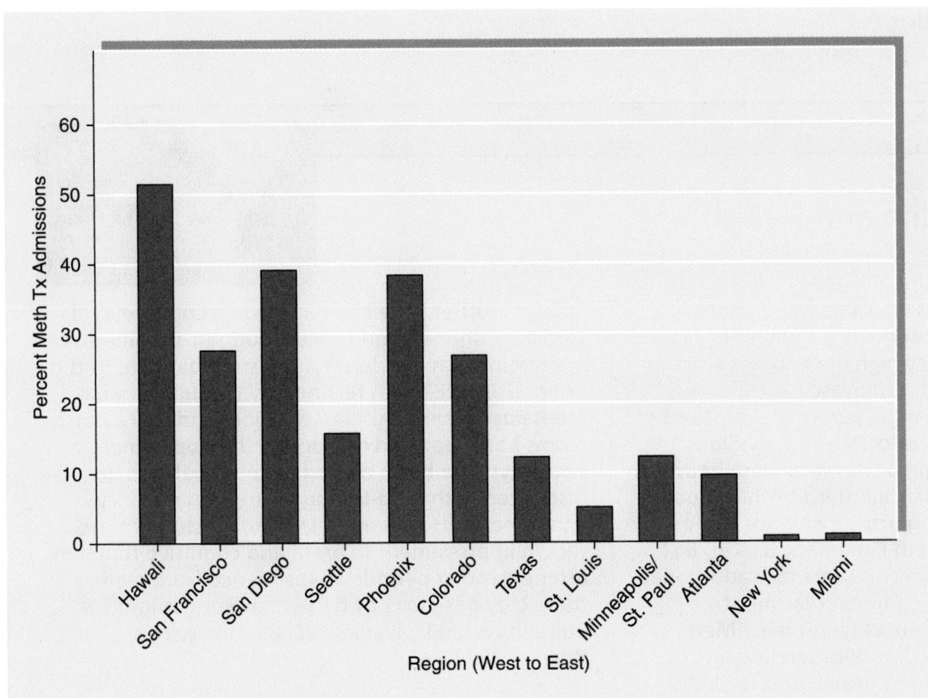

FIGURE 6.1
Primary methamphetamine treatment admissions as a percentage of total admissions (excluding alcohol admissions) across regions of the United States (Community Epidemiology Work Group, 2009)

TABLE 6.3 Number of Meth Lab Seizures in Selected States

State	2004	2008
California	2,198	346
Washington	94	137
Minnesota	123	21
Missouri	889	1,471
Illinois	363	324
Tennessee	249	553
Florida	15	125
Virginia	1	19
New York	2	9

"Meth was a call to action. . . . I felt ultrasharp. Edgy and exhilarated. Ready to roll. Equal to any task. . . . Give me enough meth and I was ready to conquer the world."

F. Owen (2007, p. 3), on meth

affected by the legislation, meth production then shifted to small "kitchen" labs, which have been much more difficult to curb (Cunningham & Liu, 2005). It does not require much space or sophisticated equipment to produce meth, and a meth lab can be set up easily in a garage, shed, or trailer. As these "kitchen" meth labs proliferated around the country, new problems emerged: The products they use pose a significant public health problem because of risk of explosion and because they produce toxic waste. Many of the chemicals used to produce meth are highly flammable, and the process also requires that the ingredients be heated with a burner; therefore, a significant risk of explosion and fire is present. Several of the chemicals used to make meth are toxic, as are some of the by-products that can cause significant health hazards wherever they are dumped; thus, meth labs represent a biohazard not only to those making the drug but to nearby residents as well (Halkitis, 2009). Meth users are also at risk for a number of health complications that we review in Contemporary Issue Box 6.3.

CONTEMPORARY ISSUE BOX 6.3

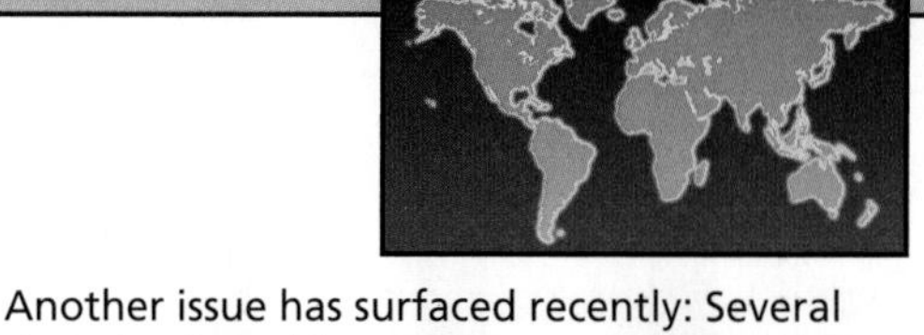

Methamphetamine and Health

In addition to the hazards associated with meth production, heavy meth users risk a number of health problems. Exposure to very high doses poses a risk of seizures, convulsions, and cardiovascular collapse. Overdose can also produce the paranoid symptoms of stimulant psychosis often associated with violent behavior. A study of young adults who were heavy meth users found that over one-third of the respondents reported committing acts of violence while under the influence of meth (Sommers, Baskin, & Baskin-Sommers, 2006). Chronic users face additional problems. Depression is a common feature of methamphetamine withdrawal syndrome. "Meth mouth," characterized by deterioration and loss of teeth, is also common among heavy users (Halkitis, 2009). Another issue has surfaced recently: Several studies in animals and humans suggest that methamphetamine may produce long-lasting damage to the brain. Using PET scan technology to study chronic methamphetamine users, two independent research teams have reported damage in the dopaminergic pathways. The brain damage may sometimes be associated with long-lasting motor and memory impairments. However, at least some studies have shown improvement in brain and cognitive function after extended periods of abstinence from meth, so these changes may not be permanent (Caligiuri & Buitenhuys, 2005; Iversen, 2008; Volkow et al., 2001; Yuan et al., 2006).

Most meth labs use pseudoephedrine (or ephedrine) as a key chemical component. Pseudoephedrine is used in a wide variety of over-the-counter cold formulations (see Chapter 14) and, until recently, was easily obtained. In an effort to shut down "kitchen" meth labs, the federal Combat Methamphetamine Epidemic Act went into effect in 2006. This act now regulates sales of any products containing pseudoephedrine and ephedrine. Sales are restricted to pharmacies, and although no prescription is required, the drugs must be kept behind the counter and pharmacists are required to record each purchase and purchaser. The amount that any individual may purchase is restricted to relatively low levels. There are indications that this act has reduced meth production. However, when meth became more difficult to produce in the United States, drug trafficking organizations in Mexico returned to the field, and it is now estimated that as much as 65% of meth consumed in the United States is produced in Mexican laboratories and smuggled across the border (Owen, 2007). This is a good illustration of the complexity of controlling drug availability when a strong demand exists for the drug.

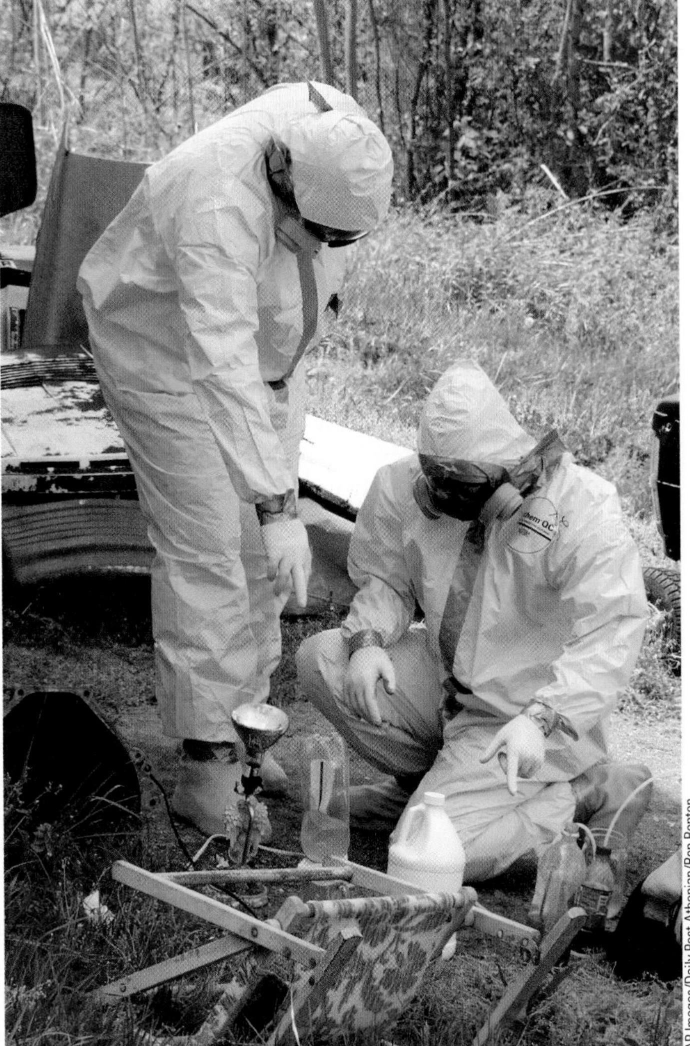
AP Images/Daily Post Athenian/Ben Benton

Law enforcement officers clean up hazardous waste from a meth lab in rural Tennessee.

Pharmacokinetics of Stimulants

As noted, stimulant drugs may be administered and absorbed in a variety of ways, and their intensity and duration of action vary accordingly. Cocaine, amphetamines, and amphetamine-like stimulants (e.g., methylphenidate) are readily absorbed after oral administration, but the onset of drug action is slower and the peak effect somewhat less than with other methods. Both cocaine and the amphetamines are commonly administered intranasally, and the absorption properties are similar to those associated with oral administration (Iversen et al., 2009). In contrast to oral or intranasal routes, which require 10 to 15 minutes for drug action to begin, intravenous injection of stimulants results in intense effects within 30 seconds. When crack cocaine and crystal methamphetamine are smoked in the form of crack or freebase, the onset of action is even faster (Jones, 1987a).

In general, the effects of the drugs considered in this chapter are quite similar. One important difference between cocaine and the amphetamines is their duration of action. Cocaine is metabolized rapidly, with most of its effects dissipating 20 to 80 minutes after administration (Newton et al. 2005). Cocaine or its metabolites (chemicals produced when the drug is broken down in the body) are detectible in human urine for two to three days after administration (Hawks & Chiang, 1986). Amphetamines are much longer acting, with effects that persist 4 to 12 hours (Newton et al., 2005), and they or their metabolites are also detectible in urine for two to three days (Hawks & Chiang, 1986).

". . . it's the best feeling you ever had. It's like your mind is running 100 miles an hour, but your feet aren't moving."

Meth user describing the effects of "slamming" (injecting) methamphetamine (Jefferson, 2005)

Mechanism of Stimulant Action

As noted in Chapter 3, stimulant drugs such as cocaine and the amphetamines are thought to affect the brain primarily through complex actions on monoamine neurotransmitters: dopamine, norepinephrine, and serotonin. For example, both cocaine and the amphetamines block reuptake of dopamine, norepinephrine, and serotonin. In addition, the amphetamines and methylphenidate also increase the release of dopamine and norepinephrine (Iversen et al., 2009). Thus, the initial effect of stimulants is to produce a storm of activity in neural pathways that are sensitive to the monoamine transmitters. Because of this increased activity, however, and particularly because reuptake is blocked so that enzymes break down the neurotransmitters, the long-term effects of stimulant use involve depletion of monoamines. If you remember that low levels of monoamines are linked to clinical depression (see Chapter 3), then you have the basis for one theory of why the aftereffects of heavy cocaine and amphetamine use involve depression (Dackis & Gold, 1985). To explain this hypothesis, we must turn briefly to data from the animal laboratory.

It has been known for a long time that animals will self-administer cocaine and amphetamines. Rats and monkeys given a choice between responses that produce cocaine and other rewards will choose cocaine over other drugs and sometimes even over food (Bozarth & Wise, 1985). The powerful reinforcing properties of cocaine and amphetamines are thought to stem from their action on dopamine-containing neurons in the mesolimbic dopaminergic pathway (Koob & LeMoal, 2006). As you may recall from Chapter 3, this brain region is thought to mediate reward, and thus use of these stimulants has been described as a chemical shortcut to the reward systems of the brain. Because a depletion of dopamine (along with other transmitters important in depression) may occur in the long run, however, users may then find that their ability to experience normal pleasure is diminished. The feeling of depression and lack of joy is so common during cocaine withdrawal that it is known as the "cocaine blues."

Figure 6.2 illustrates the relationship between mood and cocaine use for moderate and heavy use. The peak at the left shows the mood elevation that occurs upon cocaine administration; the valley at right depicts the consequent depression. The depression of mood is greater with heavy use. Note that these general observations seem to hold for the dose in a single session and longer-term use. However, the depressive abstinence syndrome is thought to be stronger and last longer in those who have been abusing the drug for an extended period. The function for amphetamines is of similar shape, but is more extended because of their longer duration of action. Of considerable concern is that some alterations in the monoamine systems after chronic stimulant use may be long-term or even permanent (Koob & Le Moal, 2006).

Acute Effects at Low and Moderate Doses

Physiological Effects

Stimulant drugs produce physiological effects that are observable outside the brain. We discuss the effects of cocaine and amphetamines together because, for all practical purposes, their measurable effects are identical. Although users often claim to notice subjective differences between stimulants, even experienced stimulant users under controlled laboratory conditions cannot discriminate among the effects of cocaine, amphetamines, and methylphenidate except for the different durations of action (Fischman, 1984; Sevak et al., 2009).

Stimulants are classic examples of sympathomimetic drugs; that is, they act to stimulate or mimic activity in the sympathetic branch of the autonomic nervous system.

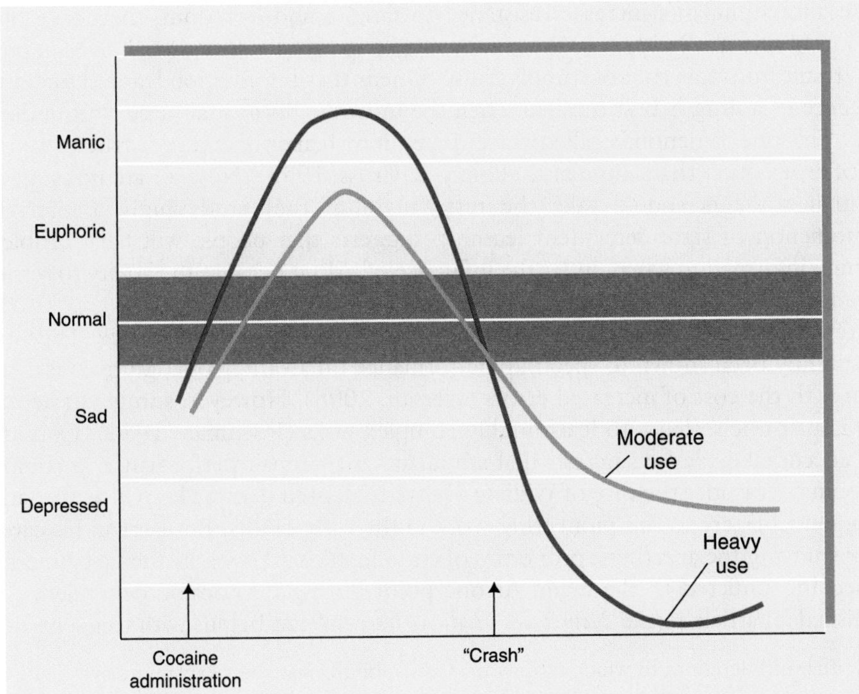

FIGURE 6.2
Relationship between cocaine dose and mood

Thus, many of their physiological effects are the same as those seen during emotional arousal: Heart rate is up, blood pressure is up, respiratory rate is up, and sweating increases. Meanwhile, blood flow decreases to the internal organs and extremities but increases to the large muscle groups and the brain. Finally, body temperature is elevated and pupils are dilated.

Cocaine and amphetamines also produce appetite-suppressant or **anorectic effects**. People simply do not feel hunger after taking these drugs. It is the anorectic effects that were sought when amphetamines were prescribed as diet pills. Although patients definitely ate less and lost weight on diet pills, they had to take larger doses to maintain the weight loss, and patients typically regained the weight when they went off the drugs. Thus, the benefits of diet pills were outweighed by the risk of dependence and other side effects. This approach to the treatment of obesity is now considered questionable at best.

anorectic effects
Causing one to lose appetite; suppression of eating.

Behavioral Effects

Moderate doses of cocaine and amphetamines produce a sense of elation and mood elevation (Hart et al., 2008; Iversen, 2008). Individuals show increased talkativeness and sociability (Higgins & Stitzer, 1988). Alertness and arousal are increased, and marked insomnia often develops. These drugs also enhance performance on a wide variety of tasks involving physical endurance, such as running and swimming, and they increase physical strength. In a review of the literature on amphetamines and sports, Laties and Weiss (1981) concluded that amphetamines confer a small but significant edge to athletes. Consider the effects, shown in Figure 6.3, of methamphetamine on performance on a stationary bicycle. Note that a control injection does little to reverse the effects of fatigue on rate of cycling, but a methamphetamine (Methadrine) injection administered at the three-hour point produces a large improvement that is sustained for several hours. Although the data on cocaine are scantier, it appears to have the same effects but is limited by its short duration of action (Grinspoon & Bakalar, 1976).

Because stimulants increase resistance to fatigue and boredom, they have often been used as a study aid, as in the amphetamine-induced "all-nighter." Several problems result from this type of stimulant use. One is that information learned under the influence of a drug is best recalled when the individual is in that same drug-induced state. This phenomenon is called **state-dependent learning**, and it is true of a number of drugs other than stimulants (Poling & Cross, 1993). Now we are not suggesting that students should take the test "high" if they study high. Rather, the phenomenon of state-dependent learning suggests that people will have problems learning information when under the influence of a drug because the ability to retrieve the information will not be as good when sober.

state-dependent learning
When learning under the influence of a drug is best recalled when one is in the same "state."

Stimulants can definitely enhance some types of cognitive performance. They have consistently been shown to speed up performance on a variety of cognitive tasks, but often with the cost of increased errors (Iversen, 2008). However, stimulants actually may impair one's ability to learn highly complex tasks (Fischman, 1984). Considerable anecdotal evidence suggests that stimulants may impair performance in complex reasoning. Consider the case of William Halsted. Halsted became known as the father of modern surgery for his pioneering work in the early 1900s. But later in his career, while studying the anesthetic properties of cocaine, he was probably the first American to become addicted to the drug. At one point during his cocaine dependency, he published an article in the *New York Medical Journal* that begins with this sentence:

> Neither indifferent as to which of how many possibilities may best explain nor yet quite at a loss to comprehend, why surgeons have, and that so many, quite without discredit, could have exhibited scarcely any interest in what, as a local anaesthetic, had been supposed, if not declared, by most so very sure to prove, especially to them, attractive, still I do not think that this circumstance, or some sense of obligation to rescue fragmentary reputation for surgeons rather than the belief that an opportunity existed for assisting others to an appreciable extent, induced me, several months ago, to write on the subject in hand the greater part of a somewhat comprehensive paper, which poor health disinclined me to complete. (Grinspoon & Bakalar, 1976, p. 32)

Given the apparent effects of cocaine on Halstead's writing style, it is frightening to imagine how his surgery was going! So the notion that cocaine enhances intellectual performance appears to be a myth.

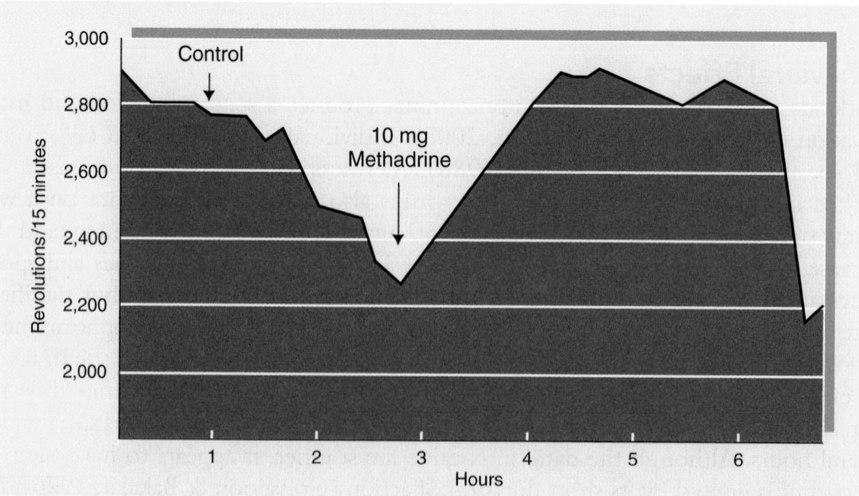

FIGURE 6.3
Performance on a bicycle machine after control and methamphetamine injections
Source: Adapted from "The Amphetamine Margin in Sports" by G. Laties and B. Weiss, in Federation Proceedings, 40(12), 1981. Reprinted by permission.

Another popular notion about cocaine and the amphetamines deals with their ability to enhance sexual prowess. The story with this one is complex. Although this has not been well studied, surveys suggest that although some report enhanced sexual feelings and performance with stimulants, most people do not. Men may experience increased sexual desire under stimulant drugs, but these drugs can also interfere with erectile function and often cause impotence (Iversen, 2008). However, in recent years, a trend has emerged in the gay community to combine methamphetamine with drugs designed to treat erectile dysfunction (e.g., Viagra). This drug combination apparently allows users to maintain an erection while under the influence of methamphetamine and has been associated with high frequencies of risky sexual behavior and an increased probability of testing HIV positive among men who have sex with men (Halkitis et al., 2009).

Acute Effects at High Doses

As we noted earlier, when people take high doses of stimulant drugs, a characteristic psychotic state emerges. This state can be produced in normal volunteers in a laboratory setting by amphetamines, cocaine, or methylphenidate (Ritalin) (Davis & Schlemmer, 1980). Such psychotic reactions are currently a serious problem with high-dose uses of methamphetamine or crack cocaine. Paranoid delusions are the most common symptom of stimulant psychosis, but a second symptom commonly noted is compulsive stereotyped behavior like rocking, hair pulling, chain smoking, or "fiddling with things." Other symptoms may include hallucinations and, as noted earlier, formication. Interestingly, stimulant psychosis may be successfully treated with chlorpromazine (Thorazine) or other drugs used in the treatment of schizophrenia (Davis & Schlemmer, 1980).

A risk of overdose death also accompanies high doses of cocaine or amphetamines. Specifying the dose that places users at risk is difficult. With cocaine in particular, when we speak of low to moderate doses, we refer to 15 to 60 milligrams (a typical "line" contains 10 to 20 mg). But cocaine overdose deaths have been reported in individuals who were given as little as 20 milligrams as a local anesthetic, apparently because they suffered from a rare deficiency in the enzyme that breaks down cocaine in the blood and liver (Weiss & Mirin, 1987). Such cases are certainly exceptional, and generally much higher doses are taken before either stimulant psychosis or death results. When very high doses of stimulant drugs are taken, several complications may produce a medical emergency or overdose death. These include convulsions or seizures that may result in respiratory collapse, myocardial infarction (heart attack) due to coronary artery spasm, and stroke (Sorer, 1992). To further complicate matters, users often combine cocaine with other drugs to produce complex and often unpredictable drug interactions (see Contemporary Issue Box 6.4).

Effects of Chronic Use

Tolerance

When stimulants are taken regularly over a long period (chronic use), several additional problems and issues arise. Users may develop a tolerance for the drug, and this turns out to be fairly complex in the case of the stimulants. First, acute tolerance develops for cocaine; that is, the effects obtained from the first administration of the

CONTEMPORARY ISSUE BOX 6.4

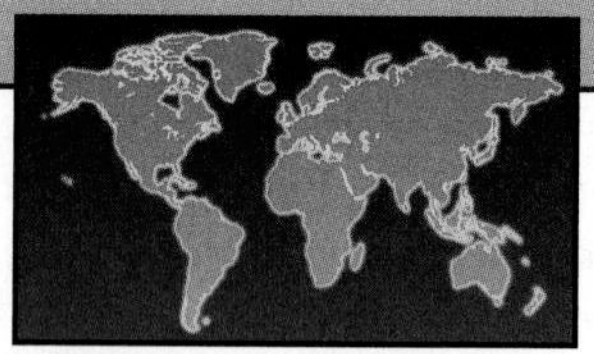

Cocaine and Other Drugs

Cocaine and other stimulant drugs are often taken in combination with other drugs, particularly alcohol and opiates. Laboratory studies in humans have shown that alcohol can enhance and prolong the subjective pleasure associated with cocaine, and this is likely the basis for their frequent association. Recent studies have revealed that when cocaine is taken with alcohol, a new compound called cocaethylene is formed in the body. Cocaethylene has pharmacological properties similar to cocaine, but it may be more toxic. Some cases of cocaine overdose may in fact involve cocaethylene toxicity caused by combining cocaine and alcohol (Raven et al., 2000; Rush, Roll, & Higgins, 1998). The combination of cocaine (or amphetamine) and heroin (or other opiate) is called a "speedball" and is particularly popular among heroin addicts. Morphine and cocaine combinations have been studied in the laboratory, and as with alcohol, morphine appeared to enhance the pleasurable effects of cocaine but also increased the cardiovascular effects. Combinations of cocaine and heroin have sometimes been blamed for drug overdose deaths (as in the deaths of comedian John Belushi and actor River Phoenix), and the synergistic effects on blood pressure and heart rate may be a factor (Foltin & Fischman, 1992; Rush et al., 1998).

drug are not produced by a second administration shortly afterward, unless a higher dose is used. This effect is described by a freebase user:

> You can do enough freebase to kill you and not realize it because the base numbs your lungs and you can keep sucking it in. After that first hit, you spend the rest of the night trying for that same rush. You keep hoping the next hit will do it, and you add more to the pipe and breathe in deeper, but it's never the same and I mean never the same. Nothing compares to that first hit. (Kirsch, 1986, p. 49)

"I need it. I need it. You couldn't possibly understand."

John Belushi on cocaine (Woodward, 1984)

Acute tolerance to the subjective effects of cocaine has been demonstrated in humans in laboratory settings (Ward et al., 1997). This acute tolerance dissipates rapidly too, usually within 24 hours. But studies of the development of long-term protracted tolerance to cocaine and amphetamines have not yielded consistent findings. Ward et al. (1997) found both acute and chronic tolerance to the heart rate increases produced by cocaine in the laboratory. That is, tolerance to the heart rate–increasing effects developed within a single session, and the tolerance persisted and developed further across sessions. However, only acute tolerance was found with the effects of cocaine on blood pressure and subjects' self-reports of stimulation and feeling high. On a given day, the effects of the first cocaine injection were not matched by subsequent injections, but strong effects could still be obtained the next day (Ward et al., 1997).

Comer et al. (2001) studied the effects of chronic methamphetamine use in a 15-day residential study with seven volunteers. The participants lived in the dormitory-style laboratory during the experiment and were given questionnaires several times each day about their subjective state as well as computer-based cognitive and performance tasks. On days 4 through 6 and 10 through 12, they were administered methamphetamine tablets, and on all other days, they received identical placebo tablets. Participants reported feeling a "good drug effect" and "high" on the first day of each methamphetamine run (days 4 and 10), but they did not report these positive effects on the second and third methamphetamine days (days 5 and 6, and days 11 and 12). Instead, on the third methamphetamine days (days 6 and 12), participants reported unpleasant effects such as dizziness and flu-like symptoms. Their food intake declined, and their sleep patterns were also disrupted across each of the methamphetamine exposure periods. In sum, Comer et al. (2001) found that tolerance developed to positive subjective effects of methamphetamine use. The increase in negative effects with repeated administration was attributed in part to the accumulation of sleep loss and reduction of caloric intake. Although there is evidence of tolerance to both cocaine and the amphetamines, some studies have shown the development of what might be termed reverse tolerance or sensitization following repeated administration. In these cases, a given dose of cocaine produces a larger effect after one or more repetitions (e.g., Kollins & Rush, 2002). In any case, the occurrence of reverse or regular tolerance may depend on complex aspects of the situation and response being studied (Hughes, Pitts, & Branch, 1996; Reed et al., 2009).

Dependence

For many years, drug dependence was defined by physical withdrawal symptoms like those produced after heroin withdrawal (see Chapter 10). As a result, the severity of cocaine and amphetamine dependence was underestimated because users do not show dramatic signs of physical illness upon withdrawing from these drugs. The broader definition of drug dependence provided by DSM-IV (see Chapter 1) has helped to change perceptions about dependence on stimulants. Although the withdrawal syndrome associated with cocaine or amphetamines does not involve life-threatening physical symptoms, it is real and compelling. The primary symptoms are depression, anxiety, changes in appetite, sleeping disturbances, and craving for the drug (Schuckit, 2000). The temptation to resume use of the drug is described by many as overpowering. Some individuals go through distinct phases of withdrawal, but variability is considerable. The "crash" occurs first and involves several days of intense craving and exhaustion alternating with agitation and depression. Particularly in methamphetamine withdrawal, users may show greatly increased sleep time and food intake during this phase (McGregor et al., 2005). For several weeks, addicts continue to feel intense cravings, moderate to severe depression, and an inability to experience normal pleasure (*anhedonia*). Although improvement gradually occurs, addicts may continue to experience intermittent cravings for months or even years. This phase has been called the *extinction phase* because the cravings seem to be caused by exposure to particular cues in the environment that were associated with cocaine use in the past and continue to "trigger" craving until eventually, perhaps via classical conditioning, the craving response is extinguished to these cues (Halkitis, 2009).

Stimulant Drugs and ADHD

Some children (and adults) have trouble sitting still and paying attention. This problem can be serious enough to interfere with a child's ability to perform in school, and such children are often diagnosed as suffering from attention deficit/hyperactivity disorder, or ADHD. Children with ADHD are not necessarily hyperactive, and many suffer primarily from symptoms of inattention. ADHD often leads to impaired academic performance, misbehavior at school, and conflict with peers, siblings, and parents. Although some children outgrow ADHD during puberty, more often these problems persist into adulthood.

In 1937, a physician named Charles Bradley discovered what appeared to be an extraordinary paradox: Hyperactive children were calmed by a dose of the stimulant drug amphetamine. Since then, many millions of children with ADHD have been treated with stimulant drugs, and methylphenidate (e.g., Concerta and Ritalin) and amphetamines (Adderall) are now the most widely prescribed treatments for ADHD. The effects of methylphenidate are by and large the same as those of amphetamines reviewed previously in this chapter. Whether stimulants are overprescribed in the United States

DRUGS AND CULTURE BOX 6.5

Cocaine Babies: Legacy of the Crack Era?

Taking drugs during pregnancy creates additional risks. Women who use cocaine during pregnancy have higher rates of spontaneous abortion, fetal death, and premature labor and birth. Infants born of cocaine-using mothers had lower birth weights and lengths and were more likely to die during infancy. There has been widespread publicity and concern that children exposed to cocaine in utero would show permanent neurological damage with attendant learning disabilities.

Many reports have indicated a higher percentage of abnormal arousal patterns and other neurological problems in "crack babies." However, these effects may be relatively short-lived. Some studies have reported long-term learning and behavior problems in children exposed to cocaine in utero, but the studies often lack an appropriate comparison or control group. Remember that "crack babies" are likely to suffer from maternal neglect and an impoverished family and social environment as well. It is difficult to separate the effects of prenatal cocaine exposure from the other problems that the child faces after birth. In studies that have controlled for such factors, "crack babies" generally do not appear to perform worse than the comparison group. Neither group does very well on intellectual tasks, however, with IQ scores well below the national average. Perhaps for children growing up under deprived environmental circumstances, adding cocaine exposure makes little long-term difference. If there is any good news here, it is that the difficulties may not involve permanent neurological damage induced by cocaine. Although well intentioned, labeling children as "crack babies" may stigmatize them and create a self-fulfilling prophecy (see Schama, Howell, & Byrd, 1998; Zuckerman, Frank, & Mayes, 2002, for reviews).

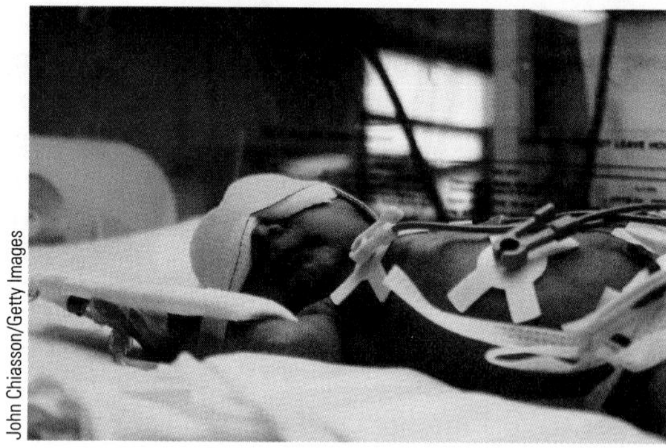
John Chiasson/Getty Images

Crack babies: Future at risk.

today has become controversial in part because of the enormous increase in prescriptions for Ritalin and other stimulants. Since 1990, use of these stimulants increased by nearly 500%, and it is estimated that over two million school-aged children in the United States take Ritalin or some other prescription stimulant drug. Prescription drug sales for ADHD exceeded $3 billion in 2004 (Cox et al., 2008; Kollins, 2005; Tyre, 2005).

One line of criticism holds that children with ADHD should not be prescribed drugs because ADHD is not truly a medical disorder:

> The collection of behaviors subsumed in the diagnosis of ADHD including squirming in a seat and talking out of turn are not symptoms and do not reflect a syndrome. They are behaviors that disrupt classrooms and can be caused by anything from normal childhood energy to boring classrooms or overstressed parents and teachers. We should not suppress these behaviors with drugs; we should instead identify and meet the needs of our children in the school and the home. (Breggin, 2001, p. 595)

But, here is another side of the issue:

> Seemingly unknown to the experts du jour and talking heads of the popular media is that ADHD handily meets the two simple yet elegant criteria for constituting a "real disorder." . . . It constitutes a failure or serious deficiency in a mental mechanism that is universal to humans (a psychological adaptation in the evolutionary sense), in this case, response inhibition

and self-regulation. And it produces harm. That is, it leads to substantial impairment in major life activities, including increased psychological and physical morbidity. (Barkley, 2001, p. ix)

We look at the diagnosis of psychological disorders in Chapter 13, but the ADHD controversy is certainly a thorny one. What seems clear is that, although many of the symptoms of ADHD (inattention, fidgeting, restlessness) are indeed common to virtually all children (and adults), these problems are far more severe and debilitating for some children.

One thing is certain: Stimulant drugs *do* improve performance in children with ADHD. Numerous studies have evaluated the effects of Ritalin and other stimulants on children's performance, and it is well documented that these drugs improve attention, time on task, and other measures of classroom performance, while decreasing disruptive behavior (see Brown et al., 2005, for a review). A recent study showed that children who received medication for ADHD scored higher on standardized tests for mathematics and reading achievement than unmedicated peers with ADHD (Scheffler et al., 2009). There are problems as well, however. Some children experience physical side effects such as insomnia, loss of appetite, and weight loss. Growth delays may occur but are usually managed by giving the child a "drug holiday," often during the summer months, and although some "catching up" may then occur, there is evidence of continued mild growth suppression (Lerner & Wigal, 2008). There are concerns about psychological effects as well. Some have argued that Ritalin is a gateway drug to other stimulants or to other drug-abuse problems, but the literature on this indicates otherwise. Children diagnosed with ADHD are more likely to develop substance-abuse problems as adults, but several studies suggest that boys with untreated ADHD are more likely to develop drug and alcohol problems than are boys with ADHD who were treated with stimulants (see Wilens et al., 2003, for a review).

The short duration of action of Ritalin can also lead to problems. Because the beneficial effects of the drug wear off in about four hours, children often experience a midday loss of functioning and have to be given another dose. This entails a visit to the school nurse or other school staff and can lead to compliance problems. An extended-release methylphenidate preparation (Concerta) with a 12-hour duration of action is now widely used to solve this problem.

Another controversial aspect of ADHD is its increasing diagnosis in adults. This has led to increases in stimulant drug prescriptions. For example, an estimated 1.5 million adults between the ages of 20 and 64 in the United States are prescribed medication for ADHD (Tyre, 2005). Although ADHD used to be thought of as a disorder that children "outgrew," the symptoms may persist into adulthood for many individuals. Another source of controversy is that prescription stimulants are increasingly being diverted (illegally sold or traded). In fact, Ritalin (vitamin R) has come to be one of the popular "club" or "dance" drugs because, like amphetamines, it makes users feel energetic and enhances mood (Hall et al., 2005).

In summary, Ritalin's advocates view it as a nearly miraculous treatment for ADHD, whereas its detractors argue that it is a greatly overprescribed drug with substantial abuse potential. This

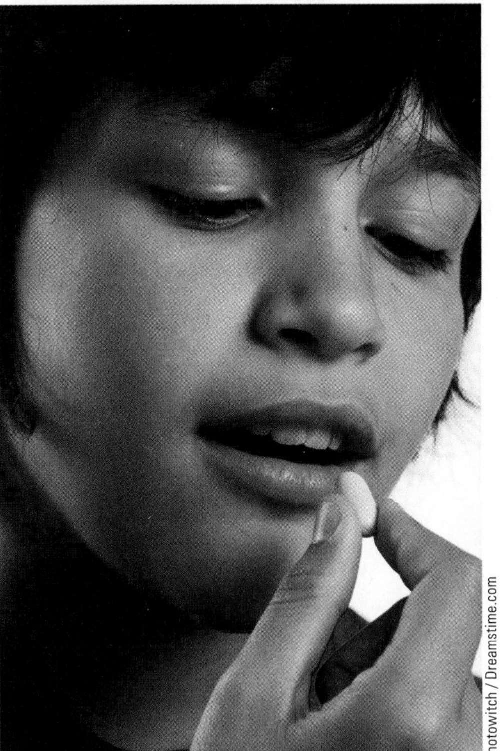
Photowitch / Dreamstime.com

Just say yes? Millions of children are given stimulant drugs to treat ADHD.

DRUGS AND CULTURE BOX 6.6

Khat: A Stimulant from the Horn of Africa

Cocaine and the amphetamines are the best known of the monoamine stimulants in North America, but the most popular stimulant from this group worldwide may be khat (pronounced "kaht"), a plant native to East Africa. Khat, or qat, is the local name for a small shrub (*Catha edulis*) that is widely cultivated in the countries of Yemen, Somalia, and Ethiopia. Among some Muslim cultures, it is considered a more acceptable drug than alcohol, and it is widely used throughout East Africa and the Arabian Peninsula. Some estimates of khat use indicate as many as 5 million daily users throughout the region (Spinella, 2001).

The most common route of khat administration is chewing the fresh leaves of the plant. The juices are swallowed and contain two stimulants: cathine and cathinone. These substances produce effects that are very similar to cocaine and amphetamine mediated by actions on the monoamine neurotransmitter systems. Users report that khat provides energy and a euphoric feeling. An initial period of several hours of stimulation and euphoria generally is followed by a period of depression. In a variety of laboratory studies, the effects of cathinone are indistinguishable from those of cocaine and amphetamine, but khat effects appear to be less intense in practice, perhaps because drug absorption is poor when khat is chewed.

With the increased U.S. military presence in the Middle East and East Africa, there has been concern that Americans may become addicted to khat and that the drug could gain a foothold in the United States. The fear that military personnel would become addicted to the drug appears to have been unfounded, but the drug has appeared in some large U.S. cities. Khat use in North America may be limited by the fact that leaves are pharmacologically active only when fresh, so unless khat is smuggled in by air, it is unlikely to be effective. Of greater concern in the United States is the increased use of methcathinone ("cat"), a potent synthetic stimulant derived from khat (Anderson et al., 2007).

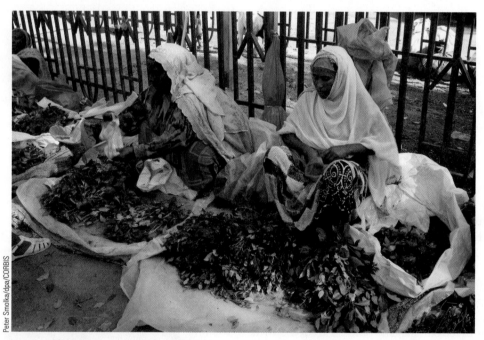

Peter Smolka/dpa/CORBIS

Women sell khat leaves at a market in Ethiopia.

controversy cannot be resolved here and is expected to be a major research focus in the next decade. Hopeful developments include the introduction of drugs such as atomoxetine (Strattera) with different mechanisms of action that appear to be effective treatments of ADHD, but that may present fewer problems to users (Prasad et al., 2009).

Summary

- Cocaine comes from the leaves of the coca bush, and the practice of chewing coca leaves by South American Indians goes back many centuries. The Spanish introduced cocaine to Europe, and when the process necessary to separate cocaine from the leaf was developed in the 19th century, a major epidemic of cocaine abuse swept the world.
- Amphetamines are synthetic stimulant drugs discovered in the 1920s. They became major drugs of abuse as well, but their popularity waned in the 1970s and 1980s as cocaine returned to favor.
- Cocaine became one of the most frequently abused drugs in the 1980s and '90s with the introduction of an inexpensive smokable form—crack.
- Methamphetamine has returned to popularity in recent years, moving from the Western United States to the East, and methamphetamine abuse and illegal production have once again become significant social problems.
- The effects of cocaine and the amphetamines are virtually identical except that cocaine is metabolized rapidly and thus has a short duration of action (20 to 80 minutes), whereas amphetamine effects are more prolonged (4 to 12 hours).
- Both cocaine and the amphetamines act through the monoamine neurotransmitter systems, particularly by enhancing dopaminergic activity. This action in the brain's reward pathways may account for the highly addictive nature of cocaine.
- Both cocaine and the amphetamines are sympathomimetic drugs that increase heart rate, blood pressure, and respiratory rate, and cause pupil dilation.
- Other effects of stimulants include anorectic effects, increased alertness and arousal, mood elevation, and at low doses, enhanced performance on a variety of tasks.
- High doses of cocaine or amphetamines may produce a paranoid state called stimulant psychosis, or death through overdose.
- Dependence may develop after chronic use of cocaine or amphetamines. The abstinence syndrome is characterized primarily by depression and craving with few measurable physiological effects. Thus, a drug that does not cause severe physical withdrawal symptoms can still be highly addictive.
- Ritalin (methylphenidate), amphetamines (Adderall), and other stimulants are widely used to treat attention deficit/hyperactivity disorder (ADHD).

Answers to "What Do You Think?"

1. Cocaine is a synthetic drug developed during World War II.
   F *Cocaine is derived from the leaves of the coca bush.*
2. Cocaine abuse was epidemic in the United States in the 1880s.
   T *Cocaine was a legal drug in the United States until the passage of the 1914 Harrison Narcotics Act and was widely abused around the turn of the century.*
3. Stimulant drugs are often used to treat children who have attention deficit/hyperactivity disorder.
   T *Ritalin (methylphenidate) and other stimulants are actually effective in the treatment of ADHD.*
4. Amphetamine effects are very similar to cocaine effects.
   T *Cocaine and amphetamine are virtually indistinguishable in their major physical and behavioral effects.*
5. Overdoses of cocaine and amphetamine may produce a psychotic state.
   T *The stimulant psychosis resembles paranoid schizophrenia.*
6. Amphetamine has been used medically as a sleeping pill.
   F *Amphetamines cause insomnia. They have been used as diet pills.*
7. Crack is a smokable form of amphetamine.
   F *Crack is smokable cocaine.*
8. The most common withdrawal symptom associated with cocaine is depression.
   T *Depression following cocaine use is referred to as the "cocaine blues."*

9. Stimulant drugs enhance learning and intellectual performance.
   F *Experimental evidence shows that stimulants may impair learning ability and complex reasoning performance.*
10. One difference between cocaine and the amphetamines is that cocaine has a longer duration of action.
   F *Amphetamine effects last from 6 to 12 hours, whereas cocaine is a relatively short-acting drug.*
11. Severe physical withdrawal symptoms follow heavy cocaine use.
   F *Cocaine produces no major physical withdrawal symptoms.*
12. Cocaine and amphetamines act by blocking the reuptake of endorphins.
   F *Cocaine and amphetamines block dopamine reuptake.*

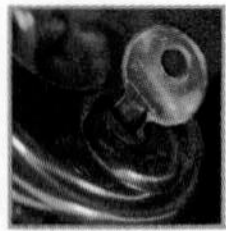

Key Terms

anorectic effects
crack
formication syndrome
state-dependent learning
stimulant psychosis

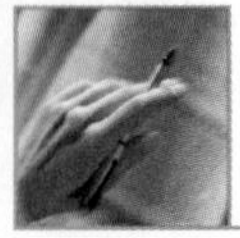

Essays/Thought Questions

1. Consider the different effects and risks associated with the various forms of cocaine (chewing the coca leaf, snorting cocaine, injecting cocaine, smoking crack). Should different laws and penalties be applied to the different forms?
2. Should drugs be prescribed to children who have ADHD? What about adults?

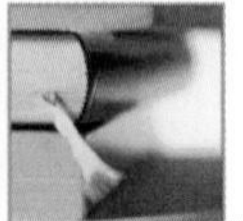

Suggested Readings

Halkitis, P. N. (2009). *Methamphetamine addiction: Biological foundations, psychological factors, and social consequences.* Washington: American Psychological Association Press.

Iversen, L. (2008). *Speed, ecstasy, Ritalin: The science of amphetamines.* Oxford: Oxford University Press.

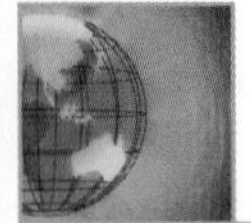

Web Resources

Visit the Book Companion Website at www.cengage.com/psychology/maisto to access study tools including a glossary, flashcards, and web quizzing. You will also find links to the following resources:

- Medline Plus: Cocaine abuse
- Cocaine Anonymous
- National Institute on Drug Abuse (NIDA): Methamphetamine
- NIDA: Crack and Cocaine
- History Channel special on cocaine video
- NIMH site on ADHD
- Video on ADHD treatment

CHAPTER 7

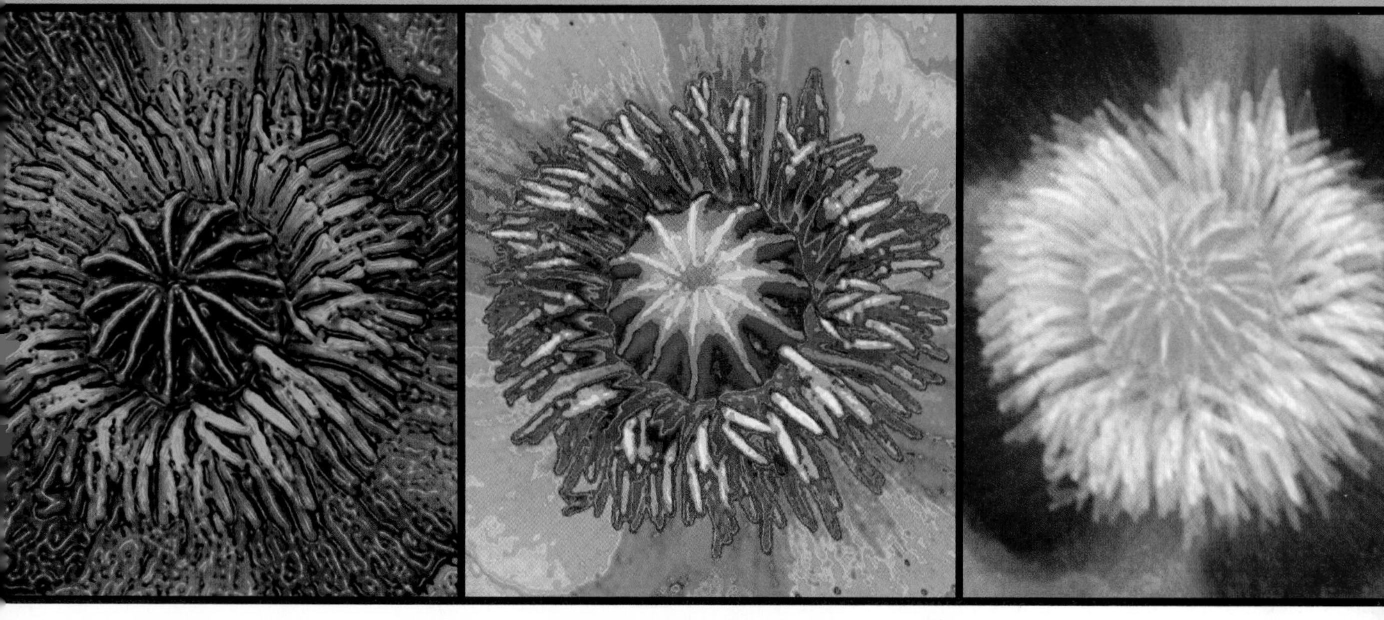

Nicotine

What Do You Think? True or False?

Answers are given at the end of the chapter.

___ 1. Tobacco was once thought to have major medical value.

___ 2. Throughout the age ranges, men have higher smoking rates than women do.

___ 3. The prevalence of smokeless tobacco use among men is about three times that of use among women.

___ 4. Nicotine can be considered both a stimulant and a depressant.

___ 5. When using commercial tobacco products, people reach the peak blood level of nicotine most quickly by using smokeless tobacco.

___ 6. Though psychological dependence is common, no cases of physical dependence on nicotine have been identified.

___ 7. Nicotine's calming effects are a main reason for its use.

___ 8. Nicotine plays a secondary role to learning and social factors in maintaining tobacco use.

___ 9. Health damage from cigarette smoking cost the U.S. economy about $25 billion in 2004.

___10. Low-tar, low-nicotine cigarettes are less damaging to health than cigarettes that do not have reduced tar and nicotine content.

___11. Despite the media hype, passive smoking actually poses a serious health risk to few Americans.

___12. A large portion of ex-smokers quit on their own.

In this chapter and in Chapter 8, we review two more stimulant drugs: nicotine and caffeine. We cover these two drugs apart from other stimulant drugs because nicotine and caffeine are used so prominently in societies around the world. Use of other stimulant drugs has a small fraction of the prevalence that use of nicotine or caffeine does.

This chapter is a review of nicotine and begins with some background information about its source and the ways that nicotine is consumed, followed by a history of tobacco use. We then discuss the prevalence of nicotine use and the mechanisms of its pharmacological action. We also review the acute and chronic effects of nicotine. The chapter concludes with a description of professional services available to help individuals stop smoking.

Nicotine is found naturally in one source: the leafy green tobacco plant. The plant belongs to the genus *Nicotiana* and has 60 species. Only two of these can be used for smoking and other human consumption: *Nicotiana rustica* and *Nicotiana tabacum*. The latter species provides all of the tobaccos typically consumed in the United States, including burley, oriental, and cigar tobaccos. Different types of tobacco result mostly from differences in cultivation and processing. In this regard, tobacco leaves are harvested when still green and then undergo curing and fermentation. The tobacco then is converted into commercial products—cigarettes, cigars, snuff, chewing tobacco, and pipe tobacco (Blum, 1984).

Tobacco has many constituents, but nicotine is singled out as having the broadest and most immediate pharmacological action. Nicotine is extremely toxic—about as toxic as cyanide (Rose, 1991)—and only 60 milligrams are needed to kill a human. When tobacco is burned, the smoke contains a small portion of nicotine, which the body metabolizes to a nontoxic substance.

The tobacco products meant for smoking—in the form of cigarettes, cigars, or pipes—are generally familiar. Not so familiar are the forms of smokeless tobacco, which include snuff and chewing tobacco (Gritz, Ksir, & McCarthy, 1985). Snuff is powdered

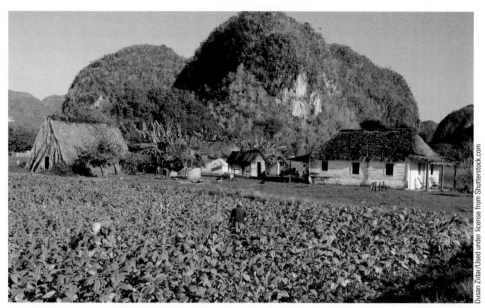

These tobacco plants await conversion to commercial products such as cigarettes and chewing tobacco.

tobacco that is mixed with salts, moisture, oils, flavorings, and other additives. It is marketed in two forms, dry and moist. Chewing tobacco is marketed in loose-leaf form, pressed as a rectangle called a plug, or in a twist or roll. As with snuff, aroma and flavoring agents are added to chewing tobacco. A quid (piece) of tobacco can be either chewed or held between the cheek and gum. "Dipping" is holding a pinch of moist snuff in the same place. In Europe, snuff is most commonly taken dry and intranasally.

History of Tobacco Use[1]

The West Discovers Tobacco

In the late 15th century, Columbus and other explorers found Native Americans in the New World smoking dried tobacco leaves. The pleasant effects of nicotine caught on like fire, and smoking quickly became popular among the Europeans. They brought home seeds of the tobacco plant and spread them to other parts of the world on their ventures. In these early years, the Spanish held a monopoly on the world tobacco market because *Nicotiana tabacum* is indigenous to South America. However, the English took a piece of the business when John Rolfe's *Nicotiana tabacum* crop flourished in the colony of Virginia.

At first, only the wealthy could afford tobacco. For example, in England, tobacco was worth its weight in silver, and people paid that price. By the early 17th century, however, tobacco use had become widespread and even the poor could afford it. In 1614, London had about 7,000 tobacco shops. By the middle of that century, tobacco use had spread throughout central Europe, and signs of the addictive nature of the drug were evident. For example, African natives would trade land, livestock, and slaves for tobacco.

[1]This section on the history of tobacco use is taken from Brecher (1972), Stewart (1967), and Blum (1984).

"A custom loathsome to the eye, hateful to the nose, harmful to the brain, dangerous to the lungs, and in the black, stinking fume thereof nearest resembling the horrible Stygian smoke of the pit that is bottomless."

James I of England, *Counterblaste to Tobacco*, 1604

Not everybody regarded tobacco so highly. In the middle 1600s, Popes Urban VIII and Innocent X issued papal bulls against tobacco use, but clergy and laymen alike continued to smoke. In 1633, in Constantinople, the Sultan Murad IV paid surprise visits to his men in combat during war. If the soldiers were caught smoking, the good sultan punished them by quartering, hanging, beheading, and worse. Yet the soldiers continued to smoke. The Russian czar in 1634 also prohibited smoking. He punished offending subjects by slitting their nostrils and by imposing other consequences that might discourage them from smoking. However, the Russians did not give up tobacco either.

Portuguese seamen gave tobacco to the Japanese in 1542. Like their Western counterparts, the Japanese quickly took to smoking—so quickly that the emperor had issued an edict against smoking by 1603. However, the Japanese did not stop. In 1639, smoking had become so established in Japan that a person was offered a smoke with a ceremonial cup of tea. "From these days until today . . . no country that has ever learned to use tobacco has given up the practice" (Brecher, 1972, p. 213). No substance has replaced tobacco in people's hearts, minds, and bodies. When tobacco smokers discovered the pleasures of smoking marijuana or opium, even these drugs did not displace tobacco; they were merely smoked in addition to it.

Tobacco as Panacea

From the time Columbus and his colleagues discovered tobacco use among the Native Americans until about 1860, the tobacco plant was accepted widely as having medical therapeutic value. Tobacco probably reached its peak of recognition as a medicinal herb at the beginning of the 17th century, even though King James I of England published his skepticisms about tobacco's curative powers at the same time. The king admonished that using tobacco for pleasure was morally wrong. To give you an idea of how its reputation exceeded its critics' influence, Table 7.1 lists some of the ways tobacco has been used medically. During the 360 years the table covers, some people believed it was literally possible to breathe life into another person as long as that breath carried tobacco smoke. Tobacco was esteemed at one time as a panacea weed.

"Just what the doctor ordered."

Advertisement, L & M Cigarettes, 1956

From Panacea to Panned

The promotion of tobacco as a therapeutic agent took a serious blow in 1828, when two Frenchmen, W. H. Posselt and L. A. Reimann, isolated nicotine. The chemical

TABLE 7.1 Uses of Tobacco as Medical Treatment, 1492–1853

- Applied externally in various forms (such as ashes, hot leaves, balm, lotion, mush, oil, and many more) for pain due to internal or external disorders and for skin diseases or injuries of any kind
- Introduced into all openings of the head to treat diseases of the ears (such as smoke blown into), eyes (juice to cleanse), mouth (such as small ball chewed), and nose (such as snuff blown up nose of patient by physician)
- Introduced into the mouth to reach other organs, such as the lungs (such as smoke introduced directly by the physician), the stomach (such as through juice, boiled or uncooked), and the teeth (such as use of ashes to clean)
- Introduced into the nostrils to reach lungs (such as inhaled odor of snuff powder)
- Introduced into the intestinal canal (such as smoke or tobacco enema)
- Introduced into the vagina by injection

Source: Adapted from Stewart (1967), Appendix 5.

was named after a man named Nicot, who was the French ambassador to Portugal and who conducted exacting experiments with tobacco as a medicinal herb. He published his purported successes worldwide. The isolation of nicotine was damaging to its medical reputation because the toxic and addictive properties of the compound began to be understood.

During the years between 1830 and 1860, the use of tobacco for medicine and pleasure in the United States was subject to a stream of attacks by clergy, educators, and some physicians. This also occurred in Europe. Sometimes the ills attributed to tobacco were not based in medical science. For example, perverted sexuality, impotency, and insanity all were attributed to tobacco. In 1849, Dr. R. T. Trall denounced the medical use of tobacco and illustrated his argument by describing a case of tobacco addiction. By the middle of the 19th century, tobacco had all but vanished from the U.S. pharmacopoeia, and the dangers of tobacco as a drug were well known. As the United States prepared for a civil war in 1860, the use of tobacco as a medical agent had virtually ended. However, people continued to use tobacco for pleasure.

"We shall not refuse tobacco the credit of being sometimes medical, when used temperately, though an acknowledged poison."

Jesse Torrey (1787–1834), *The Moral Instructor*, Part IV

Prevalence of Tobacco Use

History shows that tobacco's popularity can resist even the most severe obstacles. In the United States today, cigarette smoking is by far the most common way to use tobacco. Six of every seven pounds of tobacco grown in the United States are used for making cigarettes, and the other pound is used for making pipe and cigar tobaccos and smokeless tobacco products (USDHHS, 1987b). That ratio remained unchanged in 2000, according to the U.S. Surgeon General's report on reducing tobacco use. Furthermore, cigarette smoking demands the most attention because it is the most toxic way to smoke tobacco, followed in order by cigar and pipe smoking (Blum, 1984). Accordingly, we begin this discussion with the prevalence of cigarette smoking.

Smoking in the United States

Many national surveys of smoking among American adults have been conducted. These studies show that the percentage of men and women who smoke declined in the latter part of the 20th century. Coupled with the decline in smokers is a steady increase in the percentage of adults who identified themselves as former smokers (Hughes, 1993; Molarus et al., 2001; USDHHS, 1987b). That is, increasing numbers of people have said they quit smoking, and most of them did so on their own (Zusy, 1987). Self-quitters are thought to have been "lighter" smokers (smoking fewer than 25 cigarettes a day). Nevertheless, many current smokers say they want to quit but find it difficult to do so.

It probably is no coincidence that the peak of smoking among Americans was in 1963. In 1964, the U.S. Public Health Service's *Smoking and Health: Report of the Advisory Committee to the Surgeon General* was published. It detailed the health hazards of cigarette smoking in a way then unprecedented in scope and persuasion.

You learned in Chapter 1 that the overall prevalence of drug use masks important differences among subgroups of the population. This also applies to smoking. Table 7.2 summarizes 2007 national survey data for cigarette use in the past month by age, gender, and racial/ethnic subgroups (SAMHSA, 2008). One point that emerges from Table 7.2 is that age is an important factor, with the highest rates of current cigarette use among 18- to 25-year-olds. An interesting comparison within this age group is individuals in college versus individuals not in college. Among individuals aged 18 to 22, 25.6% who were enrolled in college full-time reported cigarette use in the last month, compared to 41.2% of those who were not full-time college students.

On the other hand, there is some alarm over the resurgence in popularity among college students and other young people of the "hookah" (or water pipe, among other names). The water pipe, which is a device to deliver nicotine by smoking, is so named because the smoke that is inhaled first passes through water (Maziak, 2008). The water pipe first appeared in Africa and Asia over four centuries ago, but has gained new popularity around the world since the 1990s. A main reason for the re-emergence seems to be the perception among young people that the hookah is a harm-free, pleasant way to smoke tobacco. Others feel this way also; according to a Tobacco Regulation Advisory Note published by the WHO in 2005, the Indian physician who invented the water pipe billed it as a safer way to smoke tobacco. In addition, a proliferation of websites promoting the water pipe and retailing it in ways that are highly appealing have fed what Maziak (2008) called a water pipe use "epidemic" (p. 1763). Unfortunately, as with other alternatives to tobacco cigarettes that have been promoted as "safe," smoking from a water pipe is a threat to health, because the smoke from a water pipe contains nicotine, tar, and carbon monoxide. We show later in this chapter how tar and carbon monoxide are especially toxic. Although few studies have addressed this question, the prevalence of use of the water pipe among college students in the United States in the past month has been estimated to be in the range of 15 percent to 20 percent (Eissenberg et al., 2008).

Note also that discrepancies between the genders in smoking prevalence vary across the age groups. Rates of smoking for men and women are less different among individuals 12 to 17 years old and among those 26 and older, compared to individuals 18 to 25 years old. It warrants mention that differences in smoking rates between men and women during the 1950s were considerably greater (around 20%) than they are now. The rates of decline in smoking prevalence since that time have been steeper for men than for women, but men started out at a considerably higher rate.

Racial/ethnic identity also relates to smoking rates. White individuals have the highest rates of the three groups in Table 7.2 in the 12- to 17- and 18- to 25-year-old age groups, but black individuals have a slightly higher rate among those who are 26 and older.

"Smoking is one of the leading causes of statistics."

Anonymous

Two factors not included in Table 7.2 are education and employment status. Although these variables are correlated, it is of interest to look at them separately. Current smoking prevalence for all respondents 18 years and older consistently was

TABLE 7.2 Percentages of Individuals in Different Age, Gender, and Racial/Ethnic Groups Who Reported Cigarette Use in the Past Month, 2007

	Age			
	12–17	**18–25**	**26 and older**	**Total**
Gender				
Male	10.0	40.5	27.1	27.1
Female	9.7	31.8	21.3	21.5
Race/Ethnicity				
White	12.2	40.8	24.8	25.6
Black	6.1	26.2	25.7	23.2
Hispanic	6.7	29.5	21.0	24.8

Source: SAMHSA (2008).

highest for individuals who were unemployed. The overall difference was about 20 percentage points between the unemployed and those employed full- or part-time. Regarding education among respondents 18 years and older, there was a negative relationship between smoking and education: As years of education went up, prevalence tended to go down. Data such as these on education and employment are the bases for arguments that the ills of smoking fall disproportionately on the least advantaged in U.S. society (Droomers, Schrijvers, & Mackenbach, 2002).

Initiation of Smoking

It is important to know who initiates smoking and the number of people who do so because people tend to become dependent on nicotine quickly and before they are 20 years old. This point takes on practical significance because, once nicotine dependence is initiated in adolescence, it tends to persist into the adult years (O'Loughlin et al., 2009). For example, close to 90% of the people who die from smoking-related causes in the United States began smoking when they were adolescents (Primack et al., 2006). Moreover, the younger the age at which a person starts to smoke, the harder it seems to be able to quit later (Breslau & Peterson, 1996). This tendency can be seen during the undergraduate college years. One study (Wetter et al., 2004) classified first-year college students as "nonsmokers," "occasional smokers," or "daily smokers." Four years later, these students were reassessed, and the findings showed that the majority of students who smoked as freshmen still smoked as seniors—this was true for 90% of the daily smokers and for 50% of the occasional smokers. Overall, it seems a lot easier to start smoking than it is to stop (Colder et al., 2001). Data on smoking initiation from the 2004 National Survey on Drug Use and Health (based on the number of individuals who said that they first used cigarettes in the last year) show that the increase registered over the decade of the 1990s masks a pattern of an initial increase followed by a decrease. Among respondents younger than 18 years old, the rate of cigarette smoking initiation from 1990 to 1995 increased 35%. From 1995 to 2001, however, the rate declined by 13%. Overall, for the period between 1990 and 2001, the rate of smoking initiation increased 14%. The data for individuals over 18 years old show a similar but less dramatic trend. From 1990 to 1995, their rate of smoking initiation increased by 11%, but from 1995 to 2001, it dropped by 15%. From 1990 to 2001, the rate increased by 0.9%. It should be noted that, as might be expected, the absolute number of smoking initiates among respondents younger than 18 consistently was about three times the number among those who were older than 18. The survey data suggest that during the years between 2002 and 2004, there was a slight reduction in smoking initiation rates among individuals younger or older than 18.

One reason the rate of smoking initiation has fallen among young people in the last few years in the United States may be changes in the practices of advertising cigarettes and other nicotine products. In this regard, historical studies show a strong relationship between advertising campaigns targeted to specific subgroups of youth (such as boys and girls) and increases in smoking prevalence among those subgroups (Pierce & Gilpin, 1995). For this reason, the tobacco settlement package (discussed later in this chapter) includes provisions for marketing tobacco products only to adults.

Despite the decline in smoking initiation in the United States that the national survey data suggest, these same data show that, in the year 2000, 5,000 adolescents tried smoking for the first time, and 2,100 adolescents became daily smokers. Given the shorter- and longer-term health consequences of smoking, which we will discuss later in this chapter, it is important to understand the high likelihood that, if smoking is initiated, it will occur during adolescence, and the reasons why it is such a difficult behavior to stop once begun. Later in this chapter, we will discuss the strong push to continue to smoke once the behavior starts and the ways people go about trying to stop smoking. However, it is instructive here to comment on the factors that might influence smoking initiation.

As you might guess, because of the enormous public health consequences of smoking, a lot of research has been devoted to explaining smoking initiation. Consistent with the approach to understanding human drug use that is taken in this text, the reasons for smoking initiation are a complex interplay of biological, psychological, and social/environmental factors. We will give you a few examples of findings that have led to this conclusion. From the biological side, recent animal research suggests a major reason why smoking tends to begin in adolescence is that teens' brains are more sensitive to the rewarding (reinforcing) effects of nicotine than are the brains of older individuals (Belluzzi et al., 2004). In this same vein, biopsychological research has used brain imaging (PET scans) to provide data suggesting that individuals who score higher on the personality characteristics of hostility and aggression are more stimulated by a dose of nicotine than are individuals who score lower on these characteristics. This finding suggests that certain people not only are more likely to begin smoking, but also are more likely to continue the behavior than are other individuals (Fallon et al., 2004).

"Have you ever experienced the snuff sensation yet? Wow, it's heady stuff. Well here's your chance to delight in the sensual pleasure of snuffing for free."

Promotion of Imperial Tobacco, England (Wilkinson, 1986, p. 62)

Psychological factors also may combine with environmental variables to affect smoking initiation. One study found that adolescents who score high on the characteristic of "novelty seeking" (they tend to be impulsive, to take risks, and to have a high need for stimulation) are more receptive to tobacco company advertisements than are people who score lower on novelty seeking (Andrain-McGovern et al., 2003).

In summary, a complex of biological, psychological, and social/environmental variables affect smoking initiation and its continuation. As we will discuss, the consequences are substantial.

Smokeless Tobacco Use

Subgroup data on smokeless tobacco use in the past month also are available from the 2007 national survey (SAMHSA, 2008) and are presented in Table 7.3. As we have seen for other drugs, smokeless tobacco use is most popular among 18- to 25-year-olds. An even more striking difference is between men and women—men's usage rates exceed those of women by almost 16-fold.

TABLE 7.3 Prevalence of Smokeless Tobacco Use in the Past Month by Age and Gender, 2007

	Prevalence (%)
Age	
12–17	2.4
18–25	5.3
26 and older	3.0
Gender	
Male	6.3
Female	0.4

Source: SAMHSA (2008).

Pharmacology of Nicotine

Sites of Action

To understand the action of nicotine, it is essential to understand the neurotransmitter acetylcholine (ACH), which we reviewed in Chapter 3. Nicotine stimulates the same receptors that are sensitive to ACH and therefore is a cholinergic agonist drug (Julien, 2005). ACH stimulates both the autonomic and central nervous systems. Table 7.4 is a summary of the effects of ACH on biology and behavior. Julien (2005) also noted that nicotine acts to raise dopamine levels in the mesocorticolimbic system.

Nicotine is called a biphasic drug because it stimulates ACH receptors at low doses but it retards neural transmission at higher doses (Taylor, 2001). This biphasic action partly explains the complex effects that humans perceive when they ingest nicotine, which we discuss shortly.

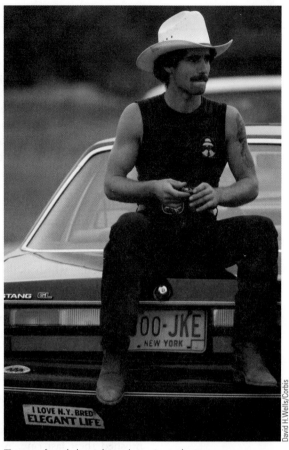

David H.Wells/Corbis

The use of smokeless tobacco is most prevalent among young men.

Pharmacokinetics

Absorption

Nicotine can be absorbed through most of the body's membranes. The drug is rapidly absorbed through the oral, buccal (the cheeks or mouth cavity), and nasal mucosa; the gastrointestinal tract; and the lungs (O'Brien, 1995). Russell (1976) related a story to illustrate how readily nicotine can be absorbed: A florist was using a pesticide spray that contained nicotine and soaked the seat of his pants with it by accident. In only 15 minutes, the florist had **nicotine poisoning** and had to be hospitalized for four days. When he recovered and was dressing to return home, the florist put on the same pants, which still had some nicotine on them. He was readmitted to the hospital an hour later with nicotine poisoning.

nicotine poisoning
A consequence of nicotine overdose characterized by palpitations, dizziness, sweating, nausea, or vomiting.

Nicotine absorption depends on both the site of absorption and how the nicotine is delivered. Nicotine is most readily absorbed from the lungs, which makes inhaling cigarette smoke an efficient way to get a dose of nicotine. Nicotine is not as readily absorbed through the oral, buccal, or nasal mucosa. The nicotine in cigar or pipe smoke, for example, is not as readily absorbed as the nicotine in cigarettes because people usually do not inhale smoke from cigars or pipes. As a result, the nicotine is

TABLE 7.4 Effects of Acetylcholine on Biology and Behavior

- Increases blood pressure
- Increases heart rate
- Stimulates release of adrenalin from adrenal glands
- Increases tone and activity of the gastrointestinal tract
- Facilitates release of dopamine and serotonin
- Affects CNS functions of arousal, attention, learning, memory storage and retrieval, mood, and rapid eye movement (REM) during sleep

Source: Adapted from *A Primer of Drug Action*, by R. M. Julien, W. H. Freeman and Company, 2005.

absorbed through the mouth. When nicotine is taken by using snuff or by chewing tobacco, it is absorbed through the mucosa of the nose and the mouth, respectively.

How nicotine is delivered also affects its absorption. You will recognize some of the factors that affect absorption from reading Chapter 4. One factor is the acidity of the medium (for example, smoke) of delivery. The more alkaline (basic) the medium, the easier the absorption. Cigar or pipe smoke is more basic than cigarette smoke, which compensates to some extent for the difference between the mouth and lungs in ease of absorption. Length of contact of the nicotine-containing substance with the absorption site also is important. The longer the contact, the greater the amount of nicotine absorbed. For example, using snuff and chewing tobacco allows considerable time for nicotine absorption at the nose and mouth (Blum, 1984).

Distribution

After nicotine is absorbed, the blood distributes it to a number of sites of pharmacological action. When a cigarette is inhaled, nicotine reaches the brain from the lungs within 7 seconds. By comparison, it takes 14 seconds for blood to flow from the arm to the brain, which is the typical route for intravenous injection. Therefore, in the delivery of nicotine, brain levels rise rapidly and then decline just as quickly as the drug is distributed to other parts of the body. The effects of nicotine can be observed rapidly because its distribution half-life is only 10 to 20 minutes (Heishman, Taylor, & Henningfield, 1994). A study using PET scan methods illustrates this phenomenon nicely. It showed that, with only one cigarette puff, almost one-third of the primary nicotine receptors (nicotinic ACH) of the brain is occupied, and with three puffs, almost three-quarters of the receptors are occupied. After smoking two and one half cigarettes, the receptors are saturated and the smoker feels satiated (Brody et al., 2006). However, because nicotine levels in the brain also fall rapidly, we have a major biological reason why smokers tend to reach for a cigarette so soon after they have finished their last one. Average smokers of a typical cigarette manufactured in the United States absorb between 0.1 and 0.4 milligram of nicotine for each cigarette they smoke (Julien, 2005).

Metabolism and Excretion

The major organ responsible for metabolizing nicotine is the liver. The lungs and kidneys also play a part in the body's chemical breakdown of nicotine (Taylor, 2001). Nicotine is eliminated primarily in the urine, and about 10% to 20% of nicotine is eliminated unchanged through the urinary tract (Blum, 1984). Less important vehicles of eliminating nicotine and its metabolites are saliva, sweat, and the milk of lactating women (Jones, 1987b; Russell, 1976). Nicotine's elimination half-life in a chronic smoker is about two hours (Julien, 2005).

One study compared blood nicotine levels over a course of two hours in 10 subjects administered comparable doses of nicotine in cigarettes, oral snuff, and chewing tobacco (Benowitz et al., 1988). The study showed that the peak nicotine blood levels reached through the three sources did not differ. However, the rise in nicotine level was steepest for smoking, with a quick and then a more gradual decline leveling off to about one-third the peak level. In contrast, with both snuff and chewing tobacco, the rise in blood level was slower, but higher levels of nicotine were maintained considerably longer. These findings follow from the quicker nicotine absorption time through inhalation but the increased nicotine exposure time in using chewing tobacco or snuff.

The course of nicotine blood levels by smoking gives additional insight into why smokers often smoke many cigarettes a day. They need to smoke often to maintain a nicotine blood level that is not below a threshold for the beginning of withdrawal symptoms. Figure 7.1 is a graph of the average level of nicotine in the blood of a cigarette smoker over the course of a full day. The level of nicotine in the blood rises during the 16-hour part of the day when people are awake, with a peak around midnight. The level then declines during sleeping hours, but there is a positive level upon wakening in the morning.

Tolerance and Dependence

Tolerance

Tolerance to nicotine develops quickly. For example, a person's first attempts at smoking usually result in palpitations, dizziness, sweating, nausea, or vomiting (Russell, 1976). These are signs of acute nicotine poisoning. However, signs of tolerance to these autonomic effects of nicotine are evident even within the time of smoking the first cigarettes. Similarly, the effects of the nicotine in the initial puffs of the first cigarette of the day are greater than those in the last few puffs of that cigarette (Jones, 1987b). The rapid development of tolerance to nicotine also is apparent in the short time it takes some people to become seasoned smokers. The time from their unpleasant first cigarette to pleasurable smoking of a pack a day or more can be as short as several weeks. Besides tolerance to the effects of nicotine, dispositional tolerance develops. For instance, smokers metabolize the drug more quickly than nonsmokers do (Edwards, 1986).

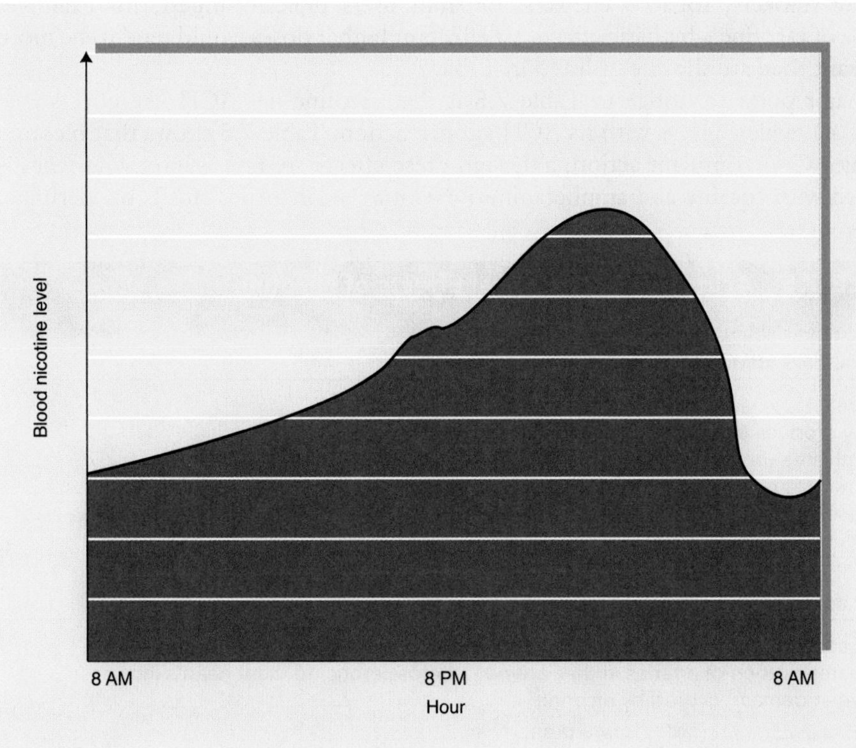

FIGURE 7.1
Blood nicotine levels in a typical cigarette smoker over a 24-hour period

"Recruits, you'll find that smoking will make you nauseous at first, but you will keep with it, and smoke a little more with each passing month until you level out your consumption, usually at about 20 cigarettes a day, and hold this pattern for years, maybe a lifetime."

Drill sergeant, describing smoking to new users of nicotine (Krogh, 1991, p. 74)

"Thank heaven, I have given up smoking again! . . . God! I feel fit. Homicidal, but fit. A different man. Irritable, moody, depressed, rude, nervy, perhaps; but the lungs are fine."

A. P. Herbert

Physical Dependence

There is no question that people can become physically dependent on nicotine. The major criterion for classification of a drug as one that induces physical dependence is what ensues when the drug is taken away for long enough that the amount of it in the blood drops considerably or is eliminated. When a consistent set of physical symptoms results, it is said that the drug induces physical dependence. The reverse side of this criterion of physical dependence is that readministration of the drug alleviates any withdrawal symptoms that are present. In 1988, the U.S. Office of the Surgeon General issued a full report with the conclusion that physical dependence on nicotine develops and that the drug is addicting. In 1989, the Royal Society of Canada came to the same conclusion.

Actually, studies have shown for some time that users of nicotine may become physically dependent on it. For example, Hughes, Grist, and Pechacek (1987) collected smokers' reports of the symptoms they experienced 24 hours after stopping smoking. The most common report (73% of the smokers) was a craving for tobacco, followed in order by irritability, anxiety, difficulty concentrating, restlessness, increased appetite, impatience, somatic complaints, and insomnia. A range of what are generally considered unpleasant symptoms results when dependent smokers stop smoking. As we noted earlier, once people begin smoking cigarettes, they have a high likelihood of becoming dependent on nicotine.

Acute Effects of Nicotine

You have seen that nicotine's effects are pervasive and complex. Table 7.5 is a summary of nicotine's acute pharmacological effects at "normal" doses, or at doses that everyday smokers, tobacco chewers, or snuff users typically ingest, for example. Because of nicotine's biphasic effects, its effects at higher doses would tend to be more depressant than are the effects listed in Table 7.5.

A major point to notice in Table 7.5 is that nicotine has ACH-like effects (see Table 7.4), which agrees with its ACH agonist action. Table 7.5 shows that nicotine has major CNS stimulant action, although these effects are not as intense as what is observed with cocaine and amphetamines. Nicotine's enhancing effects on alertness,

TABLE 7.5 Acute Pharmacological Effects of Nicotine

General CNS stimulant

- Increases behavioral activity
- May produce tremors
- Stimulates vomiting center in brain stem (tolerance to this effect develops quickly)
- Stimulates release of antidiuretic hormones from hypothalamus, increasing fluid retention
- Reduces muscle tone by reducing activity of afferent nerves from muscles
- Enhances alertness, learning, and memory

Other actions

- Increases heart rate, blood pressure, and contraction of the heart
- Initiates dilation of arteries, if they are not atherosclerotic, to meet heart's increased oxygen demand caused by nicotine

Source: Adapted from Julien (2005) and Taylor (2001).

learning, and memory are of considerable importance to us because these effects may account for part of nicotine's reinforcing effects in humans. It is important to note that nicotine deprivation in smokers tends to result in impaired performance on cognitive tasks, but administration of nicotine reverses that impairment. Reversal of cognitive impairment, therefore, could play a part in maintaining cigarette use (Heishman, Taylor, & Henningfield, 1994; Parrott, 1998).

Another point to notice in Table 7.5 is nicotine's autonomic effects, particularly on the cardiovascular system. The stimulation of the heart and its resultant increased demands for oxygen underlie the association of nicotine and heart disease. In this regard, a less-than-adequate supply of oxygen to the heart may result in chest pain (angina) or a heart attack (Julien, 2005).

Nicotine is classified as a stimulant drug, but people who use it often report decreased arousal. That is, the perception is that nicotine has a calming effect, and nicotine users find this effect reinforcing (Todd, 2004). The reasons for this perception of lowered arousal are complex. One factor may be nicotine's acute effect of relaxing the skeletal muscles (see Table 7.5; also see Jones, 1987b). Another pharmacological reason is nicotine's biphasic action: At higher doses, its effects are more depressant.

Pharmacology is only part of the explanation of how aroused people feel when they use nicotine. One of the sedating psychological effects of smoking is the smoker's perception of successfully coping with stress while smoking, which suggests that individuals' beliefs about nicotine's effects influence their reaction to smoking cigarettes (Abrams & Wilson, 1986; Juliano & Brandon, 2002). More fundamentally, personality research suggests that arousal and the perception of stress reduction are independent factors, so they are positively related on occasion, not surprisingly (Parrott, 1998). Along these same lines, nicotine use often is associated with pleasant social situations like parties. Many other secondary (associated) effects of nicotine use exist and can contribute to users' perceptions at times that the drug has calming effects.

A final acute effect of nicotine is its relationship to lower body weight. Nicotine decreases one's appetite for sweet foods and increases the amount of energy the body uses both while it is resting and while it is exercising (Jaffe, 1990; West & Russell, 1985). These effects of nicotine use help to explain the common finding that quitting smoking is associated with weight gain. The nicotine–body weight relationship is noteworthy to us for a couple of reasons. First, the association of smoking with body weight may affect adolescents' decisions to start smoking. Austin and Gortmaker (2001) found that frequency of dieting among middle-school girls (which implies concern about weight control) was directly related to the probability that they would start smoking within the next two years. In addition, among adults who already smoke, the perception that smoking controls weight is a powerful motivator for continuing to smoke and for resuming smoking after stopping for a period of time (Pomerleau & Saules, 2007). The motivation seems to be particularly strong among women (McKee et al., 2005), although weight gain also has been associated in men who resume smoking after stopping for a period of time (Borelli et al., 2001).

"Reach for a Lucky instead of a sweet."

Lucky Strike advertisement, 1920 (Krogh, 1991, p. 69)

Nicotine's Dependence Liability

The U.S. Surgeon General's 1988 conclusion that nicotine is physically addicting stunned many people, although knowledge that physical dependence on nicotine can develop had been around for years. The shock of the report probably lay in the public's failure to view nicotine as a "serious" drug like cocaine or heroin. Yet, the circumstances are most conducive for developing both psychological and physical dependence on nicotine.

Nicotine's CNS-stimulating effects, coupled with the frequent perception that it is sedating, are powerfully reinforcing to humans. Nicotine remains a highly accessible drug in spite of the numerous taxes levied on its purchase over the years. In addition, although the number of social settings where nicotine use is acceptable has decreased, enclaves of social support for its use remain in the United States.

The rapid rise and fall of nicotine blood levels creates the demand for many nicotine reinforcements a day. For smokers, each inhalation results in a drug reinforcement that must be replaced quickly because of a rapid fall in the blood level of nicotine. For two-pack-a-day smokers, estimates average 300 nicotine reinforcements a day, which equals about 110,000 a year.

Reasons such as these make psychological dependence on nicotine so likely once use of the drug starts. Many social and environmental associations with nicotine use strengthen the psychological dependence. Additionally, strong incentive to continue using the drug is added when people become physically dependent on it. Use must continue to avoid unpleasant withdrawal symptoms, or to escape such symptoms if they begin. Use of nicotine under such conditions is strengthened through negative reinforcement. Therefore, pharmacological, psychological, and social/environmental variables combine to make nicotine a drug with high-dependence liability. Indeed, it now is generally agreed that smokers smoke, tobacco chewers chew, and snuffers snuff primarily for the effects of nicotine (Jarvik et al., 2000).

Effects of Chronic Tobacco Use

Chronic or long-term use of tobacco products is associated with life-threatening diseases (see Figure 7.2). The seriousness of these consequences is reflected in precedent-setting legislation enacted in Canada in 1997. As of 2000, part of the law requires cigarette packs to display gruesome pictures of possible long-term consequences of smoking, such as a lung tumor or a mouth with oral cancer. The pictures must cover 50% of the front and back of each pack. The Canadian legislation is part of an international trend to use the cigarette (and cigar and smokeless tobacco) package itself to reduce the world's health care burdens by helping people either to stop smoking or not to initiate it (National Cancer Council of Australia, 2006).

We begin this section with a discussion of the effects of chronic cigarette smoking because that is the dominant way tobacco is used. Current estimates are that more than 430,000 people in the United States who smoke die prematurely each year—almost 1,200 people a day. Woloshin, Schwartz, and Welch (2002) made this figure

FIGURE 7.2
Four warnings that must appear on cigarette packages, according to a 1984 U.S. federal law. One warning per package appears, with each message rotated every three months. The contents of the message are based on the Reports of the Surgeon General on the Health Consequences of Smoking.

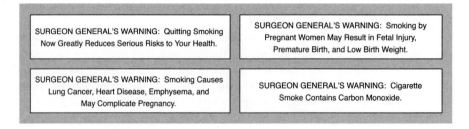

SURGEON GENERAL'S WARNING: Quitting Smoking Now Greatly Reduces Serious Risks to Your Health.

SURGEON GENERAL'S WARNING: Smoking by Pregnant Women May Result in Fetal Injury, Premature Birth, and Low Birth Weight.

SURGEON GENERAL'S WARNING: Smoking Causes Lung Cancer, Heart Disease, Emphysema, and May Complicate Pregnancy.

SURGEON GENERAL'S WARNING: Cigarette Smoke Contains Carbon Monoxide.

more personal by comparing rates of death from different diseases among adults 20 years of age and older who currently smoke or who never smoked. These researchers computed the chances of dying in the next 10 years for a given medical problem for different age groups, and used the 1998 National Center for Health Statistics Multiple Cause-of-Death Public-Use files for their computations. For women, there were some diseases for which the probability of dying in the next 10 years does not differ at any age between smokers and nonsmokers. For example, at age 30, the chance of dying of breast cancer in the next 10 years is 0.001 for both groups, and at age 45, it is 0.004 . For other diseases, however, there are big differences between the groups. At age 45, 6 of 1,000 (0.006) women smokers are likely to die of a heart attack compared with 2 of 1,000 (0.002) nonsmokers. At age 55, the counterpart numbers are 24 (0.024) and 7 (0.007). The disparity continues with further aging; at age 80, the numbers are 453 (0.453) and 90 (0.090). For all causes of death, at age 30, the numbers are 14 (0.014) for smokers and 7 (0.007) for nonsmokers; at age 45, they are 50 (0.050) and 26 (0.026); at age 55, 125 (0.125), and 66 (0.066); and at age 80, 950 (0.950), and 581 (0.581).

The picture is similar for men. Smokers and nonsmokers did not differ in projected death rates from diseases like colon or prostate cancer, and they did not differ in rates of death by accidents. However, for death by heart attack, stroke, or lung cancer, the disparities in death rates were large and evident from age 30 to old age. The proportions of

DRUGS AND CULTURE BOX 7.1

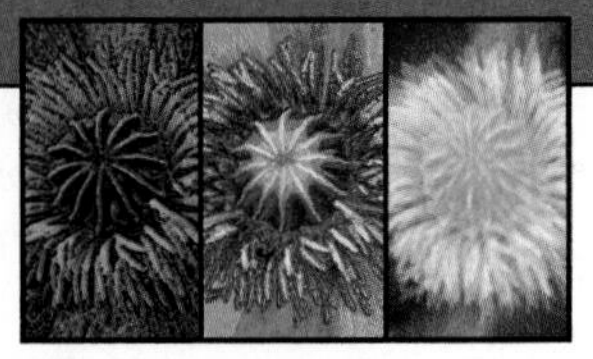

Smoking Overseas

As we discussed earlier, the prevalence of cigarette smoking among adults in the United States has gone down considerably over the last 40 years. This reduction has been attributed mainly to information about the health hazards of smoking and to government policies and laws that restrict access to smoking. In western Europe, the rates of smoking also have gone down in the past few decades, but the current prevalence of smoking still is considerably higher in some of those countries than they are in the United States. In the developing countries of Asia and elsewhere, the prevalence of smoking actually has increased in recent years.

Of course, the knowledge about the effects of smoking on health that is available to Americans is available to the governments of other countries as well. Thus, it seems that cultural, social, and financial factors account for the continued and sometimes increased popularity of smoking around the world. For example, one reason that sounds very American is that smoking is viewed as a personal choice that may cause some harm but not that much. As such, society and governments alike should tolerate smoking. In France, smoking is very much a part of café life and lends an intellectual aura to smokers. In China and Japan, smoking is a symbol of liberation from restrictive female gender roles. Finally, in countries like Italy and China, the governments are at best ambivalent about their citizens' smoking. Although these governments are aware of the health risks of smoking, they also control tobacco product distribution and sales in their respective countries. Countries with such monopolies on tobacco have a financial incentive to keep people smoking.

The financial and health implications of smoking trends overseas are profound. This is especially true for developing nations. These countries offer major new market opportunities for the American tobacco industry, which faces increasing government regulation and an uncertain adult market at home. China, which is the largest cigarette producer and consumer in the world, has an estimated 500,000 to 750,000 smoking-related deaths a year (Lam et al., 1997; Lopez, 1998). The estimate reaches 3 million deaths a year by the time today's young smokers reach middle and old age.

Given what is known about cigarette smoking, what do you see as the major ethical, social, and financial factors that must be considered in deciding on a government's smoking laws? How much weight do you think should be given to each of these factors?

death from all causes at age 30 were 0.030 for smokers and 0.013 for nonsmokers; at age 45, they were 0.091 and 0.039; at age 55, 0.125 and 0.066; and at age 80, 0.950 and 0.650. Statistics like these are represented in cost-of-illness studies: According to the American Lung Association, in 2004, the cost of smoking to the U.S. economy was $193 billion, or $4,260 for each adult who smoked.

All the data we cited on the health consequences of chronic cigarette smoking are for the United States only. However, 4.3 million men and women worldwide die prematurely due to their cigarette smoking (Ezzati & Lopez, 2003). The problem is not estimated to resolve itself. In February 2008, the World Health Organization (WHO) issued a report estimating that, in the 20th century, 100 million people around the world died prematurely due to smoking; by the year 2100, the WHO projects 10 times that number, or 1 billion premature deaths due to smoking worldwide (see the Drugs and Culture Box 7.1).

Tar, Nicotine, and Carbon Monoxide

Cigarette smoking damages health because of the constituents of tobacco smoke. The three main culprits are tar, nicotine, and carbon monoxide, and cigarette smokers face continual exposure to them for years. For example, a two-pack-a-day smoker could be seen with cigarette in hand, mouth, or ashtray 13.4 hours a day, taking about 400 puffs and inhaling as much as 1,000 milligrams of tar. Carbon monoxide appears to facilitate many of the disease processes associated with smoking. This is due to carbon monoxide's advantage over oxygen in binding to hemoglobin, which carries oxygen from the lungs to the tissues in the body. Exposure to even small amounts of carbon monoxide reduces the amount of hemoglobin available for binding to oxygen and thereby deprives the body's tissues of oxygen. The brain and heart are especially vulnerable to this action of carbon monoxide because they depend on aerobic respiration for proper functioning (Blum, 1984).

Most of the cancer-causing substances in smoke are in tar, which is the material that remains after cigarette smoke is passed through a filter. A cigarette typically contains 0.3 milligrams to 2.0 milligrams of nicotine (cigars yield 9 to 12 times more). When cigarettes are smoked and inhaled, about 20% of the nicotine is absorbed, compared with 2.5% to 5% when smoke is drawn into the mouth and then exhaled. That virtually all cigarette smokers inhale is one reason (other than sheer numbers) that cigarette smoking, as opposed to cigar or pipe smoking, is the major cause of diseases related to tobacco use.

Because of the importance of the tar and nicotine content of cigarettes, until the mid-1980s, the Federal Trade Commission (FTC) published statistics on the tar and nicotine yield of cigarette brands manufactured in the United States. The FTC used to conduct its own yield tests by using smoking machines; today, tobacco companies report the results of the same kind of tests, which the FTC requires them to do (Cotton, 1993).

The amount of tar and nicotine delivered in U.S. brand-name cigarettes has declined considerably. In 1968, the average tar and nicotine yields of cigarettes produced in the United States were 21.6 mg and 1.35 mg respectively. In 1978, these contents were 16.1 mg and 1.11 mg; in 1988, they were 13.3 mg and 0.94 mg; and in 1998, 12.0 mg and 0.88 mg (Federal Trade Commission, 2001). These averages cover a range of values for "light" versus "regular" versus "ultra" brands. For example, according to a report published by the Lorillard Tobacco Company in February 2009, each Newport Lights Box 80s cigarette has 9.0 mg of tar and 0.80 mg of nicotine, each Newport Medium Box 80s cigarette has 12.0 mg of tar and 1.00 mg of nicotine, and each Newport Regular Box 80s cigarette has 18.0 mg of tar and 1.30 mg of nicotine. A similar range is evident in cigarettes manufactured in other countries too. For example, Endo et al. (2009) reported the tar and nicotine levels of the 10 most popular cigarette brands in Japan. The tar and nicotine levels were determined by following the testing procedures of the International Organization for Standardization (ISO), whose protocol is aligned with that of the FTC. (It is interesting to note that Canadian cigarette brands published tar and nicotine levels according to far more strict protocol called "Health Canada Intense" that results in far higher estimates of tar and nicotine levels than those of either the FTC or the ISO.) The findings for the Japanese brands ranged from 0.90 mg of tar and 0.20 mg of nicotine for each "Pianissimo" cigarette, to 14.80 mg of tar and 1.11 mg of nicotine for each "Seven Stars" cigarette.

Reduced delivery of tar and nicotine from cigarettes seems like a good thing, given what we know about their contribution to serious disease. Indeed, the American public perceives that cigarette brands with low tar and nicotine yields are healthier (Cotton, 1993). However, an essential point to understand throughout this discussion is that tar and nicotine delivery is measured by a smoking machine, which puffs consistently in the same controlled way regardless of the cigarette content. Humans are not so standardized. When the nicotine content of a cigarette is reduced, smokers consciously or unconsciously either inhale the smoke more intensely or smoke more cigarettes (DeGrandpre et al., 1992). The result is exposure to similar amounts of toxic substances in the smoke from lower-yield and higher-yield cigarettes. This was confirmed empirically in a study of 298 smokers from New Mexico (Coultas, Stidley, & Samet, 1993). It is a critical finding because the risk of death from smoking goes up with increased exposure either by number of cigarettes smoked or by depth of inhalations. Therefore, any implication that low-yield nicotine and low-yield tar cigarettes are less hazardous is deceptive. Accordingly, in 2001 the National Cancer Institute issued a report proposing that Congress pass a law banning the tobacco industry's use of terms like *light, ultra light,* and *low-tar* cigarettes. Such a law never was passed in the United States, but U.S. tobacco companies do note in their public reports that lower tar and lower nicotine cigarettes, when used by humans, are not less of a health hazard than cigarettes that are of higher tar and nicotine content. Such a statement has a biological basis as well. Brody et al.'s (2008) experiment showed that, when smokers smoked a cigarette containing 0.6 mg of nicotine, which is at the lower end of the range of quantities contained in commercial "light" brands, close to 80% of the nicotinic-ACH receptors in their brains were occupied.

Diseases Linked to Cigarette Smoking

Cigarette smoking kills because it leads to the development of coronary heart disease, cancer, and chronic obstructive lung disease. Heart disease is the single biggest killer in the United States, and people who smoke have nearly twice the risk of contracting it than nonsmokers do. Cancers of the larynx, oral cavity, esophagus, bladder, pancreas, and kidney are associated with cigarette smoking—so associated that 30% of all cancer deaths are caused by it, as are 80% to 90% of all lung cancer deaths. For the first time, a study showing a link between smoking and lung cancer at the cellular level gave strong support that smoking causes lung cancer (Denissenko et al., 1996). Finally, smoking causes 80% to 90% of chronic obstructive lung diseases, such as **emphysema**. Fortunately, the risk of contracting these diseases decreases with time away from cigarettes. If smokers can manage to quit smoking, then their risk of illness and death drops considerably and continues to decline with subsequent years of abstinence from smoking (Huxley et al., 2007; Williams et al., 2002).

emphysema
Disease of the lung characterized by abnormal dilution of its air spaces and distension of its walls. Frequently, heart action is impaired.

"Cigarettes are killers that travel in packs."

Anonymous

Many of the statistics on cigarette smoking and health in the United States have been based on studies done with men. However, large numbers of women began the habit after World War II, and they soon fell prey to similar health damages (USDHHS, 1987b). This upsurge likely was due in part to the tobacco industry's specific targeting of women in their advertising campaigns and to their design of cigarettes to suit women's product preferences (Henningfield, Santora, & Stillman, 2005). The rate of death due to lung cancer in women in 1990 was more than four times higher than it was in 1960, and lung cancer displaced breast cancer as the leading cancer-related cause of death for women in the 1980s (Center for Disease Control and Prevention, 1993; Ernster, 1993). According to information that the University of Michigan's Comprehensive Cancer Center provided in 2006, the ratio of lung cancer diagnoses in men to women in the 1970s was 3.5:1, and by 2000, it was 1.5:1. In this regard, the rates of lung cancer in men in the United States began to fall in the 1980s, as the rate for women began to climb.

"SURGEON GENERAL'S WARNING: Not Quitting Smoking Now is Absurd."

Hypothetical Surgeon General's warning, Letters to the Editor page, *The New York Times*, June 13, 2009

Women also face some unique health consequences of smoking. For example, women who smoke are at higher risk of cervical cancer, unwanted side effects of using oral contraceptives, and early menopause (Ernster, 1993). Furthermore, smokers who are pregnant incur a higher risk of spontaneous abortion, preterm births, low-weight babies, and fetal and infant deaths. If the infant is born healthy, there still is risk from nicotine present in the mother's milk (USDHHS, 1987b; 2001).

Other Tobacco Products and Health

The use of other tobacco products is not risk-free. Pipe and cigar smokers also have higher death rates than nonsmokers. The differences are not as large as the comparisons we cited for cigarette smokers, however, because pipe and cigar smokers tend to consume less tobacco and tend not to inhale (World Health Organization, 1999). A review of studies conducted around the world showed some mixed evidence, but, overall, it appears that users of snuff and other kinds of smokeless tobacco are more likely to get oral cancer and types of noncancerous oral disease than are nonusers and nonsmokers (Bofetta et al., 2008). Another finding from the Bofetta et al. review was that cigarette smokers who switched from cigarettes to "spit" (chewing) tobacco still were at considerably higher risk to incur various cancers than were individuals who changed from cigarette smoking to no tobacco use at all. It seems that the risk for cancer is lower for smokeless tobacco users than for cigarette smokers, but smokeless tobacco use is not risk-free for cancer.

"They don't get your wind."
"Kent, the one cigarette that can show you proof of greater health protection."
"Less 'tar' than all leading longs."

Camels ad, 1935; Kent ad, 1953; L&M ad, 1979, respectively (Viscusi, 1992, pp. 38–39)

Passive Smoking

It once was thought that smokers were harming only themselves. However, we know now that if you merely stay in the vicinity of people smoking, then you absorb nicotine, carbon monoxide, and other elements of tobacco smoke, although in lesser amounts than if you were actively smoking. You are essentially smoking passively if your body is the recipient of the toxins of another person's tobacco smoke.

Passive smoking (also referred to as "secondhand" smoking) is an active killer. Researchers who followed 32,000 healthy nonsmoking female nurses for 10 years found that regular exposure to cigarette smoke almost doubled the nurses' chances of contracting heart disease (Kawachi et al., 1997). Indeed, one review suggested that passive smoking in households kills about 53,000 people in the United States a year—most (74%) due to heart disease (Glantz & Parmley, 1991). Notably, Glantz and Parmley's (1991) estimate matches more recent estimates (Steenland et al., 1996; University of California–Irvine Transdisciplinary Tobacco Use Research Center

[UCI TTURC], 2005). This figure (53,000 deaths) makes passive smoking the third-leading preventable cause of death in the United States, behind active smoking and alcohol. More recent data are consistent with these findings. In 1993, the U.S. Environmental Protection Agency declared environmental tobacco smoke (second-hand smoke) a "Group A" carcinogen. For reference, other Group A carcinogens include arsenic, asbestos, benzine, and radon. Such action has led to the widespread restriction of smoking in public places. Passive smoking is no less of a problem in other parts of the world. A report from the University of California–Berkeley showed that, in 2002, over 48,000 women in China died from ischemic heart disease and lung cancer caused by passive smoking (Yang, 2005). This compares to the 47,300 Chinese women who died that year from the same diseases caused by active smoking.

"If children don't like to be in a smoky room, they'll leave." When asked by a shareholder about infants, who can't leave a smoky room, Harper stated, "At some point, they begin to crawl."

David Carrig about Charles Harper (R.J. Reynolds chairman), in "RJR Wins Fight," *USA Today*, April 18, 1996

Age is no barrier to passive smoking; its effects can be felt by anyone from young children to older adults. Moreover, research has shown that the fetus is exposed to significant amounts of nicotine if a nonsmoking mother is regularly exposed to cigarette smoke during the gestation period (Eliopoulos et al., 1994), and that such exposure can harm the fetus (Grant, 2005). Children whose parents smoke are more likely than

CONTEMPORARY ISSUE BOX 7.2

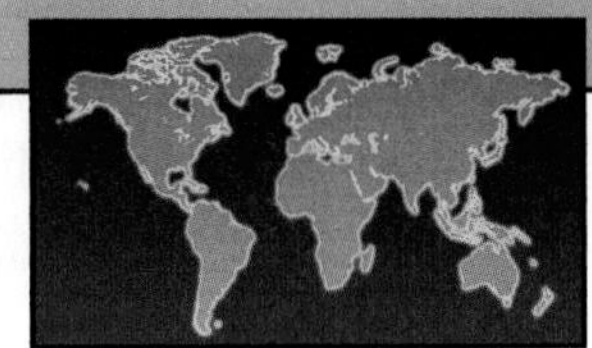

Cigarette Smoking and Health: Who's Responsible?

In the 1950s, smokers began to file hundreds of lawsuits against cigarette companies, claiming the companies were responsible for the smokers' poor health. Until the 1980s, all these cases had failed, and the tobacco industry never paid a cent in damages. Their trump card was the 1965 Federal Cigarette Labeling and Advertising Act that took effect in 1966. (This is the same act that was extended to require the rotation of four warning labels on cigarette packages.) Federal courts had always claimed that this act preempted the tobacco industry from responsibility for the health consequences of smoking, at least for any smoking done on or after January 1, 1966. Furthermore, juries had tended to perceive that smokers were responsible for their own decisions regarding smoking.

Great attention was given to a smoker's lawsuit filed in 1983 by a New Jersey woman. In 1988, a jury awarded $400,000 to the husband of the woman, who died in 1984 of lung cancer. This landmark decision was overturned in 1990 by an appeals court, which ruled that whether the woman had seen or believed tobacco industry advertisements before 1966 had not been proven. The woman's family continued to fight, but they dropped their suit in November 1992, at least partly due to the great financial cost of pursuing it. Individual smokers and their families filed other suits in the early to mid-1990s. However, legal action brought against the tobacco industry generally was unsuccessful.

Class action suits against the tobacco companies have been more successful, perhaps in part because groups of individuals tend to have more resources than any one person does. In this regard, in 1997, both Florida and Mississippi won damages ($11.3 billion and $3.3 billion, respectively) from the tobacco industry to cover the states' costs in Medicaid payments for smoking-related illnesses. In 1999, the omnibus tobacco settlement was reached as the attorneys general of 46 states and five territories signed an agreement totaling $206 billion, with tobacco companies to settle Medicaid lawsuits. This accord also has numerous other provisions aimed at preventing young people from starting smoking in the first place, as well as underwriting the costs of treating individuals who already are addicted to nicotine. The omnibus tobacco settlement likely was due primarily to revelations that the tobacco industry concealed early knowledge about the relationship between smoking and serious health problems. Overall, the consequences of legal actions related to the chronic effects of cigarette smoking have been profound for the tobacco industry, for consumers of tobacco products, and for our principles of choice and personal responsibility. For example, if tobacco companies are held liable for diseases that can be traced to the use of their products, then what does that imply about liability for the public's use of alcohol—another legal drug that could have chronic detrimental effects? What would the companies' liability imply about the principle that individuals have the freedom and responsibility for their actions?

children whose parents do not smoke to have bronchitis and pneumonia as well as some impaired pulmonary function (Rees, Gregory, & Connolly, 2006; World Health Organization, 1999); these childhood illnesses may extend into adulthood (David et al., 2005). Of further concern is "third-hand" smoke. One study showed that the toxins in tobacco smoke linger (Winickoff et al., 2009). Therefore, going outside of the home to smoke a cigarette, for example, does not eliminate the problem, because the toxins in tobacco smoke are returned with smokers in their hair or clothes, even though the cigarette has been extinguished. Third-hand smoke is especially a problem for young children, whose immune systems are not fully developed.

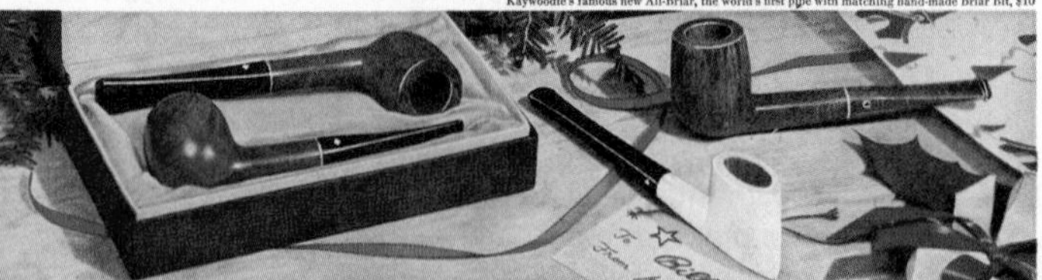
KAYWOODIE PIPES...the gift that says "Merry Christmas" to a man's taste and throat hundreds of times a year!
No matter what he smokes, light up his Christmas with a throat-easy Kaywoodie.
Only Kaywoodie Pipes are superbly crafted of the world's finest briars. Only Kaywoodie Pipes have those three exclusive throat guards that make every mellow puff cool and silky smooth to his throat. Only Kaywoodie has dozens of handsome styles to suit every man's taste. Only Kaywoodie is known the world over as "the aristocrat of fine pipes!"
So give him a Kaywoodie for Christmas. Every time he lights it—it will be a glowing reminder of your thoughtfulness.
KAYWOODIE
Look for the Kaywoodie Cloverleaf
NEW YORK–LONDON–SINCE 1851
Kaywoodie's famous new All-Briar, the world's first pipe with matching hand-made Briar Bit, $10
Kaywoodie Gift Sets, $10 to $125
Kaywoodie's new White Briar—Streamliner, $5
Other Kaywoodie Pipes from $4 to $25

Image Courtesy of Advertising Archives

Cigar and pipe smokers also have higher death rates than nonsmokers.

Treatment of Cigarette Smoking

In this section, we consider ways to stop smoking. Although stopping the use of other tobacco products also is an important topic, we again focus on cigarette smoking because it accounts for the vast majority of tobacco use and because it has been the major subject by far in the literature on ways to stop nicotine use.

Note that nicotine is the only drug for which we consider treatment, outside of Chapter 15, where we review treatment of other drugs and their abuse. This is because such a large amount has been written on the subject compared to drugs other than alcohol. Furthermore, treatments for stopping smoking have been at the center of attention for health professionals and the public due to the health hazards of smoking.

In reviewing nicotine's acute effects, you saw how easily a person might acquire and keep the habit of tobacco use. In reviewing the health consequences of chronic tobacco use, you may have wondered why anyone would continue to use tobacco products. Yet, of course, many people do continue, despite wanting to quit; others find quitting easier.

relapse
A term from physical disease; return to a previous state of illness from one of health. As applied to smoking, it means the smoker resumes smoking after having abstained for some amount of time.

Adults say they quit smoking for a variety of reasons. These reasons may be categorized broadly as "intrinsic motivation" and "extrinsic motivation" (Curry, Wagner, & Grothaus, 1990). Examples of intrinsic reasons are a fear of getting sick, feeling in control, and proving that quitting is possible (for the individual). Extrinsic reasons include stopping others from nagging, being forced by others to quit, and saving money (McBride et al., 2001). Researchers (e.g., Lichtenstein, 1982; Shiffman et al., 1996) also have summarized the determinants of smoking **relapse**, which is a major problem in smoking treatment and in treatment of the substance-use disorders in general. Smoking relapse determinants include nicotine withdrawal symptoms, stress and frustration, social pressure, alcohol use, and weight gain. Furthermore, Pomerleau (1997) suggested that people with psychiatric problems such as depression, anxiety, bulimia, and attention deficit/hyperactivity disorder have a higher prevalence of smoking and a lower rate of quitting smoking successfully than do people without such problems.

We will examine how the determinants of stopping and resuming smoking have influenced the content of formal treatments and their long-term effectiveness. Before we get to that, there is the question of whether formal treatments of cigarette smoking are needed.

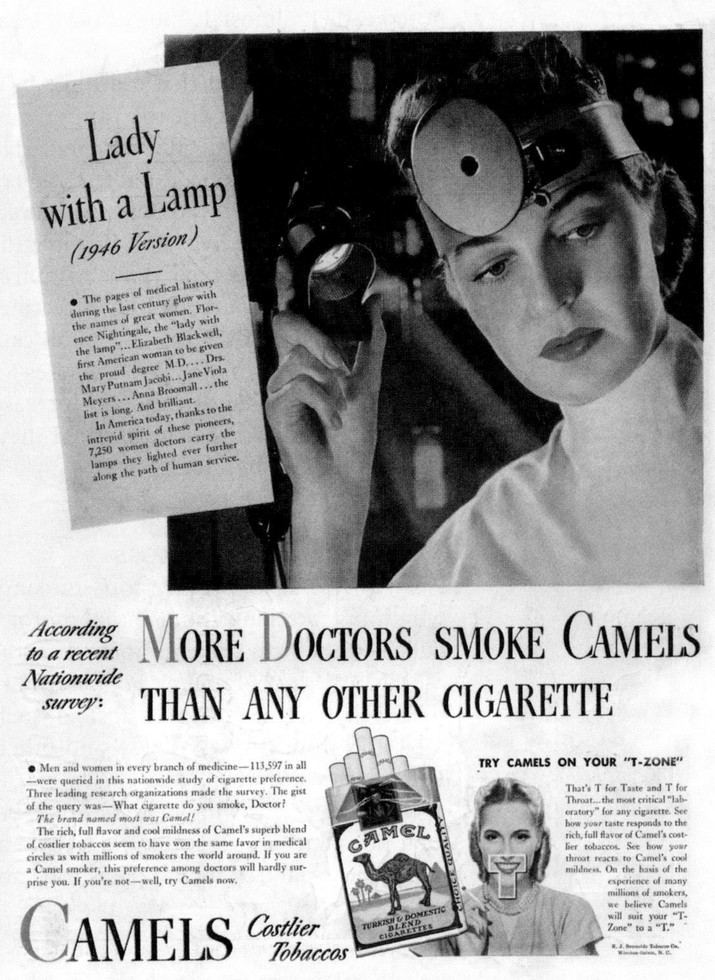

Apic/Getty images

The health message of this 1930s advertisement stands in stark contrast to current thinking.

The Necessity of Formal Treatment

The survey studies we cited earlier in this chapter show the decline in smoking rates among U.S. adults beginning in the 1960s. About half of the living adults who have said they smoked have quit (USDHHS, 1989; Wray et al., 1998). We noted that most of these people stopped smoking on their own. This raises the question of whether formal treatments for smoking are necessary.

In answering this question, we must consider several points. Although most people stop smoking without help, they tend to succeed only after multiple attempts. Perhaps you have heard the comment attributed to Mark Twain: "Quitting smoking is easy; I've done it many times." Indeed, with or without formal treatment, success at stopping smoking is more likely with more previous tries at quitting. Another important statistic, which we discuss in more detail in Chapter 15, is the rate of "spontaneous remission." Briefly, this refers to the rate of "cure" (in other words, stopping smoking) during a given time period without any formal treatment. Although data on spontaneous remission are basic to evaluating treatment effectiveness, they unfortunately are extremely hard to collect. For cigarette smoking, Abrams and Wilson (1986) estimated that the rate of spontaneous remission ranges from 3% to 14%. Formal treatments have to do better than that rate to prove their worth.

> *"To smoke or not to smoke: I can make either a life work."*
>
> Mignon McLaughlin, *The Neurotic's Notebook*, 1960

Another set of statistics to consider in deciding whether formal treatments of smoking are necessary are the economic and social costs of cigarette smoking: Earlier, we cited the figure $194 billion in the United States in 2004. This figure does not begin to reflect the human suffering of patients and their families that goes with contracting cancer, heart disease, and other diseases associated with chronic tobacco use. Also noted earlier, almost 1,200 people die each day.

Add to this the finding of a 1991 study of men and women in three different communities that showed that quitting smoking, even at a later age, prolongs life. The increased longevity is due to a quick reduction in the risk of major smoking-influenced illnesses (LaCroix et al., 1991). Similarly, Anthonisen et al. (2005) reported the findings from a follow-up of adult smokers with chronic obstructive pulmonary (lung) disease who had received intensive smoking cessation therapy 14.5 years earlier. The results showed that over 21% of the individuals who had received smoking cessation treatment sustained their status as nonsmokers, compared to about 5% of the individuals who had not received the treatment. Moreover, the percentages of individuals who had died at 14.5 years from all causes were significantly lower in the smoking treatment group compared to the rates for the group without treatment. Therefore, it seems that if smoking treatments increase the rate of smoking cessation compared to what people do on their own, then they would be more than worth their cost. We return to this point later.

Treatment Effectiveness

Programs to help people stop smoking focus on controlling nicotine withdrawal symptoms, breaking the habitual motor behavior involved in smoking, and learning skills to cope with the emotions, thoughts, and situations in which smokers say they use cigarettes to help them. People who stop smoking permanently have learned these skills well; have incentives to abstain, such as poor health; and have help in staying off cigarettes from family, friends, and others who care about them (Abrams & Wilson, 1986; Jones, 1987b).

Smoking cessation approaches may be classified into two main categories: behavioral programs and nicotine replacement therapies. Regardless of the type of treatment, the usual treatment goal is total abstinence from nicotine.

Behavioral Programs

Behavioral programs to stop smoking have changed in major ways in the last 10 years. Formerly, these programs involved ongoing, direct, often weekly contact with clinical staff in an individual or group format for a period of two or three months. The primary aims of these programs were to teach smokers to identify situations that presented a "high risk" for them to smoke, to apply techniques to weaken the habit components of smoking, to teach smokers competing (with smoking) coping responses in high-risk situations, and to teach smokers to self-monitor their smoking behavior (National Institute on Drug Abuse, 2002b).

Traditional behavioral programs still are offered and may be especially suited to more severely dependent smokers. However, the format, intensity, and duration of behavioral smoking cessation programs all have expanded from their original version in recent years. For example, behavioral programs may involve direct contact with professional staff, or they may involve telephone contact or the use of computer programs and the use of written materials. In addition, contact time may be limited to once or twice, with additional consultation as needed, or it may be more extended. Regardless of these variations, the aims of behavioral programs have stayed the same. Overall, participation in behavioral programs is an effective way to stop smoking (Hughes et al., 1999; National Institute on Drug Abuse, 2002b). It is incorporated in the American Psychiatric Association's guidelines for the treatment of cigarette smoking.

Nicotine Replacement Therapies

Although behavioral programs are effective relative to "placebo" or standard care comparison treatments, the majority of individuals who complete such programs resume smoking after six months to one year (Shiffman, 1993). This problem of relapse has been attributed to the cravings that smokers experience when they abstain from smoking or from other ways of ingesting nicotine (Naqvi et al., 2007).

"Nicotine patches are great. Stick one over each eye and you can't find your cigarettes."

Anonymous

To the extent that craving is due to physical withdrawal, a person would have a better chance of quitting for good if nicotine could somehow be used in the treatment of smoking. Based on this possibility, there has been major growth in the use of what are called nicotine replacement therapies (NRTs). These treatments involve administering nicotine to smokers as part of the effort to help them stop smoking. The vehicles of nicotine replacement that have been studied are nicotine gum, the nicotine patch, nicotine nasal spray, nicotine inhaler, and nicotine lozenges (Department of Health and Human Services, 2008; Hajek et al., 1999; Hughes et al., 1999).

"I'm telling you I wanted a cigarette so bad, I cried. I was so nervous I could hardly carry on at work, and I couldn't hide it. After a while I would just shake. People said they couldn't see it, but I could feel it."

Person trying to stay off cigarettes (Krogh, 1991, p. 71)

The growing literature on clinical trials of nicotine replacement therapies leads to the following conclusions (Hajek et al., 1999; Hughes et al., 1999; National Institute on Drug Abuse, 2002b): First, each of the nicotine replacement therapies raises the chances of quitting smoking by a factor of 2, compared to placebo. Second, the research that has compared different NRTs shows no differences in their effectiveness. Third, smokers may have initial preferences for one replacement therapy over another, but typically they come to adapt to the one that they are using. Fourth, combining NRTs with behavioral programs enhances the quit rates that typically are achieved by either type of treatment alone. The parts of behavioral programs that are particularly important, skills building and social support, make sense in view of our earlier comments on some of the characteristics of individuals who are able to stop smoking and refrain from restarting. Finally, there is little evidence of long-term negative consequences of the use of NRTs, assuming they are used as intended. The general effectiveness of these therapies led to the Federal Drug Administration's approval of the five nicotine replacement medications listed earlier for helping people quit smoking cigarettes, two by prescription of a medical provider and three (patches, gum, and lozenges) available over the counter (as opposed to prescribed by a medical provider).

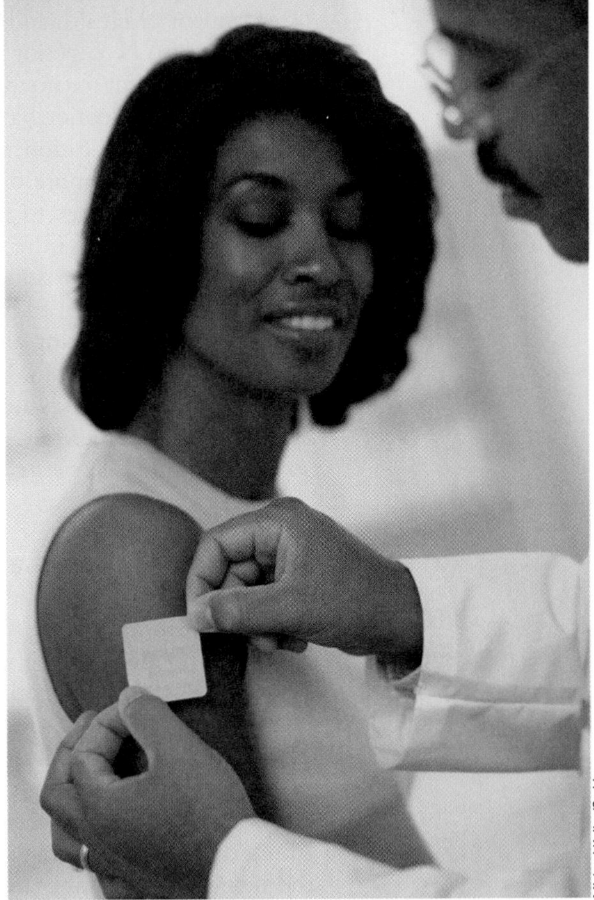

Michael Keller/Corbis

The nicotine patch is a popular type of nicotine replacement therapy.

The finding that combining behavioral and nicotine replacement treatments leads to the best outcomes raises important points about nicotine replacement treatment. Why a person experiences drug craving is extremely complex and is not just dependent on biological factors such as physical withdrawal. Craving also is a result of psychological, social, and environmental factors. In this context, it is not startling that craving for a cigarette may be reduced only to a limited degree as a result of NRT (Rose, 1991). Behavioral programs complement nicotine replacement by addressing facets of smoking behavior that administration of nicotine cannot. Behavioral programs help people to cope better with the factors that encourage them to continue to smoke or to resume smoking after stopping. Examples of these factors are social pressure to smoke, general environmental cues that are strongly associated with smoking, and psychological states like stress and frustration (Lichtenstein, 1982). As we discussed earlier, people with mental disorders may be especially vulnerable to the nonpharmacological aspects of smoking as well as to nicotine's actions on the body that may help to alleviate their psychiatric symptoms. Furthermore, Perkins's (1996) review suggests that women may have a more difficult time quitting smoking than men do, and one hypothesis is that factors other than nicotine more strongly affect their smoking . The results of a review by Cepada-Benito, Reynoso, and Erath (2004) are consistent with this hypothesis. This review of studies of the effectiveness of NRTs showed that, for men, NRTs with "low-intensity" behavioral support were effective in reducing or stopping smoking throughout the follow-up period (12 months). However, for women, NRTs with low-intensive support tended to be effective only in the short term (3 or 6 months following treatment). However, longer-term effectiveness of NRT for women tended to require more intensive behavioral support. These findings accentuate the importance of giving smokers ways other than nicotine to cope with feelings and situations that are powerfully connected to smoking.

We should add two FDA-approved pharmacological treatments for smoking that do not work by replacing nicotine: the antidepressant drug bupropion and varenicline (Department of Health and Human Services, 2008). Clinical trials have shown these medications to be superior to placebo in treating adults with nicotine dependence, and they are useful for nonpregnant individuals who request a pharmacological treatment that is not nicotine based. It is important to note that although bupropion is an antidepressant medication, and we mentioned earlier that individuals who are depressed may find it more difficult than others to stop smoking, the effectiveness of bupropion is not related to a history of depression (Lingford-Hughes, Welch, & Nutt, 2004). In this regard, other antidepressant medications, such as fluoxetine (Prozac), have been tested as a treatment for nicotine dependence but have not been shown to be effective. In contrast to buproprion, varenicline is a drug developed specifically for the treatment of smoking and works by competing with nicotine in binding to nicotine receptors in the brain. Varenicline stimulates nicotine receptors as nicotine does, so that smoking cravings are assuaged. Furthermore, if smokers smoke while on varenicline, they feel reduced nicotine effects compared to when not on the medication so that smoking is less reinforcing.

Conclusions about the Treatment of Cigarette Smoking

Nicotine is a strongly reinforcing drug to humans and can be quickly addicting. Nicotine does have some "adaptive" acute effects, such as improved sensory and cognitive functioning, but most attention has been paid to the negative health consequences of chronic nicotine use through smoking cigarettes. As a result, the emphasis today is on how to stop people from using nicotine. The best way to do this is by continuing the information campaigns and other "macro-environmental" methods, such as banning smoking in public places, which have advanced the overall decline in the prevalence of smoking and other use of tobacco among U.S. adults. Along these lines, programs aimed at youth who have not begun to use tobacco are the best investments because tobacco use is hard to stop once started. Promising tobacco-use prevention programs are being developed, but a major counterforce is tobacco industry advertising. According to the Federal Trade Commission, in 2005, the major companies in the tobacco industry spent $13.1 billion on advertising campaigns. For both adolescents and adults, advertising strengthens the positive associations that go along with smoking and other tobacco use. This is why the U.S. government continues to try to impose greater restrictions on advertising by tobacco companies, as prominently reflected in the omnibus tobacco settlement.

One direction for the future is the continued expansion of smoking treatment formats. Such treatments are the best way to capture the widest segment of the population that smokes. For example, smoking quit lines are becoming an increasingly popular and cost-effective way to reach large numbers of people who want to stop smoking but do not want to or cannot afford to access the traditional health care system (Fiori, Keller, & Curry, 2007). Their popularity is evident by going to http://www.tobaccofreehamiltoncounty.org/healthcare/resources.html, to see quit lines available in several different states of the United States, as well as references for other kinds of resources to help people quit smoking. In addition, new treatments at work sites already have proved to be an effective way to help people stop smoking. Brief behavioral or nicotine replacement treatment also may be delivered to adolescents or adults in the primary (medical) care setting (Hollis et al., 2005). Future research should continue to refine and strengthen treatments for heavily dependent smokers. A combination of behavioral and pharmacological treatments seems to work best for these individuals. Improvements in treatment efficacy can be realized, for example, by discovering what combination of treatment components works best for different types of smokers. Along these lines, a study by Uhl et al. (2008) identified several genes that marked individuals who were successful versus unsuccessful in abstaining from smoking for up to 24 weeks after the respective "quit dates" of three different clinical trials of buproprion and nicotine replacement treatment. Data such as these give information about one characteristic of individuals who are likely or not likely to have successful outcomes if they are administered buproprion or one of the nicotine replacement therapies, respectively, to stop smoking. Finally, a percentage of people will probably simply not want to stop smoking. In this regard, considerably more good research with longer-term follow-ups of patients is needed, but data suggest that a reduction in smoking may have some health benefits and may even be a step toward quitting smoking entirely for some individuals (Hughes & Carpenter, 2006; Pisinger & Godtfredsen, 2007). Developing a less hazardous cigarette or other ways of delivering nicotine would be ways to ease the serious health consequences of chronic tobacco use. Cigarettes with reduced tar and nicotine dominate today's market, but this is only part of the answer because smokers compensate for the reduction to some degree by inhaling more deeply and by smoking more cigarettes. Smokeless tobacco products are a smoke-free but controversial way to reduce the harm of using nicotine. Such an approach qualifies as "harm reduction" (see Contemporary Issue Box 7.3) because, as we noted earlier, use of smokeless tobacco incurs lower risk of cancers developing and likely a much lower risk of developing heart disease. Yet, this approach is controversial because many fear it will not encourage people to stop the use of nicotine entirely and likely would result in their return to cigarette smoking because it is a more efficient way to deliver nicotine. Nevertheless, some preliminary evidence suggests such fears may be unfounded (Tilashalski, Rodu, & Cole, 2005). The main point to take away from this discussion is that creating and testing the effectiveness of new ways to help people to stop or reduce their smoking can only advance the health of the general public.

CONTEMPORARY ISSUE BOX 7.3

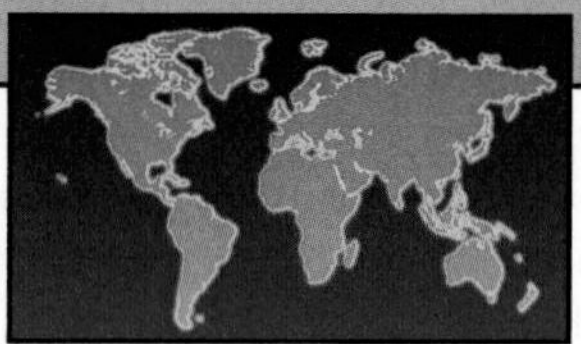

Harm Reduction and Nicotine Dependence

The traditional goal of treatments for cigarette smoking is zero tolerance for nicotine, or abstinence from any use of tobacco products. This is because most smokers have trouble maintaining a "moderate" level of cigarette consumption and because of the serious health hazards of smoking. However, the increasing availability and acceptability of nicotine replacement products, along with the continued relatively high prevalence of smoking among subgroups in society such as those who suffer from psychiatric disorders or those who are poorer and less educated, have raised the possibility of an alternative to zero tolerance called *harm reduction* (Hughes, 1996; Warner, Slade, & Sweanor, 1997). Harm-reduction approaches view as desirable any behavior change that results in the reduction, if not the elimination, of negative consequences associated with behaviors such as smoking. For those who find staying off nicotine extremely difficult or for those who do not want to, finding a safer way to ingest nicotine than cigarette smoking would be a positive step.

As you might have guessed, the nicotine replacement methods mentioned in this chapter are one way for individuals to ingest nicotine without exposing others or themselves to the toxic compounds in cigarette smoke.

Over the years, tobacco companies have pursued the smokeless path, with varying degrees of enthusiasm, in the form of inventing a "smokeless cigarette." Smokeless cigarettes have been designed to provide the nicotine and nondrug features of cigarette smoking without most or any of the toxic smoke. One of the more recent smokeless cigarettes to appear is RJR Nabisco's Eclipse, the test marketing of which began in the United States in 1996, and lasted for some time but with little success. Smokeless cigarettes traditionally have not caught on among smokers, but if the idea of harm reduction were more widely applied, then the tobacco industry would have greater incentive to continue trying to create a smokeless cigarette that is acceptable to the public. Along these lines, in 2001, the Liggett Group introduced a "lower-carcinogen" cigarette called the Omni. Like other attempts at creating a less harmful cigarette that smokers will buy, however, the Omni has had limited success. Most recently, the "electronic cigarette," was introduced and now (2009) is available for sale in several thousand retail outlets in the United States as well as on websites. Electronic cigarettes have been promoted as safer than traditional tobacco cigarettes, because tobacco is not burned as a vehicle for delivering nicotine to the body by inhalation. Instead, a battery in a holder shaped like a cigarette heats a solution of nicotine in propylene glycol and produces a fine mist that is inhaled for nicotine delivery to the lungs. The Electronic Cigarette Association estimates that sales of electronic cigarettes have grown from $10 million to $100 million in the United States between 2008 and 2009, presumably on the premise that electronic cigarettes are less of a health hazard than are tobacco cigarettes. Although there is essentially no research on the relative risks of longer-term use of electronic cigarettes, in July 2009, the FDA released a draft report of its analyses of 19 variations of electronic cigarettes that revealed that half of the brands contained nitrosamines, cancer-causing agents found in traditional cigarettes, and that a number of the brands contained diethylene glycol, an ingredient of antifreeze. Such findings deflate the idea that electronic cigarettes are safe.

The tobacco companies also have looked at tobacco products that are not cigarettes as "safer" alternatives to traditional cigarettes. Our earlier review of smokeless tobacco products suggests that they pose a lower health risk than do cigarettes but that they are hardly risk-free. Another smokeless tobacco product that has been prevalent in Sweden for 200 years and that has seen a revival in the last 20 years because of its purported lower risk to health is snus (rhymes with "loose"). Snus is moist, ground tobacco that is placed between the gum and the cheek, but it does not require spitting like chew tobacco. Tobacco companies recently have moved to test-market snus in the United States because of its great success as a "harm reduction" product in Sweden. Unfortunately, again, there are little scientific data about snus; a recent clinical trial suggests that its use is associated with higher risk of pancreatic cancer but not with oral and lung cancers as cigarettes are. Snus also delivers a potent dose of nicotine.

The harm-reduction approach to cigarette smoking is highly controversial among health professionals and other groups concerned with the consequences of cigarette smoking. Harm reduction has implications not only for nicotine use among individuals already addicted to this drug, but also for those who are not yet dependent. What do you see as the overall advantages and disadvantages of the zero-tolerance and harm-reduction approaches to changing behaviors of cigarette smoking?

Summary

- Nicotine occurs naturally in only one source: the tobacco plant. The major commercial tobacco products are cigarettes, cigars, snuff, chewing tobacco, and pipe tobacco.
- Western Europeans discovered tobacco when they saw Native Americans in the New World smoking dried tobacco leaves. The Europeans seized the idea and spread it throughout Europe and Asia.
- Until about 1860, tobacco was widely believed to have medicinal properties. Nicotine's "medical cover" was blown when it was isolated in 1828, and shown to have addictive properties.
- Cigarette smoking is the most popular way to use tobacco.
- The prevalence of smoking among U.S. adults began to decline in 1965, and continued on that trend for the rest of the 20th century. A major reduction in the number of current smokers and an increase in the number of former smokers seem to be related to the U.S. Surgeon General's 1964 report, and subsequent publications, on the negative health consequences of cigarette smoking.
- Trends in the overall prevalence of smoking vary according to age, gender, racial/ethnic identity, education, and employment status.
- Overall, from 1990 to 1999, smoking initiation among 12- to 17-year-olds increased 12.8%, but the rate of smoking initiation among teens decreased in the last five years of that decade.
- The use of smokeless tobacco products among youths is a concern. The disparity in prevalence between men and women is extremely large.
- Nicotine is a cholinergic agonist that has biphasic (stimulant and depressant) action.
- Nicotine can be absorbed transdermally through the oral, buccal, and nasal mucosa; the gastrointestinal tract; and the lungs.
- By inhalation, nicotine in tobacco smoke reaches the brain in seven seconds. Brain levels thus rise rapidly, but then they fall rapidly because nicotine is quickly distributed to other sites of action. Nicotine is metabolized primarily in the liver and eliminated mostly in urine.
- Functional tolerance to nicotine's effects is acquired quickly. Dispositional tolerance to nicotine also seems to develop.
- Nicotine induces physical dependence. In 1988, the U.S. Office of the Surgeon General's issued a report with the conclusion that nicotine is a physically addicting drug.
- Nicotine's acute effects involve the CNS and ANS. It tends to have stimulant effects at lower doses but more depressant effects at higher doses.
- Despite its classification as a stimulant, users often perceive nicotine as having calming, relaxing effects.
- Nicotine's suppressant effect on body weight is an important motivation for smoking, especially in women.
- Pharmacological, psychological, and social/environmental factors combine to make nicotine a drug with high dependence liability. The major motivator in continuing tobacco use is nicotine.
- Smoking kills because of the smoker's chronic exposure to carbon monoxide, tar, and nicotine in tobacco smoke.
- Cigarettes with reduced tar and nicotine levels are not "healthier" because smokers make up for the reduction either by smoking more cigarettes or by inhaling them more deeply.
- Major diseases linked to smoking are heart disease, chronic obstructive lung disease, and cancers of various types.
- In the last three decades, women have had rates of smoking-related diseases similar to those of men. Some smoking-related health risks are unique to women.
- Because of the negative health consequences of passive smoking, there has been an increase in banning and restricting smoking in public places.
- Smoking treatment programs focus on stopping nicotine-withdrawal symptoms, breaking the behavioral or habit part of smoking, and teaching stress-reduction skills.
- In general, treatment approaches may be classified into two main types: behavioral programs and nicotine replacement therapies.

- Quitting smoking is one thing; "staying quit" is another.
- A high rate of relapse follows smoking treatment.
- A major reason for relapse is that smokers continue to crave nicotine long after they have stopped smoking.
- Nicotine replacement treatments and other pharmacotherapies for cigarette smoking seem to be most effective when used in combination with behavioral treatments, especially for heavily dependent smokers.

Answers to "What Do You Think?"

1. Tobacco was once thought to have major medical value.
  T *From the time of Columbus until about 1860, tobacco was widely thought to be a panacea for medical problems.*

2. Throughout the age ranges, men have higher smoking rates than women do.
  F *Rates are higher for men in the 18- to 25-year-old range and (less so) among those 26 and older. Rates for boys and girls in the 12- to 17-year-old range differ little.*

3. The prevalence of smokeless tobacco use among men is about three times that of use among women.
  F *The discrepancy is almost 16-fold; men use smokeless tobacco products far more than women do.*

4. Nicotine can be considered both a stimulant and a depressant.
  T *Nicotine is called a biphasic drug because it tends to act as a stimulant at lower doses, but it acts as a depressant at higher doses.*

5. When using commercial tobacco products, people reach the peak blood level of nicotine most quickly by using smokeless tobacco.
  F *The quickest way to reach the peak blood level for a dose of nicotine is by inhalation or smoking.*

6. Though psychological dependence is common, no cases of physical dependence on nicotine have been identified.
  F *Nicotine has been identified clearly as a drug on which users can become physically dependent.*

7. Nicotine's calming effects are a main reason for its use.
  T *Even at doses associated with stimulant action in the body, users often perceive nicotine to have calming effects. Such effects are identified as major reasons for continuing to use nicotine.*

8. Nicotine plays a secondary role to learning and social factors in maintaining tobacco use.
  F *Nicotine plays a substantial, and some think a major, role; learning and social factors are important too.*

9. Health damage from cigarette smoking cost the U.S. economy about $25 billion in 2004.
  F *The health care cost estimate is $193 billion.*

10. Low-tar, low-nicotine cigarettes are less damaging to health than cigarettes that do not have reduced tar and nicotine content.
  F *Although theoretically this is true, in practice, smokers tend to increase the intensity of inhaling or the number of cigarettes when they smoke cigarettes of reduced tar and nicotine content. Therefore, exposure to these compounds is similar to what it would be with cigarettes of unreduced content.*

11. Despite the media hype, passive smoking actually poses a serious health risk to few Americans.
  F *One review in 1991, which more recent data has supported, estimated that passive smoking in households kills about 53,000 Americans every year, mostly due to heart disease.*

12. A large portion of ex-smokers quit on their own.
  T *Many people who quit smoking do so on their own after three or four tries. Self-quitters are thought to have been "lighter" smokers.*

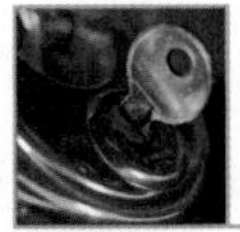

Key Terms

emphysema **nicotine poisoning** **relapse**

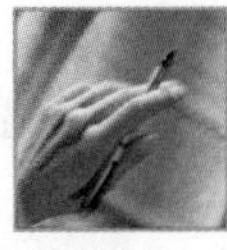

Essays/Thought Questions

1. Considering that adults in the lower socioeconomic classes have a disproportionately high rate of smoking, what do you think about the equity of the high tax rates that the federal and local governments impose on tobacco products? For example, as of this writing, a pack of cigarettes in New York City costs in the neighborhood of $10.
2. Nicotine's dependence liability is high, and how its chronic use affects health is widely known. Why, then, do you think that use of this drug remains legal in much of the world?
3. Based on our knowledge about the effects of secondhand smoke, would a total ban on smoking cigarettes in public places violate the individual's rights and freedoms in the United States?
4. In June 2009, President Obama signed landmark legislation passed by both houses of Congress that gives the U.S. Food and Drug Administration the authority to regulate tobacco products. Why do you think that this legislation is considered historic in the United States? If the FDA approached you for advice, what would your priorities be for the regulation of tobacco products? Why?

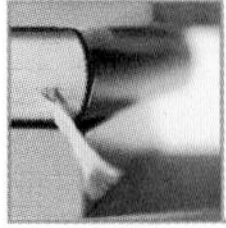

Suggested Readings

Brecher, E. M. (1972). *Licit and illicit drugs*. Mount Vernon, NY: Consumers Union.

Cotton, P. (1993). Low tar cigarettes come under fire. *Journal of the American Medical Association, 270,* 1399.

Fiori, M. C., Keller, P. A., & Curry, S. J. (2007). Health system changes to facilitate the delivery of tobacco dependence treatment. *American Journal of Preventive Medicine*, 33, S349–S356.

U.S. Department of Health and Human Services. (2008). *Treating tobacco use and dependence*. Clinical practice guideline. Rockville, MD: Author.

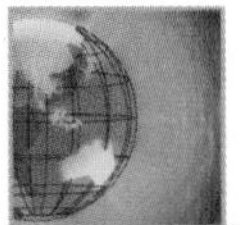

Web Resources

Visit the Book Companion Website at www.cengage.com/psychology/maisto to access study tools including a glossary, flashcards, and web quizzing. You will also find links to the following resources:

- Quitnet: This site is dedicated to providing information and resources to help people stop smoking.
- Tobacco Control Supersite: This website contains links that provide extensive information on a large number of topics relating to tobacco use in the United States, Canada, Australia, England, and other countries.
- U.S. Centers for Disease Control and Prevention: This link offers a wealth of current research and other information on smoking and other major public health problems.

CHAPTER 8

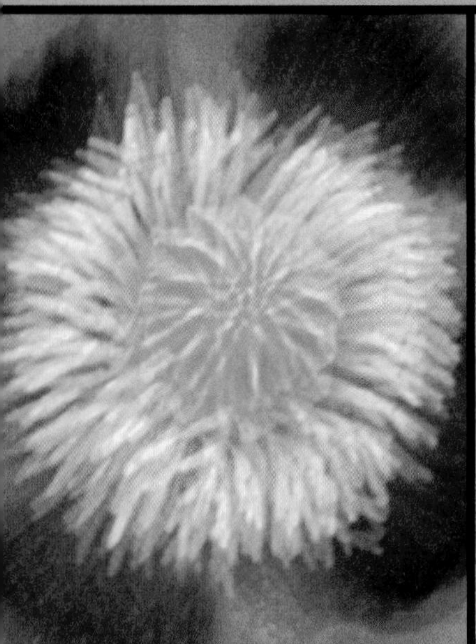
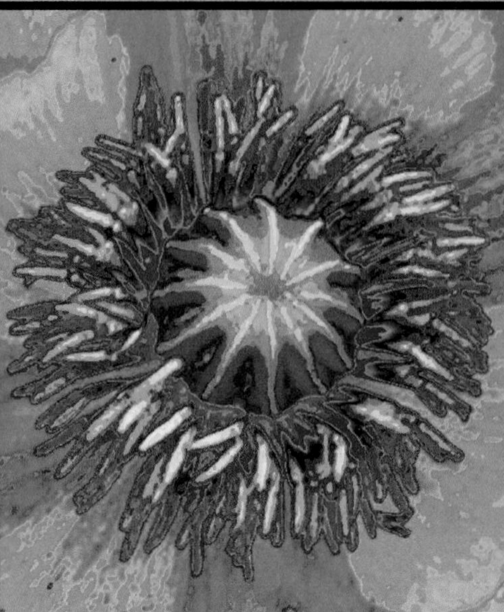
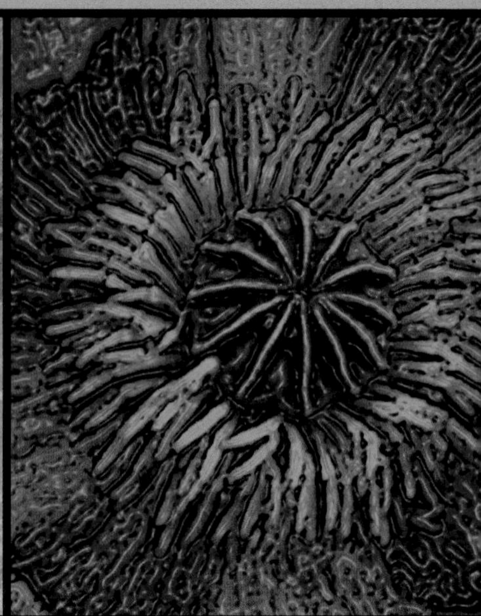

Caffeine

What Do You Think? True or False?

Answers are given at the end of the chapter.

___ 1. About half the world's population consumes caffeine regularly.

___ 2. There are major subgroup differences in caffeine use in the United States.

___ 3. In dose of caffeine consumed, young children have the highest exposure to caffeine, after adults 18 years and older.

___ 4. Caffeine is a drug that, when consumed, is distributed equally throughout the body.

___ 5. Smokers tend to metabolize caffeine more slowly than do nonsmokers.

___ 6. So many people use coffee and tea without apparent difficulty that people obviously do not become physically dependent on caffeine.

___ 7. Caffeine's stimulant effects seem to be reinforcing in humans.

___ 8. There is evidence that people can get intoxicated on caffeine.

___ 9. Caffeine crosses the placenta and poses a danger to the health of a fetus.

___10. Overall, caffeine seems to be a safe drug for everybody.

___11. Caffeine has little medical value.

___12. Caffeine's long-term effects on children are well understood.

Caffeine, theophylline, and theobromine are three chemically related compounds that occur naturally in more than 60 species of plants. These compounds are called the methylxanthines and are classified as alkaloids. An alkaloid is a compound that is of botanical origin, contains nitrogen, and is physiologically active (Levenson & Bick, 1977; Syed, 1976). Because of its overwhelming popularity, we emphasize caffeine in our discussion. This should not be taken to suggest that the other methylxanthine drugs are of no importance, however. Like caffeine, theophylline is a mild central nervous system (CNS) stimulant, although it is less active than caffeine. Theobromine is the least active of the three drugs as a CNS stimulant. Popular products that contain caffeine may also contain different amounts of the other methylxanthines. Tea contains theophylline, though in considerably smaller proportion than caffeine. Milk chocolate actually contains a higher proportion of theobromine than of caffeine. Table 8.1 gives the caffeine concentrations in coffee, tea, energy drinks, chocolate, and other foods and products.

We begin our review of caffeine by presenting the sources of caffeine and a brief history of its use. We then discuss current prevalence statistics. Following that, we describe caffeine's pharmacological action, development of tolerance to and physical dependence on caffeine, and caffeine's acute and chronic effects. We conclude with a review of some therapeutic uses of caffeine and other major methylxanthine drugs.

"Coffee is the common man's gold, and like gold, it brings to every man the feeling of luxury and nobility."

Abd-al-Kadir,
In Praise of Coffee (1587)

Sources of Caffeine

Most people take their caffeine orally, as is apparent in Table 8.1, which highlights the wide range of caffeine products that adults and children consume regularly. Compounds synthesized to treat some medical problems also contain caffeine, even though caffeine is not always of direct benefit in alleviating the problem symptoms. Table 8.1 does not present another source of caffeine—illicit street drugs (Gilbert, 1984). For example, over-the-counter pain medications such as Anacin and Excedrin contain caffeine and frequently are used as filler to adulterate street drugs like heroin and cocaine.

TABLE 8.1 Caffeine Concentration in Beverages, Energy Drinks, Foods, and Medications

Source	Caffeine Concentration (mg/oz)	Total Caffeine (mg)
Beverages		
Coffee, brewed (8 oz)	13.5	108
Coffee, drip (8 oz)	18	144
Coffee, instant (8 oz)	7	56
Coffee, espresso (1.5 oz)	51	77
Tea, brewed (8 oz)	6	48
Tea, green (8 oz)	3	24
Coca-Cola Classic (12 oz)	2.9	35
Pepsi-Cola (12 oz)	3.2	38
Mountain Dew (12 oz)	4.5	54
Dr. Pepper (12 oz)	3.4	41
Canada Dry Ginger Ale (12 oz)	0	0
Energy Drinks		
Red Bull (8.3 oz)	9.6	80
Monster (16 oz)	10	160
Rockstar (16 oz)	10	160
Full Throttle (16 oz)	9	144
No Fear (16 oz)	10.9	174
Amp (8.4 oz)	8.9	75
SoBe Adrenaline Rush (8.3 oz)	9.5	79
Tab Energy (10.5 oz)	9.1	95
Higher Caffeine Energy Drinks		
Wired X505 (24 oz)	21	505
Fixx (20 oz)	25	500
BooKoo Energy (24 oz)	15	360
Wired X344 (16 oz)	21.5	344
SPIKE Shooter (8.4 oz)	35.7	300
Cocaine Energy Drink (8.4 oz)	33.3	280
Jolt Cola (23.5 oz)	11.9	280
Lower Caffeine Energy Drinks		
Bomba Energy (8.4 oz)	8.9	75
Whoop Ass (8.5 oz)	5.9	50
High-Concentration Energy Drinks		
Ammo (1 oz)	171	171
Powershot (1 oz)	100	100
Foods		
Milk chocolate (1 oz)	6	6
Cooking chocolate (1 oz)	35	35
Prescription Medications (1 tablet)		
APCs (aspirin, phenacetin, caffeine)		32
Cafergot		100
Darvon Compound		32
Fiorinal		40
Migral		50
Over-the-Counter Preparations (1 tablet)		
Anacin		32
Aspirin		0
Tylenol		0
Cope, Easy-Mens, Midol		32

Vanquish	32
Excedrin	65
Pre-Mens	66
Dristan	30
Vivarin	200
No-Doz	100
No-Doz Maximum Strength	200
Dexatrim	200
Stay Awake	200
Ultra Pep-Back	200
Awake	100

Source: Adapted from multiple sources, including MedicineNet.com, the Vaults of Erowid (www.erowid.org), Energy Fiend (www.energyfiend.com), and Reissig, Strain, & Griffiths (2009).

History of Caffeine Use

The plants that contain the methylxanthines have been used to make popular beverages since ancient times. "Ancient" probably means at least back to the Stone Age (Rall, 1990a). Many stories, some mythical, attempt to explain how these beverages were created. For example, coffee supposedly was discovered in Arabia by a holy man. It seems that goats in a herd had been jumping around at night instead of sleeping, apparently because they had been nibbling on the beans of the coffee plant. The holy man got a brilliant idea that beans from the same plant could help him endure his long nights of prayer. It was a small next step to the first cup of coffee (Blum, 1984). Tea, on the other hand, supposedly dates back to 2737 B.C. Legend has it that Chinese Emperor Shen Nung was boiling water when the leaves from a nearby bush fell into the pot, producing the first pot of tea.

Table 8.1 shows that caffeine is found in some of our most popular beverages and foods. In Chapter 7, we noted that, during the time of Columbus, Europe knew nothing of these caffeine-containing substances. In fact, the only psychoactive substance that 15th-century Europeans did seem to know about was alcohol. All this changed with the ventures of the explorers and others from Europe. Explorers found coffee in Arabia, Turkey, and Ethiopia. In China, they found tea. In West Africa, they found the kola nut. In Mexico and much of Central and South America, they found the cacao plant, which is the source of chocolate. Other sources of teas were discovered in parts of North and South America. Travelers brought their discoveries home to Europe and then spread them across other continents.

Like other drugs, caffeine was not always well received by societies when it was introduced. For example, when the Mohammedans tried caffeine to stay awake during their long vigils, the orthodox priests were not pleased with the innovation. However, official punishments and attempts to kill coffee trees were not enough to stop coffee from becoming as popular among Arabian Moslems as tea is among the Chinese. Similar negative sanctions against coffee drinking in Egypt and Europe met with the same failure.

Caffeine, nicotine, and alcohol have been seen as having a greater effect on human civilization than all other nonmedical psychoactive substances combined (Levenson & Bick, 1977). Caffeine stands out among these three drugs because of its ubiquitous use around the world and because it is a "cradle-to-grave drug" (Kenny & Darragh, 1985, p. 278). That is, caffeine commonly is used nonmedically by young children and adults alike, which is true of no other psychoactive substance.

Prevalence of Caffeine Consumption

> *"... The coffee habit had become so strong, that the people continued, notwithstanding all prohibitions, to drink it in their own houses. ... [I]t was drunk in particular places, with the doors shut, or in the back rooms of some of the shopkeepers' houses."*
>
> 16th-century text (Greden & Walters, 1992, p. 358)

Good estimates of caffeine consumption around the world are not nearly as available as estimates for other drug use, even though caffeine use is more widespread (Barone & Roberts, 1996). Finding good worldwide estimates is difficult for several reasons. For one, due to the fact that people consume caffeine in many different products, they find it hard—say, in a survey—to provide accurate data on all their caffeine use over a given time period. The surveys that have been done are, accordingly, expensive to conduct and thus are limited in numbers of respondents. Furthermore, finding good caffeine consumption survey data outside of North America and Europe is hard (James, 1991). Collecting good estimates of caffeine consumption is also difficult because some products are prepared in ways that can differ the caffeine content. For example, coffee-brewing method affects caffeine content. The caffeine content is higher for boiled than for percolated coffee (D'Amicis & Viani, 1993).

Despite these problems, estimates of caffeine consumption have been derived, typically based on survey data or on a country's import figures for a given caffeine-containing product. The estimated average consumption of caffeine per capita worldwide is around 70 milligrams (mg) per day (Gilbert, 1984). However, countries vary considerably in per capita caffeine consumption and in the sources of that consumption. Table 8.2 shows per capita caffeine consumption estimates for a number of countries. In the United States, for example, people average nearly 170 mg per day of caffeine consumption, with the vast majority of that amount accounted for by coffee consumption. This figure is possibly on the rise: Using a national survey of food intake in the U.S. population, Frary, Johnson, and Wang (2005) found a per capita caffeine consumption rate of 193 mg per day. Although the U.S. per capita rate is well over double the worldwide per capita rate, the world's top per capita rates of caffeine consumption are the Scandinavian countries—Finland, Sweden, Denmark, and Norway—along with the Netherlands, which ranks number one at 414 mg per person per day, predominantly via coffee consumption.

Tea is the dominant source of caffeine in the United Kingdom, and the same is true for its close neighbor, Ireland. Kuwait and the United Arab Emirates also rank high on per capita caffeine consumption through their tea consumption. Brazil is the world's leading producer of coffee (more than 25% of the total), but its citizens' primary caffeine source is maté, a type of tea grown in South America (James, 1991).

Cocoa is produced primarily in Africa, but the world's biggest consumer (by overall volume) is the United States. Germany and Russia are the next nearest consumers by overall volume, at less than one-third the amount of the United States (Fredholm et al., 1999). Looking at per capita caffeine consumption via cocoa, the highest rate is reported by Denmark, at 21 mg per person per day. Switzerland, a country often

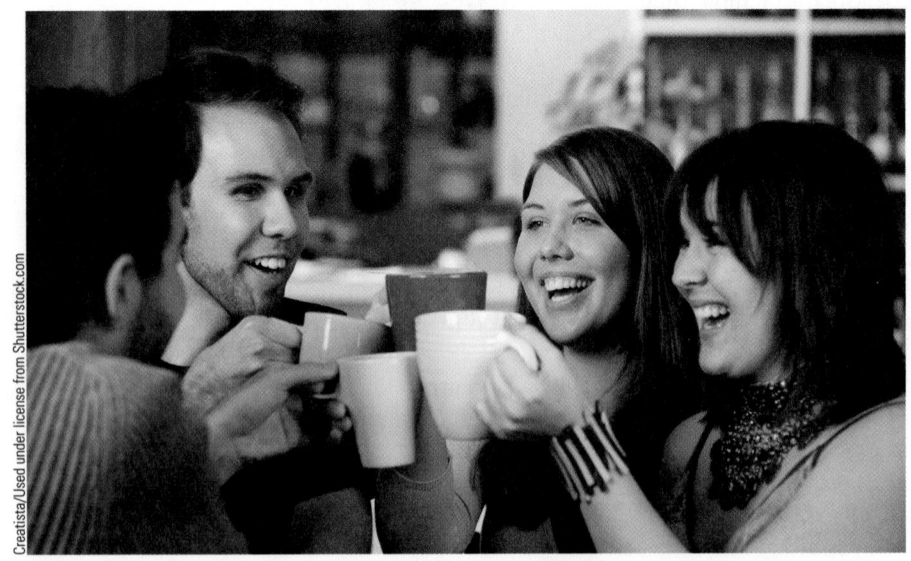

Coffee is the most popular source of caffeine in the United States.

associated with chocolate, has a very low rate of caffeine consumption through cocoa (approximately 1 mg per person per day).

Since the early 1980s, the level of caffeinated coffee consumption has risen only slightly. Therefore, whatever decline in caffeine consumption may have occurred from drinking less caffeinated coffee was compensated for to some degree by drinking more soft drinks. The contribution of soft drinks to total caffeine consumption is significant: One study showed that, in 1962, one-third of the population said they had consumed soft drinks the day before, but currently, around two-thirds said they had. Nevertheless, it will be important in future surveys on caffeine consumption to focus greater attention to soft drink and energy drink consumption so as to obtain the most accurate estimates. For example, the Frary, Johnson, and Wang (2005) study mentioned earlier included the contribution of soft drink consumption to their estimates of per capita caffeine consumption and found a rate of 193 mg per person per day, 25 mg per person per day higher than the rate provided in Table 8.2.

Caffeine consumption does not vary much in the United States among different subgroups of the population. One exception is age. Caffeine consumption increases

TABLE 8.2 General Estimates of Caffeine Use from around the World

	(in mg/person/day)			
Country	**Caffeine from Coffee**	**Caffeine from Tea**	**Caffeine from Cocoa**	**Caffeine from All These Sources**
Argentina	43	1	5	49
Australia	202	29	0	232
Brazil	26	1	4	31
Canada	180	18	12	210
Denmark	354	15	21	390
Egypt	5	53	1	58
Finland	322	6	1	329
France	215	8	16	239
Germany	292	9	12	313
India	1	26	0	27
Ireland	81	127	5	213
Kuwait	49	112	13	173
Netherlands	369	38	6	414
Nigeria	1	2	1	4
Norway	379	8	13	400
Paraguay	51	1	3	55
Poland	100	33	8	141
Russian Federation	26	40	7	72
Saudi Arabia	14	13	2	28
South Africa	15	23	1	40
Sweden	388	12	7	407
Switzerland	275	11	1	288
United Arab Emirates	74	87	5	167
United Kingdom	92	96	14	202
United States	143	12	12	168
Venezuela	135	0	4	139

Not included in this table is caffeine consumption from maté, a tealike beverage consumed mainly in several South American countries. It is prepared by steeping dried leaves of the yerba maté plant in hot water. With regards to the listed estimates of caffeine consumption, the following amounts should be added for the following countries: Argentina, 52 mgs/person/day; Brazil, 10 mgs/person/day; and Paraguay, 101 mgs/person/day.

Source: Adapted from Fredholm et al. (1999), p. 85.

CONTEMPORARY ISSUE BOX 8.1

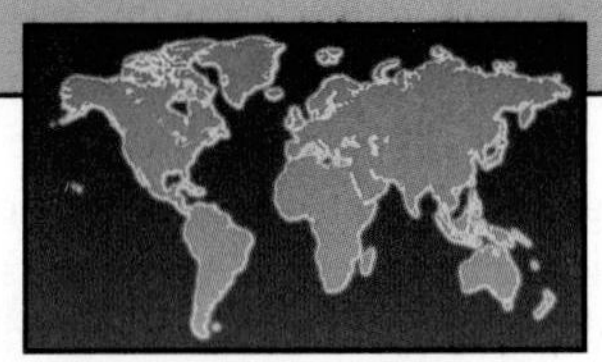

Caffeine and Children

Studies show that children all over the world regularly consume pharmacologically active amounts of caffeine. This pattern of use combines with our knowledge about the high degree of caffeine exposure in young children (because of their lower body weights) to raise serious concerns about children's use of caffeine. Despite the potential seriousness of this problem, little is known about caffeine effects in children (Hughes & Hale, 1998; Temple, 2009). What research is available suggests that children are not more or less sensitive than adults to caffeine's action in the body (James, 1991).

Children's use of caffeine is a major concern for two reasons. First, caffeine is very popular among young people, as reflected in the surge in children's consumption of "high-energy" (high-caffeine) beverages. Goldstein and Wallace's (1997) exploratory study provided evidence for what may be a caffeine withdrawal syndrome in children (ages 11 to 12). The children's major source of caffeine was soft drinks. Second, caffeine exposure in children is high compared to that of adults. In addition, little is known about the long-term effects of children's caffeine use.

Given these circumstances, would you, for example, require soft drink or candy makers to eliminate caffeine from their products? Children are major consumers of caffeine-containing soft drinks and chocolate. Would you require warning or caution labels on caffeine products, as are required for tobacco products and alcoholic beverages? Why or why not?

"Coffee leads men to trifle away their time, scald their chops, and spend their money, all for a little base, black, thick, nasty, bitter, stinking nauseous puddle water."

The Women's Petition Against Coffee, 1674

with age, until the elderly years (65 and older), when it declines somewhat (Barone & Roberts, 1996; Frary, Johnson, & Wang, 2005). However, for "dose" of caffeine consumed, which takes into account body weight (see Chapter 4), children aged 1 to 5 have the highest exposure to caffeine after adults aged 18 and older (Greden & Walters, 1992). Coffee is the major source of caffeine for adults, and soft drinks are the major source for children and adolescents (Frary, Johnson, & Wang, 2005) (see also Contemporary Issue Box 8.1).

In summary, people of all races and social classes worldwide consume caffeine. Estimates are that about 90% of the world's population regularly consumes products that contain caffeine, with coffee, tea, and soft drinks being the most common sources (James, 1991). Trends in recent years in overall caffeine use are difficult to specify because of the measurement problems we referred to earlier, along with limited attention to the consumption of products such as soft drinks, energy drinks, caffeinated water, and caffeine-containing herbal supplements. Nevertheless, there is no question that caffeine is the world's most preferred drug.

Pharmacology of Caffeine

Sites of Action

For many years, caffeine's effects were thought to be a result of the drug's inhibition of the enzyme phosphodiesterase. However, the phosphodiesterase theory fell out of favor following the realization that caffeine acts only at doses much higher than the typical dose required for pharmacological effects in humans, which is about 200 milligrams (Snyder & Sklar, 1984). The explanation for caffeine's acute effects most accepted now is the adenosine hypothesis (Daly & Fredholm, 2004; Fisone, Borgkvist, & Usiello, 2004). Adenosine is a chemical that the body produces; it is an inhibitory neurotransmitter (see Chapter 3). Adenosine receptors are in the central and peripheral nervous systems. Adenosine leads to behavioral sedation, regulation of oxygen delivery to cells, dilation of cerebral and coronary blood vessels, and production of asthma

(Julien, 1996). Caffeine and the other methylxanthines occupy adenosine receptors and then block the action of that transmitter.

Pharmacokinetics

Absorption

Caffeine is rapidly absorbed from the gastrointestinal tract. The drug quickly reaches the brain because it can pass through the blood-brain barrier. The half-life of caffeine in the blood varies widely among people and ranges from about 2½ to 7½ hours (Blum, 1984; Julien, 1998; Leonard, Watson, & Mohs, 1987; Lorist & Tops, 2003). Peak levels of caffeine occur 15 to 45 minutes after the drug is taken and sometimes depend on the source (Snel, Tieges, & Lorist, 2004). For example, one study (Marks & Kelly, 1973) involved three healthy men who were given an average of 155 milligrams of caffeine in the form of Coca-Cola, tea, or coffee. The men's plasma levels of caffeine were then charted for two hours. The peak levels of caffeine were higher for tea and coffee and were reached within 30 minutes of ingestion. The peak for Coca-Cola was lower and did not occur for about an hour. After two hours, the plasma level of caffeine for the cola was higher than for tea or coffee and was still at a level comparable to its peak. In a later study of 13 individuals who averaged more than 450 milligrams of caffeine consumption a day, however, no differences in peak caffeine level reached or in time to reach peak level were found among coffee, cola drinks, and caffeine capsules (Liguori, Hughes, & Grass, 1997).

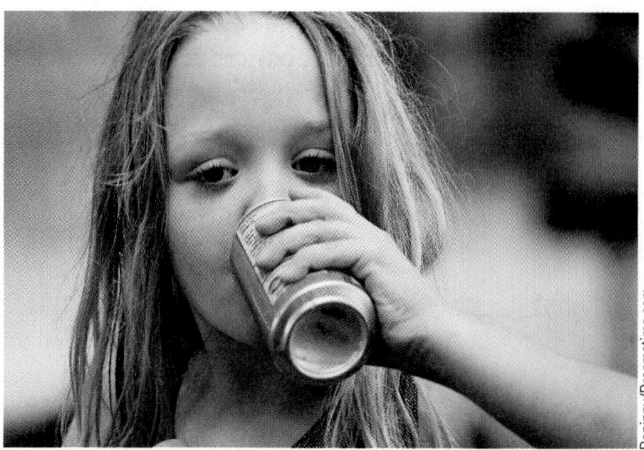
Doninny/Dreamstime.com

Children 1 to 5 years of age have the highest exposure to caffeine by dose, next to adults aged 18 and older.

Distribution

Caffeine is equally distributed in total body water and freely crosses the placenta to the fetus (Julien, 1998). Therefore, after consumption, the concentration of caffeine is similar throughout the body.

Metabolism and Excretion

The liver does most of the metabolizing of caffeine. The drug is excreted almost entirely by the kidneys—less than 10% in pure form and the rest in metabolites. Very small proportions of caffeine are also excreted in feces, saliva, semen, and breast milk. Of interest is the variance among people in caffeine metabolism and excretion from the body. For example, the rates of these processes are slower in people who have been using caffeine over a shorter period of time (Leonard, Watson, & Mohs, 1987). Other differences in metabolism and excretion are caused by liver disease (it slows the process), pregnancy (slows), and use of oral contraceptives (slows). On the other hand, those who smoke cigarettes metabolize caffeine more quickly (Julien, 1998). One study showed that ex-smokers' blood levels of caffeine more than doubled from what they were when they drank the same amount of coffee before they quit smoking (Benowitz, Hall, & Modin, 1989). Other therapeutic drugs interact with caffeine to increase or decrease its metabolism and excretion.

Tolerance and Dependence

Caffeine long was considered a strange drug because of its unorthodox potential for inducing tolerance and physical dependence (Gilbert, 1976). Evidence of a distinct caffeine withdrawal syndrome has been available for some time; indeed, an individual's pattern of using caffeine can meet the DSM-IV criteria for drug dependence that we described in Chapter 1 (Strain et al., 1994). The evidence for tolerance to caffeine is far less clear, however. The usual picture for drugs is the reverse: They can induce tolerance without dependence but rarely dependence without tolerance.

Caffeine Withdrawal

The caffeine withdrawal symptoms most consistently reported are headache and fatigue (Juliano & Griffiths, 2001). Other withdrawal symptoms have been documented in studies by Goldstein, Kaizer, & Whitby (1969), and are summarized in reviews by Dews, O'Brian, and Bergman (2002) and Juliano and Griffiths (2004). Their subjects reported symptoms of caffeine abstinence that included depression, decreased alertness, less contentment and relaxed mood, decreased activity and energy, greater sleepiness and drowsiness, and increased irritability. These findings have been replicated in experimental studies (Evans & Griffiths, 1999). Furthermore, these experiments show that physical dependence can develop with an exposure of 300 milligrams of caffeine a day for only three consecutive days. Withdrawal symptoms can range from mild to severe and begin within 12 to 24 hours of cessation of caffeine use (Comer et al., 1997; Nehlig, 2004). They may last about a week (Griffiths & Woodson, 1988a; Hughes et al., 1992). A large survey of people who ingest caffeine on a daily basis found that 11% report withdrawal symptoms upon cessation of caffeine use (Dews et al., 1999).

Tolerance

The contradictions about tolerance to caffeine that abound in the experimental findings are probably a result of poor research methods, such as not specifying caffeine use patterns in subjects (Curatolo & Robertson, 1983). In general, tolerance probably does develop to caffeine's effects on renal function, sleep, and other physiological functions, such as blood pressure and heart rate. On the other hand, little tolerance seems to develop to caffeine's stimulant effects (Hogan, Hornick, & Bouchoux, 2002).

Confusion about caffeine tolerance also results from ignoring differences among people in what is an "acceptable" level of caffeine. Differences between high- and low-caffeine users in the acute effects of a dose of caffeine in children and adults have been attributed to differences in the degree of acquired tolerance. However, some better-controlled studies offer another explanation: One reason people are heavier or lighter caffeine users is their individual ability to tolerate caffeine. This interpretation is always an alternative in studies that fail to specify long-term patterns of caffeine consumption in the experimental participants. The best strategy is to measure caffeine use and effects in the same people over a period of time.

Acute Effects of Caffeine

Caffeine's primary action is stimulation of CNS activity but, as we saw, caffeine is distributed freely throughout the body. Such distribution is evidenced by caffeine's actions outside the CNS: contraction of striated muscle, including the heart; relaxation of smooth muscle, especially the coronary arteries, uterus, and bronchi; diuretic effects on the kidneys; a stimulating effect on respiration at higher doses; elevation of basal metabolism; and various endocrine and enzymatic effects (Levenson & Bick, 1977; Rall, 1990a). Caffeine's effects on the body's systems provide good evidence for the blockade of adenosine receptors as its mechanism of action because caffeine's effects essentially are opposite to those of adenosine (Leonard, Watson, & Mohs, 1987).

Behavioral and Psychological Effects

Mood

The CNS-stimulation action of caffeine elevates mood. A large amount of research has shown that moderate doses of caffeine are reliably associated with feeling energized, creative, efficient, confident, and alert (Fredholm et al., 1999; Temple, 2009). This effect was anecdotally documented in a quote from the will of Dr. William Dunlap, who died in 1848: "I leave John Caddle a silver teapot, to the end that he may drink tea therefrom to comfort him under the affliction of a slatternly wife" (Gilbert, 1976, p. 77). The acute mood-elevating effects of caffeine account for much of the popularity that coffee and tea have as morning wake-up beverages. It also has been speculated that many people who are afflicted with significant depression "medicate" themselves by using caffeine products.

"Among the numerous luxuries of the table . . . coffee may be considered as one of the most valuable. It excites cheerfulness without intoxication; and the pleasing flow of spirits which it occasions . . . is never followed by sadness, languor or debility."

Benjamin Franklin

Performance

Caffeine's effects on human task performance are complicated. Table 8.3 lists some of the major performance effects of caffeine. The table shows that the range of caffeine

TABLE 8.3 Caffeine's Acute Effects on Human Performance

Performance Variable	Effect of Caffeine
Physical endurance	
Bicycle ergometer	
—Fixed load	Increases
—Progressive load	No effect
Motor skills	
Rapidity and accuracy	Decreases at higher doses; increases at lower doses
Eye-hand coordination	Decreases
Vigilance	
Visual	
—Night driving analogue	Increases
—Target scanning:	
low coffee users	Decreases
high coffee users	No effect
Reaction time	
Simple reaction time	Decreases (speeds up)
Choice reaction time	
—Decision time	Increases (slows down)
—Motor time	Decreases
Verbal tests	
Graduate Record Exam practice test	
—Speed and accuracy:	
extroverts	Increases with higher doses
introverts	First increases and then decreases with higher doses
Time stress accuracy	
—Extroverts	Increases
—Introverts	Decreases
Accuracy	
—Low impulsives	Increases (in the a.m.), decreases (in the p.m.)
—High impulsives	Decreases (in the a.m.), increases (in the p.m.)

Source: Adapted with permission from D. A. Sawyer, H. L. Julia, and A. C. Turin (1982), Caffeine and human behavior: Arousal, anxiety, and performance effects, Journal of Behavioral Medicine, 5, 415–439. © 1982 Plenum Publishing.

CONTEMPORARY ISSUE BOX 8.2

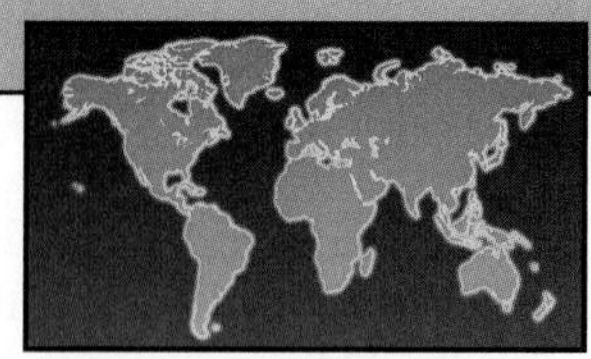

On the Issue of Energy Drinks

Energy drinks are canned or bottled beverages that contain large doses of caffeine. Other ingredients often include sugar, B vitamins, amino acids (e.g., taurine), and herbal stimulants such as guarana and ginseng. At present, literally hundreds of brands of energy drinks are being distributed worldwide.

The amount of caffeine in energy drinks varies considerably. The top-selling brands (including Red Bull, Monster, Rockstar, Full Throttle, No Fear, Amp, SoBe Adrenaline Rush, and Tab Energy) have comparable caffeine concentrations (ranging from around 9 mg/oz to 11 mg/oz) (Reissig, Strain, & Griffiths, 2009). However, the amount of caffeine contained in a can or bottle of these brands has more variability because they contain anywhere from 8.3 ounces (Red Bull, with 80 mg of total caffeine) to 16 ounces (No Fear, with 174 mg of total caffeine). Also being marketed are energy drinks with considerably higher levels of caffeine, ranging in caffeine concentrations of 11.9 mg/oz (in the 23.5 oz Jolt Cola, resulting in 280 mg of total caffeine) to 35.7 mg/oz (in the 8.4 oz SPIKE Shooter, resulting in 300 mg of total caffeine) (Ibid.). The energy drink leaders in terms of total caffeine are the 24 oz Wired X505 (at 505 mg) and the 20 oz Fixx (at 500 mg).

For the most part, energy drinks contain considerably higher concentrations of caffeine than coffee or tea (beverages that are typically consumed at a much slower pace than energy drinks), or soft drinks such as Coca-Cola, Pepsi-Cola, or even Mountain Dew (which contains 54 mg of caffeine).

Regulation

Given the high amounts of caffeine in energy drinks, it is perhaps surprising that the U.S. Food and Drug Administration (FDA) has not exerted oversight or regulation, as has been the case in a limited number of other countries. (Norway and Denmark have banned energy drinks, Canada requires warning labels, and Sweden only allows energy drinks to be sold in pharmacies for medicinal purposes.) Curiously, by way of contrast, the FDA does monitor caffeine-containing over-the-counter products such as NoDoz (containing 100 mg caffeine per tablet), requiring warning labels despite the total caffeine content being much lower than that contained in the majority of energy drinks. The lack of oversight is also surprising because the health consequences of energy drink consumption (including long-term consequences) are not known. (Keep in mind that consumers of energy drinks include adolescents and even children!) Also unknown are the potential impact of the other ingredients in energy drinks, alone or in conjunction with the caffeine.

Marketing

Energy drinks are predominantly marketed to adolescents and young adults, with claims of enhancing alertness and providing an energy boost. In some cases, energy drinks have been marketed in the context of improving endurance and performance (including athletic performance) and even weight loss. Many such claims appear to be offered without much in the way of substantiation.

A considerable amount of the advertising of energy drinks is geared toward young males, with the suggestion that the beverages will enhance strength, vigor, and virility. Recent research by Dr. Kathleen Miller on energy drink consumption has provided some interesting insights on this topic. Her research suggests a relationship between drinking energy drinks and "toxic jock behavior," characterized with hypermasculine attitudes and excessive risk taking. Miller (2008) found that frequent energy drink consumers (drinking energy drinks six or more days per month) were considerably more likely to have smoked cigarettes, abused prescription drugs, or been in a serious physical fight in the past year. The frequent consumers also reported drinking alcohol, have alcohol-related problems, and using marijuana about twice as often as nonconsumers. In addition, they were more likely to engage in other risk taking, including unsafe sex, not using a seatbelt, participating in extreme sports, and doing something dangerous on a dare. The associations with smoking, drinking, alcohol problems, and illicit prescriptions were found for white students but not black students. According to Miller, these findings overall suggest that frequent energy drink consumption may serve as a useful screening indicator to identify students at risk for a broader "problem behavior syndrome."

Combining Energy Drinks and Alcohol

Mixing energy drinks such as Red Bull with alcohol has become increasingly popular among young people, who often believe that this combination will improve their stamina while partying, or their physical performance more generally. Indeed, a popular drink today in a number of clubs is Red Bull and vodka. This popularity led several alcohol beverage producers to market alcoholic energy drinks, although these companies recently ceased this practice.

A research team in Brazil recently studied the effects of combining alcohol with Red Bull (Ferreira et al., 2006). In an interview reported in *Science Daily* (March 30, 2006), Oliveira de Souza-Formigoni, one of the study authors, stated that "[y]oung people believe that Red Bull and other energy drinks avoid the sleepiness caused by alcoholic beverages and increase their capacity to dance all night." In their study, they assessed the effects of ingesting alcohol alone, an energy drink alone, or alcohol and an energy drink (Red Bull) combined. For each participant, sensations of intoxication and measures of motor coordination and visual reaction time were assessed.

Two key findings emerged. First, drinking alcohol and Red Bull together reduced the *perception* of headache, weakness, dry mouth, and motor coordination impairment. Second, Red Bull did not significantly reduce alcohol-related deficits on the measures of motor coordination and visual reaction time.

The take-home message is clear: The combined use of Red Bull and alcohol decreases sensations of sleepiness and tiredness, but it does not reduce the harmful effects of alcohol on motor performance. In fact, the combined use of these beverages might be harmful, as some drinkers may believe they are less impaired than they actually are.

effects is wide, and many of them are stimulative (also see Smit & Rogers, 2000; Smith, 2002). It should be noted that one of the major ways caffeine improves task performance is by decreasing fatigue and increasing vigilance so that, over time, performance does not drop below what is typical for a person (Institute of Medicine, 2001). Such action is in contrast to pushing performance above what is normal for a person. In addition, the complexity of caffeine's effects is illustrated in the choice reaction time task. Caffeine impairs the decision-making part of the task but improves the motor component. The drug's effects are different even for different components of the same task. The inconsistency in the findings about caffeine effects is probably due in part to the different methods experimenters have used. Also, caffeine's effects depend not only on the drug's pharmacological action but also on the dose of the drug, the setting in which it is used, and the personality of the user. This is represented in Table 8.3 by findings such as verbal test accuracy (the last entry in the table), which caffeine affects according to the personality of the subject (impulsiveness) and the setting (time of day) (Sawyer, Julia, & Turin, 1982). Finally, there is evidence that caffeine enhances athletic performance, including perceived exertion and endurance (Burke, 2008; Ganio et al., 2009; Hogervorst et al., 2008; Hudson et al., 2008; Jones, 2008).

"It makes the body active and alert . . . it banishes tiredness and cleanses bodily fluids and the liver . . . it eases the brain and strengthens the memory. It is especially good for sustaining wakefulness."

English text, 1660, on the properties of tea (Schivelbusch, 1992, pp. 83–84)

Overall, it seems that caffeine's acute effects at lower doses are what sustain the world's use of beverages such as coffee and tea (Griffiths & Woodson, 1988a; James, 1991). Although caffeine's effects at low doses are not so intense as, say, cocaine's, its reinforcing properties are strong enough to make it the world's most popular drug.

Interactions among Caffeine, Nicotine, and Alcohol

Caffeine, nicotine, and alcohol are the world's most popular drugs, and many people use them in combination (Koslowski et al., 1993; Steptoe & Wardle, 1999). An important question, therefore, is what the interactive effects of these compounds are. It seems, for example, that smokers smoke fewer cigarettes after they drink coffee compared with when they have not had coffee (Hepple & Robson, 1996). This effect is stronger for lighter caffeine users. Another effect of nicotine is in the excretion of caffeine from the body, which occurs more than 50% faster in smokers than in nonsmokers (Benowitz, Hall, & Modin, 1989; Sawyer, Julia, & Turin, 1982). Furthermore, how individuals react to nicotine may be associated with how they react to caffeine and alcohol (Perkins et al., 2001).

One study (Lowe, 1988) suggests that everyday forgetfulness has something to do with the state-dependent effects of caffeine, nicotine, and alcohol in combination. In the first study, 24 men and women college undergraduates who were smokers and drinkers were given a moderate dose of vodka and two cigarettes to smoke. They were exposed to a list of 19 items about a route on a map and then had to recall the items in successive tests until they achieved 14 correct items. On the day of their next session, the participants were randomly assigned to one of four drug conditions: alcohol and nicotine (control condition), alcohol and nicotine placebo, alcohol placebo and nicotine, or alcohol placebo and nicotine placebo. The participants then were asked to recall as many of the 19 items as they could from their first experimental session. The results showed no recall decrement (between the Day 1 and the Day 2 score) for those who had alcohol and nicotine on both days. However, recall scores decreased significantly for participants in the other three groups. These "dissociative" or state-dependent effects seemed attributable to alcohol and, to a lesser extent, nicotine.

The next study by Lowe (1988) was the same as the first except that 16 undergraduates who drink coffee and alcohol participated, and caffeine was substituted for nicotine. The results of this study showed state-dependent effects for alcohol and caffeine. Because the major recall decrements occurred in people who had no caffeine the second day, even if they drank alcohol, it seems the state-dependent effect was mostly due to caffeine.

Acute Toxic Effects of Caffeine

Health professionals have recently given a lot of attention to caffeine intoxication, or caffeinism (Hogan, Hornick, & Bouchoux, 2002). An example of a case of caffeinism will give you an idea of the phenomenon (adapted from Greden, 1974, pp. 1, 090–1,091):

> A 27-year-old nurse requested an evaluation at an outpatient medical clinic because of lightheadedness, tremulousness, breathlessness, headache, and irregular heartbeat occurring sporadically about two to three times a day. The symptoms had developed gradually over a three-week period. The nurse said there were no precipitating stresses. The physical exam was within normal limits, except that an electrocardiogram showed premature ventricular contractions.
>
> At her final session with the evaluating internist the nurse was referred to an outpatient psychiatric clinic with the diagnosis of anxiety reaction, probably due to fear that her husband would be transferred by the military to be stationed in Vietnam. However, the nurse did not accept this diagnosis and searched for a dietary cause of her symptoms. After about 10 days she had linked her symptoms to coffee consumption.
>
> With the recent purchase of a new coffee pot the nurse had been drinking 10 to 12 cups of strong black coffee a day—more than 1,000 mg of caffeine. She stopped drinking coffee, and within 36 hours virtually all of her symptoms disappeared, including the cardiovascular irregularities.[1]

"Caffeine's effect at high doses is like having a chronic anxiety condition. It exaggerates the perception of stress and the body's response to it, and I think could be contributing to the stress we all experience in daily life."

Dr. James D. Lane, professor of medical psychology, Duke University (*New York Times*, December 12, 2006)

Note that the symptoms occurred in the nurse apparently as a result of her consuming more than 1,000 mg of caffeine a day. As with other caffeine effects, however, people differ in how much caffeine they can ingest before they experience symptoms of intoxication. For example, caffeinism has been reported following consumption of as little as 250 mg of caffeine in a day, which is not much more than the average for adults in the United States. Generally, ingesting 600 mg of caffeine a day greatly increases the chances of developing caffeinism (Kenny & Darragh, 1985).

Consuming more than 1,000 mg of caffeine a day increases the risk of experiencing even more severe toxic symptoms, including muscle twitching, rambling flow of

[1]Published with permission of American Psychiatric Press, Inc.

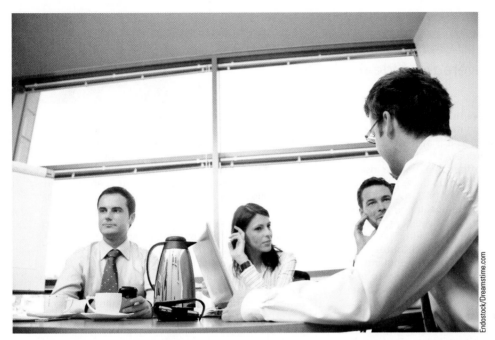

Caffeine's enhancing effects on the performance of various cognitive and motor tasks make it a popular drug in the workplace.

thought and speech, cardiac arrhythmia, periods of inexhaustibility, and psychomotor agitation (American Psychiatric Association, 1987). Other symptoms that have been reported are ringing in the ears and seeing flashes of light. The lethal dose of caffeine when it is taken orally is about 10 grams for adults and 100 mg/kg for children (Leonard, Watson, & Mohs, 1987). The adult lethal dose is equal to about 75 cups of coffee, 125 cups of tea, 200 colas, or 100 NoDoz tablets. Reports of death due to caffeine overdose are rare. Much more common is people appearing for treatment of acute overexposure to caffeine. In fact, caffeinism may be viewed as a more extreme case of acute overexposure to caffeine (James, 1991). Keep in mind, however, caffeine overexposure occurs most infrequently given the commonality of its use.

Chronic Effects of Caffeine Use

The chronic effects of caffeine have been studied primarily for major medical problems, and the research has produced some inconsistent findings. For example, a retrospective study (Infante-Rivard et al., 1993) found a positive relationship between reported caffeine intake one month before and during pregnancy and loss of the fetus. In another longitudinal study, however, no relationship was found between caffeine consumption during the first three months of pregnancy and damage to the fetus, including spontaneous abortion (Mills et al., 1993). Overall, the FDA's position is that moderate doses of caffeine do not have negative effects on reproduction (Hogan, Hornick, & Bouchoux, 2002), although high levels of caffeine intake among women attempting to become pregnant can be associated with lower rates of conception (Temple, 2009). Research on other medical problems has suggested there is no consistent relationship between caffeine consumption and cancer, myocardial infarction, or cardiovascular disease (Abbott, 1986; Grobbee et al., 1990; Nkondjock, 2009; Temple, 2009; van Dam, 2008). An exception might exist among people with slow

DRUGS AND CULTURE BOX 8.3

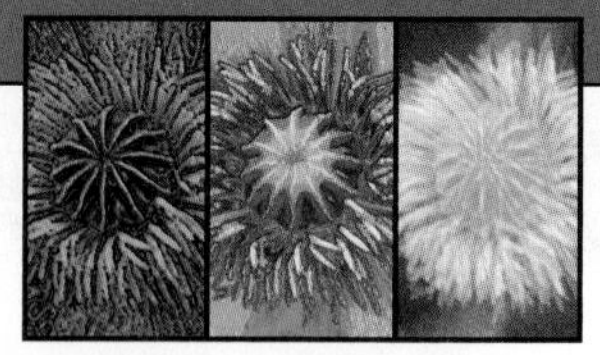

Coffee as the Beverage of Ideals

Many people today believe that coffee helps them sober up after drinking too much alcohol. This belief, actually, is far from new, as it is at least as old as 17th-century western Europe. At that time, a book on beverages noted that "coffee sobers you up instantaneously, or in any event sobers up those who are not fully intoxicated" (Schivelbusch, 1992, p. 35). Coffee was regarded as an ideal beverage. In the 19th century, the poet and historian Jules Michelet praised coffee because it "heightens purity and lucidity" (Ibid.).

Coffee was credited with other attributes during those years in Europe. In 18th-century England, for example, coffee was seen as an alternative to sex. To some people, coffee was a way that erotic arousal could be replaced by stimulation of the mind.

Of course, the ideas that coffee is a sobering agent and a displacer of erotic desires have long since been discredited scientifically, yet the belief of coffee aiding in sobering up persists. These ideas may have originated in the pharmacology of caffeine—a CNS stimulant—and in the cultural and ideological factors that prevailed in Europe from the 17th to the 19th centuries (Schivelbusch, 1992). During that time, more and more emphasis was placed on achievement in an increasingly industrialized society, with which caffeine's pharmacology is highly consistent. Because coffee had been a popular drink anyway, it was an ideal candidate to help foster the ideals of the time and to show disapproval of behaviors thought to be inconsistent with them, such as alcohol use and sex.

Why many continue to view coffee as a sobering agent is open to discussion. Caffeine's CNS stimulant action probably gives consumers the illusion of coming out of the drowsiness and lethargy that alcohol causes. Yet, alcohol's CNS depressant action remains relatively untouched by caffeine.

caffeine metabolism, based on a recent report indicating that coffee intake was associated with an increased risk of nonfatal myocardial infarction in this subgroup of coffee drinkers (Cornelis et al., 2006).

One study on postmenopausal women discovered a positive relationship between the lifetime amount of caffeinated coffee consumed and osteoporosis (Barrett-Connor, Chang, & Edelstein, 1994). In this study, drinking two cups of coffee a day was associated with decreased bone mineral density, a measure of osteoporosis. However, the relationship between coffee and osteoporosis was negated in women who said they drank at least one glass of milk a day during the ages between 20 and 50. More recent research also suggests that the little effect that caffeine consumption might have on bone density can be reversed or counteracted by including small amounts of milk in the diet (Lloyd et al., 2000).

Some studies have shown an association between serum cholesterol levels and caffeine consumption: As one level goes up, the other one also tends to rise. Level of serum cholesterol is related to atherosclerosis. The caffeine–cholesterol research illustrates the complexity of linking chronic drug use to medical problems and is one reason caffeine research in particular has yielded so many inconsistent findings. When researchers consider coffee intake as the source of caffeine, the caffeine–cholesterol relationship seems to depend on how the coffee is brewed. It appears that when coffee is boiled—as is common, for example, in Norway—the caffeine–cholesterol link holds up. The link disappears when the coffee is made by drip-filtering (Bak & Grobbee, 1989; Urgert et al., 1996).

Caffeine consumption seems to be associated with other symptoms that are less major but are experienced more commonly. Abbott (1986) cited a survey of 4,558 Australians that concerned caffeine ingestion and the occurrence of indigestion, palpitations, tremor, headache, and insomnia. The more caffeine respondents ingested, the more likely they were to report these symptoms (the average consumption for the sample was 240 mg a day).

In terms of potential health benefits of coffee, there are indications that coffee consumption may help prevent several chronic diseases, including liver disease, Parkinson's disease, and type 2 diabetes mellitus (Higdon & Frei, 2006). In one study, Klatsky et al. (2006) found an ingredient in coffee that appears to protect against liver cirrhosis, especially alcoholic cirrhosis. The cause of the apparent protective effect was not clear. There is some speculation that caffeine is playing a central role. However, the protective effect was not found among tea drinkers (although there were fewer tea drinkers relative to coffee drinkers). In another domain, no clear evidence exists for a causal relationship between caffeine consumption and peptic ulcer (Council on Scientific Affairs, 1984). Recently, a large study of women found that coffee consumption was not associated with an increased risk of hypertension (in fact, it appeared to be protective among the heaviest coffee consumers studied) (Winkelmayer et al., 2005). Interestingly, though, the women who consumed caffeine via soft drinks did have an increased risk for hypertension, although how much of this effect is attributable to the caffeine was not clear. In other research, coffee consumption has regularly been found to reduce risk of type 2 diabetes mellitus (Temple, 2009), although caffeine itself does not appear to be the mechanism accounting for this benefit. Finally, there are some indications that caffeine may provide some protections to the development of Alzheimer's disease (Eskelinen et al., 2009; Rosso, Mossey, & Lippa, 2008).

In summary, based on the apparent infrequency of acute caffeine overexposure and research on its chronic effects, caffeine is considered a relatively safe drug. However, because more minor symptoms occur with higher levels of caffeine consumption (but still within the range of typical use patterns, as indicated earlier in the Australian study), it has been recommended that caffeine consumption be moderated. Furthermore, some individuals, such as pregnant women, particularly benefit by keeping their caffeine consumption at a low to moderate level. In addition, there is an ongoing concern over the caffeine intake associated with energy drinks, particularly among children and teenagers. The absence of data on the effects of such intake, especially in the longer term, has led to calls for adding warning labels to energy drinks or even regulating the amount of caffeine they can contain. Another example is people who suffer from certain psychiatric disorders characterized by high levels of anxiety (see Chapter 13). It appears, for instance, that people who have been diagnosed as having generalized anxiety disorder are hypersensitive to the effects of caffeine, and the drug may exacerbate the anxiety symptoms (Bruce et al., 1992). You can connect this finding with the case study we cited that involved mistaking caffeinism for an anxiety reaction.

"Sometimes when I had drunk a lot of coffee, and the least little thing would startle me, I noticed quite clearly that I had jumped before I had heard any noise."

Georg Christoph Lichtenberg (Schivelbusch, 1992, inside front cover)

Therapeutic Uses of Caffeine

Table 8.1 shows that caffeine is also used in a variety of prescription and over-the-counter medications. Caffeine is very much a part of the medications used to treat a range of ailments. In fact, other methylxanthines also have therapeutic value. You can better appreciate this by looking at Table 8.4, which lists the xanthine used to achieve a preferred pharmacological action. The differences among the xanthines in their effects are based on slight differences in their chemical structure. For example, aminophylline, a cardiac and bronchial dilator that contains theophylline, is used to treat both

TABLE 8.4 Methylxanthine Compounds and Desired Pharmacological Action

Desired Action	Preferred Compound
Cerebral stimulation	Caffeine (coffee)
Coronary dilation	Theophylline (tea)
Diuresis	Theobromine (cocoa)
Respiratory stimulant for premature infants	Caffeine

Note: Products in parentheses are sources of the indicated compound.
Source: From D. M. Graham (1978), Caffeine: Its identity, dietary sources, intake and biological effects, *Nutrition Reviews*, 36, 101. Used with permission of John Wiley & Sons, Inc.

cardiac and bronchial asthma. Caffeine is the most common drug, as it is part of many remedies for headaches and colds. Its mild stimulant properties help to counteract some of the side effects of medications for those ailments (Gilbert, 1976). Caffeine also is in appetite-suppressant medications because of its diuretic effects (Snyder & Sklar, 1984).

Conclusions

Caffeine is an extremely important drug because of its widespread use. Overall, it also seems to be a relatively safe drug. Despite the many years of research that have been devoted to caffeine, however, we still have a lot to learn about it. Probably the most essential research concerns developing better ways to obtain accurate measures of caffeine consumption. Such advances would help us answer important research questions. For example, we need to know more about the long-term effects of caffeine use in children, the development of tolerance to caffeine, and the prevalence of more minor symptoms of higher, but not extreme, levels of caffeine use. Another question is how caffeine affects people in special populations, such as those who are medically or psychiatrically ill.

Finally, Sawyer, Julia, and Turin (1982) made the excellent point that much of the research on caffeine has been done with healthy volunteers who have consumed only well-specified single doses of caffeine. Little information exists on the cumulative effects on task performance during, say, one day of caffeine use, although studies are beginning to address this question (Hindmarch et al., 2000). Such information is important because that is most people's pattern of caffeine use. Similarly, caffeine effects in combination with other commonly used drugs need more attention. Lowe's (1988) findings on state-dependent learning and alcohol, caffeine, and nicotine suggest that significant practical questions can be answered by such research.

Summary

- Caffeine and other methylxanthine drugs occur naturally in more than 60 species of plants. Caffeine is the world's most popular drug, and humans have used it since ancient times. Many everyday products that children or adults consume contain caffeine.
- Overall, coffee is the major source of caffeine, but tea is the dominant source for many countries. In the last 20 years, soft drinks and energy drinks have emerged as other significant sources of caffeine.
- Total caffeine consumption does not seem to vary by characteristics of people, except for age.
- When we factor in body weight, children aged 1 to 5 have the highest exposure to caffeine, after adults aged 18 and older.

- Caffeine's mechanism of action seems to be blocking of adenosine receptor sites.
- Caffeine is rapidly absorbed from the gastrointestinal tract and is distributed throughout the body. Its half-life in the blood ranges from 2 1/2 to 7 1/2 hours.
- Caffeine is metabolized primarily in the liver and is almost entirely excreted in the urine.
- A clear withdrawal syndrome has been identified for caffeine, and there is evidence for the development of tolerance to some of caffeine's effects.
- The acute effects of caffeine include diuresis, stimulation of the heart and CNS, relaxation of smooth muscles, and stimulation of gastric acid.
- Because many people use caffeine, nicotine, and alcohol in some combination, knowing how each of these drugs interacts with the other two is important.
- Acute caffeine intoxication is called caffeinism. Caffeinism is most likely to occur with a dose of 600 mg or higher. The higher the dose of caffeine, the more severe the symptoms.
- Overall, caffeine is a relatively safe drug, but important research questions remain about long-term caffeine use and health.

Answers to "What Do You Think?"

1. About half the world's population consumes caffeine regularly.
   F *An estimated 90% of the world's population consumes caffeine regularly.*
2. There are major subgroup differences in caffeine use in the United States.
   F *There are few subgroup differences in caffeine consumption, except for age.*
3. In dose of caffeine consumed, young children have the highest exposure to caffeine, after adults 18 and older.
   T *When body weight is taken into account, children aged 1 to 5 have the highest caffeine exposure after adults.*
4. Caffeine is a drug that, when consumed, is distributed equally throughout the body.
   T *Because caffeine is equally distributed in total body water, it has similar concentrations throughout the body.*
5. Smokers tend to metabolize caffeine more slowly than do nonsmokers.
   F *Studies show that smokers metabolize caffeine more quickly than do nonsmokers.*
6. So many people use coffee and tea without apparent difficulty that people obviously do not become physically dependent on caffeine.
   F *Caffeine withdrawal syndrome has been clearly identified.*
7. Caffeine's stimulant effects seem to be reinforcing in humans.
   T *Caffeine's acute effects of mood elevation and overall improvement in task performance seem to be reinforcing to humans.*
8. There is evidence that people can get intoxicated on caffeine.
   T *Acute caffeine intoxication, also called caffeinism, has been well documented. It is most likely to occur when 600 mg or more of caffeine are consumed in a day.*
9. Caffeine crosses the placenta and poses a danger to the health of a fetus.
   F *The latest evidence is that typical doses of caffeine consumption by mothers pose little health risk to the fetus.*
10. Overall, caffeine seems to be a safe drug for everybody.
    F *Although caffeine is a relatively safe drug overall, some individuals are advised to reduce its use. One example is people with anxiety disorders.*
11. Caffeine has little medical value.
    F *Caffeine and the other methylxanthine drugs are in medications used to treat a variety of medical problems.*
12. Caffeine's long-term effects on children are well understood.
    F *Despite the high consumption of caffeine in children, little is known about the chronic effects of their use of this drug. It is a major research area for the future.*

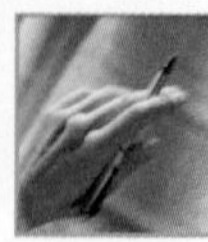

Essays/Thought Questions

1. Research provides us with good evidence that individuals may build a physical dependence on caffeine. Is this a reason to impose any restrictions, warning labels, or other controls on caffeine use? Why or why not?
2. Why has it proved difficult to obtain reliable information on caffeine consumption in the general population by use of survey research methods?

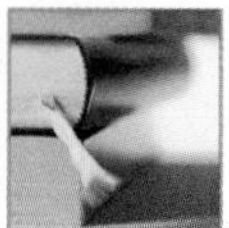

Suggested Readings

Coe, S. D., & Coe, M. D. (1996). *The true history of chocolate*. London: Thames & Hudson.

Hogan, E. H., Hornick, B. A., & Bouchoux, A. (2002). Communicating the message: Clarifying the controversies about caffeine. *Nutrition Today*, 37, 28–36.

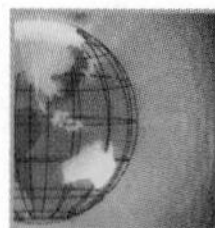

Web Resources

Visit the Book Companion Website at www.cengage.com/psychology/maisto to access study tools including a glossary, flashcards, and web quizzing. You will also find links to the following resources:

- Medline Plus: Caffeine
- Energy Fiend
- Vaults of Erowid

CHAPTER 9

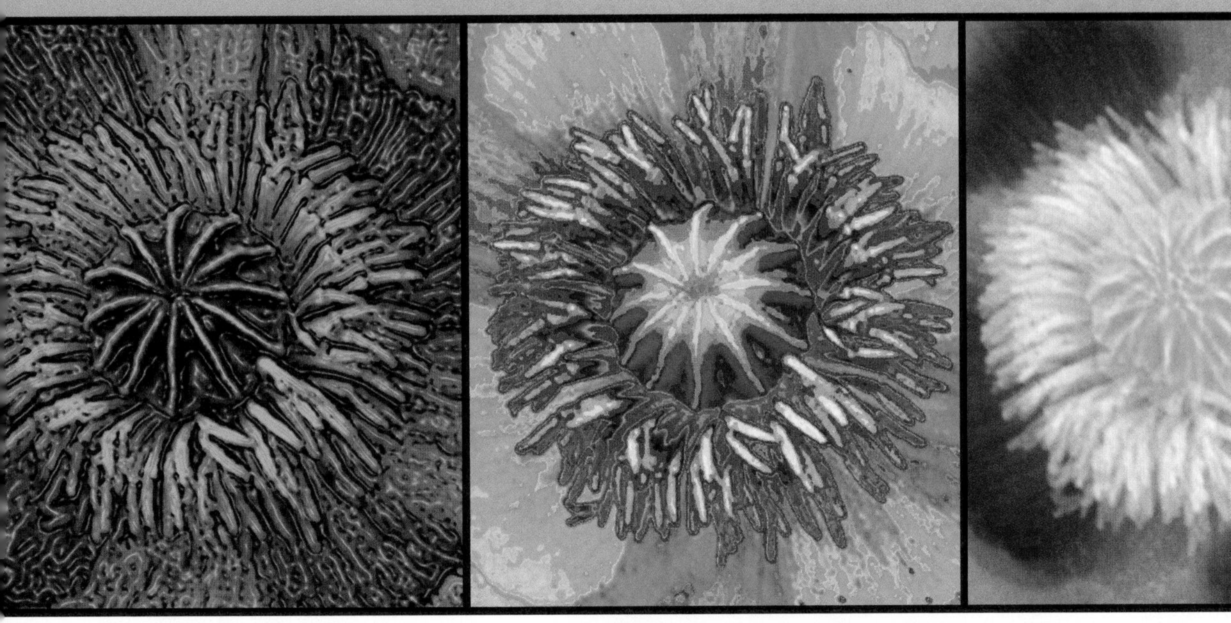

Alcohol

What Do You Think? True or False?

Answers are given at the end of the chapter.

___ 1. Humans have consumed alcohol since between 6000 B.C. and 5000 B.C.

___ 2. In the United States of 1830, adults' average alcohol consumption was about five drinks a day.

___ 3. The highest rates of heavy drinking, and thus the greatest vulnerability to drinking problems, are in men between the ages of 40 and 45.

___ 4. It is difficult to consume a lethal dose of alcohol.

___ 5. If not treated properly, alcohol withdrawal syndrome can be fatal.

___ 6. Alcohol is a drug that has no legitimate medical value.

___ 7. If you drink a lot and black out, it means you have lost consciousness.

___ 8. Alcohol causes violent behavior.

___ 9. Alcohol improves sexual performance.

___10. The cognitive deficits that seem to occur in some people as a result of years of heavy drinking are reversible.

___11. The majority of alcoholics eventually develop cirrhosis of the liver.

___12. Moderate drinking (one to three drinks a day) is associated with reduced risk of heart disease.

In the preceding chapter, we said alcohol, nicotine, and caffeine are the most popular psychoactive drugs. Of the three, alcohol has been known, manufactured, and used the longest by far. Most important, this drug has had profound influences on the societies around the world in which it is used. "Alcohol" actually refers to several substances—for example, isopropyl alcohol (rubbing alcohol), methyl alcohol (wood alcohol), and ethanol. Ethanol is the alcohol we drink, and the word *alcohol* in this text means ethanol unless otherwise specified.

In this chapter, we give you an overview of the many facets of alcohol use. We begin with information on the major alcoholic beverages, how they are manufactured, and some history of the use of alcohol in human societies. We follow with a discussion of trends in alcohol consumption in the United States, including a discussion of heavy drinking. We also explore more detailed information about alcohol use and patterns of alcohol consumption. With this general background, we then examine the pharmacology of alcohol, including site of action, processing of the drug in the human body, and the development of tolerance and dependence. Then we examine the acute and chronic physiological, psychological, and social consequences of alcohol use in humans. The chapter ends with a discussion of the causes of alcohol dependence.

Alcoholic Beverages

Fermentation and Distillation

distillation
The process by which the heating of a fermented mixture increases its alcohol content.

Alcohol virtually always is drunk in one of the three major classes of alcoholic beverages: beer, wine, and hard liquor (also called distilled spirits). For their manufacture, all these beverages depend on the process of fermentation, and on the further process of **distillation** for hard liquor. Fermentation begins when sugar is dissolved in water and exposed to air, which creates the perfect environment for living microorganisms called yeasts. In this environment, yeasts multiply rapidly by eating the sugar, which is then converted to ethanol and carbon dioxide by the yeasts' metabolic processes. The carbon dioxide bubbles to the top of the mixture, leaving ethanol. As the yeasts grow, so does the percentage of ethanol—as much as 10% to 15%. At this highest point, the yeasts cease their work. Therefore, fermented beverages do not have an alcohol content higher than 15%. Which kind of beverage results from fermentation depends on what sugar-containing substance is used. When grapes are used, the grape juice ferments to form wine; when grains are used, fermentation produces beer.

"Fermentation may have been a greater discovery than fire."

David Rains Wallace

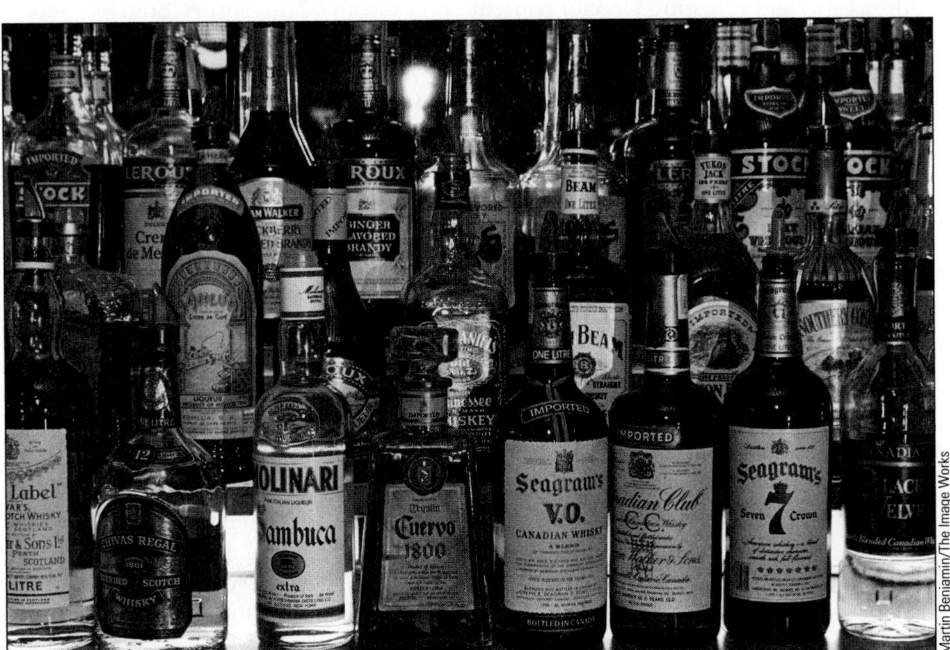

Martin Benjamin/The Image Works

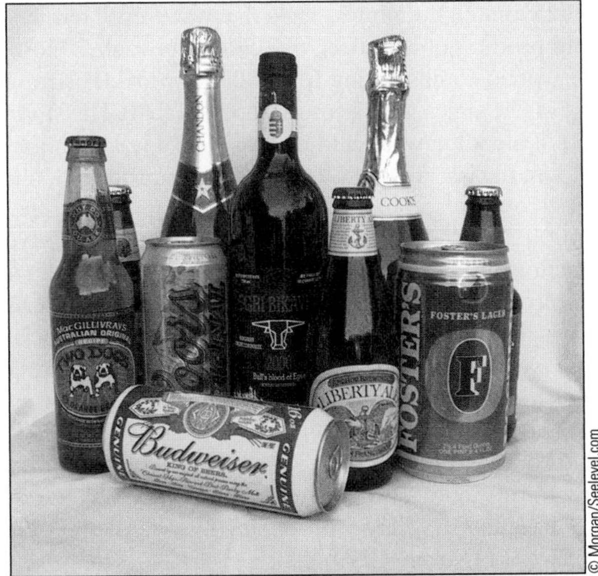

© Morgan/Seelevel.com

A variety of alcoholic beverages is available to interested consumers.

Distillation was developed to increase the ethanol content of fermented beverages. Distillation first involves heating a fermented mixture. Because alcohol has a lower boiling point than water, the steam emitted through boiling has a higher alcohol content than does the original fermented mixture. The vapor then is condensed through cooling, and the resulting liquid has a higher alcohol content than the original fermented mixture. By repeating this cycle, it is possible to raise the alcohol content of a beverage to progressively higher levels.

Expressing the Alcohol Content of a Beverage

In the United States, alcohol percentage is denoted by volume. This calculation is straightforward: 16 ounces of a beverage that is 50% ethanol contains 8 ounces of alcohol. Another way of expressing alcohol content is by weight, which is done, for example, in Britain.

proof
The proportion of alcohol in a beverage, by volume. Proof typically is used in reference to distilled spirits and equals twice the percentage of alcohol.

The alcohol content of a beverage is also designated by **proof**. Proof is used primarily for distilled spirits and is equal to twice the percentage of alcohol by volume. Accordingly, a beverage that is 43% alcohol by volume is 86 proof. This somewhat indirect way of expressing alcohol content comes from 17th-century England, where it was determined that a mixture that was 57% alcohol by volume, if poured over gunpowder, would cause its ignition in an open flame. The English still refer to their beverages as "over proof" (.57% alcohol by volume) or "under proof" (.57% alcohol by volume) (Becker, Roe, & Scott, 1975).

Table 9.1 is a summary of the major types of alcoholic beverages commercially available. Varying the substances that form the base of the beverage and varying the alcohol concentration produce different alcoholic beverages.

History of Alcohol Use

Humans have used alcohol for thousands of years. Keller (1979, p. 2,822) reflected this fact in his comment, "in the beginning there was alcohol." The first nondistilled alcoholic beverages were made inadvertently by natural fermentation. The first wines, which probably were drunk several thousand years ago, were likely made from fruit juice. The juices obtained from most types of fruit are contaminated with microbes, including yeasts, which constitute the flora on the fruit (Rose, 1977). Alcoholic fermentation results when the environmental temperature is right. Authorities believe the first beers were produced in Egypt as long ago as between 6000 B.C. and 5000 B.C. Traditionally, it has been thought that the first beer production was similar to baking bread. An earthenware vessel filled with barley was placed in the ground until germination occurred. At that point, the barley was crushed, made into dough, and then baked until a crust formed. This cake of dehydrated dough was soaked in water until fermentation was complete. The resulting product of acid beer was called "boozah." However, a study of beer residue in Egyptian tombs dating to 2000 B.C. provides strong evidence that the brewing process of the times was far more sophisticated. The study suggests that the process consisted of blending water and malt to yield a refined liquid (Williams, 1996). Distilled spirits were the last alcoholic beverages to be produced, but they are by no means recent entries on the scene. The earliest reference to distilled spirits appeared in China about 1000 B.C. Western Europe apparently does not have any record of distilled spirit production and consumption until about A.D. 800.

"I like alcohol. It is a powerful drug and, God knows, for some people a hellish one, but, if used carefully it can give great pleasure."

62-year-old man (Weil & Rosen, 1983, p. 190)

Since the beginning of its use, alcohol has been a double-edged sword to human societies. On the one hand, alcoholic beverages have played a role in important social occasions, such as births, religious ceremonies, marriages, and funerals. Such drinking was viewed as not harmful to individuals and as positive to societies. On the other hand, alcohol seemingly always has been consumed in excess by some, with consequent problems to individuals and to the society in which they lived. The definition of "problem" has varied according to time and culture (Warner, 1997). Nevertheless, such negative social consequences have led the clergy, prophets, physicians, and philosophers to repeatedly condemn alcohol (Keller, 1979).

The two faces of alcohol were seen clearly when distilled spirits hit western Europe. Europeans sang the praises of this drug. For example, a French professor in the 13th

TABLE 9.1 Major Kinds of Alcoholic Beverages, How They Are Made, and Their Alcohol Content

Beverage	How Made	Percentage of Alcohol (by volume)
Beer (includes lager, carbohydrate ale, malt, stout)	Lager 3–6, extracted from barley malt (or rice or corn) by cooling with water. The product is boiled with hops, cooled, and fermented. Types of beer vary in malt, hops, and alcohol content	Fermentation of others 4–8
Wine		
Red (table wine)	Fermentation of red grapes in skins	
White (table wine)	Fermentation of skinless grapes	Average 12
Champagne	Same as white wine, with carbon dioxide	
Fortified (dessert) wines	Ordinary table wines with alcohol content raised	Up to 20
Distilled spirits		
Brandy	Distilled from any sugar-containing fruit. Brandy was probably first to be produced commercially.	About 40
Whiskeys	Grains brewed with water to form a beer of 5% to 10% alcohol. Beer is distilled and aged in new or used charred oak barrels for two to eight years before blending.	40–50
Bourbon	Corn with rye and malted barley	
Scotch	Malted barley and corn	
Irish whiskey	Corn and malted and unmalted barley	
Rye whiskey	Rye and malted barley	
Other spirits		
Rum	Distilled from fermented molasses; aged about three years	40–75
Gin	Distilled from any fermentable carbohydrate (barley, potato, corn, wheat, rye); flavored by a second distillation with juniper berries	35–50
Vodka	Distilled from potato or almost any other carbohydrate source; kept free of flavors	35–50

Source: Abstracted from C. E. Becker, R. L. Roe, and R. A. Scott (1975), *Alcohol as a Drug*, New York: Medcom Press.

century dubbed alcohol *aqua vitae,* which means "water of life." The Danes expressed the same sentiment with their *akkevitt;* the Swedes, with *akvavit.* European societies also attributed many of their problems to alcoholic beverages, especially distilled spirits. For instance, the social problems in 18th-century England were represented in works of art such as William Hogarth's "Gin Lane."

Colonial America adopted alcoholic beverages and many drinking customs from western Europe. In one story, the Pilgrims were believed to have landed at Plymouth Rock because they were out of alcohol. The double-edged nature of alcohol was manifested again in colonial America. The tavern was the center of town politics, business, trade, and pleasure. These Americans drank beer, wine, cider, and distilled spirits in considerable quantities. The practice of drinking was pervasive: Colonial American

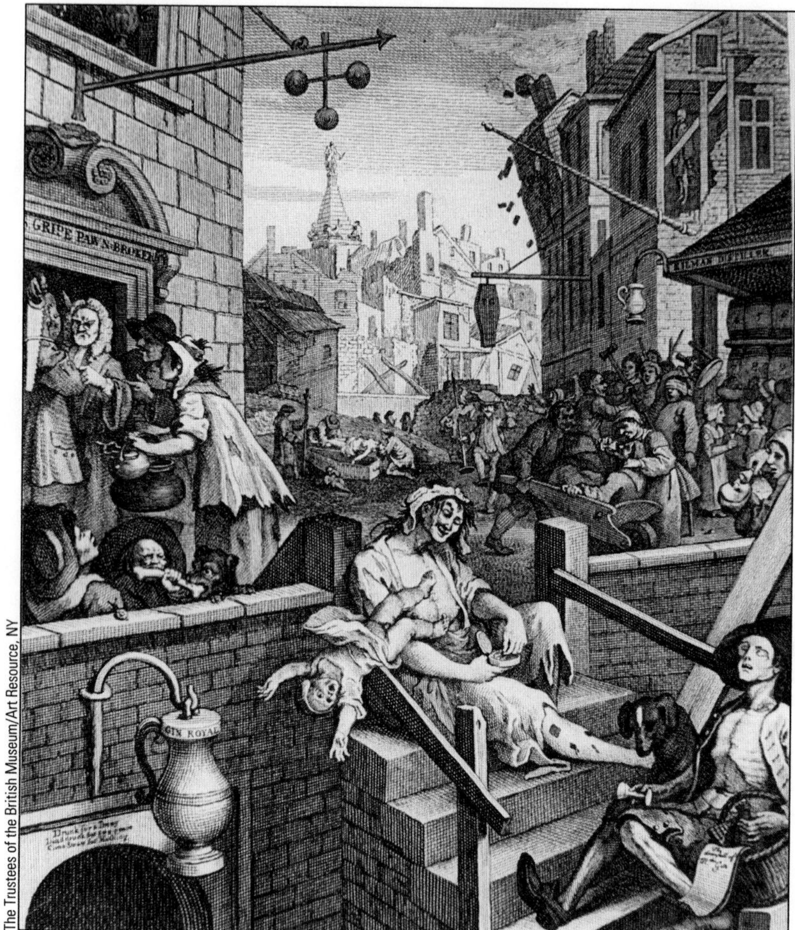
The Trustees of the British Museum/Art Resource, NY

Eighteenth-century Europeans tended to attribute many of their social problems to alcoholic beverages, particularly distilled spirits.

drinking showed no distinction among time, place, or person. The attitudes toward alcohol consumption were positive, and alcohol was viewed as meeting an array of physical, psychological, and social needs. The importance of alcohol to colonial Americans was also represented in language. In 1737, Benjamin Franklin published a "Drinkers Dictionary," which included more than 235 terms to describe the drunkard. Included among these were "Loaded his cart," "Cock ey'd," "Moon-ey'd," "Tipsy," and "He carries too much sail" (Mendelson & Mello, 1985).

With such supporting attitudes and customs, America became known as a country of drunkards. In 1790, adult citizens of the young country annually drank 6 gallons of pure alcohol per capita, and by 1830, per capita alcohol consumption had risen to 7 gallons. That amounts to almost five alcoholic beverage drinks a day for each adult! With this consumption, the ills of heavy drinking became more evident, especially in a society that was moving increasingly toward urbanization and industrialization. Some people began to speak out against the ravages of alcohol, again mostly in reference to distilled spirits. The most influential among these critics, and a pillar of the temperance movement that was to gain strength in the 19th century, was the physician Benjamin Rush. Dr. Rush's 1785 treatise, "Inquiring into the Effects of Distilled Spirits on the Human Body and Mind," delineated the effects of distilled spirits on humans. It also was the basis of the idea that alcoholism is a disease.

In the 19th century, America expanded westward, and with that came the saloon. The word *saloon* comes from the French word *salon,* which refers to a public meeting place and entertainment hall. The saloon did serve a social function for the frontier people, but it quickly moved away from a center of civilized interchange to a reflection of the rural community of the American West (Mendelson & Mello, 1985). The first saloons were not exactly pictures of fine carpentry; as little as a tent and a few barrels might make up the bar. The decor was the era's version of macho and may have consisted of pictures of naked women, well-known boxers of the time such as John L. Sullivan, and famous events such as Custer's Last Stand (Mendelson & Mello, 1985). This decor was in tune with the typical clientele: aggressive men who were inclined to exploit other men, women, and nature. These explorers, soldiers, Native Americans, trappers, settlers, and cowboys had few of the attachments to family or community that might have helped to limit excessive drinking. Instead, their drinking in the saloon was characterized by downing large quantities of whiskey for the purpose of engaging in explosive behavior (Keller, 1979). The whiskey was plentiful and usually wretched—consider common names for it such as "extract of scorpions" and "San Juan paralyzer."

The behavior associated with the saloon led to a rebirth of the temperance movement, which had been quieted somewhat by the American Civil War. The saloon was the focal scapegoat of the temperance movement and was blamed for social ills such as thievery, gambling, prostitution, and political corruption. The temperance movement also changed its stand from support of moderate use of nondistilled beverages to total abstinence from alcohol. The captains of industry of the late 19th and early 20th centuries, such as John D. Rockefeller, Andrew Carnegie, and Henry Ford, supported the temperance movement. They believed that abstemious employees would be better employees. These industrial giants also gave money to back their moral support.

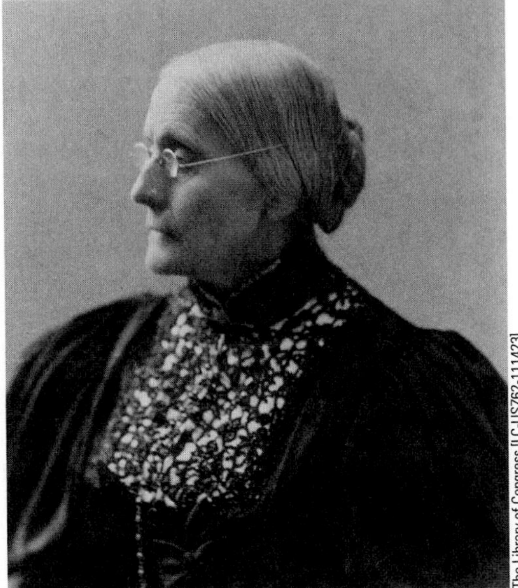
The Library of Congress [LC-USZ62-111423]

Susan B. Anthony (1820–1906) was an early and active leader in the temperance movement.

As World War I approached, the antialcohol drive had gained considerable financial, social, and political power. As mentioned in Chapter 2, this drive led to Prohibition and then to passage of the Volstead Act. The short life of Prohibition in the United States is well known; Prohibition was repealed nationally in 1933. However, the states still had much discretion in regulating the sale and consumption of alcohol. The stew of local laws that has evolved since illustrates America's ambivalence about the use of alcoholic beverages. For example, some laws required the windows of drinking establishments to be curtained, and others forbade it; some laws forbade women to drink standing at the bar, and others granted women the right to drink standing anywhere that a man could. The laws were consistent in their restriction of youths purchasing alcoholic beverages and in the channeling of alcohol tax revenues to local, state, and federal treasuries (Keller, 1979).

The public remains ambivalent about alcohol. This is reflected in the saying, "everybody enjoys a drink, but nobody enjoys a drunk." Since the 1980s, the general trend in the United States has been toward limiting alcohol's use through changes in social attitudes and tighter governmental controls. Drinking remains a major part of many social rituals, however, and many people hail the benefits of moderate alcohol consumption. The negative consequences of excessive alcohol use are probably more apparent than ever because of activists with access to sophisticated communications techniques, yet they and government regulations are far from successful in stopping or limiting alcohol consumption. This seems to be especially true among people who have alcohol dependence. We are still working to understand the mystery of how alcohol problems develop, are maintained, and can be prevented and treated.

Consumption of Alcohol and Heavy Drinking in the United States

In this section, we consider trends in alcohol use in the United States. Because we covered data on the prevalence of alcohol and other drug use in Chapter 1, we limit this discussion to trends we did not review earlier, including the prevalence of specific alcoholic beverages and the prevalence and correlates of heavy drinking.

Per Capita Consumption

The U.S. federal government compiles many statistics on the consumption of alcoholic beverages. One statistic, per capita consumption, gives a good general summary of how much the "average" person in the United States drinks. Before we present this information, you should know that the population is all individuals (both drinkers and nondrinkers) at least 14 years old. The age of 14 might seem young to some and is undoubtedly below the legal age for purchasing alcoholic beverages. It is used because survey data suggest that many 14-year-olds are drinking beverages that contain alcohol. U.S. Census figures are used to estimate the number of people aged 14 and older for a given year in computing per capita consumption. The "quantity of alcohol" part of the computation is based on beverage sales figures for each of the states or, if those data are not available, on shipments and tax receipts data (combining the three data sources does not affect the conclusions significantly). The quantities of different types of beverages (beer, wine, hard liquor) are translated to amounts (in gallons) of pure alcohol according to standard alcohol equivalence formulas. For example, 12 ounces of regular domestic beer is computed as containing about 0.48 ounce or .045 gallon of pure alcohol. With these estimates, quantity of alcohol in gallons is divided by population number to yield per capita alcohol consumption in gallons.

Figure 9.1 graphs the estimated per capita consumption of all alcoholic beverages combined from 1935 to 2006 (Lakins et al., 2008). One minor point to recognize in interpreting the information in Figure 9.1 is that, until 1970, 15 was the lower age limit in computing population numbers. Figure 9.1 shows a few general trends. Per capita consumption showed a constant increase from 1935, shortly after the end of Prohibition, into the 1940s. There also was a considerable increase in consumption from 1960 through the 1970s. Then, 1980 marked the beginning of a decline in consumption that was slightly reversed in 1990. Consumption then declined again and, from 1995–2006, rose slightly to about 2.27 gallons. To give you some reference, 2.2 gallons of pure alcohol equals about 563 12-ounce cans or bottles of regular domestic beer.

Combining data for all three types of alcoholic beverages masks some important differences, however. A more precise look at the per capita consumption decline in the 1980s to the mid-1990s reveals that it was due largely to a reduction in the use of hard liquor. In fact, the Lakins et al. (2008) report showed that, in 1995, the per

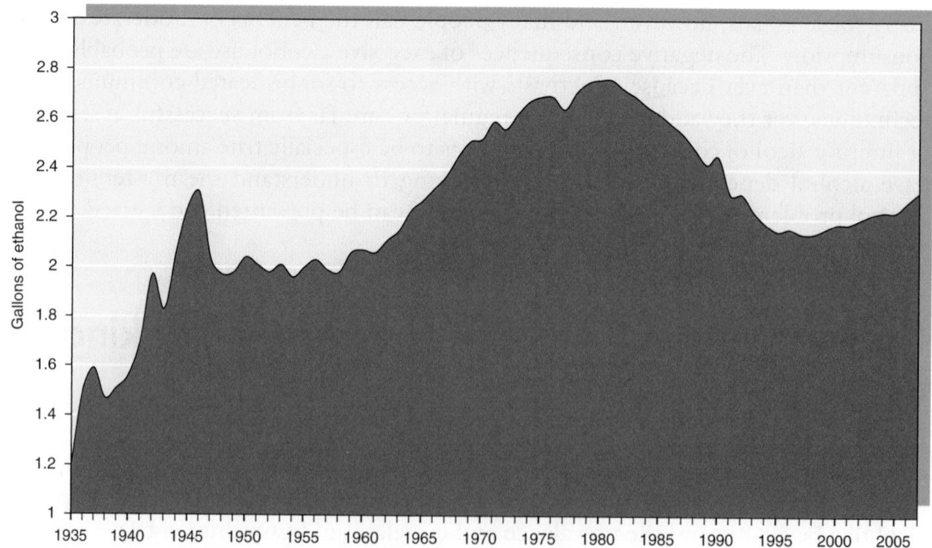

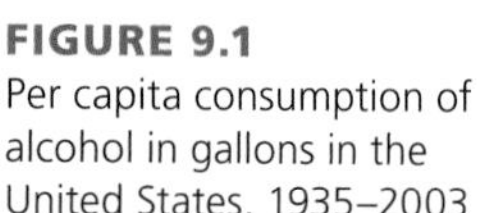

FIGURE 9.1
Per capita consumption of alcohol in gallons in the United States, 1935–2003

Note: Data prior to 1977 are from Hyman, M., Zimmerman, M., Gurioli, C. and Helrich, A. (1980), *Drinkers, drinking, and alcohol-related mortality and hospitalizations: A statistical compendium, 1980 edition,* New Brunswick, NJ: Rutgers University.

Source: http://pubs.niaaa.nih.gov/publications/surveillance73/tab1_03.htm

capita consumption of alcohol from hard liquor was at its lowest point since 1939. From 1995 to 2006, the consumption of wine and hard liquor increased slightly, and beer showed a slight decrease.

The data on per capita alcohol consumption tell us how much the "average" drinker in the United States consumes. This statistic alone can be deceptive, however, because the average value masks the large variation in drinking quantities and patterns among Americans. For example, as we saw in Chapter 1, national survey studies have shown consistently that drinking differs according to factors such as age, gender, and racial/ethnic background.

Essential to any discussion of alcohol is the rate of "heavy" drinking. Of course, what is "heavy" is open to wide interpretation and is highly dependent on the setting where the drinking occurs. From a public health point of view, however, what is called "heavy" is drinking that is associated with negative consequences: accidents, job and family problems, and symptoms of dependence on alcohol (such as an inability to cut down on drinking and memory loss associated with drinking). What seems to be important is the volume consumed on one drinking occasion, even if these occasions do not occur with great frequency (Midanik & Room, 1992).

Table 9.2 is a summary of data collected in the National Survey on Drug Use and Health conducted in 2007. The table presents reported heavy alcohol use—the consumption most highly associated with problems—in the 30 days preceding the interview. The data are highly consistent with earlier surveys and reveal that current heavy drinking is by no means a rarity in the American population aged 12 and older. Almost 7% of the national sample reported heavy drinking in the last month in 2007. However, major differences are hidden in that total percentage. Men reported a rate of heavy drinking over three times higher than women reported. Age also was a powerful factor: Almost 15% of 18- to 25-year-olds reported heavy drinking (remember the 6.9% overall rate). Again, gender within this age group is critical, as the rate for men was 19.9% and for women 9.9%. Also striking in Table 9.2 are the differences among the racial/ethnic groups for 18- to 25-year-olds. Whites reported a higher rate (18.5%) than did either blacks (5.7%) or Hispanics (10.7%).

In summary, the data on prevalence of drinking patterns and problems show that the average U.S. drinker consumes a considerable amount of alcohol in a year. Many personal, social, and environmental factors are associated with drinking patterns and

TABLE 9.2 Percentages of Individuals in Different Age, Gender, and Racial/Ethnic Groups Who Reported Heavy Alcohol Use in the Past Month, 2007

	Age			
	12–17	**18–25**	**≥26**	**Total**
Gender				
Male	2.8	19.9	10.1	10.6
Female	1.8	9.5	2.5	3.3
Race/Ethnicity				
White	3.1	18.5	6.8	7.8
Black	0.5	5.7	4.5	4.1
Hispanic	1.7	10.7	4.9	5.5
Total	2.3	14.7	6.1	6.9

Note: "Heavy" alcohol use is five or more drinks per occasion on five or more days in the past 30 days. Data are based on the 2007 national survey of drug use conducted by the National Institute on Drug Abuse.
Source: SAMHSA (2008).

drinking problems. Particularly vulnerable in this regard are young adult men (18 to 25 years old).

Consumption of Alcohol and Heavy Drinking among College Students

A topic that has received a lot of attention from the media and national politicians in the United States in recent years—alcohol consumption among college undergraduates—actually has been discussed for a long time. Indeed, drinking has been such a large part of life at most colleges that many believe there is a campus "culture of alcohol" (National Institute on Alcohol Abuse and Alcoholism [NIAAA], 2002; 2008). That is, on many campuses, a tradition of customs and beliefs regarding alcohol permeates campus social life, and each generation of students passes it on to the next.

The typical college undergraduate is in the young adult age range. Therefore, according to the national survey data, you would expect a majority of college students to drink alcohol, and a large proportion of these students have days when they drink heavily. That prediction has been confirmed in a series of national surveys of U.S. colleges and universities (about 120 of them and well over 20,000 students for each survey) that have been conducted since 1993 (Wechsler et al., 2002). One of these surveys found that, in 2001, 81.3% of the women and 79.0% of the men who responded to the mailed questionnaires said they drank alcohol in the last year. The 2001 survey also showed that 40.9% of the women and 48.6% of the men were "binge drinkers," which means consuming at least five (for men) or four (for women) drinks on at least one occasion in the last two weeks.

CONTEMPORARY ISSUE BOX 9.1

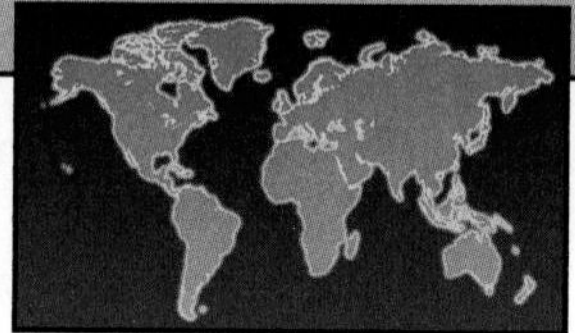

Ends of the Age Spectrum and Drinking

U.S. national surveys of drinking patterns and practices have paid relatively little attention to the elderly (generally, 65 and older) and no attention to young children. The reason in the case of the elderly probably is that this group has consistently shown a low prevalence of heavy drinking and drinking problems. Young children simply have not been sampled.

Some factors unique to the elderly are now thought to put them at higher risk of negative consequences when they drink. One factor is an age-related decrease in physical tolerance for alcohol so that smaller quantities can have considerable effects on an older person. Another factor is that many of the elderly are taking prescribed medications that are synergistic with alcohol, again magnifying the effects of a given quantity of alcohol. The higher risk of alcohol problems among the elderly who do drink is receiving a lot more attention than in previous years because of the increasing number of elderly: In 1983, the elderly were 11% of the U.S. population; in 2025, they are expected to be 17.2%. Other research shows a higher rate of alcohol-related hospitalizations among the elderly than once thought (Adams et al., 1993). Accordingly, there is a strong need to learn about the development of drinking patterns and problems among the elderly, and any special needs for treatment of those individuals who do experience problems.

On the other end of the age range, knowledge of young children's drinking is limited at best. There has been some research on this age group's knowledge about alcohol and attitudes toward its use. For example, children as young as 4 years old can identify alcoholic beverages, and 6-year-olds show some knowledge of the customs surrounding adult drinking. Unfortunately, much less is known about young children's actual alcohol consumption. The reason we know so little is that the extent of children's drinking is difficult to study scientifically—say, by the survey methods that have been used to study adults' drinking. Can you think of some problems you would face if you wanted to research drinking among young children?

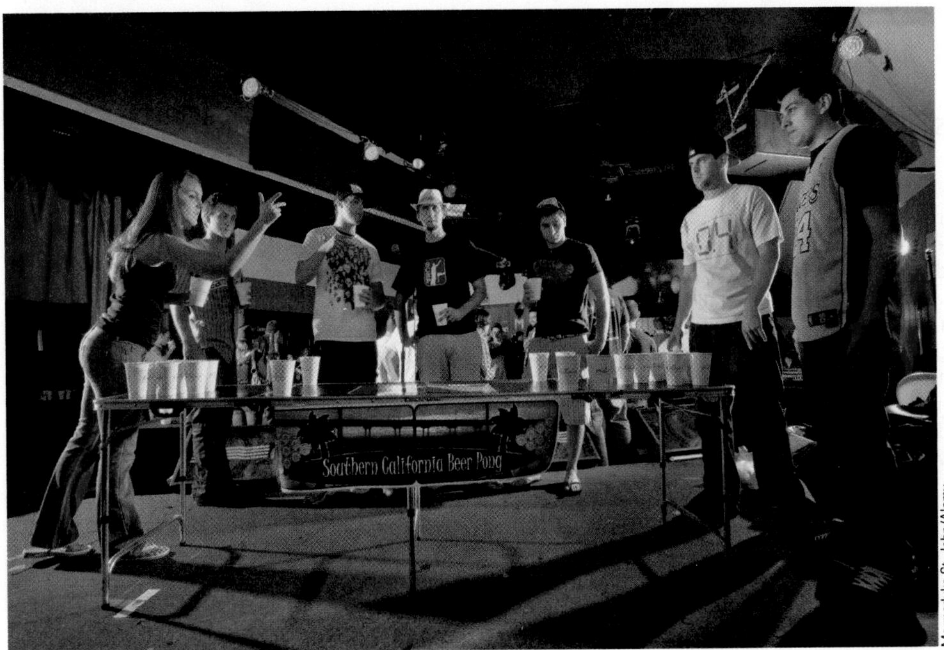

Drinking games, such as beer pong, are popular among college students and promote heavy drinking.

Calling heavier drinking episodes "binge drinking" is in some ways unfortunate, because people who are acquainted with treatment settings tend to associate that term with extended periods (days or weeks) of very heavy alcohol consumption. However, semantics should not distract us from the main point: Heavy drinking among undergraduates attracts national attention because it is associated with accidental death, injury, assault, unwanted and unprotected sex, drunk driving, vandalism, suicide, and academic problems (Neal & Fromme, 2007).

As we have seen in reviewing the findings of other surveys, the average or typical results do not apply to all campuses or to all students. Various studies have found that students who drink the least attend religious schools, commuter schools, and historically black colleges and universities. The students who drink the most are first-year students, whites, members of fraternities and sororities, and athletes (NIAAA, 2002).

The college surveys also have shown some important trends since 1993. The percentage of students classified as binge drinkers has remained the same statistically over time, but the percentage of students classified as abstainers (did not drink in the last year) increased in 2001, compared with 1993. In addition, the number of students who asked other students to reduce their alcohol use increased, as did the number of students who supported policies such as prohibiting kegs, banning alcohol advertisements, and offering alcohol-free residences (Wechsler et al., 2002).

Colleges also have increased their alcohol prevention efforts, according to the surveys. Most of these prevention programs target beliefs about alcohol and try to increase students' awareness of the negative consequences of heavy drinking. In other words, prevention programs try to change the alcohol culture on campuses. Other possible ways to reduce heavy alcohol use involve environmental change. Examples are decreasing alcohol's availability to underage drinkers, raising alcohol prices and taxes, introducing responsible beverage service, limiting the number of places where alcohol can be purchased, and changing the hours of service and days of sale (NIAAA, 2008; Wechsler et al., 2002). You might recognize that environmental adjustments

CONTEMPORARY ISSUE BOX 9.2

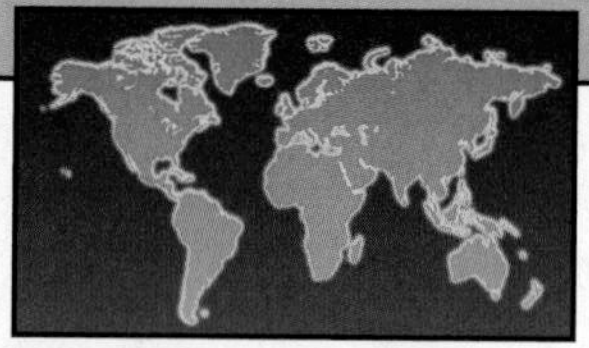

Drinking Games and Alcohol Advertising

Drinking games such as beer pong are notorious for promoting heavy drinking. They also have been around for centuries and are popular among current college students. The association between heavy alcohol consumption on an occasion and the occurrence of negative consequences raises the question of what role beer manufacturers should play in promoting drinking games through advertisement campaigns. In this regard, major beer manufacturers in the United States have entered the business of marketing accessories to drinking games like beer pong. Is such promotion legitimate?

Technically, it is. This marketing strategy is not legally prohibited, and the beer manufacturers argue that they are targeting people who are 21 years of age and older. Moreover, the manufacturers claim that their promotions always encourage "responsible drinking." The counterargument is that, regardless of the manufacturers' intent, their promotions increase the popularity of drinking games among college students and other young adults and, with it, heavy drinking on a given occasion.

Do you think that beer manufacturers should be legally able to promote drinking games? Should the alcohol beverage industry be as restricted in its advertising as the tobacco industry?

such as these go beyond the college campus and can be initiated by the governments of the localities where campuses are situated.

In conclusion, heavy drinking among college students has drawn attention not because it predicts that students will have alcohol problems after they leave college. Research has shown that significant percentages of people who do have alcohol problems as adults drank heavily in college, but most people who drink heavily in college do not have later alcohol problems. Rather, heavy drinking among college students gets attention because it is associated with serious consequences for students while they are students—that is, right now.

Pharmacology of Alcohol

Sites of Action

Alcohol is a drug that depresses the CNS. Alcohol may exert its effects by dissolving in lipid membranes, which disturbs the normal chemical actions that occur there (Rall, 1990b). That is, alcohol alters the cell membranes' anatomy by entering their internal structure. The result is reduced efficiency of conduction of neural impulses along axons, which reduces the action potential amplitude that reaches the synapse. As a consequence, neurotransmitter release and transmission of impulses across the synapse are inhibited. There is good evidence that alcohol acts on GABA-benzodiazepine receptors, and there is increasing evidence that alcohol enhances serotoninergic and dopaminergic activity (Julien, 2005). Actually, pinpointing a site of action or a single mechanism of alcohol effects is difficult because the drug affects cell membranes, all neurochemical systems, and all endocrine systems (Abel, 1985). However, specific information does exist about the pharmacokinetics of alcohol.

"What contemptible scoundrel has stolen the cork to my lunch?"
W. C. Fields

Pharmacokinetics of Alcohol

Absorption

Because it provides calories, alcohol is formally classified as a food. Unlike other foods, however, alcohol does not have to be digested before the body absorbs it. Nevertheless, most of the alcohol that is consumed must pass from the stomach to the small intestine for rapid absorption to occur. This is by far the most common way humans absorb alcohol. If alcohol is vaporized, however, it can be absorbed through the lungs and subcutaneous sites (Ritchie, 1985).

As you saw in Chapter 4, the rate at which a drug is absorbed varies widely among people, depending on individual differences in physiology and situational factors. Alcohol is no exception to this rule. The major factors influencing absorption are those that alter the rate of alcohol's passage from the stomach to the intestines. Drinkers can considerably slow absorption by eating while drinking, because the presence of food in the stomach retards absorption. Milk is especially effective for slowing alcohol absorption. Another factor is the rate at which an alcoholic beverage is consumed; faster drinking means faster absorption. Drinks that have a higher concentration of alcohol, such as whiskey on the rocks, are absorbed more quickly than those with a lower concentration, such as a scotch and water. The food substances in beer slow its absorption. Carbonated beverages are absorbed more quickly than noncarbonated ones; this explains why people may feel a quick kick from a glass of champagne on an empty stomach, when they may not get the same effect from drinking a comparable amount of table wine. Given these factors, the time between stopping drinking and the peak concentration of alcohol in the blood may range from 30 to 90 minutes (Rall, 1990b).

Some people exhibit a reflexive action of the body that works to prevent the drinking of large quantities of alcohol. The pylorus, which is the muscular valve that separates the stomach from the intestines, shuts when a large amount of alcohol has been ingested. This action is called **pylorospasm** and prevents whatever is in the stomach from passing to the intestines. This is an important safeguard because only 10% to 20% of the alcohol in the stomach is absorbed (Julien, 2005); therefore, large amounts of alcohol may remain in the stomach unabsorbed when pylorospasm occurs. This mechanism is a natural defense against an individual's becoming a very heavy drinker.

pylorospasm
The shutting of the pylorus valve that occurs in some people when they drink very large quantities of alcohol.

Distribution

After absorption, the blood distributes alcohol to all of the body's tissues. Because alcohol is easily dissolved in water, the proportion of water in a tissue determines the concentration of alcohol in it. Blood is about 70% water and therefore gets a high concentration of alcohol. Muscle and bone contain smaller percentages of water and have correspondingly smaller percentages of alcohol.

Alcohol affects primarily the CNS, especially the brain. The concentration of alcohol in the brain approximates that in the blood because of the brain's large blood supply and because alcohol freely passes through the blood-brain barrier. Alcohol's LD 50 varies as a function of different factors. The average adult would reach alcohol's LD 50 after drinking about 25 standard drinks in an hour or so. Of course, saying this estimate is an average means that many people would die from drinking considerably fewer than 25 drinks in an hour. A **standard drink** may be defined as 0.5 ounce of alcohol, which is about the amount in 1 ounce of 90- to 100-proof whiskey, 12 ounces of 4% alcohol beer, or 4 ounces of table wine (12% alcohol).

standard drink
The alcohol equivalent in a drink of beer, wine, or distilled spirits. A standard drink equals 0.5 ounce of alcohol—about the alcohol content in 12 ounces of beer, 4 ounces of table wine, or 1 ounce of 90- to 100-proof whiskey.

Because all humans have the same proportions of the different tissues and water, it is possible to estimate the concentration of alcohol in the body from its concentration in the blood. The blood alcohol concentration (BAC), as the name implies, is the amount of alcohol in the bloodstream. It is expressed as a percentage of weight of alcohol per 100 units of blood volume (Sobell & Sobell, 1981). Typically, the ratio is expressed as milligrams (mg) of alcohol per 100 milliliters (ml) of blood. Therefore, one drop of alcohol (about 10 mg) in 1,000 drops of blood (about 100 ml) gives a BAC of 0.01% (100 ml of blood weighs about 100 g). For your reference, the legal level for intoxication in all 50 states, the District of Columbia, and Puerto Rico is 0.08%. The legal level is also 0.08% in all of Canada; the level is 0.08% in Great Britain, 0.05% in Norway, and 0.02% in Finland and

Sweden. Alcohol's LD 50 is a BAC of between 0.45% and 0.50%, although there have been case reports of people surviving BACs up to a little more than 1.0% (Berild & Hasselbalch, 1981).

You can translate these numbers into an approximation of the number of drinks consumed over time. We emphasize approximation because, as you saw earlier, a person's BAC depends in part on the different factors that influence absorption. However, knowing approximately what your BAC is at a given time can have practical value.

When a healthy 160-pound man consumes a standard drink, his BAC is raised by 0.02% to 0.03% within 45 to 60 minutes of drinking. Factors besides dose of alcohol determine the peak BAC that is reached. Again, the information in Chapter 4 will help you to understand this. Total body mass is a major factor because alcohol is distributed in both muscle and fat. As a result, heavier people will have a lower BAC than lighter ones after drinking the same amount of alcohol. Another factor is how much of a person's body consists of fat and muscle. Alcohol is soluble in fat but is even more soluble in water. Everything being equal, a drink will result in a lower BAC for a leaner person than for a drinker who has a higher percentage of body fat. This is the reason a woman tends to reach higher BACs from drinking a given amount of alcohol than does a man of the same body weight. Women tend to have a higher percentage of body fat than men do. Also, one study suggests that women have less of the enzyme alcohol dehydrogenase in their stomachs, which prevents them from metabolizing as much alcohol in their stomachs. More alcohol enters a woman's bloodstream and eventually the brain and other organs (Frezza et al., 1990). This finding suggests that, for a man and a woman of equal weight, the same amount of alcohol affects the woman more (this is one reason "binge drinking" is defined as five drinks for men and as four drinks for women).

Aspirin also may affect the amount of alcohol that is metabolized in the stomach. If a person who has recently eaten takes a moderate dose of aspirin as drinking begins, the resulting BAC will be higher than it would be if the aspirin were not taken (Roine et al., 1990). It seems that aspirin suppresses alcohol dehydrogenase in the stomach, so less alcohol is metabolized there. The "recently eaten" part of this finding is important because aspirin makes no difference when alcohol enters an empty stomach. In that circumstance, alcohol enters the intestines so rapidly that there is no time for aspirin's effect on alcohol dehydrogenase.

Individual differences in the rate at which the body metabolizes alcohol are also variables that influence what peak BAC is reached. For these and other reasons, the following formula for computing BAC gives only an approximation. The formula estimates the BAC that would result at a given time in our hypothetical 160-pound man who drank a given number of standard drinks. In the formula, BAC = blood alcohol content, NSD = number of standard drinks, and NHD = number of hours since drinking began:

$$\text{Estimated BAC} = \text{NSD} \times (0.025\%) - \text{NHD} \times (0.015\%)$$

In the formula, NSD is multiplied by 0.025% because that is the midpoint of our estimated range of increase in BAC that results when the 160-pound drinker has a standard drink. NHD is multiplied by 0.015% because that is the BAC equivalent of the estimated hourly rate that the liver metabolizes alcohol (Rall, 1990b). The metabolic rate is independent of body weight, unlike the rise in BAC for a given amount of alcohol that is drunk.

Based on our approximation formula, a 160-pound man who drinks three 12-ounce regular beers in an hour will have a BAC of about 0.06%. That result would be adjusted up or down depending on the important factor of body weight; many conversion charts like Figure 9.2 are available to make such corrections. Also, as discussed earlier, some adjustment up in the BAC gives a better estimate for women.

The estimation formula reflects that the BAC essentially depends on the dose of alcohol that is consumed and the time that it takes to drink it. Figure 9.3 shows the

Weight	Drinks (two-hour period) 1 1/2 oz. 80-proof hard liquor or 12 oz. beer or 5 oz. wine							
100	1	2	3	4	5	6	7	8
120	1	2	3	4	5	6	7	8
140	1	2	3	4	5	6	7	8
160	1	2	3	4	5	6	7	8
180	1	2	3	4	5	6	7	8
200	1	2	3	4	5	6	7	8
220	1	2	3	4	5	6	7	8
240	1	2	3	4	5	6	7	8

Caution
BAC to .05

Driving Impaired
.05 or higher

Figures are averages. Alcohol effects may vary with each individual.

FIGURE 9.2
A conversion chart for approximating blood alcohol concentration as a function of number of drinks, time, and body weight

BAC–time relationship. The figure illustrates that the BAC rises quickly and then more gradually returns to zero after drinking stops. Therefore, time is an important factor in determining BAC. Time enters the formula independent of the number of standard drinks because of the way the liver metabolizes alcohol—generally, at a constant amount over a given time, regardless of the amount that is drunk.

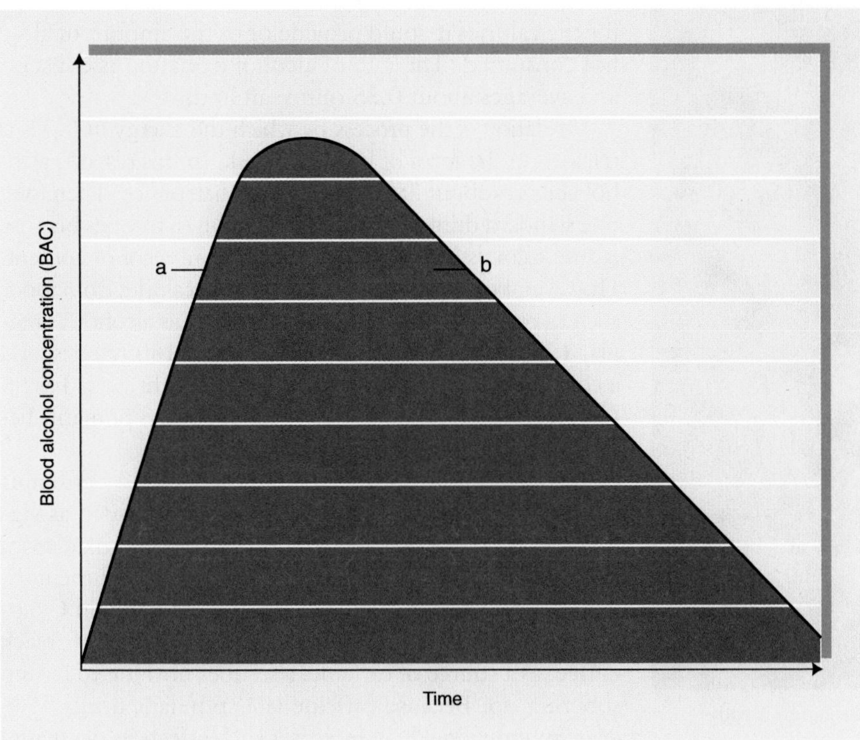

FIGURE 9.3
Acute tolerance to alcohol's effects—the effects of alcohol at time a are greater than the effects at time b

For medical or legal purposes, BAC is not estimated by formula but as precisely as possible by standardized procedures. Blood and urine samples are taken frequently for medical and medical/legal reasons to measure BAC. For example, blood samples often determine the BACs of drivers killed in motor vehicle accidents. BAC is commonly measured by breath sample because of the known ratio (1:2,100) between the amount of alcohol in the lungs and the amount in the blood. The police departments of many U.S. cities measure BAC by breath analysis. Gas chromatography is used to obtain excellent estimates of BAC, so good they are considered legally admissible evidence. Gas chromatographic methods are expensive, however, and until recently, cost has prohibited the precise measurement of BAC in settings where it would be very useful, such as outpatient alcohol treatment programs. Substantial improvements in electronic technology have made possible breath-testing devices that give good BAC estimates and cost only a few hundred dollars.

disulfiram
A drug that interferes with the metabolism of alcohol so that people soon feel very ill if they drink while on a regimen of disulfiram. The drug may be used as part of a treatment program for alcohol dependence.

Metabolism and Excretion

More than 90% of the alcohol that is absorbed is metabolized by the body, mainly in the liver. (We saw earlier that the stomach also plays a part in metabolizing alcohol.) The small percentage of alcohol that is not metabolized is excreted in pure form through the kidneys and the lungs. When alcohol is metabolized in the liver, it is broken down to acetaldehyde by the enzyme alcohol dehydrogenase. This step is the basis of using the drug **disulfiram** (trade name Antabuse) in the treatment of alcohol dependence. We have more to say about this in Chapter 15. Acetaldehyde eventually is broken down to carbon dioxide and water. At this point, there is a release of energy, or calories (Julien, 1996). The carbon dioxide is excreted from the body through air exchange in the lungs, and the water is excreted in urine. Unlike other foods, such as proteins and carbohydrates, the rate that alcohol is metabolized is independent of the body's need for the calories it could provide or of the amount of alcohol consumed. The rate of alcohol oxidation is constant and averages about 0.35 ounce an hour.

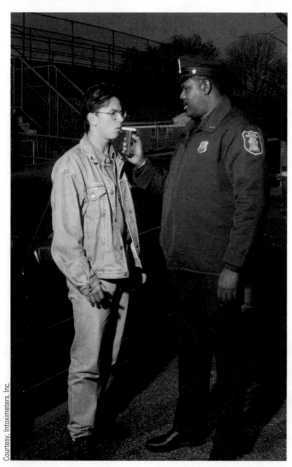
Courtesy, Intoximeters, Inc.

Blood alcohol concentration can be measured by breath analysis, as shown here.

Oxidation is the process by which the energy in foods is released in the form of heat and work. In this respect, alcohol liberates about 75 calories in each half ounce. Therefore, one standard drink of whiskey has about 75 calories because all the calories in distilled spirits are from alcohol content. However, beverages such as beer provide calories from foods such as proteins and carbohydrates as well as alcohol. A regular 12-ounce, 4% alcohol beer has about 150 calories, and a comparable amount of the commercial light beers has 95 to 135 calories. Light beers have fewer calories primarily because they contain less alcohol.

Alcohol is notorious for being unaffected by attempts to hasten its removal from the body. Efforts such as vigorous exercise do nothing to speed up alcohol oxidation, except to the extent that exercise takes time and the individual does not drink while exercising. As noted in Chapter 8, the long-used intoxication "remedy" of black coffee, as a source of caffeine, also does nothing to hasten sobering up. Because caffeine is a stimulant drug, however, an individual may interpret such effects as decreased alcohol intoxication. In fact, little can be done to hasten sobriety except to wait for the liver to do its work in its own constant time. Therefore, if you go to bed on Saturday at 2 A.M. with a BAC of 0.15%, you will still be legally drunk three hours later at 5 A.M. (your BAC will be 0.105%) and will not be alcohol-free until noon.

Tolerance and Dependence

Tolerance

Regular use of alcohol results in some dispositional tolerance (see Chapter 5 for a detailed discussion of tolerance). Therefore, a drinker must consume greater quantities of alcohol to maintain a certain BAC. Dispositional tolerance can be reversed with a period of abstinence from alcohol. Functional tolerance has a greater practical influence than does dispositional tolerance in altering how alcohol affects a person with repeated use. Tolerance to alcohol may be both acute and protracted. Because of acute tolerance, the effects of alcohol at a given BAC are greater when the BAC curve is rising than on the descending limb of the curve. For example, at a BAC of 0.10% as it is ascending, an individual may show considerably impaired performance on tasks related to driving. If the BAC peaks at, say, 0.15% and then hits 0.10% as it is falling, however, an individual's performance on those same driving-related tasks would be improved, although still probably far from its level with no alcohol in the blood. Of course, such improvement would make no difference to the police. A person with a BAC of 0.10% is legally drunk in every state that has per se intoxication laws, regardless of what direction the BAC is heading when it is measured. Acute tolerance is illustrated in Figure 9.3.

As with dispositional tolerance, the development of protracted tolerance requires that the individual drink greater amounts of alcohol to achieve an effect once achieved with less alcohol. Because protracted functional tolerance far outpaces dispositional tolerance, the person becomes more susceptible to serious health and other consequences of heavy alcohol consumption. For example, a person may drink large quantities of alcohol to achieve a mood change that was once reached with much less alcohol. However, the BAC does not behave in the same way. Drinking large quantities of alcohol still results in a high BAC. With higher BACs, the body is more vulnerable to suffering alcohol's toxic effects, which we review shortly. Similarly, chronic heavy drinkers may not feel drunk or even impaired at BACs greater than 0.08%, but they still are defined legally as drunk. Such a designation leaves people liable to arrests for drunk driving and other alcohol-related charges.

As we noted in Chapter 5, there is cross-tolerance between alcohol and other CNS depressant drugs. We also noted how cross-tolerance might cause difficulties for an anesthesiologist preparing a patient for surgery. Sometimes the problem is acute in the emergency room, where surgery must be performed immediately following a serious accident. You will see later how alcohol intoxication is associated with the occurrence of accidents, and as you might expect, the heaviest users (most tolerant) of alcohol are the people who are most likely to have the accidents (USDHHS, 1993).

Alcohol also shows cross-dependence with CNS depressant drugs. This means that taking one drug can suppress withdrawal symptoms of the other. For example, alcohol and the benzodiazepine drugs such as Valium and Librium show cross-dependence. This phenomenon has proved valuable in managing withdrawal from alcohol in individuals who are physically dependent on it.

Physical Dependence

With chronic heavy drinking, individuals can develop physical dependence on alcohol. Symptoms of physical dependence can be severe and may be classified into three phases,

TABLE 9.3 Symptoms of Alcohol Withdrawal Syndrome

Phase	Onset	Symptoms
1	As soon as a few hours after drinking stopped; BACs may still be .0%	Tremulousness (shakes), profuse perspiration, weakness, alcohol and other drug seeking. Also may include agitation, headache, anorexia, nausea and vomiting, abdominal cramps, high heart rate, and exaggerated and rapid reflexes. Visual and auditory hallucinations may follow in increased intensity. Hallucinations may also occur when the individual is severely intoxicated (called acute alcoholic hallucinosis).
2	Within 24 hours of drinking cessation	Grand mal seizures, ranging from one seizure to continuous severe seizure activity with little or no interruption
3	About 30 hours after drinking cessation. This is the most protracted phase, and may last 3 to 4 days; commonly called delirium tremens (DTs).	Severe agitation, often appearance of confusion and disorientation; almost continual activity; very high body temperature and abnormally rapid heart beat; terrifying hallucinations, may be visual, auditory, or tactile. The latter is most often felt as bugs or little animals crawling on the skin. Hallucinations are accompanied by delusions, with a high potential for violent behavior without medical management. Deaths during DTs still occur due to high fever, cardiovascular collapse, or traumatic injury.
End of withdrawal course	About 5 to 7 days after drinking stopped	Exhaustion and severe dehydration

Source: From M. R. Jacobs and K. O'Brien Fehr (1987), *Drugs and Drug Abuse: A Reference Text* (2nd ed.). Copyright © 1987 Addiction Research Foundation. Used with permission.

as outlined in Table 9.3. As you can see, a wide range of symptoms is associated with time of onset after drinking cessation, although some symptoms overlap in the different phases. You should note that not all people who are physically dependent on alcohol experience all three phases of symptoms. For example, Phase 2 symptoms probably appear least frequently, and individuals may go directly from Phase 1 to Phase 3 symptoms. Another important point: Withdrawal symptoms may appear when the BAC is falling but still at a fairly high level, such as 0.15%. The BAC does not need to have fallen all the way to zero for withdrawal to begin. Before its management by use of drugs associated with cross-dependence with alcohol, alcohol withdrawal often ended in death. More recently, less severe alcohol withdrawal has been managed without the use of drugs (**social detoxification**) or with drugs in an outpatient setting.

social detoxification Treatment of alcohol withdrawal without the use of medicine.

The following account, based on a case described in the *DSM-III Casebook* (Spitzer et al., 1981, pp. 104–105), gives a good description of an individual experiencing alcohol withdrawal.

The patient was a 43-year-old divorced carpenter. His sister reported that the patient had been drinking more than a fifth of cheap wine every day for the past five years. The patient also had not eaten well, maybe only one meal a day, and had relied on wine as his main source of nourishment. The patient stopped drinking three days ago, and the morning after, he awoke with his hands shaking so badly that he could barely light a cigarette. He also had a feeling of inner panic that made sleep almost impossible. A neighbor called the patient's sister in concern because he was not making any sense and seemed as if he could not take care of himself.

When he was examined at the hospital, the patient alternated between superficial, chatty warmth and apprehension. He went back and forth from recognizing the doctor to thinking he was the patient's brother. Twice during the interview, the patient called the doctor by his brother's name and asked him when he had arrived, apparently losing track of the interview. When the patient is at rest, he shows a gross tremor and picks "bugs" off the bedsheets. The patient has no **orientation to time** and thinks that he is in the parking lot of a supermarket. The patient says that he is fighting against his feeling that the world is about to end in a holocaust. The patient is startled every few minutes from what he says are sounds and sights of fiery car crashes. These perceptions apparently are retriggered by sounds of rolling carts in the hall. Memory testing is not possible because the patient's attention shifts too rapidly. (Reprinted with permission from the *Diagnostic and Statistical Manual of Mental Disorders*. Copyright 1981 and 1989 American Psychiatric Association.)

orientation to time
Awareness of temporal specification, such as time of day, day of the week, or year. Orientation to time is one of the functions assessed in a psychiatric mental status exam.

Therapeutic Uses

Alcohol might have been thought to be the panacea for all of life's ills, but we now know its medical value is probably outdistanced by its social value (Ritchie, 1985). In fact, there was a hint of this knowledge some time ago based on a remedy for treating colds taken from an old English book: At first inkling of a cold, hang your hat on the bedpost, drink from a bottle of good whiskey until two hats appear, and then get into bed and stay there. The therapeutic value of alcohol in this case was in keeping the cold victim in bed.

"Drink no longer water, but use a little wine for thine stomach's sake and thine often infirmities."
The Bible, I Timothy 5:23

Alcohol does have a few actual therapeutic uses. For example, it is an ingredient in several legitimate medical products (Jacobs & Fehr, 1987). Because alcohol is an excellent solvent, small amounts are combined with other ingredients in cough syrups and other products taken orally. Furthermore, alcohol is an ingredient in mouthwashes and shaving lotions. If the individuals like them, alcoholic beverages may be recommended in moderate amounts to convalescent or elderly patients to be taken before meals to stimulate appetite and digestion. Alcohol also is included in compounds created to treat skin problems. Because alcohol cools when it evaporates, ethanol sponges are used to treat fevers. In addition, alcohol is part of mixtures that serve as liniments (Rall, 1990b). Finally, dehydrated alcohol may be injected close to nerves or sympathetic ganglia to relieve chronic pain that may occur, for example, in patients with inoperable cancer (Ritchie, 1985).

Acute Effects of Alcohol

In this section, we review both the acute and chronic effects of alcohol consumption. We first go over alcohol's many acute physiological, sensory-motor (sensorimotor), and psychological effects. We also discuss several topics of special societal concern related to alcohol's acute effects, including aggression, sexual behavior, and driving.

One point about alcohol's acute effects is that alcohol generally acts on the body as a depressant, and its acute effects are proportional to the magnitude of the BAC. Simply put, as the BAC increases, acute effects increase in number and intensity. However, how humans experience some degree of **intoxication** and behave under different doses of alcohol may be modified by psychological and situational factors as well as alcohol dose and tolerance to this drug. For some behaviors, these nondrug factors may be even more powerful determinants of alcohol's acute effects than drug factors.

intoxication
A transient state of physical and psychological disruption caused by the presence of a toxic substance, such as alcohol, in the CNS.

Physiological Effects

Alcohol taken at low doses has several physiological effects.[1] Alcohol inhibits the secretion of the antidiuretic hormone, which causes increased urination. The effect happens when the BAC is rising but not when it is falling. Alcohol also reduces the amount of body fat that is oxidized. This acute effect of alcohol accumulates to result in long-term increased body fat and weight gain when alcohol is used in addition to normal food intake (Suter, Schutz, & Jequier, 1992). Such weight gain is commonly called a "beer belly." Alcohol is a peripheral dilator and causes the skin to feel warm and turn red. A number of authors have cautioned against using alcoholic beverages to warm up in cold environments. This advice is counterintuitive to many drinkers, who experience the warmth that occurs with peripheral dilation and know of the Saint Bernard and its keg of brandy rescuing victims in snow-covered mountains. Alcohol's dilating effect on peripheral blood vessels causes some loss of body heat, however, and such action was thought to ultimately decrease protection against the cold. It turns out the problem is not a serious one, as experimental studies have shown that alcohol does not significantly tilt the balance of the body's temperature regulation in cold environments.

An acute alcohol effect with wide practical application is that it increases gastric secretion, which is one basis for the U.S. cocktail hour. The increase in gastric secretion stimulates the appetite. Unfortunately, alcohol at high doses harms the stomach mucosa and causes gastric distress. Nausea and vomiting may occur at BACs greater than 0.15%. Another physiological effect of alcohol when taken in high doses and when the BAC increases rapidly is a release of corticosteroids, part of the body's general reaction to stress. In this case, the stressor is a high dose of alcohol, which is toxic to the body.

An important acute effect of alcohol is disruption of sleep patterns. Even at lower doses, alcohol suppresses **REM sleep**, which is the stage of the sleep cycle when most dreaming occurs (REM stands for "rapid eye movements," which characterize this stage of sleep). When the dose is low, REM sleep is suppressed only in the first half of the night, but REM time rebounds and increases in the second half. At larger doses of alcohol, REM sleep is suppressed throughout the night.

REM sleep
Acronym for "rapid eye movements," which are associated with dream activity and are one stage in a cycle of sleep.

Alcohol impairs memory. Its acute effects are on short-term memory, and when high BACs are reached rapidly, a **blackout** may occur. Blackouts are an individual's amnesia about events when drinking, even though there was no loss of consciousness. For example, a person who had a lot to drink the night before may wake up and have absolutely no recollection of where he or she parked the car. Blackouts are thought to result from a failure in the transfer of information in **short-term memory** to **long-term memory**. People also have "grayouts," in which they can partially recall events that occurred in full consciousness during a drinking occasion. Grayouts probably reflect state-dependent learning. Blackouts and grayouts do not happen consistently in the same individuals with a given dose of alcohol, and the factors that specifically determine their occurrence have not been identified.

blackout
Failure to recall events that occurred while drinking even though there is no loss of consciousness.

short-term memory
Memory for recent events; thought to differ from long-term memory in several important ways.

long-term memory
Memory for remote events. According to one theory of memory, information enters long-term memory through short-term memory.

[1] Much of the discussion of alcohol's acute effects is based on Becker et al. (1975), Jacobs and Fehr (1987), McKim (2000), and Sobell and Sobell (1981).

Every drinker probably has had at least one somewhat-delayed consequence of an episode of overindulgence—the hangover. Hangovers may be thought of as a minor withdrawal syndrome because they are the body's readjustment to a nonalcohol state. Hangovers begin to appear about 4 to 12 hours after reaching the peak BAC and generally are not considered a pleasant alcohol effect. Symptoms may include headache, dizziness, nausea, vomiting, increased heart rate, fatigue, and thirst (Gauvin, Cheng, & Holloway, 1993). Furthermore, although the BAC is zero, hangovers are associated with a reduced ability to perform the complex skills required to drive a motor vehicle (Franck, 1983). Although people usually do not think of hangovers as a serious negative consequence of overindulging in drinking alcohol beyond not feeling well temporarily, the cumulative effect of hangovers for a society are considerable. For example, in England, hangovers cost the economy about two billion pounds a year, primarily because of people skipping work (Pittler, Verster, & Ernst, 2005).

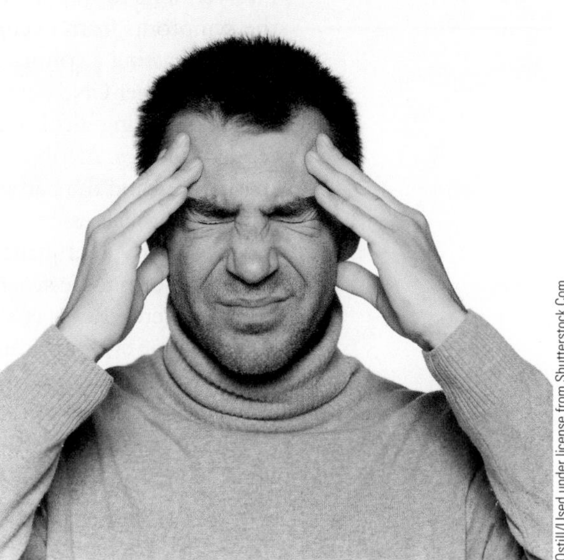

Headache is one symptom of a hangover, which is a common consequence of alcohol overindulgence.

Remedies galore, from folk medicine and medical science alike, have been sought to cure the hangover (see Contemporary Issue Box 9.3). Perhaps the one heard most often is the "hair of the dog that bit you," and in this case, the dog is alcohol. It is true that alcohol erases its own hangover symptoms, just as drinking stops alcohol withdrawal symptoms. This solution is far from perfect, however, because all that is being accomplished is postponing the inevitable. Of course, a real danger in using alcohol in this way is that it is courting a pattern of frequent, heavy drinking, because alcohol is used to remove an unpleasant effect of drinking in high quantities. Many studies have shown this effect to be highly reinforcing to humans and other animals alike.

Therefore, it seems that the only dependable and safe cure for the hangover is time or, of course, drinking in moderation or not at all. The Pittler, Verster, and Ernst (2005) article cited earlier confirmed this conclusion, as its review of clinical trials of

CONTEMPORARY ISSUE BOX 9.3

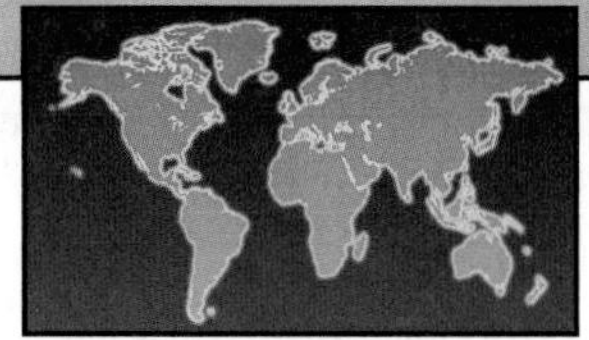

The Hangover's Many "Cures"

Besides the "hair of the dog that bit you," other purported hangover cures have made the circuit among drinkers from around the world for millennia. Here are some of them:

1. Take megadoses of vitamins, so your body will have the strength to ward off the hangover.
2. Eat solyanka (a Russian soup made with pickle juice).
3. Inhale pure oxygen to quicken the body's oxidation of alcohol.
4. Run 6 miles.
5. Drink sports drinks.
6. Drink a repulsive concoction, so the disgusting taste will help you to forget the hangover.
7. Eat pickled herring (from Germany).
8. Stay in bed and lie still.

Some of these remedies sound as though people desperately suffering from hangovers created them. None of them has a basis in medical science or practice. Hangovers are "cured" in only two ways: time and not getting too intoxicated in the first place.

interventions to treat hangover showed nothing to be nearly as effective as preventing the symptoms from occurring in the first place.

In discussing alcohol's acute effects, we must reemphasize that it interacts synergistically with other CNS depressants. The point is worth repeating because of the dangerous effects of mixing alcohol and barbiturates—a common method of intended and unintended suicides. Alcohol and the benzodiazepines do not have the potential for suicide that alcohol and the barbiturates have, but they can cause serious decrements in the performance of skills essential to survival, such as driving a car or staying awake while driving a car. Similarly, marijuana and alcohol are frequently consumed on the same occasion, and there seem to be synergistic effects of these two drugs on skills related to driving (for example, Perez-Reyes et al., 1988). Antihistamines, which are available over the counter, also combine synergistically with alcohol. Another point about combining alcohol with other drugs: Alcohol decreases the effects of certain prescribed medications, such as antibiotics, anticonvulsants, anticoagulants, and **monoamine oxidase (MAO) inhibitors**.

monoamine oxidase (MAO) inhibitors Drugs used to treat depressions that inhibit the activity of the enzyme monoamine oxidase, which degrades the neurotransmitters of norepinephrine and serotonin.

Alcohol causes slight respiratory depression at lower doses, but this effect does not reach dangerous levels in healthy people unless they consume very high doses. Higher doses also are associated with the induction of sleep, stupor, and in extremely high doses, coma. In the overdose range of consumption, cardiovascular depression can occur. Earlier, we noted that a dose of alcohol could be lethal (lethal dose 50, or "LD 50" BAC of 0.45% to 0.50%) due to dysfunction of the more primitive areas of the brain like the medulla that control breathing and heartbeat.

Sensorimotor Effects

At moderate (0.05%) to higher BACs, alcohol has several acute effects on the senses. Vision decreases in acuity, and taste and smell are not so sensitive. Pain sensitivity decreases when the BAC is in the 0.08% to 0.10% range. Simple reaction time begins to slow significantly at a BAC of 0.10%. An example of a simple reaction time task is to press a key as quickly as possible when a single light on a panel shines. In a complex reaction time task, research participants are asked to integrate two or more stimuli and then respond to them as quickly as possible. An example is to press a key when a white and a red light shine but not to press it when only the white light shines. Complex reaction time may be impaired in both speed and accuracy at BACs of 0.05% or even lower.

"Before I'd know it (while drinking), I'd be stumbling around, being loud and jovial, insensitive to pain. I'd feel great at the time, and I'd also know what was in store for me. And the next day I'd be totally out of action, feeling as if I'd been poisoned, which I guess I had. I got really scared one time when I woke up like that and couldn't remember anything of the night before."

37-year-old man describing his drinking during college (Weil & Rosen, 1983, p. 191)

Alcohol strongly affects body sway, which is measured by asking people to stand steady with their eyes closed. The body's deviation from a "steady state" is then recorded. At a BAC of 0.06%, body sway is impaired by about 40%. At a high BAC, we see alcohol's effect on body sway manifested as staggering and, eventually, as an inability to walk independently at all. The sensitivity of body sway to alcohol is the reason for the "walk a straight line" test that police use to decide whether a suspect is drunk. Alcohol's influence on body sway is due to its effects on balance controls in the inner ear. This also is why the room may spin when partygoers lie down and close their eyes to sleep after a night of heavy drinking.

Alcohol impairs psychomotor skills. In tasks designed to measure these skills, participants are asked to make controlled muscular movements to adjust or position a machine or some mechanism on an experimental apparatus in response to changes in the speed or direction of a moving object (for example, see Levine, Kramer, & Levine, 1975, p. 288). A common example is the mechanical or computerized version of the pursuit rotor task, in which participants must keep a stylus on a target that moves circularly on an automated disk.

Psychomotor task performance on the average shows deterioration at BACs of about 0.03% and higher (Levine, Kramer, & Levine, 1975). These tasks commonly require relatively fine motor dexterity. At high BACs, 0.15% or more, there is clear abnormality in gross motor functions like standing and walking. At these levels, alcohol has impaired the brain centers responsible for motor activity and balance to such a degree that the neural messages are not being sent to the muscles.

Alcohol and Driving Ability

Sensorimotor skills constitute a major part of driving ability. During the early 1980s, public awareness of drinking and driving a motor vehicle increased enormously. Probably most influential in opening the public's eyes and ears about drunk driving were citizens' organizations such as Mothers Against Drunk Driving (MADD) and Students Against Drunk Driving (SADD). These movements contributed to and were strengthened by the more conservative attitudes toward alcohol and drug use that marked the 1980s in the United States. Part of this trend was increased enforcement of stricter legal penalties for driving under the influence (DUI) of alcohol (or other drugs). As one example, the large majority of the United States has administrative license revocation for anyone who fails or refuses to take a BAC test (NIAAA, 2000; U.S. National Highway Traffic Safety Administration [USNHTSA], 1997).

"I'm in NO condition to be driving . . . wait a minute! I shouldn't be listening to myself—I'M DRUNK!"

Homer Simpson

Attention regarding the dangers of alcohol use has focused on motor vehicles, particularly cars. There is ample cause for concern. Motor vehicle crashes are the most common nonnatural cause of death in the United States; they are the leading cause of death overall of people aged 1 to 24 (NIAAA, 2000). Alcohol is implicated as a causal factor in traffic fatalities, but statistics are not conclusive because we have only correlational studies. The argument for alcohol as a cause is strengthened, however, by data on the relationship between relative risk of involvement in a traffic accident (fatal or not) and BAC. The relative risk of a fatal single-vehicle crash at different BACs is especially striking. At a BAC of 0.02% to 0.03%, such a crash is 1.4 times as likely as it is at a BAC of 0%. At a BAC of 0.05% to 0.09%, it is 11.1 times as likely. At a BAC of 0.10% to 0.14%, it is 48 times as likely, and at BACs of 0.15% and higher, it is 380 times as likely (Zador, 1991).

The case for alcohol as a causal factor in traffic fatalities becomes even more solid with experimental data on how alcohol affects performance on tasks that require

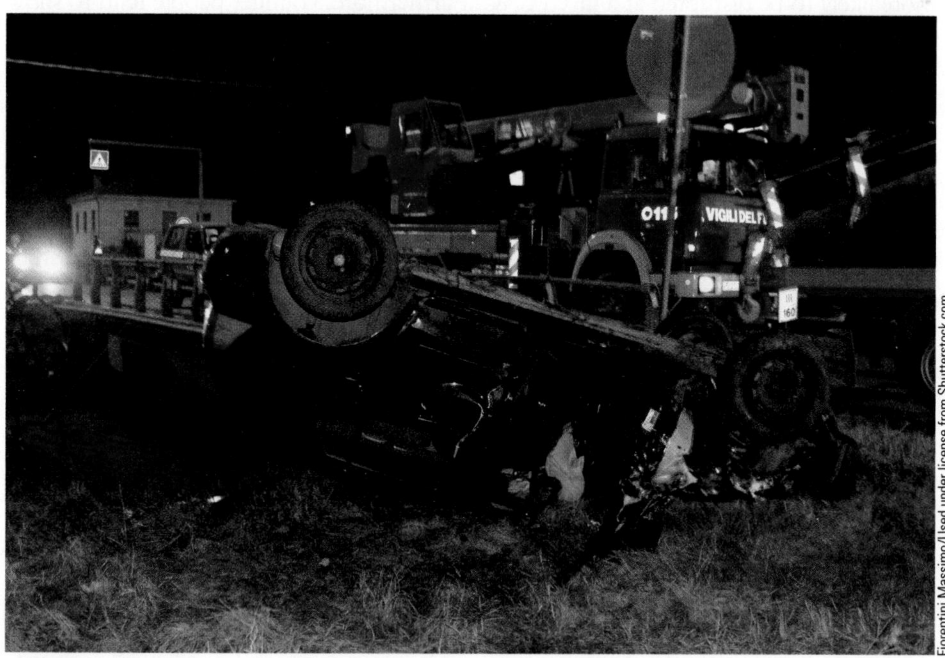

Motor vehicle accidents are the single most common nonnatural causes of death in the United States.

psychomotor skills and an integration of sensory information. An example, called a "divided-attention" task, is combining the pursuit rotor and complex reaction time tasks into one experimental task. Participants are required to keep the stylus on target (pursuit rotor) while they are simultaneously responding to the two light stimuli on a panel (complex reaction time). Driving a car requires the same motor control and sensory integration abilities that are necessary to perform such a divided-attention task. Alcohol impairs performance on divided-attention tasks at BACs of 0.05% or lower. In fact, this is one basis of the recommendation of several groups, such as the American College of Emergency Physicians, the Associates for the Advancement of Emergency Medicine, and the American Medical Association, that the legal level of intoxication be uniform across the United States at a BAC of 0.05%. In many states, arrest still is possible at BACs below their respective legal levels of intoxication for "driving while impaired."

"In Amarillo, Texas, I participate in a community coalition dedicated to fighting drunken driving and underage drinking. Our motto: All it takes is everyone. Only community-wide efforts around the country can defeat the problem of alcohol abuse."

Bernadette Teichmann (*USA Today*, August 30, 1993, p. 11A)

Alcohol therefore seems to be a primary factor that raises the risk of involvement in fatal and nonfatal motor vehicle accidents. Other factors interact with alcohol to affect risk, and two of the more important ones are gender and age. Young drivers are disproportionately more likely to be involved in alcohol-related accidents. For example, one study showed that, in 1980, 18-year-olds constituted 2.2% of the driver population and drove 2% of the total number of miles traveled, yet they were involved in 5.5% of the alcohol-related accidents. By comparison, 45- to 54-year-olds drove nine times as many miles as the 18-year-olds but had only one and one-third as many alcohol-related accidents. Young people seem to be at higher risk for motor vehicle accidents across the range of BACs. For example, in the study of fatal single-vehicle crashes by Zador (1991) cited earlier, men and women aged 16 to 20 were more at risk for such accidents at every BAC from 0.02% to 0.15% and higher. Zador's study also showed that the risk for single-vehicle fatal crashes was highest for 16- to 20-year-olds when the BAC was in the lowest range of 0.00% to 0.01%.

Taken together, these data suggest that the higher risk found consistently for young people is due in part to their relative inexperience in both drinking and driving (USDHHS, 1987a). This means driving is not as well learned a skill in younger people and is more likely to be disrupted at a given BAC. Furthermore, younger people tend to show less protracted tolerance in general at a given BAC because of their shorter period of use of alcoholic beverages. These reasons, along with the designation of 21 years as the minimum age for legal purchase and possession of beverages containing alcohol, underlie the enactment of "zero-tolerance" laws in most of the United States. These laws make it illegal for people under age 21 to drive with measurable amounts of alcohol in their bodies (USNHTSA, 1997). Many states have called "measurable" BACs higher than 0.02%.

Young men (18 to 34 years old) seem to be the group most likely to be intoxicated, driving, and in traffic accidents (Chou et al., 2006). This coincides with the consistent finding in surveys that young men are the ones most likely to drink heavily (say, five or more drinks) on an occasion. Data published in 1983 show that 38% of the young men drivers who were involved in fatal accidents had a BAC of 0.10% or higher, compared to 30% for all other age and gender groups (USDHHS, 1987a). Young men are more likely to be legally intoxicated and the drivers in fatal accidents because of their tendency to drink heavily on occasion and because they drive a relatively higher percentage of miles on weekend nights, when all drivers are most likely to be intoxicated. In this regard, one study suggests that young men take more risks when in a group and intoxicated, which could affect their decision to drink and drive in the first place and to be more reckless if they do drive (Sayette et al., 2004).

In summary, drunk driving is a serious problem in the United States. It is also important to say that action taken against drunk driving in recent years may be paying off. From 1982 to 1997, alcohol-related traffic fatalities fell 36%, and the greatest reduction (59%) was among individuals 15 to 20 years old (NIAAA, 2000). This finding is consistent with more recent U.S. national survey data, which show a 22% reduction in the rate of driving after drinking "too much" in the last year between 1991 and 1992 and 2001 and 2002 (Chou et al., 2006). These changes may be due to several factors, but research has shown that strict drunk-driving laws and the driver's perception that arrest and conviction are likely if they are broken are critical to reducing the drunk-driving problem.

Psychological Effects

Alcohol combines with other factors to change emotion and mood. Different people report a range of psychological effects at a given BAC, and the same drinker may report different effects at a given BAC on different occasions. The influences of nondrug factors, particularly situational and cognitive variables (for example, expectancies and attitudes), are perhaps most powerful in this domain. The person's mood state before starting to drink also is an important factor.

"Always do sober what you said you'd do drunk. That will teach you to keep your mouth shut."

Ernest Hemingway

At lower BACs, drinkers report feeling elated and friendly when the BAC is rising, but when it is falling, common feelings are anger and fatigue. Other reports when the BAC is rising have been expansiveness, joviality, relaxation, and self-confidence. The importance of nondrug factors is accented in the finding that during the ascending phase of these same BACs, other subjects have reported feeling hostile, depressed, and withdrawn. When BACs go above 0.10%, drinkers commonly become more labile and may change abruptly from friendly to hostile. Often the level of tolerance for frustration is lowered.

Alcohol's effects on thinking and perception are less influenced by nondrug factors and are influenced more by BAC. Alcohol significantly impairs short-term memory at BACs higher than 0.05%. At a BAC of 0.05%, the ability to estimate time is impaired. Drinkers seem to overestimate the passage of time at a BAC of 0.05%; they might estimate a time passage of 8 minutes to be 12 minutes. The ability to estimate distance (depth perception) also is disrupted at lower BACs, as are attention and concentration. At higher BACs, these cognitive effects are intensified and are compounded by more disorganized thinking.

Alcohol and Behavior

Among alcohol's effects, those involving interpersonal behavior are of great social interest. As the word implies, *interpersonal* means "between people." The interpersonal behaviors of sex and aggression in combination with alcohol have garnered the greatest interest and concern.

Alcohol and Aggression

Aggression is behavior intended to harm a person who would prefer not to receive such treatment (Bushman & Cooper, 1990). Violence is a type of aggression that is a major social concern. As you saw in Contemporary Issue Box 1.5 in Chapter 1, studies suggest that when people commit violent crimes, they tend to be under the influence of alcohol. Violent crimes include murder or attempted murder, manslaughter, rape or sexual assault, robbery, assault, and others such as kidnapping, purse snatching, hit-and-run driving, and child abuse. The same findings hold for Canada and western Europe (Collins, 1980; see http://info.ki.se/index_se.html for a collection of articles on alcohol and crime in western Europe). The co-occurrence of alcohol use and violent crime is especially prevalent among men 18 to 30 years old, who have a relatively high rate of both heavy drinking and criminal activity. Another problem of national concern is physical abuse of spouses (predominantly husbands abusing wives), and alcohol has been estimated to be involved (offender or victim) in 25% to 50% of spousal abuse incidents (Collins, 1980).

National statistics show associations between alcohol and violence toward others and also violence toward oneself. For example, suicide is one of the three leading causes of death (the other two are homicide and accidental death) among men 15 to 34 years old and one of the 10 leading causes of death among all people 34 to 54 years old. One study of the causes of violent death focused on 3,400 individuals who had had their BACs tested at the time of their deaths. Among those people who died by suicide, 35% had been drinking alcohol when they took their lives (USDHHS, 1987a). Another study of 100,000 deaths in 1989 showed positive BACs in 35% of the suicide victims (NIAAA, 1993).

During the late 1980s, national attention was directed at alcohol and behavior at baseball games and other professional sports events and in fraternities. In both cases, aggressive behavior was the focus, and alcohol was singled out as a major culprit. One example is the fans' rowdy reactions during an April 1988 game at Cincinnati's Riverfront Stadium, when an umpire made a call unfavorable to the home-team Reds. Alcohol was viewed by league officials to be at the heart of the "deterioration" of the situation. This and similar events led many major league baseball teams to restrict alcohol sales (primarily beer) and even to have alcohol-free sections in the stands, similar to smoke-free areas in public places. Such restrictions continue to be in effect at virtually all ballparks where professional teams play. Alcohol also has been identified as a major problem in the behavior of members of fraternities on college campuses. The misconduct and violence against property and people that some fraternities are known for have been highly correlated with the occurrence of popular frat functions such as beer bashes.

The consistency of the co-occurrence of drinking and violent behavior tempts us to conclude that alcohol causes such behavior. Data such as government statistics are only descriptive and correlational, however, and cannot be the bases of valid causal statements about alcohol and aggression. Nevertheless, the adult drinking public believes that alcohol does indeed cause aggression. A consistent finding in many studies of beliefs about the effects of alcohol is that it increases power and aggression (Goldman, Darkes, & Del Boca, 1999). Perhaps these beliefs underlie officials' statements that alcohol causes disorderly conduct at ballparks and fraternities.

Of course, aggressive behavior is a highly significant social concern, and it is important to find the reasons for the association between drinking and violent behavior. A traditional explanation is the disinhibition theory, which was first proposed in the early 20th century. This theory holds that alcohol releases behavior normally inhibited by society, such as aggression and sex, as a result of its depressant action on the brain. Essentially the theory suggests that whatever anxieties we have about the social consequences of behavior such as aggression vanish as a result of alcohol's pharmacological action. Thus, people who have been drinking should be more aggressive than people who have not.

Controlled laboratory experiments involving human subjects do not support the disinhibition theory, however. Some epidemiological studies have shown a correlation between alcohol and aggression, but this was not a simple matter of alcohol's pharmacological action, as disinhibition theory predicts. Rather, alcohol combines with situational factors, such as social pressure and threat of retaliation (Adesso, 1985; Graham et al., 1998), as well as personal factors, such as how angry a person is characteristically (Parrot & Giancola, 2004). Furthermore, drinkers' expectancies about alcohol and aggression also seem to contribute to aggression, sometimes considerably more than actually drinking alcohol does (Bartholow & Heinz, 2006).

It seems, therefore, that alcohol does not simply cause aggression, despite the beliefs of some public officials and the general population. Instead, aggression is a complex social behavior affected by the characteristics of the aggressor and situational factors, only one of which is alcohol consumption (Exum, 2006). Theories about aggression must accommodate this complexity to be useful.

Alcohol and Sex

For the last 500 years, Shakespeare probably has been the author most frequently cited on the acute effects of alcohol on human sexual response. The specific reference is from *Macbeth,* act 2, scene 2: "It [alcohol] provokes and unprovokes; it provokes the desire, but it takes away from the performance." It turns out that the results of experimental studies are in part consistent with Shakespeare's observations.

Alcohol and sexual response in men and women has been a favorite subject of writers for thousands of years. Much of the writing has been like Shakespeare's comments, based on informal personal observations. With regard to male sexual response, the folklore leads to dose-dependent conclusions. Alcohol has been thought to be an aphrodisiac in men at lower doses but an impediment to sexual performance at higher doses. An example is a quote of the Greek poet Euenas, from the 5th century B.C.:

> The best measure of wine is neither much nor very little; For 'tis the cause of either grief or madness.
> Then too, 'tis most suited for the bridal chamber and love.
> And if it breathe too fiercely, it puts love to flight.
> And plunges men in a sleep, neighbor to death. (in Abel, 1985)

Efforts have been made to systematically study human sexual response to a dose of alcohol, but it has only been possible to do well-controlled research on this topic in the past 30 years or so. The significant breakthroughs have been the invention of the penile strain gauge to measure penile erectile response and the photoplethysmograph to measure vaginal blood volume and pressure. These advances paved the way for experimental study of human sexual response and alcohol.

Experimental studies of men have consistently shown that, at BACs of 0.05% to 0.10%, alcohol pharmacologically retards sexual arousal. When the BAC climbs to more than 0.10%, erection and ejaculatory competence are inhibited or eliminated. These results have been found repeatedly in samples of college students who were not problem drinkers and in those with alcoholism. Alcohol does not stimulate men's libido, especially at moderate or higher BACs.

At lower BACs, alcohol effects are not so dominant. It appears that cognitive factors, such as expectancies about alcohol effects, may work to increase men's libido. Indeed, studies of alcohol expectancies suggest that the drinking public generally believes alcohol enhances sexual experience (Brown, Christiansen, & Goldman, 1987). Consistent with this finding, balanced placebo design studies (see Contemporary Issue Box 9.4) suggest that men's sexual arousal is increased when they believe they are drinking a dose of alcohol that brings them to a BAC less than 0.05%. Alcohol itself, however, has no effect on measured arousal at such BACs, which agrees with many other studies of the pharmacology of alcohol (Peugh & Belenko, 2001). Another characteristic of male drinkers that seems to affect their sexual arousal at BACs lower than 0.05% is personality. One study showed increased sexual response was especially evident in subjects who thought they were drinking alcohol and who scored high on a measure of guilt about sex (Lang et al., 1980).

A reasonable conclusion about the acute effects of alcohol on male sexual response is that, similar to aggression, the disinhibition theory falls far short of explaining the information that is available. Rather, social and psychological factors seem to be important determinants of sexual response in men at low BACs and often work to increase libido. However, the pharmacology of alcohol begins to dominate at BACs greater than 0.05%, which cause a decrease in arousal and sexual competence.

The folklore about the acute effects of alcohol on sexual behavior in women is that it promotes promiscuity, a belief that even adolescents in the middle school and high school range in the United States report (Young, McCabe, & Boyd, 2007). For example, Chaucer wrote in "The Wife of Bath's Tale" in his *Canterbury Tales*: "After wine, I think mostly of venue for just as it's true that cold engenders hail a liquor mouth must have a liquorous tail. Women have no defense against wine as lechers know from experience."

CONTEMPORARY ISSUE BOX 9.4

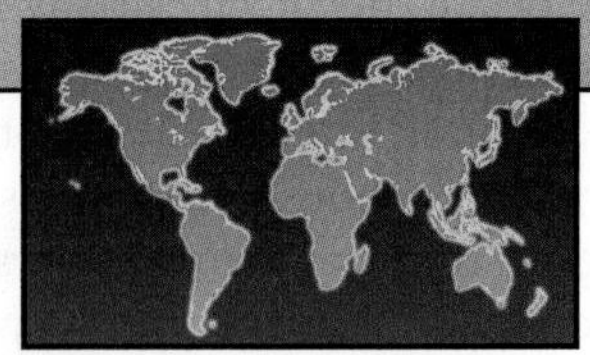

The Balanced Placebo Design

To control for placebo effects (see Chapter 5), experimental studies of drug effects in humans and other animals usually include a placebo control group. In studies of alcohol effects in humans, control subjects are told they are drinking an alcoholic beverage when, in fact, they are not given one. Instead, they are given a nonalcoholic drink that resembles the alcoholic beverage in every way except alcohol content. So, in the traditional placebo group design, all people in two groups of subjects are told they will drink an alcoholic beverage, but only one group's beverage actually contains alcohol. Studies that use this design have varied in their success of making the alcoholic and placebo beverages indistinguishable on cues such as taste and smell and therefore in the validity of their findings. How do you think failure to make the alcohol and placebo beverages indiscriminable would affect the interpretation of study results?

A significant advance in studying the effects of drugs on human behavior was made over four decades ago in what has been named the balanced placebo design (BPD), which is illustrated in Table 9.4. The design has helped to advance knowledge about alcohol's effects on aggression and sex, among other human behaviors. In the BPD, two groups are added to the traditional two-group placebo group design. The participants in each of the two additional groups are told they will not receive a drug; then those in one group get the drug and those in the other group do not. Therefore, comparisons may be made with a group of subjects who believe they are not getting and do not get a drug (the sober control group). It also is possible to make comparisons with a group of subjects who believe they are not receiving a drug but really do get one. The design offers the advantage of separating a pure drug effect, an "expectancy" (about drug actions) effect, and their interaction. Under the best conditions of control, the traditional placebo design provides a comparison of drug plus expectancy and expectancy conditions, which permits conclusions about drug action. In investigations of the effects of lower doses of alcohol, the BPD seems much better suited than the traditional placebo design for studying the complexity of drugs and human behavior.

TABLE 9.4 Balanced Placebo Design

		Beverage Received	
		Alcohol	**Placebo**
Beverage Told	**Alcohol**	Group 1	Group 2
	Placebo	Group 3	Group 4

(An outline of the balanced placebo design in studying alcohol effects. The traditional design includes groups 1 and 2 only.)

Previous nonexperimental studies, as well as studies of alcohol expectancies we cited earlier, suggest that alcohol increases sexual arousal in women and that women believe alcohol has that effect. The recent experimental evidence is that, as in men, women's physiological sexual response decreases with increasing alcohol dose. Unlike men, however, women continue to perceive increased sexual arousal and sexual pleasure even as the physiological indexes of their response and arousal are declining. It seems that Shakespeare's observation most clearly applies to women, even though he was referring to men. It also is important not to conclude that the disinhibition theory accounts for the data on alcohol effects in women. Despite their perceived increased sexual arousal when they drink, whether women act on such perception depends on characteristics in the drinking setting and what the drinker has learned is acceptable sexual behavior in that setting. Therefore, again, a theory about the acute effects of alcohol on women's sexual behavior should incorporate social and psychological factors as well as the pharmacology of alcohol.

To conclude this section, Table 9.5 provides a summary of the acute effects of alcohol at different BACs. The table succinctly shows how pervasive alcohol's effects are. It is essential to remember, however, that the effects listed for given BACs are what might be observed in "typical" drinkers. Alcohol's effects are notorious for their variability among people and in the same person on different drinking occasions. And,

TABLE 9.5 Typical Acute Effects of Alcohol Associated with Different Ascending Blood Alcohol Concentrations (BACs)

BAC (%)	Effects
0.01–0.02	Slight changes in feeling; sense of warmth and well-being
0.03–0.04	Feelings of relaxation, slight exhilaration, happiness; skin may flush; mild impairment in motor skills
0.05–0.06	Effects become more noticeable; more exaggerated changes in emotion, impaired judgment, and lowered inhibitions; coordination may be altered
0.08–0.09	Reaction time is increased, muscle coordination is impaired; sensory feelings of numbness in cheeks, lips, and extremities; further impairment in judgment; legal level of intoxication is .08% in all 50 of the United States, Puerto Rico, and the District of Columbia.
0.10	Deterioration in motor coordination and reaction time; person may stagger and slow speech
0.15	Major impairment in balance and movement; large increase in reaction time; large impairment in judgment and perception
0.20	Difficulty staying awake; substantial reduction of motor and sensory capabilities; slurred speech, double vision, difficulty standing or walking without assistance
0.30	Confusion and stupor; difficulty comprehending what is going on; possible loss of consciousness (passing out)
0.40	Typically unconsciousness; sweatiness and clamminess of the skin; alcohol has become an anesthetic
0.45–0.50	Circulatory and respiratory functions may become totally depressed; LD 50 in humans

as our discussion of alcohol and aggression and sex most clearly illustrated, situational and psychological factors also influence what behaviors occur in people when they drink as well as the effects they perceive alcohol is having on them.

Effects of Chronic Heavy Drinking

Chronic heavy use of alcohol may have numerous physiological and psychological effects. All the effects involve increased dysfunction, and some may be fatal. Some chronic alcohol effects are caused directly by alcohol's toxicity to the body, such as damage to the liver. Other effects are indirectly related to long-term heavy drinking. For example, Wernicke's disease, which involves impaired cognitive functioning, is caused by nutritional deficiencies that tend to occur in people who are dependent on alcohol (Brands, Sproule, & Marshman, 1998).

Chronic heavy drinking is difficult to define precisely. Suffice it to say, many of alcohol's long-term effects take years to become evident, and heavy drinkers vary greatly in their susceptibility to alcohol-related impairments.

A standard for what is heavy, or at least "unsafe," drinking has been proposed. However, long-term drinking of a given quantity of alcohol affects different drinkers in different ways, in both number and severity of symptoms. Furthermore, the standard could vary according to what risk (for example, liver disease, pancreatitis, or brain damage) we are concerned about (Bradley, Donovan, & Larson, 1993). Nevertheless, it is useful to have a guide to what is a "safe" level of alcohol consumption for the average drinker. One estimate is to set an upper limit of four drinks a day for men and three drinks a day for women, with a frequency of no more than four times a week for both genders (Dawson, 2000; Sanchez-Craig, Wilkinson, & Davila, 1995).

CONTEMPORARY ISSUE BOX 9.5

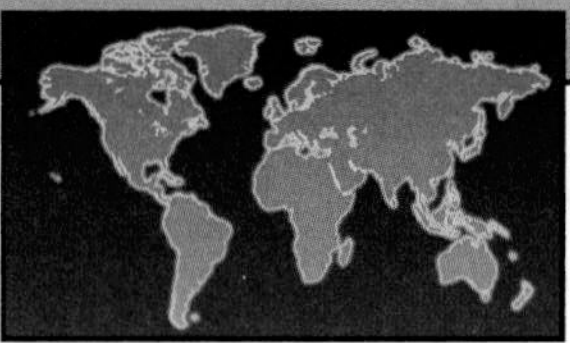

Accuracy of Self-Reports of Alcohol Consumption

Our review of information on alcohol's acute effects highlights that a lot of research has been done on how much alcohol humans drink, why they drink it, and what effects it has on them. As you might have noticed, many of these studies used the survey method to obtain information about humans' use of alcohol. Surveys on alcohol almost always ask research participants to tell the researcher how much alcohol was consumed over some period of time (a day, a week, a month, a year), occurring at different points back from the survey date (yesterday, last week, last month, last year). The first question that most people ask about such "retrospective self-reports" of drinking is, "How accurate are they?"

This is an excellent question, because a lot of factors may affect the accuracy of self-reports of drinking, the most fundamental of which is the limitations of human memory. However, other factors could affect accuracy, even if memory were perfect. One of these is knowledge about how much a drinker is drinking when out in a bar or restaurant. It seems that the way bartenders vary in how they define a "shot" of whiskey or a "glass" of wine has more to do with their personal habits, inclinations, or mood than it does with any measurement system. Bartenders, even experienced ones, however, also seem to be vulnerable to a well-known perceptual illusion. Along these lines, a study by Wansink and van Ittersum (2005) showed that, when instructed to pour a "shot" (defined as 1.5 oz.) of whiskey into a glass, bartenders poured more liquid into a tall, narrow glass than they did into a short, wide glass. Nonbartender college students were subject to the same illusion as the experienced bartenders were.

Many other factors besides perceptual illusions could also affect the accuracy of retrospective self-reports. On the other hand, research has identified the conditions that increase the likelihood of accurate self-report data. The ultimate reason why survey studies of alcohol use have advanced knowledge is that scientists have looked to converging evidence within studies (Do the different sources of data that I've collected in this study lead me to the same, reasonable conclusions?) and replication across studies (Do different researchers doing the same study under different conditions get similar results?) as the main criteria for confidence in their results.

Table 9.6 lists the major effects of chronic heavy drinking on body systems. Worldwide, the effects are devastating: In 2004, a total of 6.3% of global deaths for men were attributable to alcohol (death by cancer, cardiovascular disease, liver cirrhosis, and injury), as were 1.1% of the deaths among women. The large discrepancy in rates between men and women characterized the data from all countries of the world. These rates varied wide, ranging across both sexes from 0.5% in the eastern Mediterranean countries, to 6.5% in the countries of Europe. The rate for the Americas was 5.6%, second to Europe (Rehm et al., 2009). It is important to note that the estimates that Rehm et al. provided consider or "partial out" the possible beneficial effects that moderate alcohol consumption has on disease and disability, which we discuss later in this chapter.

These global mortality data reflect what Table 9.6 shows, that alcohol can be highly toxic to the human body and can cause extensive damage in a variety of ways. Two prominent body systems that alcohol harms are the brain and the liver. We will look at alcohol's chronic effects on these systems in more detail. Alcohol's chronic effects also extend to human reproductive functioning, which has to do with alcohol's altering effect on the functioning of the hypothalamic-pituitary-gonadal endocrine axis and with fetal alcohol syndrome (FAS).

Alcohol and Brain Functioning

The acute effects of alcohol on memory and other cognitive functioning are manifest at moderate BACs and are reversible. However, alcohol— if drunk long enough and heavily enough—affects these same functions in the long term in some people. Such chronic effects

TABLE 9.6 Effects of Chronic, Heavy Drinking on Body Systems

System	Effects
Central Nervous	Specific and general impairment in cognitive functioning
Liver	Minor reversible (with abstinence) damage to irreversible, sometimes fatal damage
Cardiovascular	Increased mortality from coronary heart disease and increased risk for cardiovascular diseases in general; alcohol-induced wasting of the heart muscle (alcohol cardiomyopathy)
Endocrine	Effects on the secretion of hormones in different hormone hierarchies, or "axes"—for example, the hypothalamic-pituitary-adrenal axis and the hypothalamic-pituitary-gonadal axis
Immune	Increased susceptibility to several infectious diseases
Gastrointestinal	Cause of gastritis and increased risk of pancreatitis
Multiple	Increased risk of contracting the following cancers: oral cavity, tongue, pharynx, larynx, esophagus, stomach, liver, lung, pancreas, colon, rectum

Source: The information in this table is based on USDHHS (1987a) and Brands, Sproule, and Marshman (1998).

vary in severity, evidenced from mildly impaired performance on **neuropsychological tests,** to severe, irreversible brain structural and functional damage shown as severe memory impairment in people who have Korsakoff's syndrome (Charness, 1993; Parsons, 1986).

neuropsychological tests
Formal ways of measuring behavioral functions that may be impaired by brain lesions.

The average alcohol-dependent individual who has been studied, when abstinent from alcohol or other psychoactive drugs, performs more poorly than nonalcoholic control groups on tests of abstracting, problem solving, memory, learning, and perceptual-motor speed. Reviews of research have shown consistently that such impairments are associated with alcohol dependence. Other characteristics of the drinkers also influence their vulnerability to alcohol's effects on brain function. A major one is the individual's drinking history. Although the evidence is mixed, in general, the longer a person drinks and the greater the quantity consumed, the greater the impairment in cognitive functioning (NIAAA, 2001).

Fortunately, with long-term abstinence from alcohol, most alcohol-related neuropsychological impairment once evidenced can be virtually reversed, with only mild deficits left compared with control subjects. This conclusion is based on studies that followed participants' test performance during periods of abstinence lasting from one month to five years (Fein et al., 2006; Sullivan, Rosenbloom, & Pfefferbaum, 2000).

The reversibility of cognitive deficits may be due to several factors, including increased cerebral blood flow, better nutrition, the reorganization of brain-cell networks, and some recovery of brain atrophy (Mello, 1987; Nace & Isbell, 1991; NIAAA, 2001; USDHHS, 1990). The more recent findings on changes in the brain and recovery of cognitive function are the result of technology that allows noninvasive study of brain structure and activity, such as computerized axial tomography (CT).

Wernicke-Korsakoff Syndrome

This severe CNS disorder results from the combination of extreme nutritional deficiency, specifically vitamin B_1 or thiamine, and chronic heavy drinking. Basically there are two diseases.

Wernicke's disease is characterized by confusion, loss of memory, staggering gait, and an inability to focus the eye (USDHHS, 1987a; 1990). In the absence of permanent brain damage, Wernicke's disease is reversible by giving the patient vitamin B_1.

confabulation A fabrication of events, when asked questions concerning them, because of an inability to recall.

Korsakoff's syndrome may have a nutritional component but is primarily due to alcohol. It is associated with damage to brain structure and most affects memory. The impairments in short-term memory and learning are serious. Because of these dysfunctions, there often is considerable confusion and **confabulation**. There also is a lesser degree of impairment in memory for events in longer-term memory. The following case, based on one discussed in the *DSM-III Casebook* (Spitzer et al., 1981, pp. 56–57), is a good illustration of some of the major symptoms of Korsakoff's syndrome:

> The patient was a 40-year-old man who in the interview claimed to be an accountant. He said that he had some business troubles and had come to the hospital to get help. His story was coherent, but there was a lack of consistency and details to it. As regards his hospitalization, the patient said that he had been in for only a few days but a few minutes later he said several weeks. He could not recall his doctor's name.
>
> Formal testing showed that the patient could not recall the names of three objects that he had seen five minutes earlier, or repeat a story that was told to him. However, the patient could perform simple calculations, define words and concepts, and find similarities and differences among objects and concepts. The patient's medical record showed that he had a long history of alcohol dependence and had been living in a nursing home for the last three years until he was admitted to the hospital a week ago. He was admitted after several incidents of his wandering from the nursing home and being returned there by police. (Reprinted with permission from the *Diagnostic and Statistical Manual of Mental Disorders.* Copyright 1981 and 1989 American Psychiatric Association.)

Alcohol and the Liver

As the major metabolic site of alcohol, the liver is highly vulnerable to alcohol's toxic effects. The damage that alcohol can cause to the liver occurs in three ways: fatty liver, alcohol hepatitis, and cirrhosis. Fatty liver is characterized by fat accumulating in the liver and is the earliest, most benign effect of alcohol on the liver. This condition is reversible with abstinence from alcohol, and there is no evidence that it is a precursor of cirrhosis. Alcohol hepatitis is more serious and involves the inflammation and death of liver cells. Often jaundice occurs because of the accumulation of bile. This condition is reversible with abstinence and medical treatment but can cause death if it is severe enough and not treated. Liver hepatitis can be caused by means other than heavy drinking. Evidence of such drinking must be obtained to diagnose alcohol hepatitis.

The most serious and life-threatening of alcohol's liver assaults is cirrhosis. Alcohol dependence is the leading cause of cirrhosis, which is the eighth leading cause of death by disease in the United States and kills about 25,000 people a year (National Institutes of Health, 2000; Stinson, Grant, & Dufour, 2001). Drinking must be prodigious and long-term for someone to develop cirrhosis. For example, one survey showed that people with alcohol dependence who developed cirrhosis drank an average of 13 drinks a day for about 20 years! It did not matter what beverage form the alcohol was consumed in. It should be noted that a minority of people with alcohol dependence develop cirrhosis—between 10% and 20%. Individuals with alcohol dependence who are diagnosed with cirrhosis often have other liver diseases at the same time, such as alcohol hepatitis (NIAAA, 2000).

For those who do get cirrhosis, the condition is not reversible, and only half are still alive five years after receiving the initial diagnosis. Cirrhosis is a chronic inflammatory disease of the liver involving cell death and the formation of scar tissue. Alcohol hepatitis may or may not precede it. Death results from cirrhosis because the liver fails to metabolize various toxins, such as ammonia, and these toxins accumulate in the body.

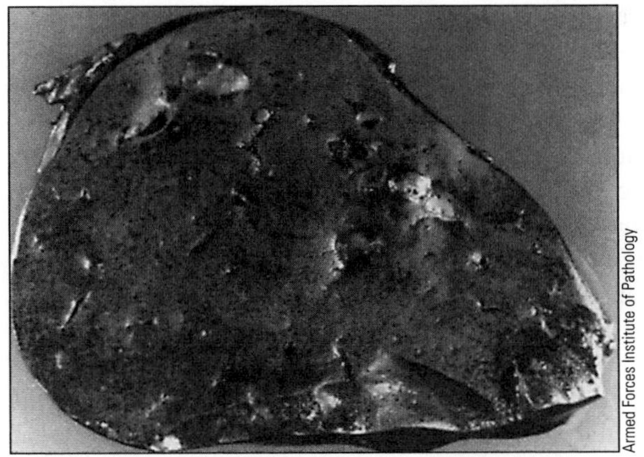

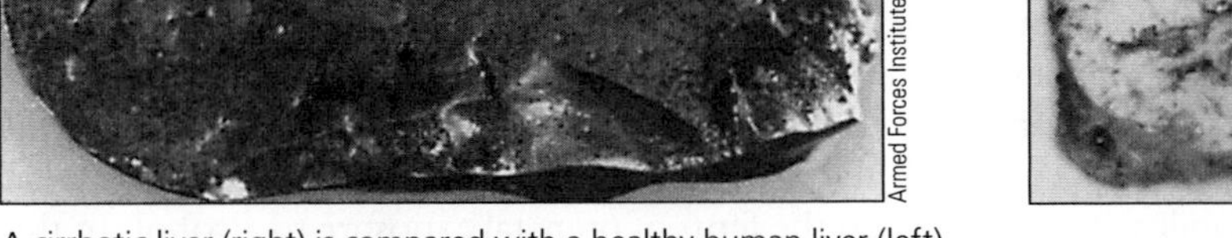

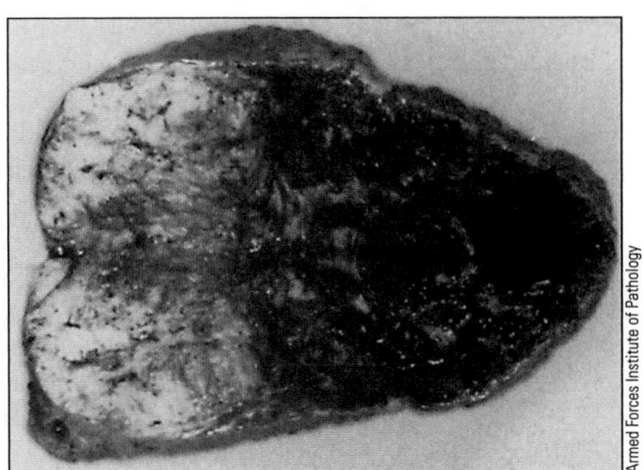

A cirrhotic liver (right) is compared with a healthy human liver (left).

Alcohol and Reproductive Functioning

Both men and women suffer impaired reproductive functioning as a result of chronic heavy drinking. In men, such drinking affects the male sex hormones, reflexive responses of the nervous system relating to sexual performance, and sperm production. First, men often experience gynecomastia (formation of breasts in men), which is a result of alcohol altering the balance of the female sex hormone (estrogen) and the male sex hormone (testosterone). The shift in balance is due to damage to the liver from alcohol and resorption of estrogens into the blood. Another result of changing the balance in the sex hormones is a loss in sexual desire. Along with a loss in desire is a drop in sexual performance, manifested as ejaculatory incompetence and impotence. These latter effects are due to alcohol's inhibition of reflexive responses in the nervous system. Finally, chronic heavy drinking may result in hypogonadism and eventual sterility. There is also some possibility that sperm production is so impaired that defective offspring could be conceived (Abel, 1985; Mello, 1987; Peugh & Belenko, 2001).

As with most alcohol effects, we know less about the chronic effects of alcohol on reproductive functioning in women. The scientific information available suggests alcohol dependence in women is associated with dysfunction of the ovaries, disruption of the luteal phase of fertilization, and amenorrhea (cessation of the menstrual period) (Brands, Sproule, & Marshman, 1998; Mello, 1987; Nolen-Hoeksema, 2004; USDHHS, 1990). A household survey suggests that a woman does not have to be diagnosed as having alcohol dependence to experience impaired sexual function related to alcohol use. A survey of more than 900 women living in households showed a positive correlation between alcohol consumption and the occurrence of different menstrual disorders (Wilsnack, Klassen, & Wilsnack, 1984).

Fetal Alcohol Syndrome

In this section, we discuss a chronic alcohol effect that does not focus on a specific body system or on the drinker. Rather, it focuses on the fetus and what alcohol consumption may do to it if its mother drinks during pregnancy. A characteristic set of symptoms that appear in some newborns of mothers who drink during pregnancy has become known as the fetal alcohol syndrome (FAS). FAS falls into the class of alcohol teratology. **Teratology** is defined in biology as the study of monsters or deformities.

teratology
In biology, the study of monsters, or distortions in growth.

FAS has been written about since the time of Aristotle but began to receive scientists' attention much more recently. Since 1973, the literature on it has grown geometrically. FAS involves gross physical deformities that were first identified in eight very young children who had severely alcohol-dependent mothers who drank during pregnancy. These deformities were described in a 1973 clinical report, and include the following: small eyes and small eye openings, drooping eyelids, underdeveloped mid-face, skin folds across the inner corners of the eyes (which were abnormal in this sample of 11 white children), underdevelopment of the depression above the upper lip, and a small head circumference. Furthermore, abnormal creases in the palm were reported, along with abnormalities in the joints. Some of the children had cardiac defects, benign tumors consisting of dilated blood vessels, and minor ear abnormalities (Jones et al., 1973). A 10-year follow-up of these children showed low-normal to severely retarded intellectual functioning, physical deformities similar to those originally reported, and the development of additional physical problems.

Although estimates vary, FAS occurs in one to three of every 1,000 live births (USDHHS, 1990). As you think about these statistics, remember that there is great individual variability in the effects on the fetus of prenatal exposure to alcohol. In this regard, the rate of occurrence of FAS is much lower than the rate of women who use alcohol while they are pregnant. Furthermore, rates of FAS vary with the population in question. For example, rates of FAS seem to be much higher among Native American and African American mothers of low socioeconomic status, who have been the participants in most FAS studies conducted in the United States, than they are among white, middle-class mothers (USDHHS, 1993).

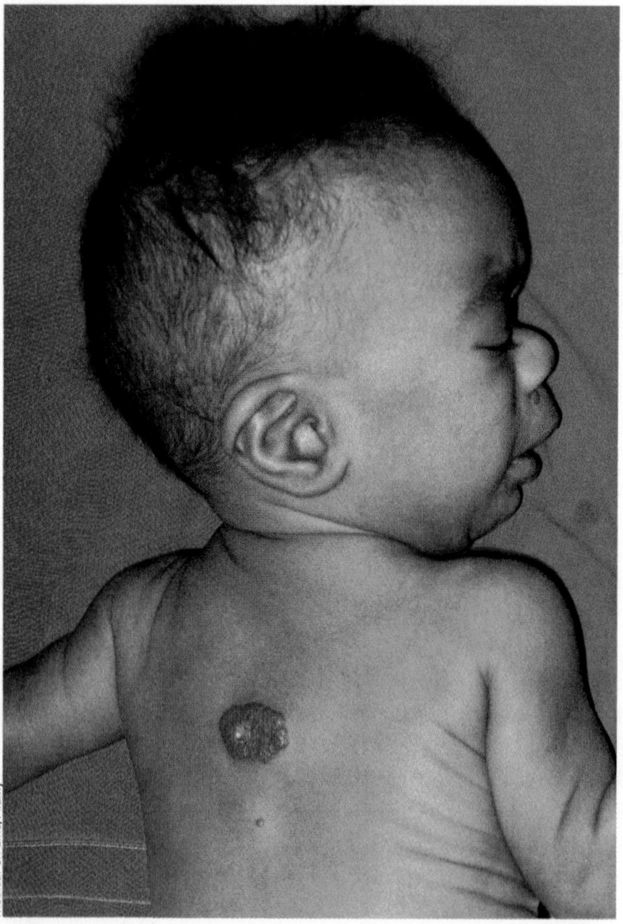

The variability in rates of FAS hints at the complexity in conducting human studies of this serious public health problem. For one reason, it is extremely difficult to get accurate self-reports from pregnant women about their drinking; this seems to be particularly true for women who are heavier, with a drinking problem (Alvik, Haldorsen, & Lindermann, 2005). Why do you think this is the case? Because FAS can be detected only after a child is born, postpartum environmental and other factors cloud an interpretation of what part prenatal alcohol exposure played in the resulting FAS. It is sometimes even difficult to determine whether alcohol was the only prenatal substance that may have resulted in FAS. For example, other drug use during pregnancy is possible, and this would be most likely to occur among the heaviest drinkers (Erenhart, 1991). When other drugs are taken during pregnancy, they may harm the fetus in ways similar to alcohol.

Everybody wants to know the "safe" level of drinking during pregnancy. As our brief discussion of FAS suggests, no simple answer is available. Actually, it is best to think of FAS as the most severe result of a continuum of effects of prenatal exposure to alcohol (Rasmussen, 2005). Subtle behavioral or cognitive effects may be observed on the other end of the continuum. Each abnormal outcome may have its own yardstick of amount of alcohol exposure and timing of exposure (Jacobson et al., 1993; USDHHS, 1990).

Medical-on-Line/Alamy

This child was diagnosed as being affected by fetal alcohol syndrome.

Although a straightforward answer about safe drinking during pregnancy is not available, there is one rule to go by. FAS or milder degrees of abnormality in newborns have not been observed without prenatal exposure to alcohol or other drugs. Therefore, the safest course remains the most conservative: If you are pregnant, do not use alcohol or other drugs (Barr & Streissguth, 2001).

This section on the chronic effects of heavy alcohol consumption has highlighted the idea of alcohol as a double-edged sword. On the one side, as we showed you in Chapter 1, the economic costs of alcohol abuse to the United States and the rest of the world are tremendous and come from many sources. The toll of chronic, heavy alcohol use on the body results in major health care expenses. Furthermore, if you consider some of the social consequences that contribute to the costs, they may become even more real to you. We already discussed how alcohol is implicated in traffic accidents, crime, and violence. Its use also is associated with accidental falls, drownings, fires and burns, traumatic injuries like broken bones, and family violence (spouse abuse or child abuse, for example) (Gutjahr, Gmel, & Rehm, 2001).

The other edge of the sword is the economic gain afforded by alcohol, not to mention the high regard many people have for it as a social and psychological booster. The alcoholic beverage industry creates and maintains a lot of jobs and contributes a lot of revenue to governments. The alcoholic beverage industry publication *Beverage Dynamics* estimated that, in 2001, retail sales of alcohol in the United States totaled $127.3 billion.

So, perhaps you can see why there seems to be never-ending discussion about how to regulate alcohol, with opinions ranging from reinstating Prohibition to allowing freer use. What arguments on each side can you think of? What policy would you end up with if given the responsibility to write one?

Moderate Drinking and Health

As we suppose you are convinced at this point, long-term heavy use of alcohol could seriously damage the body. However, what about long-term abstinence from alcohol and long-term lighter drinking? A number of studies has suggested that the moderate drinkers turn out to be the healthiest, followed by the abstainers, and dead last are the heavy drinkers. "Health" most often has been measured by risk of cardiovascular disease and mortality.

The surprise here, of course, is that drinking can be healthful, although the medical community has considered this possibility since the 19th century (Doll, 1998). The first question is: What is 'moderate'? Generally, moderation with alcohol has been defined as one to three drinks a day. How could such drinking possibly aid health? One hypothesis is that light alcohol consumption increases the production of high-density lipoproteins (HDLs), which take damaging cholesterol away from artery walls (Gaziano et al., 1993). Alcohol also appears to affect other biological indicators of risk of cardiovascular disease (Dejousse et al., 2009; Rimm, 2000).

Most experts have concluded that moderate drinking is associated with lower risk of coronary disease (Lee et al., 2009; Marmot, 2001). Until recently, many people doubted this conclusion, however, because some studies failed to consider factors that correlate with drinking patterns and that also are associated with risk of cardiovascular disease. One of these factors is income; more of the abstainers than the moderate drinkers were defined as poor, and income is negatively related to health. There also has been a question of whether many "light/moderate daily drinkers" exist. Most light drinkers do not drink every day, and most people who drink every day do not drink lightly. Moreover, a review by Fillmore et al. (2006) suggests that the abstainers in these studies may have included many people who recently stopped

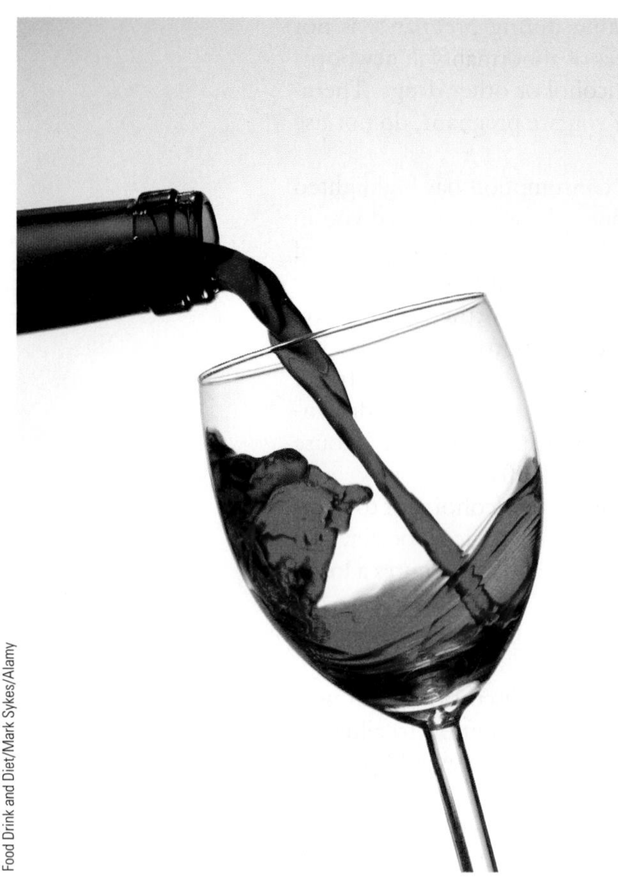

Food Drink and Diet/Mark Sykes/Alamy

The discovery that moderate use of red wine is associated with a lower incidence of heart disease stimulated research on the effects of moderate alcohol use on health.

drinking because they had become ill. On the other hand, recent better-designed correlational studies have shown an association between moderate alcohol use and cardiovascular health. Furthermore, experiments have demonstrated a reduction in biological indicators of risk of cardiovascular disease following administration of a moderate dose of alcohol (one to three drinks).

In conclusion, it seems that the connection between moderate drinking and cardiac health question still would benefit from additional research; for example, a large longitudinal study from Denmark suggests that the moderate drinking–heart health relationship is evident in men who have 7 to 35 drinks a week, and it is evident in women who have as little as one drink a week (Tolstrup et al., 2006). This is the first study that suggests that whatever the relationship between alcohol use and cardiac health, its mechanism may be different for men and women and may be triggered by different amounts of alcohol between the sexes, with as little as a drink a week for women. However, the weight of the evidence is that moderate alcohol use in general is associated with cardiovascular health.

The French Paradox

The moderate drinking–health hypothesis relates to a research finding that has been called the French paradox, or the co-occurrence of a diet high in saturated fats and a low incidence of coronary heart disease (Frunkel et al., 1993). This biological paradox was first identified among people who live in Touraine, France. Again, we are talking about moderate drinking, and the focus is on red wine; the French consume wine in relatively high amounts. The equivalent of one to two 4-ounce glasses of wine a day is associated with improved health effects (Renaud & deLorgerd, 1992). In fact, some researchers have argued that the apparent relationship between moderate alcohol use and lowered risk of heart disease is specific to wine (Gronbaek et al., 1995), although experimental studies suggest that the effect is due to alcohol and is not specific to wine. A lot of attention is being given to resveratrol, a nonalcohol constituent of red wine, as a main reason for the health benefits of its moderate consumption (Baur & Sinclair, 2006; Brown et al., 2009).

In summary, research on the interesting question of whether and why moderate alcohol use is associated with cardiovascular health is needed and will likely continue. It is important to note here that our discussion of "health" has primarily concerned cardiovascular function and does not include other indicators, such as liver function, cancers, or cognitive functioning. In addition, this question needs much more information on what is "moderate consumption" for different subgroups, such as the elderly or individuals with coexisting illness (Karlmangla et al., 2009; Saitz, 2005).

The Development of Alcohol Abuse and Dependence

The National Survey on Drug Use and Health data we covered in this chapter and in Chapter 1 showed that well over 60% of Americans drink alcohol and that a minority of them drink heavily. Some of those who drink heavily develop problems with alcohol to different degrees. When they do, the effects on themselves, their families, and their society are devastating. Accordingly, this question has preoccupied many for many years: How do alcohol abuse and dependence develop, or what is their etiology? In this last section, we briefly present approaches taken to address this question and describe the current thinking.

Traditional Approaches to Etiology

Until recently, researchers and clinicians alike usually sought a single-factor explanation of what causes alcohol problems. Theories frequently outpaced data available to evaluate them and can be classified as biological, psychological, or sociological.

Biological approaches have waxed and waned in popularity over the years. Such theories hold that a physiological or structural anomaly causes the individual to become alcohol dependent. Earlier single-factor biological approaches, which have not received experimental support, have included hypotheses that the source of the structural deficit is metabolic, glandular, due to body chemistry, or due to an allergic condition. The most prevalent position among U.S. treatment providers is that alcohol dependence is a physical disease (see Contemporary Issue Box 9.6). Although the cause of the disease process is not specified, disease model adherents use the process of a physical disease, such as a fever, as an analogy to understand alcohol dependence. As a result, the disease model is classified as a biological model.

Biological explanations of alcohol problems have regained popularity among scientists because of findings that suggest there is a genetic predisposition at least to some "types" of alcohol dependence (Kendler et al., 1992; Schuckit, 1987). The evidence comes primarily from family, twin, and adoption studies. In summary, family studies show that sons and daughters of alcohol-dependent parents are four times more likely to develop the disorder themselves, relative to people whose parents are not dependent on alcohol. In addition, studies of twins show a greater likelihood of both members of identical twin pairs having alcohol dependence ("concordance") than of concordance in fraternal twins. This finding is significant because identical twins are genetic matches, whereas members of fraternal twin pairs have only 50% of their genes in common. Another finding pertains to adopted children of alcohol-dependent parents. These studies show that the development of alcohol problems in the offspring is far more influenced by having an alcoholic parent than by the adoptive home environment. This conclusion is especially strong for males. Based on this body of research, the argument for a biological predisposition to alcohol dependence has gained considerable strength. In this regard, genetic factors may account for up to a half of the variance in the etiology of alcohol dependence (Schuckit, Smith, & Kalmijn, 2004). Moreover, the mapping of the human genome has made the identification of specific gene candidates far more accessible that it was formerly (Johnson et al., 2006).

Psychological explanations of etiology have centered on identifying the "alcoholic personality," which means a psychological trait or set of traits that predispose someone to having alcohol dependence. Failure to find such a high-risk profile has not been due to lack of trying, as evidenced by the number of publications on the topic. However, recent research has revealed that the personality dimensions of neuroticism–emotionality,

CONTEMPORARY ISSUE BOX 9.6

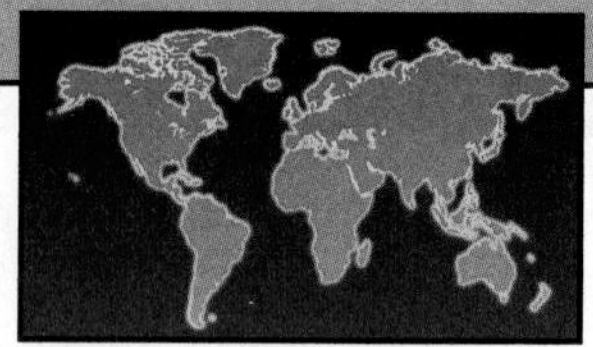

Is Alcohol Dependence a Disease?

Periodically, controversy flares over whether alcohol dependence is a disease. *Disease* may be defined broadly, but in the strict medical sense, it refers to a clearly identified physical process that is pathological. A critical feature of the definition is that once a disease is contracted, the afflicted individual has no control, or is not responsible, for the disease running its course. Typically when alcohol dependence is called a disease, the traditional medical model of disease is the referent.

Treatment providers and other citizens fought long and hard in the early 20th century to get alcohol dependence acknowledged as a disease in order to take "treatment" of alcohol dependence out of the legal system and into the medical profession. The campaign has been more than successful. In 1957, the American Medical Association formally recognized alcohol dependence as a disease and still does. Other professional organizations that followed include the American Hospital Association, American Academy of Pediatrics, American Dental Association, American College Health Association, American Chiropractic Association, the U.S. Congress, and the U.S. Surgeon General. Public opinion polls consistently have shown that a large majority of Americans say they believe that alcohol dependence is a disease. Moreover, advances in neuroscience research have bolstered this widespread support with more direct studies of drug action on the brain than were once possible (Peele, 1996).

The controversy is over whether the symptoms we call alcohol dependence are not more accurately thought of as a result of behavior that is learned and voluntary rather than as a manifestation of some disease process. The question is based on research and clinical findings over the last 30 years that have sparked much discussion in scientific journals (see Chapter 15).

The question is not just an academic one. It has important implications for how alcohol-dependent people are given treatment, for one thing. In this respect, the dominant position among U.S. treatment professionals, as well as Alcoholics Anonymous, is that alcohol dependence is a disease. It also has legal ramifications. For example, in a 1988 Supreme Court case, two U.S. military veterans argued unsuccessfully that they should have an extension of the time to take advantage of their benefits because they were "afflicted" with alcoholism within the usual benefit period. The gist of their argument was that, because alcoholism is a disease, they should not be punished for having something they have no control over. The Department of Veterans Affairs instead asserted alcoholism is the result of "willful misconduct."

With this example, what might be some ramifications of adherence to a strict position that alcohol dependence is the result of a biological disease process?

extraversion–sociability, and impulsivity–disinhibition predispose people to alcohol dependence (McCarthy, Kroll, & Smith, 2001). In Chapter 5, we also discussed some earlier research on psychological characteristics that may predispose an individual to alcohol dependence.

Sociological models of etiology were proposed partly in response to the failure to discover the unique alcoholic personality. The models are supported by findings of cross-cultural differences in drinking patterns (the benchmark citation is MacAndrew & Edgerton, 1969) as well as demographic factors that you have seen are correlated with drinking patterns and problems. Studies that take them into account have shown consistently that sociological factors help to explain the development of alcohol dependence.

"Biopsychosocial" Approaches to Etiology

Although each type of single-factor explanation has merit, each alone ultimately fails to explain how alcohol abuse and dependence develop. For example, a minority of children of parents with alcoholism develop alcohol dependence themselves. What happens to the rest? A set of psychological characteristics may be associated with developing alcohol dependence, but those same characteristics could be correlated with other outcomes. Demographic factors are correlated with drinking problems, but the factors themselves are often associated with biological and psychological variables, too. It seems that single-factor researchers design their studies so that one type of factor—say, psychological—is emphasized and other types are underplayed or not represented at all. Indeed, the fact that there are seeds of support for each type of approach, but not strong support for any one alone, suggests that multiple types of factors influence the development of alcohol dependence. At least among scientists, this is the most current thinking: Alcohol, as well as drug dependence, is caused and maintained by a combination of biological, psychological, and sociological factors (see, for example, Galizio & Maisto, 1985). As we discuss further in Chapter 15 on treatment, the three types of factors together in "shorthand" are called *biopsychosocial.*

What this means in practice is that scientists and practitioners alike cannot hope to understand alcohol dependence unless they consider together all the types of influencing variables. A good example is some of the exciting research done with sons of alcoholics who do not have alcohol dependence. One finding is from electrophysiological studies of the brain that show preadolescent sons of fathers with alcoholism may have a deficit that is expressed as a lesser ability to focus on stimuli in the environment (Porjesz & Begleiter, 1995). This difference from boys who do not have alcohol-dependent parents is presumably inherited and cannot be a consequence of the person's own drinking. In theory, such a deficit could increase the risk of developing alcohol dependence because of, say, a decreased ability to discriminate degree of intoxication when drinking moderately. Additionally, discrimination deficits could affect performance on various cognitive tasks and how individuals relate to other people (Schuckit, 1987). Whether risk actually is translated into alcohol dependence, however, depends in large part on how the environment (say, the family and school systems) "reacts" to any deficit in discrimination. Another example is a magnetic resonance imaging study of adolescents

DRUGS AND CULTURE BOX 9.7

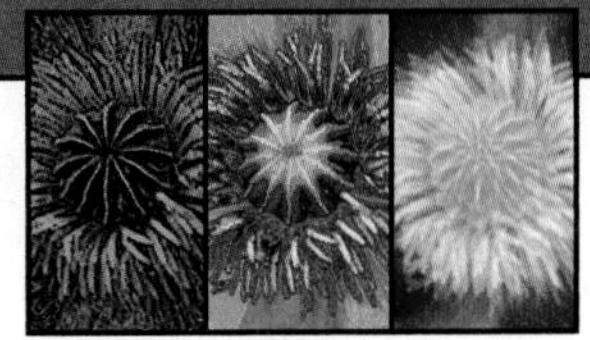

Alcohol and the Japanese

One of many countries that lend support to sociological/cultural theories of alcohol use is Japan. Dr. Dwight Heath, then a cultural anthropologist at Brown University, noted in a 1984 article that alcohol consumption increased steadily after World War II in Japan, as in many countries. Patterns of drinking also showed some major changes. For example, men who worked together often drank together nightly at loud parties. This contrasted sharply with the more traditional social and religious drinking contexts of the Japanese. The changes triggered predictions of increasing alcohol abuse and dependence, but the expectations never were realized.

A major reason drinking did not have large-scale negative consequences was cultural. In Japan and throughout Asia, moderate alcohol use is valued, and excessive drinking is not. Alcohol still is linked to social and religious rituals, customs that tend to discourage an individual's abuse of alcohol. According to Heath, alcohol dependence is relatively rare in Asia.

Another reason the Japanese did not develop an epidemic of alcohol problems may be biological. The phenomenon of importance here is the "Asian flushing response"—a physical reaction that occurs with drinking alcohol; it consists of cutaneous flushing and sometimes other symptoms, including palpitations, tachycardia, perspiration, and headache. As the name implies, the reaction occurs in Asians but not in people of other races. It appears to be due to a deficiency in aldehyde isozyme, which leads to a buildup of acetaldehyde when drinking, as alcohol metabolism is disrupted. The acetaldehyde causes the flushing response. The important point is that this response is assumed to be unpleasant to most people and thus may set a biological limit on the amount of alcohol that is drunk on an occasion (Kitano, 1989).

Not all Asians show the flushing response, and those who do show it to different degrees (Higuchi et al., 1992). However, this biological reaction, coupled with cultural customs for alcohol use in the Japanese, provides an excellent example of how different types of factors work together to influence alcohol use.

that Hill et al. (2009) reported. In this study, adolescents who were "high risk" for developing alcohol use disorders, because of the multiple "layer" presence of that disorder in their family histories, showed lower volume of brain orbital frontal cortex (OFC) matter than did adolescents who were "low risk" because they did not have a family history of alcohol use disorders. The OFC is an area of the brain that is associated with emotional processing and impulsivity. Furthermore, the differences in right-brain OFC matter seemed to be due to genetic variation between the high- and low-risk groups.

Saying that multiple factors combine to cause alcohol dependence is, after all, an extension of a theme we have followed since Chapter 1: Human experience and behavior under the influence of drugs can be understood only by considering multiple types of factors in combination. The research suggests that the same thinking should be applied to understanding alcohol dependence.

Summary

- Alcohol virtually always is drunk in the form of three major classes of alcoholic beverages: beer, wine, and hard liquor (also called distilled spirits).
- Alcoholic beverages are produced through fermentation and distillation.
- The alcohol content of a beverage may be expressed by volume or by weight.
- The proof of an alcoholic beverage refers to its percentage of alcohol content.
- People have used alcohol for thousands of years, but societies always have viewed alcoholic beverages as mixed blessings.
- In the United States, per capita alcohol consumption increased from the end of Prohibition into the 1940s. There was another increase from 1960 into the 1970s. In 1980, a decline in consumption began that was slightly reversed in 1990, but that continued to the mid-late 1990s. Since then, there has been a slight increase.
- Overall consumption figures mask beverage differences. Consumption of hard liquor has dropped the most overall since 1980, with slight reductions in beer and wine consumption.
- Social and environmental factors, such as urban versus rural residence, gender, age, and racial/ethnic background, are associated with alcohol consumption rates. The same is true for the prevalence of heavy drinking.
- Alcohol is a drug that depresses the CNS. It may exert its effects by dissolving in lipid membranes.
- The GABA receptors are one locus that likely is a specific neural site of alcohol's action in the body. Identifying a specific receptor mechanism is difficult, however, because alcohol's effects on the body are so diffuse.
- Alcohol is a food primarily absorbed from the small intestine. The rate of alcohol absorption can vary widely according to an individual's physiological and situational factors.
- Following its absorption, alcohol is distributed to all of the body's tissues. Blood gets an especially high concentration of alcohol.
- Alcohol primarily affects the CNS, particularly the brain. The LD 50 for alcohol is a BAC of 0.45% to 0.50%.
- BAC is approximated by a simple equation that includes alcohol dose and time. Other factors that influence BAC are percentage of body fat, gender, and rate of alcohol metabolization.
- Breath analysis is a practical, precise way of measuring the BAC.
- The body metabolizes more than 90% of the alcohol it absorbs, primarily in the liver.
- The liver metabolizes alcohol at a constant rate of about 0.35 ounce of alcohol an hour, and little can be done to quicken the pace.
- Alcohol use leads to dispositional tolerance and, more important, to both acute and protracted functional tolerance.
- Chronic heavy use of alcohol can lead to physical dependence on it. The alcohol withdrawal

syndrome is a serious medical problem that can result in death if not treated properly.

- Alcohol has few direct medical uses but is an ingredient in several legitimate medical products.
- Alcohol's acute action is evident in a wide variety of physiological, sensorimotor, and behavioral effects. In general, as the BAC increases, acute effects increase in number and intensity. However, how humans experience degree of intoxication and behave under different doses of alcohol are modified by psychological and situational factors as well as alcohol dose and tolerance to this drug.
- Sensorimotor skills, which alcohol impairs, are crucial in driving motor vehicles.
- Alcohol seems to be a major contributor to fatal and nonfatal automobile accidents. Gender and age combine with alcohol to influence risk of involvement in an automobile accident.
- Stemming the drunk-driving problem seems to be a matter of sustained attention and action by law enforcement and citizens' action groups. Drivers' perceptions that arrest and conviction are likely consequences of drunk driving also are important.
- Alcohol's effects on sex and aggression are major topics of social interest and concern. To understand alcohol's association with aggressive behavior, it is necessary to take into account characteristics of the aggressor and situational factors, only one of which is alcohol.
- Alcohol's effects on sexual behavior are similarly complex. It is necessary to know the physiological basis of alcohol's effect on sexual function, as well as situational and psychological factors, to explain its effects on sexual behavior.
- A history of chronic heavy drinking is associated with damage to most of the body's organs and systems. Two of the most prominent ones are the liver and the brain.
- A chronic effect of alcohol use is impaired memory and other cognitive functions. Some of these effects are virtually reversible with abstinence from alcohol. However, when the brain has structural damage, as in Korsakoff's syndrome, the effects are permanent.
- As the major metabolic site of alcohol, the liver is vulnerable to the chronic effect of heavy alcohol use.
- Three liver disorders that are attributable to drinking are fatty liver, alcohol hepatitis, and cirrhosis. The first two disorders are reversible with abstinence; cirrhosis, a leading killer in the United States, is not.
- Chronic heavy drinking is associated with impaired sexual functioning in both men and women.
- A mother's drinking during pregnancy may result in fetal alcohol syndrome (FAS) in the newborn child. FAS consists of gross physical deformities that are identifiable at birth. FAS is associated with continued physical problems as well as below-average intellectual functioning later in childhood.
- The idea that moderate alcohol consumption is associated with lowered risk of cardiovascular disease and mortality has good research support, but this conclusion remains controversial.
- The development of alcohol dependence is an unsolved problem. It does seem that "single-cause" theories are inadequate to explain the etiology of alcohol dependence. Instead, it is necessary to incorporate biological, psychological, and sociological factors.

Answers to "What Do You Think?"

1. Humans have consumed alcohol since between 6000 B.C. and 5000 B.C.

   T *Humans indeed have consumed alcohol since between 5,000 and 6,000 years before the time of Christ.*

2. In the United States of 1830, adults' average alcohol consumption was about five drinks a day.

   T *Americans in the early 19th century were prodigious consumers of alcohol.*

3. The highest rates of heavy drinking, and thus the greatest vulnerability to drinking problems, are in men between the ages of 40 and 45.

   F *The highest rates are in younger men, ages 18 to 25.*

4. It is difficult to consume a lethal dose of alcohol.
   F *It is all too easy. The LD 50 of alcohol in humans is about equal to drinking a fifth (25.3 oz) of whiskey in an hour. This is not too hard to do, and it has been done with dire consequences during events such as fraternity hazings.*
5. If not treated properly, alcohol withdrawal syndrome can be fatal.
   T *Because of the availability of drugs that show cross-dependence with alcohol, medical management of alcohol withdrawal is generally straightforward. Nevertheless, it is a serious medical condition; if not treated properly or at all, alcohol withdrawal can be fatal.*
6. Alcohol is a drug that has no legitimate medical value.
   F *Although alcohol is hardly the elixir people once thought it was, it does have legitimate therapeutic uses, such as in medicinal compounds taken orally or applied externally.*
7. If you drink a lot and black out, it means you have lost consciousness.
   F *Blackouts are the loss of memory for events that occur while under the influence of a drug (in this case, alcohol). A drinker who experiences a blackout is fully conscious when nonrecalled events happen.*
8. Alcohol causes violent behavior.
   F *Alcohol is correlated with the occurrence of violent behavior, but cognitive, social, and environmental factors must also be used to explain the alcohol–violence association.*
9. Alcohol improves sexual performance.
   F *Pharmacologically, alcohol impairs sexual performance, particularly when BACs reach 0.05% and higher. However, people may perceive that the use of alcohol is associated with greater sexual arousal and better sexual performance.*
10. The cognitive deficits that seem to occur in some people as a result of years of heavy drinking are reversible.
    T *At least when there is not severe structural damage to the brain, as in Korsakoff's syndrome, many of the cognitive deficits that may occur are reversible with prolonged abstinence from alcohol.*
11. The majority of alcoholics eventually develop cirrhosis of the liver.
    F *Some, but only a minority of about 10% to 20% of chronic heavy drinkers, certainly do develop cirrhosis.*
12. Moderate drinking (one to three drinks a day) is associated with reduced risk of heart disease.
    T *Research has shown that moderate use of alcohol is correlated with reduced risk of heart disease.*

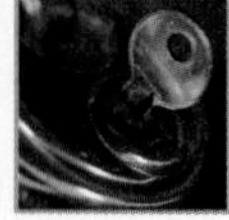

Key Terms

blackout
confabulation
distillation
disulfiram
intoxication
long-term memory
monoamine oxidase (MAO) inhibitors
neuropsychological tests
orientation to time
proof
pylorospasm
REM sleep
short-term memory
social detoxification
standard drink
teratology

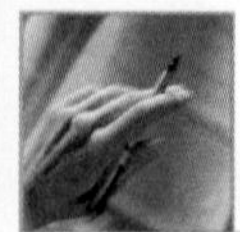

Essays/Thought Questions

1. What is your opinion of the efforts at college campuses to have an "alcohol-free" environment? How is this policy similar to or different from banning tobacco smoking in public places?
2. Since the mid-1980s, the legal minimum drinking age in all states of the United States has been 21 years old, a result of federal legislation passed in 1984 that imposed a 10% penalty on highway

appropriations funds from the federal government to any state that retained a minimum drinking age younger than 21. A number of university and college presidents and chancellors recently have signed onto the "Amethyst" movement, which has a goal of open and impassionate discussion of the advantages and disadvantages of having a minimum legal drinking age of younger than 21 and of 21 and older. University and college administrators are taking a public stance on this question because of their view of patterns of alcohol use among today's undergraduate students. Given the research and other literature on the effects of having different minimum legal drinking ages, what side of the argument do you think you would support? Why?

3. What would be the advantages and disadvantages of creating a definition of "legal intoxication" that considers an individual's protracted functional tolerance to alcohol?
4. Would requiring alcohol warning labels on alcoholic beverage containers be effective in moderating alcohol consumption? Why or why not?
5. In the section on FAS, we discussed that the typical advice given to pregnant women is that the only safe level of alcohol consumption is no consumption at all. However, although the evidence is clear that a mother's heavy consumption is dangerous to the fetus, the effects, if any, of light alcohol consumption on the fetus are far more ambiguous. In view of the current state of knowledge, do you think it is ethical to give blanket, prescriptive-like advice to women to not drink alcohol if they are pregnant? In considering your answer, consult the articles by Gavaghan (2009) and by Kelly et al. (2009).

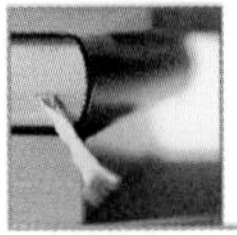

Suggested Readings

Heath, D. B. (2000). *Drinking occasions. Comparative perspectives on alcohol and culture*. New York: Brunner/Mazel.

National Institute on Alcohol Abuse and Alcoholism. (2000). *Tenth special report to the U.S. Congress on alcohol and health*. Washington, DC: U.S. Department of Health and Human Services.

National Institute on Alcohol Abuse and Alcoholism. (2002). *A call to action: Changing the culture of drinking at U.S. colleges*. Washington, DC: U.S. Department of Health and Human Services.

(See also the 2008 update on the NIAAA website, link available at the Book Companion Website.)

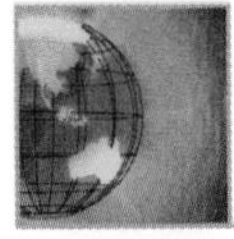

Web Resources

Visit the Book Companion Website at www.cengage.com/psychology/maisto to access study tools including a glossary, flashcards, and web quizzing. You will also find links to the following resources:

- Mothers Against Drunk Driving
- Stanton Peele Addiction: Cultural factors have a major influence on drinking patterns and their interpretation in a given society. See this site for an extreme cultural perspective with links to scholarly references.
- University of Virginia: Based on research that Dr. James Turner and his colleagues completed, the University of Virginia has charts that indicate the number of drinks, time of drinking, and estimated BACs for both men and women by body weight. This by itself is not unusual. However, on the back of the BAC chart are negative consequences of special relevance to college students for a range of BACs. Students at the University of Virginia have reported that the charts, which are wallet-sized, are a big help in their decision making about alcohol use.

CHAPTER 10

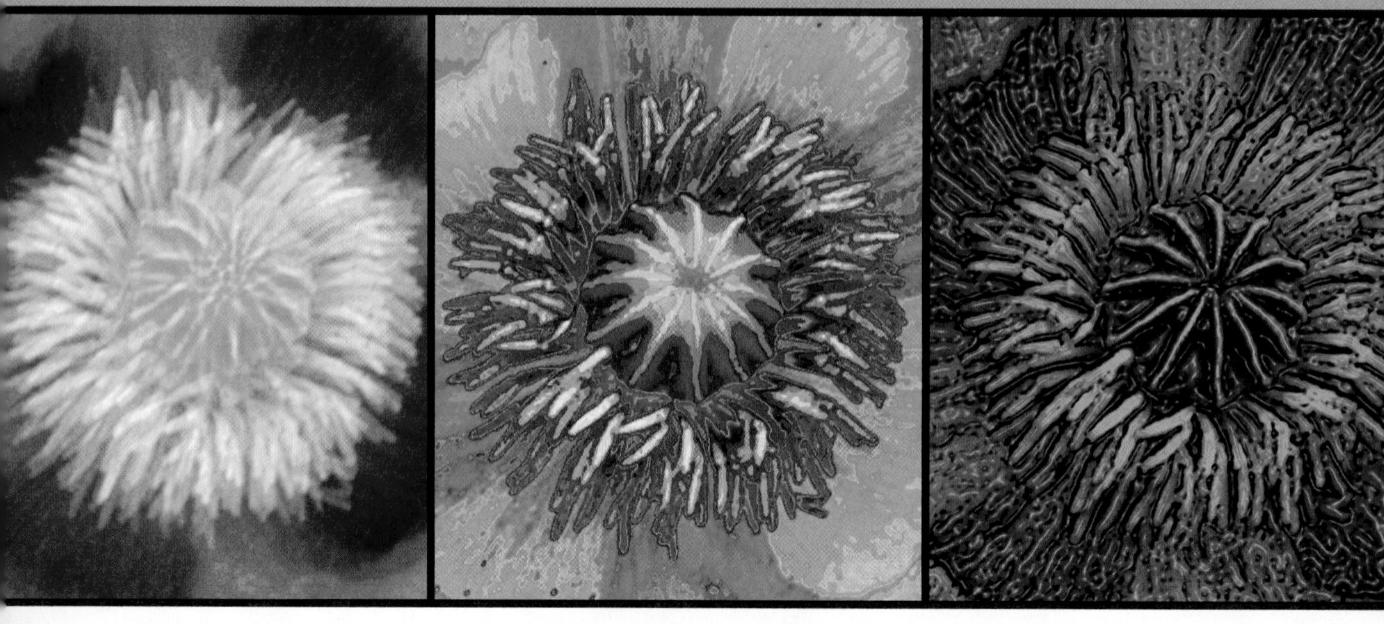

Opiates

What Do You Think? True or False?

Answers are given at the end of the chapter.

___ 1. Opium comes from the plant *Cannabis sativa.*

___ 2. Morphine is one of the active ingredients in opium.

___ 3. Heroin was first made illegal by the 1965 Drug Abuse Control Amendment.

___ 4. Use of "dirty" needles is now one of the major causes of AIDS.

___ 5. Most designer heroin compounds are less potent than pure heroin.

___ 6. The opiates are among the most powerful analgesic drugs.

___ 7. Heroin enhances sexual desire and activity.

___ 8. Opiate drugs show cross-dependence with alcohol.

___ 9. Heroin withdrawal is much like alcohol withdrawal.

___10. Veterans of the Vietnam War had a high rate of heroin addiction and were unable to kick the habit when they returned to the United States.

___11. The effects of opiates are synergistic with those of alcohol.

___12. The expression "cold turkey" comes from the "goose bumps" seen in addicts withdrawing from heroin.

As indicated in historical overviews in earlier chapters, psychoactive drugs can be double-edged swords in their potential for improving the human condition, on one hand, and their capacity to cause destruction to individuals and society on the other. No group of drugs captures this paradox more dramatically than the class of drugs we call opiates, which includes opium, morphine, heroin, and related compounds. Opiate drugs have been used for centuries to relieve pain and, when introduced to Europe, were hailed by physicians as a godsend. One of the first European physicians to use opium to relieve pain and suffering in his patients, Thomas Sydenham, wrote in 1680: "Among the remedies which it has pleased Almighty God to give man to relieve his sufferings, none is so universal and so efficacious as opium" (Gay & Way, 1972, p. 47). Even today, opiate drugs remain the most potent painkillers available to physicians, yet we now recognize the other edge of the opiate sword—the ability of opiates to produce severe dependence. Heroin is viewed as the prototype addictive drug, and illegal use and traffic in heroin are major international problems. Thus, many of the general concerns regarding psychoactive drugs emerge in bold relief in a consideration of opiates.

History of the Opiates

Early History

Opium comes from *Papaver somniferum,* one of the many species of the poppy plant. The opium poppy is native to the Middle East, in the areas that border the Mediterranean Sea, but it is now cultivated extensively throughout Asia and the Middle East. Contrary to the experiences of Dorothy in *The Wizard of Oz,* however, simply walking through a poppy field will not cause sleep or euphoria. Rather, special procedures must be followed to extract opium from the poppy. The petals fall after the poppy blooms, leaving a round seedpod the size of an egg. If the seedpod is scored lightly

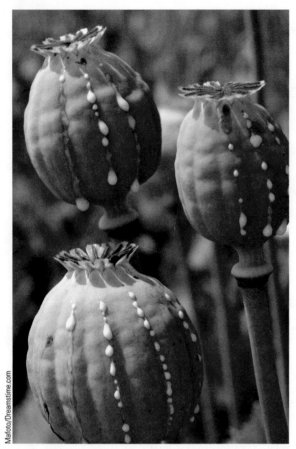
Mafoto/Dreamstime.com

Opium exudes from incisions of the poppy pod.

with a knife, it secretes a milky white sap. After drying, this sap forms a thick, gummy, brown substance that is called **opium**. A person experiences the effects of opium by consuming the substance orally or by smoking it.

The use of crude opium preparations is truly an ancient practice. There is evidence that the Sumerian and Assyrian civilizations cultivated and used opium as long ago as 6,000 years. The ancient Egyptians had discovered medical uses for opiates 3,500 years ago, as documented in the "Therapeutic Papyrus of Thebes" (Scott, 1969). The Greek and Roman civilizations also used opium for a variety of medical purposes. The great Greek physician Galen (A.D. 130–201) noted the following uses for opium:

> [Opium] . . . resists poison and venomous bites, cures chronic headache, vertigo, deafness, epilepsy, apoplexy, dimness of sight, loss of voice, asthma, coughs of all kinds, spitting of blood, tightness of breath, colic, the iliac poison, jaundice, hardness of the spleen, stone, urinary complaints, fevers, dropsies, leprosies, the troubles to which women are subject, melancholy and all pestilences. (Scott, 1969, p. 111)

Although this quote may seem more a testament to the ignorance of medical problems of this age, certainly the remarkable **analgesia** (pain relief) of opium must have made it seem helpful for many disease states. In fact, opiate drugs do have special cough-suppressant and antidiarrheal properties in addition to their analgesic actions, and they are used in modern medicine for these purposes.

opium
The dried sap produced by the poppy plant.

analgesia
Pain relief produced without a loss of consciousness.

The use of opium for medical and recreational purposes became widespread among the Islamic peoples of the Middle East. This may have been because the Koran's explicit prohibition of the use of alcohol and some other drugs did not include opiate use (Latimer & Goldberg, 1981). To this day, the use of opiates is less censored than that of alcohol among many Muslims. By the 9th century, Arab traders spread the use of opium to India and China, where the practice of smoking opium developed. Dependence on opium was first recognized as a problem in China as well, with the first edict against opium issued in 1729. However, China already had so many opium addicts that the demand remained very high. In spite of the ban on importing opium into China, British ships continued to trade opium grown in India for Chinese tea, and this activity was the basis for the Opium Wars between China and Great Britain in the middle of the 19th century (see Chapter 2).

Opiate Use in the 19th Century

Opium dependence was a serious problem in China by the beginning of the 19th century, but it was not yet seen as such in Europe or America. Although opium was readily available in laudanum and various patent medicines, it almost always was in liquid form and taken orally (a practice called opium eating, even though it was really opium drinking) rather than smoked. It was used mostly for medical purposes. Developments during the century brought the addictive properties of opiate drugs to the awareness of Western societies. As noted in Chapter 2, opium preparations were readily available and completely legal in 19th-century Europe and the United States. The pleasurable properties of opium soon led to its widespread use for nonmedical reasons. The pleasures of opium were extolled in a book written by the British poet Thomas De Quincey, *The Confessions of an English Opium-Eater,* published in 1822. De Quincey's book praised the effects of opium and included several famous quotes, including ". . . thou hast the keys of Paradise, O just, subtle and mighty opium!" (Scott, 1969, p. 52). Westerners were slow to recognize that "eating" opium could prove just as addictive as smoking it, but concern about opium became more widespread, as tomes such as De Quincey's fueled its use. By the late 1800s, opium use had spread throughout society, affecting such noted literary and scientific figures as Elizabeth Barrett Browning, Samuel Coleridge, William Halstead, Walter Scott, and Percy Shelley, to name a few. It was becoming recognized that opium dependence was not limited to the Chinese.

Pharmacological developments added to the problems. In 1803, the German pharmacist F. W. Serturner developed a process that separated morphine from opium. Morphine is the major active chemical in opium (codeine is another opiate drug found in opium) and is about 10 times more potent than crude opium. Serturner experimented with morphine and was so impressed with the blissful, dreamlike state it induced that he named the chemical after Morpheus, the Greek god of dreams. Morphine became widely available in the mid-1800s, and with the concomitant development of the hypodermic syringe, injected morphine became a major dependence problem in Europe and the United States. Because of the rapid and potent

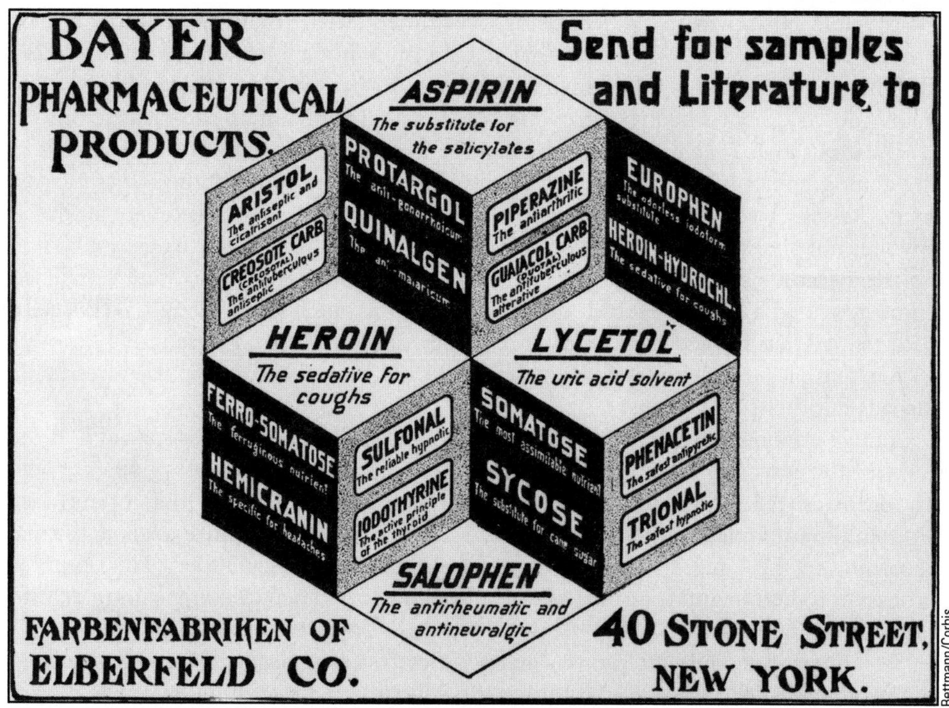

Bettmann/Corbis

Patent medicines of the 19th century frequently contained opiates such as heroin.

pain-relieving properties of injectable morphine, it was the treatment of choice during recovery from severe wounds. However, withdrawal from the morphine was often more difficult than recovery from the wound. As noted in Chapter 2, morphine dependence was so common among soldiers on both sides during the Civil War in America that it was often called "soldier's disease."

In 1874, British chemist Alder Wright published reports of experiments that produced a new chemical compound based on an alteration of morphine: diacetylmorphine. Wright's discovery went unnoticed until 1898, when the great German pharmacologist Heinrich Dreser (who also discovered aspirin; see Chapter 14) rediscovered the compound and noted that it was twice as potent as morphine. Because this new compound was so powerful, it was viewed as a new treatment with "heroic" possibilities and was christened **heroin**. Heroin was used immediately as a cough suppressant and pain reliever. Not until many years later was it recognized that heroin was even more likely than morphine to produce dependence.

heroin
A drug produced by chemically processing morphine. It is more potent than morphine and has become the major opiate drug of abuse.

Opiate Use in the 20th Century and Today

The growing awareness of the danger and pervasiveness of opiate dependence led to a number of legal changes reviewed in detail in Chapter 2. In the United States, these culminated in the 1914 Harrison Narcotics Act. Of course, the Harrison Act did not completely eliminate the nonmedical use of opiates and, in fact, it marked the beginning of drug crime in America. Illegal opiate use meant opium and heroin were smuggled into the country. This resulted in an escalation of prices and a change in the type of person who became or remained addicted to opiates. The Harrison Act placed the control of opiate drugs in the hands of physicians; determination of whether an addict had a valid medical need for opiates was exclusively the physician's decision. However, legislative interpretations ruled that a physician must not prescribe opiates unless doses could be shown to be decreasing over time (1915), that opiates must not be prescribed to addicts (1917), and that heroin must not be prescribed at all (1924) (Kramer, 1972). After the legitimate channels for obtaining drugs were blocked for many addicts, they turned to a growing black market to maintain their addiction.

Opiate use has certainly changed since the Harrison Act. One major change is in the demographics of opiate use. Before the Harrison Act, opiate addiction cut across social classes. A wealthy, middle-aged woman was as likely to be an opiate addict as anyone, but she would be addicted to laudanum purchased at her drugstore. When opiates became illegal, they began to be used mainly in large cities where organized crime provided a supply. Heroin quickly emerged as the addict's drug of choice. In addition, addicts tended more and more to be young, poorly educated men of lower socioeconomic status (James & Johnson, 1996), although heroin use has since made inroads in other populations.

A huge criminal apparatus for producing and supplying heroin was spawned in the wake of the Harrison Narcotics Act. Today, most heroin comes from poppies grown in Southwest Asia. Afghanistan produces more than 90% of the world's opium (see Contemporary Issue Box 10.1), with lesser amounts coming from Laos and Burma, according to the United Nations Office on Drugs and Crime (2009). The opium is processed to heroin and transported to Europe or Mexico before being smuggled into the United States.

Street heroin is adulterated or cut many times as it changes hands on the way from the producer to the importer to those who sell to individual users, and it may vary enormously in quality. If sophisticated chemical production and refining techniques are used, uncut heroin can be quite pure and appears as a white odorless powder

CONTEMPORARY ISSUE BOX 10.1

Poppies in Afghanistan: The Taliban and the Heroin Trade

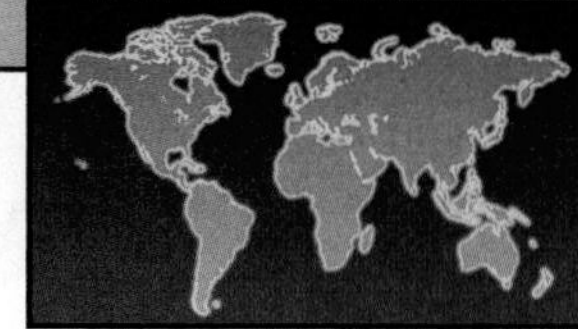

Most Americans knew little about Afghanistan or the Taliban prior to September 11, 2001, but those who follow the heroin trade have focused on Afghanistan for decades. Afghanistan has long been a major area of opium production, but the "golden triangle" of Southeast Asia (Burma, Laos, and Thailand) historically dominated opium production. By 1999, though, Afghanistan had become the undisputed world leader in opium production despite being an Islamic state ruled by the Taliban, which publicly opposed opium use. In 1999, the Taliban representative to the United States, Abdul Hakeem Mujahid, said, "We are against poppy cultivation, narcotics production and drugs, but we cannot fight our own people" (Bartolet & Levine, 2001, p. 85). Even before 9/11, the United States accused the Taliban of profiting from opium and heroin production, and using those profits to fund terrorist activities. Under pressure from the United Nations, the Taliban announced bans on poppy cultivation in 1997, 1998, and 2000, but there was little evidence of any decreased production. In 2001, though, a ban was put into place that apparently really did reduce poppy production. Cynics have pointed out that the Taliban was simply trying to increase prices by temporarily cutting the supply; whatever the reason, when the Taliban lost control of Afghanistan, the poppy made a comeback. In this war-ravaged and economically depressed nation, growing opium is one of the few ways that farmers can make a living. Afghan President Hamid Karzai has urged his people to declare jihad (holy war) on drug production, but opium farming still accounts for nearly half of the domestic economy, and Afghanistan supplies over 90% of the world's heroin (United Nations Office on Drugs and Crime, 2009a). In recent years, the resurgent Taliban has gained control of poppy production again, and it is estimated that hundreds of millions of dollars from opium sales are being used to fund the insurgency against U.S. forces and the Karzai government (Moreau, 2009).

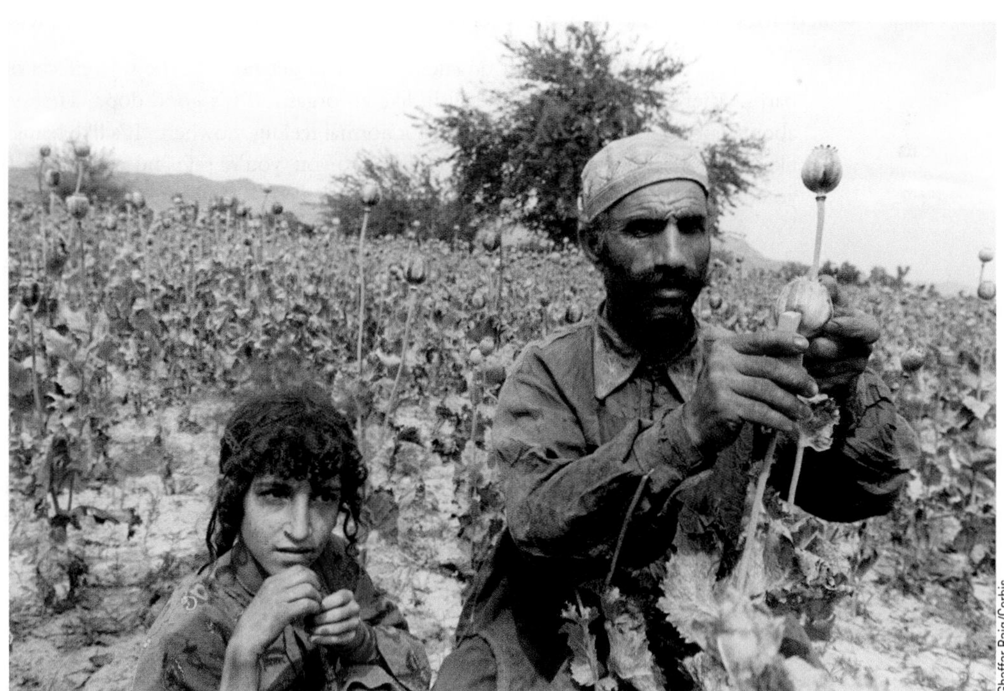

Harvesting opium in Afghanistan

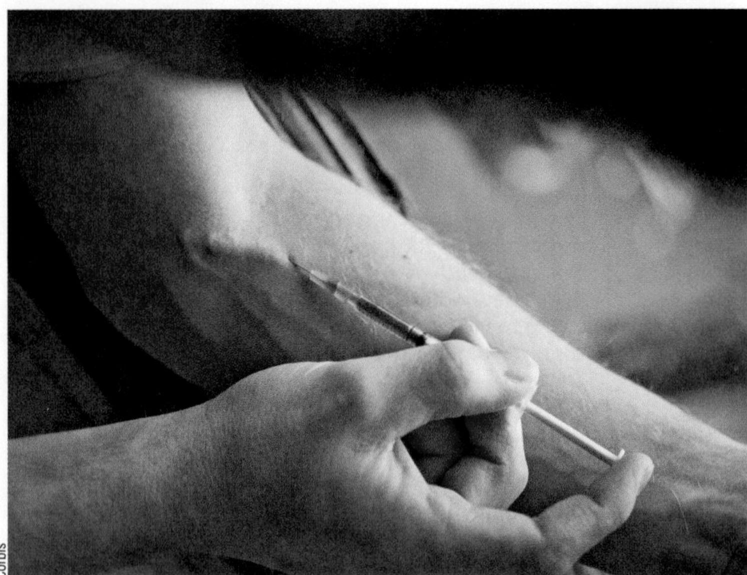
Corbis

Heroin is often administered via intravenous injection.

that can be injected, smoked ("chasing the dragon"), or taken intranasally (snorted). On the other hand, crude processing techniques may yield much lower-quality heroin. For example, black tar heroin, produced in Mexico, is a dark brown or black substance that may be tarlike or hard. It is generally too impure to be smoked or even to dissolve in water and has to be melted to be injected (Ashton, 2002). Even high-quality heroin may be adulterated (cut) with cheap adulterants such as baking powder, caffeine, quinine, or even talcum powder to increase the dealer's profit. Heroin remains a large and important source of illegal revenue, which helps recruit participants in organized crime.

Many heroin addicts become involved in criminal activity to support their habit. At first, the cost of heroin may appear relatively low to addicts who use the drug occasionally for "kicks." But in the words of an addict interviewed by Smith and Gay (1972): "It's so good, don't even try it once." Many users find that they take the drug more and more frequently, and because tolerance develops rapidly to heroin and other opiates, higher doses are soon required to produce the desired effect. Soon the cost of maintaining the growing habit virtually forces addicts to engage in criminal activities. Here is part of an interview with a street addict from San Francisco:

> [Heroin] . . . is the mellowest downer of all. You get none of the side effects of speed and barbs. After you fix, you feel the rush, like an orgasm if it's good dope. Then you float for about four hours; nothing positive, just a normal feeling, nowhere. It's like being half asleep, like watching a movie; nothing gets through to you, you're safe and warm. The big thing is, you don't hurt. You can walk around with rotting teeth and a busted appendix and not feel it. You don't need sex, you don't need food, you don't need people, you don't care. It's like death without permanence, life without pain. For me, the only hard part is keeping in H, paying my connection, man. I know these rich cats who can get good smack and shoot it for years and nothing happens, but me, you know, it's a hustle to stay alive. I run about a $100, $150-a-day habit, so I have to cop twice that much to keep my fence happy. . . . (Luce, 1972, p. 145)

In another testimonial on heroin, the great guitarist, Eric Clapton, describes his fall into addiction this way:

> I assumed I was in some way immune to it and wouldn't get hooked. But addiction doesn't negotiate and it gradually crept up on me like a fog. . . . It was so insidious. It took over my life without my really noticing. (Clapton, 2007)

In fact, heroin addiction is a hard way to live. Consider the findings of a study that followed 581 heroin addicts over a period of 33 years (Hser et al., 2001). Half of these individuals died during the study period, 50 to 100 times the death rate in the general population of the same age. Of the surviving addicts at the end of the period, 20% were still using heroin (and another 10% refused to be tested) and 14% were in

CONTEMPORARY ISSUE BOX 10.2

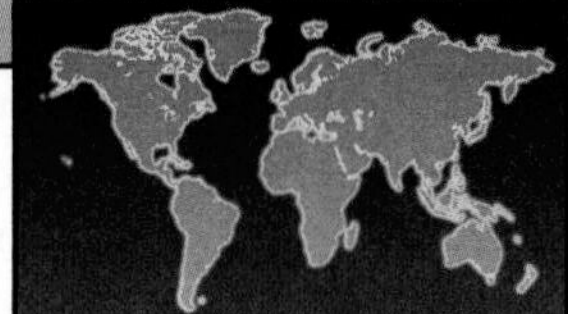

Fatal Attraction: Intravenous Drug Use and AIDS

Intravenous (IV) drug users may inject cocaine or methamphetamine, but the majority are heroin addicts. They may be young or old, black or white, male or female, but one thing they have in common is a great risk for developing acquired immune deficiency syndrome, or AIDS. In the early 1980s, male homosexuals were the major group at high risk for AIDS, but the number of drug-related AIDS cases has risen so sharply that they now account for more than 25% of all AIDS cases (NIDA, 2005). The magnitude of the problem is substantial. A recent study of IV drug users in New York City (Davis et al., 2006) found that nearly a quarter (23.9%) was infected with the human immunodeficiency virus (HIV). Moreover, it is not just the users who are involved. The virus does spread among heterosexuals, and the babies born of HIV-positive mothers will usually develop AIDS as well.

An ironic aspect of this tragedy is that it is so avoidable. IV drug users are at dual risk for HIV infection because they are likely to engage in both risky sex and the common practice of sharing needles. Using a needle contaminated with the blood of someone who has HIV leads to direct blood-to-blood transmission, which involves a very high risk of infection. If sterile needles were used, this risk would be eliminated. Health care workers are striving to send the message out to IV drug users that they should avoid sharing needles, or clean them with bleach if sharing is necessary. Some cities have developed needle exchange programs, where clean needles are given to users in exchange for dirty ones. In most areas in the country, however, hypodermic syringes are controlled legally and remain difficult for addicts to obtain. In addition, sharing needles has become part of the "culture" for users. IV drug use often occurs in "shooting galleries," places where people gather to inject and enjoy the effects of the drug. A single needle may be used to deliver dozens of injections in such a place. Unless these practices can be stopped, the desire to use IV drugs will remain a fatal attraction.

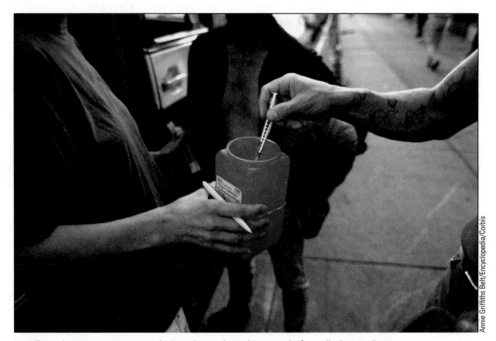

Annie Griffiths Belt/Encyclopedia/Corbis

Needle exchange programs are designed to reduce the spread of needle-borne diseases.

prison. Why is the life span of a heroin addict so short? Addicts are at great risk for disease and death from AIDS, hepatitis, and other diseases spread by sharing contaminated needles (see Contemporary Issue Box 10.2). The National Institute on Drug Abuse estimates that heroin overdose is responsible for more than 1,000 deaths every year. Overdose deaths most commonly occur when heroin or another opiate drug is combined with alcohol or another depressant drug due to synergy, but another factor is that different concoctions of street heroin can vary enormously in potency. Between 2006 and 2007, a rash of overdose deaths in the Eastern and Midwestern United States were traced to a mixture of heroin and fentanyl, a short-acting but highly potent opioid combination called "fefe," that has recently appeared in these parts of the country (Shenfeld, 2006). Between 2007 and 2008, a combination of heroin and cold medications called "cheese" resulted in numerous overdose deaths in Texas.

Another issue involving opiate drug use is "designer" heroin. Designer heroin is produced illicitly by chemists who design or develop chemical analogues to heroin. These new compounds are untested but usually produce effects similar to those of heroin or other opiates. Until the passage of the Controlled Substances Analogue Enforcement Act of 1986 (see Chapter 2), dealers also had the advantage in that federal law did not control these new compounds because some of them are new to science. Most designer heroin compounds are derivatives of the powerful opioid, fentanyl. One problem with these fentanyl derivatives (often sold on the street as "China white") is that they may be 10 to 1,000 times more potent than heroin. Thus, the risk of overdose death is greater. Another problem posed by designer compounds is chillingly illustrated by an episode from the 1980s, when an underground chemist in the San Francisco Bay area began to produce a designer heroin called MPPP. Apparently, due to poor laboratory technique, some portion of his product was a closely related but highly toxic compound called MPTP. The error was discovered when a number of young drug users were hospitalized with complete paralysis. At first the cause of this epidemic of paralysis was a mystery. The symptoms were similar to those of advanced Parkinson's disease. However, because Parkinson's is a disease of the elderly, only an inspired guess by a physician named William Langston solved the puzzle. He tried to use L-dopa with these "frozen" addicts. The L-dopa was successful enough that the paralyzed patients were able to at least talk a little. Eventually, they were identified as heroin addicts who had tried the misdesigned heroin, MPTP.

We now know that MPTP selectively attacks and rapidly destroys the substantia nigra, which leads to symptoms of advanced Parkinson's disease (see Chapter 3). The addicts who became victims of MPTP have sustained permanent damage, although L-dopa has reduced some symptoms (Langston, 2002). A couple of important points: First, the tremendous hazard associated with designer drugs is obvious. Because these drugs are not tested in animals or screened by the FDA, they pose serious risks to users. Second, designer drugs can produce brain damage without overt symptoms. Many people who were exposed to MPTP only once or twice probably do not show any Parkinson's symptoms at present. Nonetheless, some damage to the substantia nigra has occurred. As these people lose more cells during the normal aging process, they may reach the 80% threshold and may yet pay the price by developing premature Parkinson's disease (see Ibid.).

Not all heroin casualties are due to overdose or toxicity from designer drugs. As an example, Jerry Garcia of the Grateful Dead died of poor health complicated by years of heroin addiction in a drug detox center in 1996. Many believed Nirvana singer Kurt Cobain's 1994 suicide was related to his inability to kick his heroin habit. His journal, published posthumously in 2002, is a chronicle of his struggle to get off heroin during the final years of his life. He wrote:

> I remember someone saying if you try heroine [sic] once you'll become hooked. Of course I laughed and scoffed at the idea but I now believe this to be very true. Not literally, I mean if you do dope once you don't instantly become addicted, it usually takes about one month of everyday use to physically become addicted. But after the first time your mind says ahh that was very pleasant as long as I don't do it every day I won't have a problem. The problem is it happens over time. . . . (Cobain, 2002)

Despite the well-publicized dangers, heroin use increased dramatically in the United States throughout the 1990s, and has leveled off at relatively high levels in the 2000s. One reason is that the abundance of relatively pure and very potent heroin on the street has made the drug available to be snorted or smoked as well as injected. In fact, snorting or smoking heroin has become the method of choice for administering heroin among a generation of users who are younger and have a higher socioeconomic status than was once the case (Durrant & Thakker, 2003). Some estimates indicate that the United States may have as many as 900,000 heroin addicts. Although this number may seem small relative to more widespread drug problems like alcoholism and nicotine dependence, heroin has a significant impact on society (Inciardi, 2002).

Prescription Opiate Abuse

Although heroin use has leveled off over the past decade, overall abuse of opiate drugs went up dramatically during this period. The reason is the explosive increase in prescription opiate drug use (Compton & Volkow, 2006). Illicit use of prescription opiates more than tripled from the 1990s to the present. Along with increased use of prescription opiates has come an increased number of drug treatment admissions and emergency room mentions involving these drugs (Subramaniam & Stitzer, 2009). The rate of overdose deaths involving prescription opiates has also gone up and has actually been higher than rates associated with heroin in recent years (Wu, Pilowsky, & Patkar, 2008). Several prescription opiate painkillers have been part of this trend, but the most publicized of these has been OxyContin. OxyContin was introduced by the pharmaceutical firm Purdue Pharma in the mid-1990s. There was no particular reason to expect it to become a significant abuse problem. The generic drug in OxyContin, oxycodone, is not new. It is a synthetic opiate found in Percodan and other prescription painkillers that have been on the market for decades. The difference is that OxyContin was designed to treat severe and chronic pain, and so it contains a higher dose of oxycodone. Whereas Percodan might contain 5 milligrams of oxycodone and has a relatively short duration of action, OxyContin formulations contain 20 to 160 milligrams of oxycodone in time-release form so that a single pill has a duration of action up to 12 hours. This formulation makes OxyContin a highly effective pain reliever, but illicit users discovered that they could crush the OxyContin tablet to produce a powder they could inject or snort. This practice releases all of the oxycodone at once and thus delivers a large dose of opiate immediately to the user.

These large doses available in a single tablet are particularly dangerous. OxyContin abuse, addiction, and lethal overdose all skyrocketed in the early 2000s. In 2001, the DEA announced a national strategy to crack down on OxyContin use. Under pressure, Purdue Pharma, which made more than $4 billion on OxyContin sales between 2001 and 2003 (Tolman, 2005), discontinued the high-dose (160 mg) OxyContin pill in 2001 but continues to market 20-, 40-, and 80-mg tablets, and widespread diversion and abuse of the drug continues. In September, 2007, Purdue Pharma paid

$20 million in civil penalties to 26 states and the District of Columbia and $600 million in fines for misrepresenting the abuse liability of OxyContin.

The demographics of prescription opiate misuse are somewhat different than those we noted with heroin. One important feature is that nonmedical use of prescription opiates is far more widespread among young people. As an illustration, consider that although recent national high school senior surveys noted decreases in most illicit drug use over the past several years, use of OxyContin and other prescription opiates actually went up (see Figure 10.1; Johnston et al., 2009a). In fact, as Figure 10.1 shows, overall use of prescription opiates by high school seniors rose dramatically from 1991 to the present, and similar trends were noted in surveys of adults as well (Compton & Volkow, 2006). Although some of this trend is due to OxyContin use (which was not asked about specifically on the survey until 2002), use of other prescription opiates increased as well, notably hydrocodone (Vicodin) (Cicero, Inciardi, & Munoz, 2005). Other demographic trends are interesting as well. For example, heroin use is more widespread among males, whereas prescription opiate use is slightly more common among females (Green et al., 2009). In a large scale study, Wu, Pilowsky, & Patkar (2008) found that nearly 10% of U.S. adolescents between the ages of 12 and 17 reported nonprescribed use of prescription opiates. There were no differences between African Americans, Hispanics, Asians, and non-Hispanic white populations in frequency of use. The drugs used included in order of frequency: Darvocet/Darvon, Vicodin/Lortab, codeine, Percocet/Percodan, and OxyContin, with other opiates less frequently reported. Although illicit use of opiates was part of a pattern of use of alcohol and other drugs for some adolescents, fully 25% of the

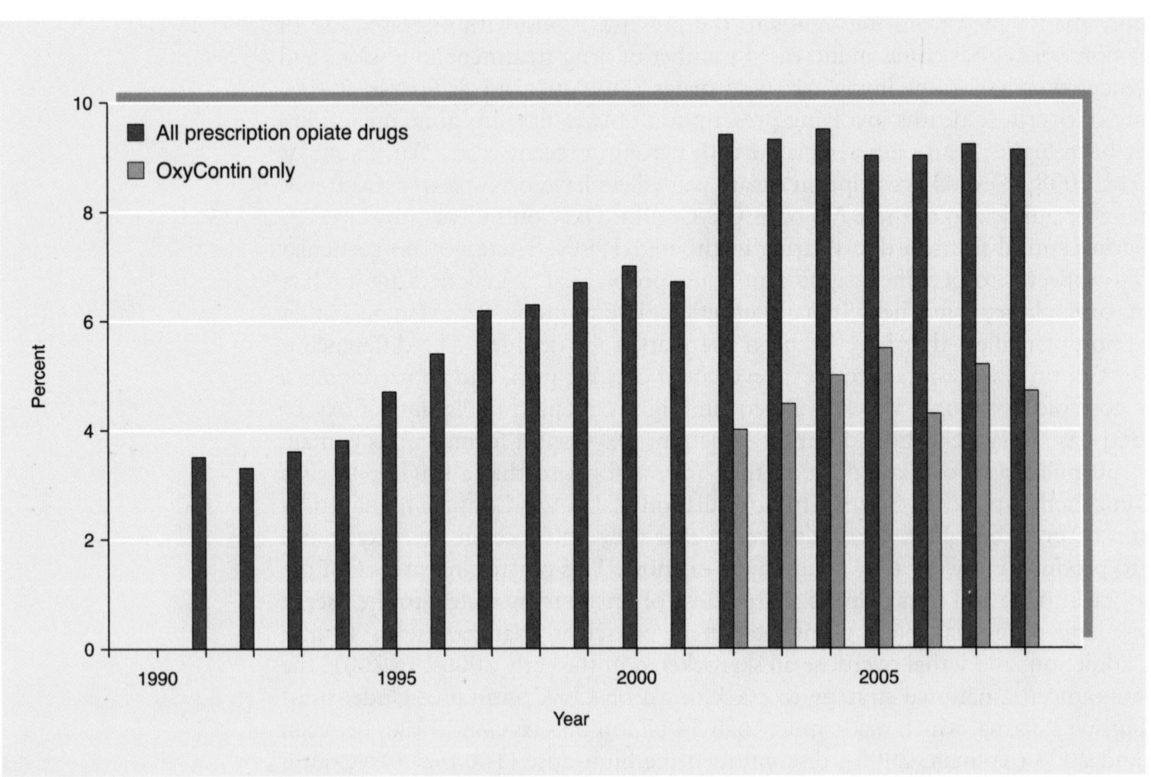

FIGURE 10.1
Percentage of high school seniors reporting illicit/nonmedical use in the past year (from Johnston et al., 2009a)

sample reported only using prescription opiate drugs. Thus, illicit use of prescription opiate drugs has emerged as a major new drug issue in the late 2000s. We will return to this topic later in this chapter in the section on Medical Use of Opiate Drugs.

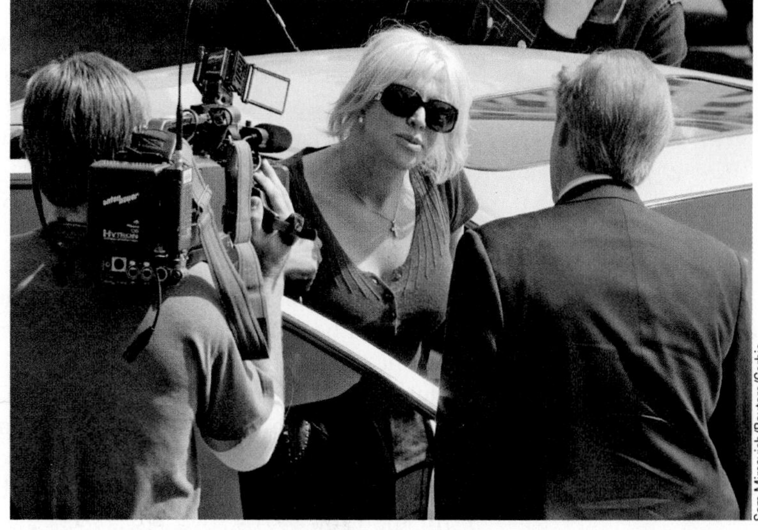

Sam Mircovich/Reuters/Corbis

Rock singer Courtney Love was sentenced to rehabilitation to recover from opiate addiction.

Pharmacokinetics

Absorption

As noted, opiate drugs may be taken into the body in a variety of ways. Most are readily absorbed from the gastrointestinal tract, although a given dose has a greater effect if it is injected intravenously. Most opioids also are absorbed through the nasal mucosa and lungs. Thus, opium and pure forms of heroin are often smoked, and heroin frequently is taken intranasally. Opiates are also absorbed after intramuscular or subcutaneous administration. On the street, for example, heroin may be injected intravenously ("mainlining") or subcutaneously.

Distribution, Metabolism, and Excretion

Once in the bloodstream, opioids are distributed throughout the body and accumulate in the kidneys, lungs, liver, spleen, digestive tract, and muscles, as well as the brain. With some opiates, such as morphine, only a small amount penetrates the blood-brain barrier. In fact, the main difference between morphine and the more potent drug heroin is that heroin is more lipid-soluble and thus more readily penetrates the blood-brain barrier. Once in the brain, heroin is converted to morphine. So heroin is essentially a more effective package for delivering morphine to the brain than is morphine itself.

Most opiate drugs are rapidly metabolized in the liver and excreted by the kidneys. Excretion of opiates is fairly rapid, with 90% excretion within a day after taking the drug. However, traces of morphine may remain in urine for two to four days after use (Hawks & Chiang, 1986).

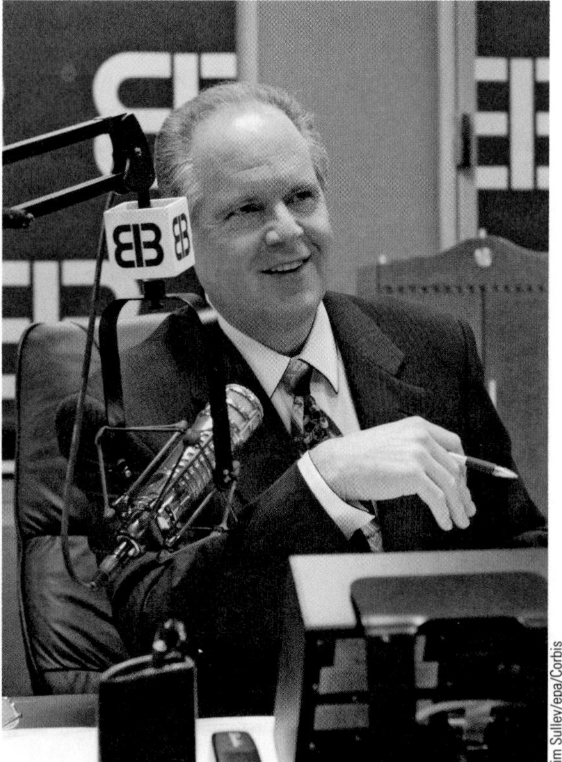

Jim Sulley/epa/Corbis

Conservative talk show host Rush Limbaugh completed rehab after developing an addiction to OxyContin.

Mechanisms of Opiate Action

Discovery of Endorphins

One of the most exciting developments in the neurosciences was the breakthrough in the understanding of the neural mechanisms of action of opiate drugs in the 1970s. Research on this topic led to the discovery of a class of brain chemicals called the endorphins, which function as neurotransmitters. It is now believed that heroin, morphine, and other opiate drugs produce their effects by triggering activity in the brain's endorphin systems (Meyer & Quenzer, 2005; Goldstein, 2001). We will review the events that led to these discoveries and consider how these developments have helped us understand the effects of opiate drugs.

In the 1960s, chemists discovered that making a slight change in the morphine molecule resulted in a chemical that did not produce any of the standard opiate drug effects (pain relief, euphoria) but instead reversed or blocked the effects of morphine and other opiate drugs. This compound is called **naloxone** and may be described as an opiate antagonist. When naloxone is given to a patient who is suffering from an overdose of heroin or morphine, it completely reverses the effects of those drugs. If naloxone is given to someone who then takes heroin, the heroin has no effect. Obviously naloxone has practical applications in the treatment of opiate overdose, but it also has theoretical implications. Because naloxone's chemical structure is similar to morphine, researchers thought that the two drugs might be acting at some common brain receptor site and that the naloxone is blocking the morphine's action at that site.

naloxone
A short-acting opiate antagonist.

In the early 1970s, two researchers at Johns Hopkins University in Baltimore—Candace Pert and Solomon Snyder—reported they had discovered brain receptors that responded selectively to opiate drugs; these were dubbed "opiate receptors" (Pert & Snyder, 1973). The existence of opiate receptors was of great interest. One might reasonably wonder why there would be neurons in the brain that responded to such drugs. Did nature somehow intend us to be heroin addicts? Neuroscientists had a different notion. They believed the presence of such receptors must mean that some natural brain chemicals have morphine-like structure and properties. The search was on for the "brain's own opiates," and, in 1975, several such chemicals were discovered (Snyder, 1989). Although several morphine-like substances (beta-endorphin, enkephalin, and dynorphin are the most important compounds) are found in the brain, these complex peptide molecules are referred to collectively as endorphins, a contraction of *endogenous morphine*.

What Do Endorphins Do?

The scientific questions that arose from the discovery of the endorphins have focused on just why the brain is endowed with its own morphine: What do endorphins do? Ongoing research started with the premise that, because opiate drugs apparently mimic endorphin activity by stimulating the opiate or endorphin receptor sites in the brain, endorphins might share many properties with opiate drugs, such as pain relief and production of pleasure. One idea is that endorphins are part of a natural pain-relief system. It has been argued that endorphins are released and produce analgesia or pain relief after certain kinds of pain or stress (Goldstein, 2001). This may help explain why, under certain circumstances such as on the battlefield or in athletic events, a person may sustain severe injury but not feel pain, at least for a time. Pain relief

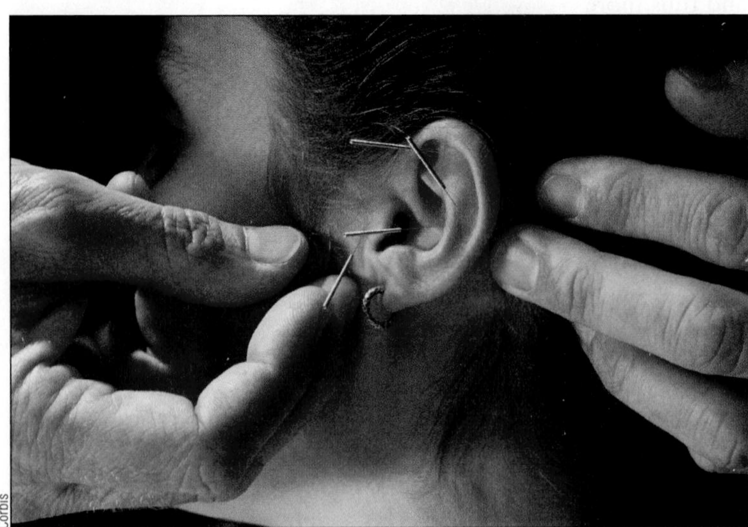

Corbis

Acupuncture may relieve pain by releasing endorphins.

produced by acupuncture may be related to endorphin release because naloxone can reverse acupuncture-induced analgesia (Han & Terenius, 1982). Because the major action of naloxone is to block the endorphin receptors, naloxone-reversible analgesia is strong evidence that the acupuncture needles are triggering the release of endorphins and relieving pain through this system. Other evidence shows that pain relief induced by placebo can activate endorphin receptors in several brain regions (Zubieta & Stohler, 2009). This suggests an endorphinergic basis for at least some cases in which simply "expecting" that you have taken a pain-relieving drug is sufficient to relieve pain. Furthermore, a PET study compared brain activity in individuals who experienced pain relief produced by placebo and by opiate drugs and found similar patterns in the brain regions that were activated (Petrovic et al., 2002). So there is good evidence that endorphin systems are involved in some of the brain's natural pain-control mechanisms. Over the years, many other claims have been made about the endorphins, but this literature has conflicting results, and other functions of the endorphins remain unclear.

Medical Use of Opiate Drugs

The major medical use of opiate drugs is for their analgesic or pain-relieving effects. As noted, opiates have been used for this purpose for centuries and remain the most potent and selective pain relievers known to medicine. Unlike the depressant-type anesthetic drugs discussed earlier, opiate analgesics relieve pain without causing unconsciousness. After receiving moderate doses of opiates, patients remain conscious and are able to report painful sensations but do not suffer from the pain.

The other major drugs that possess such analgesic properties are the over-the-counter painkillers: aspirin, acetaminophen, and ibuprofen, but none of these are as effective at relieving pain as the opiates (see Chapter 14). Table 10.1 lists some of the major opiate drugs used as analgesics along with their potency and their duration of action. Recall that *potency* refers to the dose required for a drug to produce a given effect. In Table 10.1, potency is given relative to an effective dose of morphine, which is given a value of 1. For example, heroin has a value of 2 in Table 10.1 because heroin is approximately twice as potent as morphine. This means that if 10 milligrams of morphine were required to relieve pain in a given patient, then only 5 milligrams of heroin would be required.

Morphine is the prototype opiate analgesic and is the standard by which others are measured. It is used primarily for severe pain. As we have noted, although heroin is more potent than morphine, it is not used medically in the United States because it is a Schedule I drug. Addiction is a risk in using opiate drugs for pain relief, but it should be noted that relatively few patients who use the drugs as directed develop problems. To reduce the risk, less potent opiates are used whenever possible, and treatment is as brief as possible. When pain is severe and chronic, however, as with terminal cancer patients, tolerance inevitably develops, and higher doses of more potent drugs must follow to relieve the patient's pain. Ultimately, high doses of morphine may be the only way to relieve the suffering, and eventually, even this may not be enough. In Great Britain, physicians then may use the potent opiate heroin but, because heroin is a Schedule I drug, doctors in the United States may not administer it.

". . . heroin was like a warmth that envelops you. It's an automatic warmth that encompasses your whole being as soon as it enters your body."

Female heroin addict (Goode, 1993)

Should physicians in the United States be permitted to administer heroin? One argument against heroin is that heroin is more addicting than morphine because of its

TABLE 10.1 Comparison of the Major Opiate Drugs

Generic Name	Brand Name	Potency	Duration of Action (hours)
Morphine		1	4–5
Heroin		2	3–4
Hydrocodone	Vicodin	1	5–7
Hydromorphone	Dilaudid	5	4–5
Codeine		0.1	4–6
Oxycodone	Percodan, OxyContin	1.5	4–5
Methadone	Dolophine	1	12–24
Meperidine	Demerol	0.1	2–4
Propoxyphene	Darvon	0.05	6
Fentanyl	Sublimaze	100	1–3
Pentazocine	Talwin	0.2	2–3

Note: Potency estimates are presented relative to an effective dose of morphine (1).
Source: Based in part on Jaffe and Martin (1990) and Zacny (1995).

potency. Yet, in the treatment of severe pain of terminally ill patients, addiction seems irrelevant. Besides, patients are normally receiving high and frequent doses of morphine, so they certainly are addicted to morphine by the time heroin treatment is begun. Heroin is converted to morphine in the brain, and thus morphine is the active chemical in producing pain relief in both cases (heroin is more potent because it penetrates the blood-brain barrier more efficiently). One could accomplish the same degree of pain relief by giving larger and larger doses of morphine, but terminal cancer patients often become very thin and may lose tone in their veins with repeated injections. Thus, it may become difficult to administer enough morphine solution to be effective. Here is where the more potent heroin can be of value, because less solution is required. Moving heroin to a Schedule II drug would allow physicians to elect to administer heroin but should not make it any more difficult to control heroin addiction. The move remains controversial, though, perhaps because it is seen as a softening of the heroin laws. A potential solution may come with the development of more potent opiate drugs that have not acquired the stigma associated with heroin. For example, fentanyl, a synthetic opiate drug, is at least 50 times more potent than heroin and is used primarily to produce anesthesia. However, the potent and long-acting drug OxyContin was designed and marketed for patients with severe chronic pain, and as we noted above, it has already been associated with a wave of abuse and addiction.

Unless pain is very severe, prescription opiate preparations are used that are less potent or given in lower doses than morphine. Thus codeine, hydrocodone (Vicodin), propoxyphene (Darvon), lower doses of oxycodone (OxyContin, Percodan), and pentazocine (Talwin) often are prescribed for pain (see Table 10.1). In general, opiate drugs are the most potent and effective drugs available to medicine in the treatment of pain. The limitations of their use as analgesics are primarily their abuse liability: their tendency to produce tolerance and dependence. Tolerance and dependence develop for all these drugs, although some, such as pentazocine (Talwin), for example, are thought to be less liable for abuse than others. It is hoped that safer analgesic

CONTEMPORARY ISSUE BOX 10.3

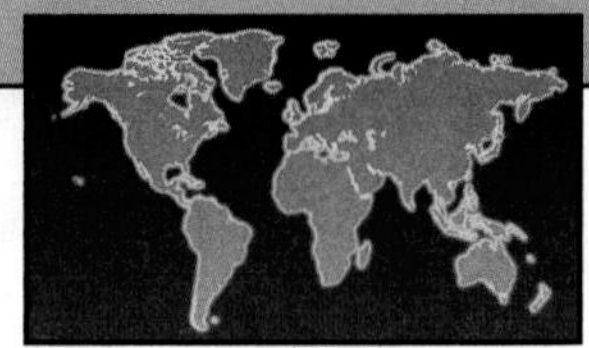

Ultralow-Dose Naltrexone and NMDA Antagonists: New Approaches to Make Prescription Opiates Safer

Opiate drugs remain the most valuable medications available for the relief of severe pain, but we have noted the many problems associated with their use and misuse. New strategies are being developed to help reduce some of these problems that involve the combination of the prescription opiate painkiller with some other drug. One such strategy involves the combination of an ultralow dose of the opiate antagonist naltrexone with the opiate agonist. Apparently, if the naltrexone dose is sufficiently low, it can actually enhance the pain-relieving effects of the opiate agonist but may still block the rewarding effects of the drug, retard the development of tolerance, and lessen withdrawal severity. These results have mainly been reported from nonhuman experiments (e.g., Largent-Milnes et al., 2008), but early trials in human patients with pain using a combination of oxycodone (OxyContin) and ultralow-dose naltrexone (Oxytrex) have been promising (Webster, 2007). Similarly, combinations of drugs that block n-methyl d-aspartate (NMDA) receptors and opiate agonists have been reported to enhance pain relief and block tolerance development and may have therapeutic potential (Craft & Lee, 2005; Fischer et al., 2008). Hopefully, the development of new compounds such as these will increase the safety of pain medication and lessen the problem of diversion and abuse of prescription opiate drugs.

drugs will be developed as we learn more about endorphins and their ability to produce natural analgesia.

Opiate drugs have other medical uses. Opiates have a constipating effect that can be a problem for addicts but is of value in treating diarrhea. Opiates still are used to treat coughs. The drug most commonly used for this purpose is dextromethorphan, which is a synthetic opiate that has no analgesic or addictive properties but is an effective cough suppressant (Jaffe & Martin, 1990). A final medical use for opiates such as methadone is in the treatment of heroin addicts in withdrawal and in maintenance programs designed to help addicts stay off heroin (see Chapter 15).

Given the long-standing and widespread medical use of opiate drugs for the treatment of pain, the recent epidemic of prescription opiate use noted previously took substance abuse professionals by surprise. Conventional wisdom was that these drugs were relatively low in abuse liability when used as directed for pain, and the basis for the sudden increase in illicit use is not completely understood. Nora Volkow, director of the National Institute on Drug Abuse, noted three potential reasons for the increases (Compton & Volkow, 2006). First, the number of prescriptions written for opiate painkillers increased, and the increase in illicit use may be a by-product of the increased availability that resulted. A second reason may involve the ready availability of prescription opiates via the Internet. The emergence of Internet access to prescription drugs has made them available without physician supervision. Third, changes in prescribing practices with more prescriptions by primary care physicians who are not necessarily expert in pain management may be related to increased diversion and abuse (Compton & Volkow, 2006). Although diversion of prescription opiate drugs has clearly become a significant national problem, leading to legislative proposals to ban some of these drugs (Tolman, 2005), it is important to remember that they are of critical importance in the medical treatment of pain and are thus of significant societal value. As Cicero, Inciardi, & Munoz (2005) put it: "Steps need to be taken to reduce prescription drug abuse, but very great care needs to be exercised in the nature of these actions so that legitimate and appropriate use of these drugs in the treatment of pain is not compromised as a result" (p. 662).

Acute Psychological and Physiological Effects of Opiates

Opiate drugs have acute effects in addition to analgesia. Subjective reports of the euphoria produced by opiates mention drowsiness, body warmth, and a heavy feeling of the limbs (Jaffe & Martin, 1990). William S. Burroughs (1953) describes the feeling in his autobiographical novel *Junky:* "Morphine hits the backs of the legs first, then the back of the neck, a spreading wave of relaxation slackening the muscles away from the bones so that you seem to float without outlines, like lying in warm salt water" (p. 7). Both the naturally occurring and synthetic opiates are capable of producing these pleasurable effects in most individuals; however, in laboratory studies, opiate abusers appear to generally report more positive effects and liking than nonabusers (see Comer & Zacny, 2005, for a review), but the basis for this is unclear. The pleasure experienced under the influence of opiates seems to interfere with the user's other interests. Burroughs described it as follows: "Junk shortcircuits sex. The drive to nonsexual sociability comes from the same place sex comes from, so when I have an H(eroin) or M(orphine) shooting habit I am non-sociable. If someone wants to talk, OK. But there is no drive to get acquainted" (p. 124). In fact, there is good evidence that opiate drugs reduce sexual drive or interest and often produce impotence in men (Quaglio et al., 2008). Consistent with Burroughs's anecdotal reports, laboratory studies show that opiates impair social interactions (Meyer & Mirin, 1979). People who smoke opium or take other opiate drugs often report vivid dreamlike experiences. These are the basis for the expression "pipe dreams." Opiates may also interfere with cognitive function. Animal studies indicate impairments in learning and memory (e.g., Galizio et al., 2003), and research with clients on methadone maintenance suggests that some methadone doses may produce cognitive impairment as well (Mintzer, Copersino, & Stitzer, 2005).

The acute physiological effects of opiate drugs resemble those of depressant drugs, with some differences. Like depressants, opiates cause respiratory depression and lowered body temperature (Grilly, 2002; see Table 10.2 in this chapter). Nausea and vomiting often occur immediately after taking opiates. Perhaps the most visible sign of opiate drug use is constriction of the pupils. This effect is so pronounced in overdose that "pinpoint pupils" are a diagnostic sign of opiate poisoning. When a high dose of heroin is fatal, the immediate cause is usually respiratory failure. The lethal dose of heroin is surprisingly high, however. As Brecher (1972) noted, many overdose victims on the street are found on autopsy to have injected less than would be expected to be lethal. These cases involve not simply an overdose of heroin but also a lethal drug interaction between heroin and alcohol or another depressant drug. Opiates and depressant drugs potentiate one another (Ho & Allen, 1981). This synergy can often be lethal, and many of the most publicized "heroin" overdoses actually involve synergy, such as the death of Janis Joplin in 1970, as reported in *Time:*

"I have seen life measured out in eyedroppers of morphine solution. I experienced the agonizing deprivation of junk sickness, and the pleasure of relief when junkthirsty cells drank from the needle."
William Burroughs (1953)

> The quart bottle of Southern Comfort (whiskey) that she held aloft onstage was at once a symbol of her load, and her way of lightening it. As she emptied the bottle, she grew happier, more radiant and more freaked out. . . . Last week on a day that superficially at least seemed to be less lonely than most, Janis Joplin died on the lowest and saddest of notes. Returning to her Hollywood motel room after a late-night recording session and some hard drinking with friends at a nearby bar, she apparently filled a hypodermic needle with heroin and shot it into her left arm. The injection killed her. (Brecher, 1972, p. 113)

TABLE 10.2 Effects of Administration and Withdrawal of Opiate Drugs

Administration	Withdrawal
Decreased body temperature	Increased body temperature
Decreased blood pressure	Increased blood pressure
Pupil constriction	Pupil dilation
Drying of secretions	Tearing, runny nose
Constipation	Diarrhea
Decreased sex drive, impotence	Spontaneous ejaculation/orgasm
Respiratory depression	Yawning
Analgesia	Pain
Euphoria	Depression/anxiety

We now recognize that the alcohol was as responsible for her death as the heroin. Synergy between depressant drugs and prescription opiates is also a dangerous possibility when these drugs are combined. The recent death of actor Heath Ledger (from a combination of prescription opiate OxyContin and benzodiazepine depressants) illustrates such synergy.

Chronic Effects of Opiates

Tolerance

The effects of opiate drugs are somewhat different when they are taken chronically. As we noted, tolerance develops to opiates, so their effects are generally diminished unless the user escalates the dose, which often occurs. Figure 10.2 shows the pattern of opiate intake in both a human and a rhesus monkey of continuous drug availability studied under laboratory conditions. Each graph shows the drug intake plotted over consecutive days in the experiment. The human data come from an experiment in which a volunteer with a history of extensive drug abuse was studied under laboratory conditions in which he could regulate his daily intravenous morphine dose. Note the gradual increase in dose he chooses over time. For the first month, the participant never administered more than 500 milligrams per day. By the fourth month, however, he frequently took more than 1,000 milligrams. Also note the bottom panel of Figure 10.2, which reveals a similar pattern of heroin self-administration by monkeys that could obtain intravenous heroin by pressing a lever. Clearly, the emergence of tolerance to the rewarding consequences of opiate drugs is a phenomenon of great generality.

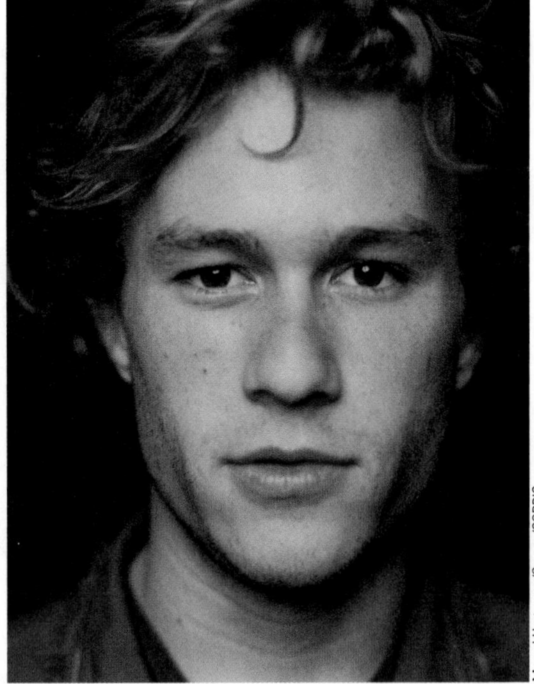

Marcel Hartmann/Sygma/CORBIS

Heath Ledger died from the synergy produced by a combination of prescription opiates and depressant drugs.

Withdrawal and Dependence

The motives for the continued use of opiates over time may change. Although repeated use is initially motivated by a desire to re-experience the pleasant rush associated with taking the drug, addicts report that continued use of a drug does not make them nearly as high as before. They continue to use the drug to avoid the unpleasant symptoms of abstinence. Thus, the processes that maintain heroin use change from positive to negative reinforcement. The withdrawal symptoms associated with opiate dependence may appear after only one to two weeks of chronic use of heroin, morphine, or a synthetic opiate drug. The symptoms become more severe with longer-term use of higher doses. Early indications of withdrawal begin 8 to 12 hours after the last dose and include flu-like symptoms such as runny nose, tearing, sweating, irritability, and tremor. As time passes, these symptoms become more severe and others appear, including pupil dilation, anorexia, and piloerection (goose bumps). This last symptom leaves an addict looking a bit like a plucked turkey and may be the basis for the expression "cold turkey." These symptoms continue to worsen and reach a peak after 48 to 72 hours. At this time, heart rate and blood pressure are elevated, and the addict experiences severe flu-like symptoms such as nausea, diarrhea, sneezing, excessive sweating, and pain in the bones. In addition, an addict may show spastic movements of the arms and legs that may appear similar to kicking. This is thought to be the basis for the expression "kicking the habit." Other somewhat bizarre symptoms, which apparently indicate a rebound of the addict's sexual system, include spontaneous erection and ejaculation in men and orgasm in women. The loss of fluids and failure of addicts to eat or drink much during withdrawal can leave addicts physically and emotionally drained and occasionally can be fatal (Jaffe & Martin, 1990).

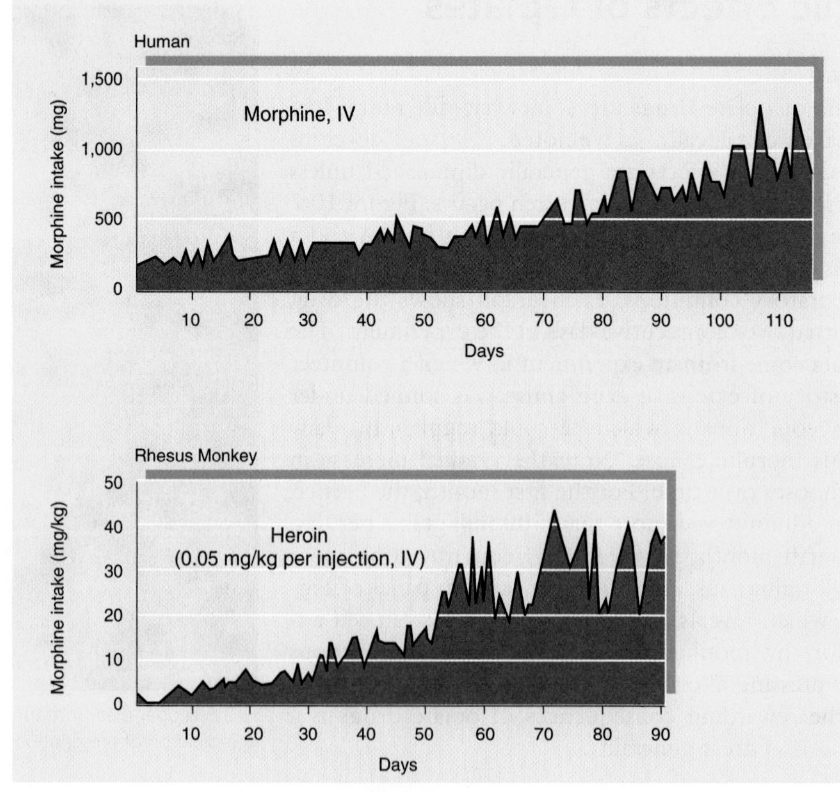

FIGURE 10.2
Patterns of opioid intake in a human and a rhesus monkey under conditions of continuous drug availability

Source: From *Behavioral Analysis of Drug Dependence* by Henningfield, Lukas, and Bigelow," eds. Goldberg and Stoleman. Copyright 1986. Used with permission from Elsevier.

It is worth noting that a suitable dose of any opiate drug (but not depressant drugs) will reverse the abstinence symptoms and restore a feeling of well-being to addicts. Hospital detoxification procedures take advantage of this fact by treating addicts in withdrawal with low doses of a synthetic opiate drug such as methadone. The dose of methadone given is sufficient to reduce the severity of the addicts' withdrawal symptoms but not enough to produce much of a high. Gradually over a period of several weeks, the dose of methadone is tapered off until finally addicts show no further signs of physical dependence. If physical withdrawal symptoms were the only factors maintaining heroin addiction, detoxification would be a cure. However, after detoxification procedures, an estimated 90% relapse within two years after leaving the hospital, and most of these relapses occur during the first six months after detoxification (see Chapter 15). Thus, returning addicts to the environment in which they became addicted is most likely to result in relapse, even in the absence of physical withdrawal symptoms.

That heroin (and other drug) addiction depends on more than just physical withdrawal symptoms is illustrated nicely by the heroin addiction epidemic that failed to occur. During the early 1970s, as the Vietnam War was drawing to a close, heroin addiction rates were high among returning American soldiers, with some estimates reaching 21%. These soldiers were required to go through a detoxification before their return to the United States, but given a 90% relapse rate, one would have expected most would return to heroin use at home. Thus, an epidemic of heroin addiction in the United States was expected. Follow-up studies showed that very few soldiers did relapse (less than 15%), however, which illustrates clearly that environmental and psychosocial factors associated with Vietnam were apparently responsible for the development of the dependence. Upon returning to the United States, Vietnam veterans found heroin far less available. That, added to the changes in lifestyle and social environment in the United States, apparently eased the pressures that led to their initial dependence (Robins, Helzer, & Davis, 1975). The radical change in environment from Vietnam to the United States cannot be duplicated in the typical treatment setting. This is one reason that treating heroin addiction is so difficult, although a number of different types of treatment have been developed. We review them in Chapter 15.

Summary

- Opium is produced from the sap of the poppy plant, and it has been used for medicinal purposes for centuries.
- In the 19th century, the major active agent in opium, morphine, was isolated. More potent than opium, morphine was prized for its analgesic effects but also became a major addiction problem.
- Heroin was developed as an alternative to morphine but soon became the addict's drug of choice. Although opiate drugs remained important in medicine, after the passage of the 1914 Harrison Narcotics Act, heroin became a major criminal drug.
- Opiate drugs act in the brain by mimicking endorphins, natural neurotransmitters that are involved in the regulation of pain.
- The major medical use for opiate drugs is in the treatment of severe pain.
- Opiates depress respiration, lower body temperature, and cause capillary constriction. They induce a pleasurable euphoria as well as relieve pain.
- Regular use of opiates results in tolerance and an abstinence syndrome characterized by flu-like symptoms and intense drug craving. Heroin addiction is more complex than simple avoidance of withdrawal symptoms.

Answers to "What Do You Think?"

1. Opium comes from the plant *Cannabis sativa.*
   F *Opium comes from the poppy plant Papaver somniferum.*
2. Morphine is one of the active ingredients in opium.
   T *Morphine and codeine are chemicals directly derived from opium.*
3. Heroin was first made illegal by the 1965 Drug Abuse Control Amendment.
   F *All opiates were brought under legal control by the 1914 Harrison Narcotics Act.*
4. Use of "dirty" needles is now one of the major causes of AIDS.
   T *In more than 20% of cases, the use of contaminated needles is suspected as the source of infection.*
5. Most designer heroin compounds are less potent than pure heroin.
   F *Designer heroin compounds may be 10 to 1,000 times more potent than pure heroin. Thus, the risk of overdose is greater.*
6. The opiates are among the most powerful analgesic drugs.
   T *The principal medical use for opiates is to relieve pain.*
7. Heroin enhances sexual desire and activity.
   F *Heroin inhibits sexual arousal.*
8. Opiate drugs show cross-dependence with alcohol.
   F *Alcohol does not eliminate the symptoms of opiate withdrawal.*
9. Heroin withdrawal is much like alcohol withdrawal.
   F *Opiate withdrawal does not include delirium tremens but rather is characterized by flu and cold symptoms.*
10. Veterans of the Vietnam War had a high rate of heroin addiction and were unable to kick the habit when they returned to the United States.
    F *Most veterans were able to quit using heroin when they returned to their home environment.*
11. The effects of opiates are synergistic with those of alcohol.
    T *Alcohol and other depressant drugs act synergistically with heroin and other opiates, and these combinations are often fatal.*
12. The expression "cold turkey" comes from the "goose bumps" seen in addicts withdrawing from heroin.
    T *The resemblance is thought to be the basis for that expression.*

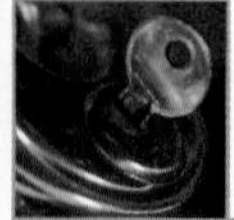

Key Terms

analgesia
heroin
naloxone
opium

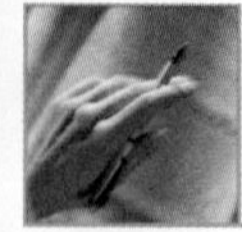

Essays/Thought Questions

1. Heroin is often considered to be the prototype addictive drug. Why do you think this is so?
2. Medical management of pain with opiates has often been controversial because of the risks of diversion and abuse. Considering the recent problems with OxyContin in this regard, what do you think about public policy, pain management, and opiate drugs?

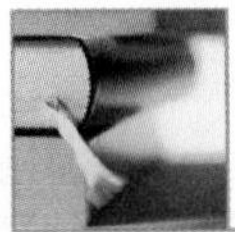

Suggested Readings

Ashton, R. (2002). *This is heroin.* London: Sanctuary Publishing LTD.

Inciardi, J. A. (2002). *The war on drugs III: The continuing saga of the mysteries and miseries of intoxication, addiction, crime, and public policy.* Boston: Allyn & Bacon.

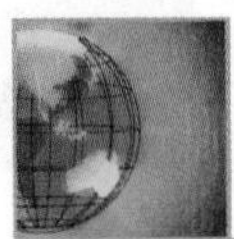

Web Resources

Visit the Book Companion Website at www.cengage.com/psychology/maisto to access study tools including a glossary, flashcards, and web quizzing. You will also find links to the following resources:

- Heroin Addiction Drug Rehab
- Heroin Times
- HIV prevention in IV drug users
- NIDA on heroin
- National Geographic special on hero in users

CHAPTER 11

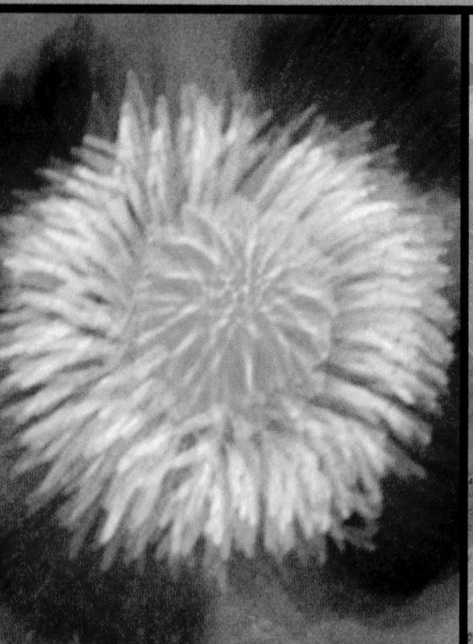
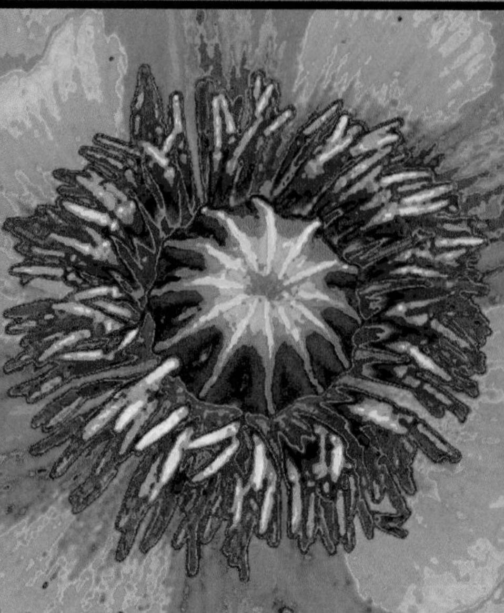
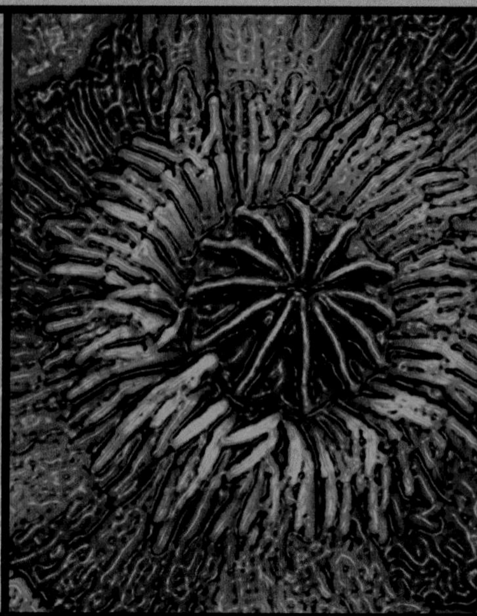

Marijuana

What Do You Think? True or False?

Answers are given at the end of the chapter.

___ 1. The cannabis plant was raised for its psychoactive properties by the settlers at Jamestown and later by George Washington.

___ 2. The Eighteenth Amendment prohibiting the use of alcohol had the paradoxical effect of increasing the prevalence of marijuana use in the United States.

___ 3. Criminal penalties in the United States for the possession and use of marijuana have increased steadily since the 1960s.

___ 4. Data recently gathered both in national household surveys and in annual surveys of high school seniors demonstrate a lower prevalence of marijuana use relative to the 1970s.

___ 5. The marijuana smoked in the United States today is more potent than that smoked 20 years ago.

___ 6. Drug effects following oral ingestion of marijuana last longer than after the drug is smoked.

___ 7. Tolerance to cannabis has been well-documented in animal studies.

___ 8. Marijuana has been used effectively to treat the nausea and vomiting often associated with chemotherapy in the treatment of cancer.

___ 9. Marijuana cigarettes contain more tar than tobacco cigarettes.

___ 10. Marijuana use often causes long-term damage to the cardiovascular system.

___ 11. One consequence of cannabis intoxication is the impairment of short-term memory.

___ 12. The most commonly reported emotional effects of cannabis use are suspiciousness and paranoid ideation.

___ 13. An area of concern regarding marijuana use is that it often causes users to be aggressive and violent.

Cannabis sativa, more commonly known as marijuana, is a hemp plant that grows freely throughout the world. The cannabis plant is known most commonly today as a potent psychoactive substance, but for many years, it was harvested primarily for its fiber. These strong hemp fibers were employed in the production of rope, clothes, and ship sails. Although cannabis was used for several centuries in other parts of the world for its mind-altering properties, its psychoactive properties were not recognized in the United States until the first third of this century. Then the hemp plant was more often harvested for its psychoactive effects.

The term *marijuana* is thought to be based on the Portuguese word *mariguango,* which translates as "intoxicant." Marijuana, incidentally, is not the same as hashish, although both are derived from the *Cannabis sativa* plant. Marijuana is the leafy top portion of the plant, whereas hashish is made from the dust of the resin that the hemp plant produces for protection from the sun and heat and for maintaining hydration. Plants that grow in warmer climates produce greater amounts of the resin, which generally has stronger psychoactive effects.

We begin this chapter with a historical overview of marijuana and its use through the centuries. This is followed by a section on the epidemiology of current marijuana use. Next, we provide information on absorption, distribution, metabolism, and excretion; mechanisms of action; and tolerance and dependence. Following this is an overview of the medical and psychotherapeutic uses of marijuana. The chapter's final sections concern the physical, psychological, and social/environmental effects of marijuana.

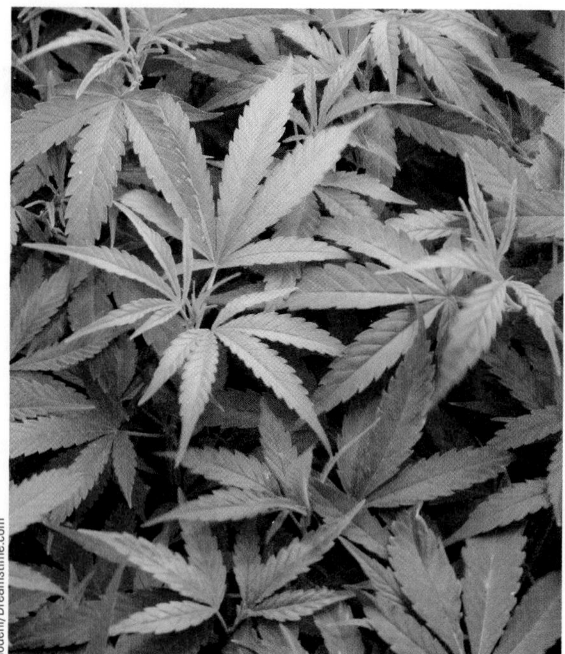
Rodehi/Dreamstime.com

The marijuana plant

Historical Overview

According to Ernest Abel in his book *Marihuana: The First Twelve Thousand Years* (1980), the earliest known evidence of the use of cannabis occurred more than 10,000 years ago during the Stone Age. Archeologists at a Taiwanese site discovered pots made of fibers presumed to be from the cannabis plant. The earliest known references to the use of cannabis for its pharmacological properties are attributed to Shen Nung in about 2800 B.C. Shen Nung was a mythical Chinese emperor and pharmacist who purportedly shared knowledge of the medicinal uses of cannabis with his subjects. It has been speculated that cannabis was used in this period in China for sedating, treating pain and illness, countering the influences of evil spirits, and gaining its general psychoactive effects (Abel, 1980; Nahas, 1973).

Cannabis use gradually spread from China to surrounding Asian countries. Of particular note was its adoption in India, where cannabis served a religious function. The *Atharva Veda*, one of the oldest books of Hinduism, includes it as one of the five sacred plants (Aldrich, 1977). This gave cannabis the protection and reverence engendered by cultural or religious acceptance. Not until much later did cannabis use spread to the Middle East and then on to North Africa. During this expansion, hashish was first identified. The use of hashish dates to around the 10th century among the Arabs and to the 11th century in Egypt (Abel, 1980).

"[The Scythians] have discovered other trees that produce fruit of a peculiar kind, which the inhabitants, when they meet together in companies, and have lit a fire, throw on the fire, as they sit round in a circle; and that by inhaling the fumes of the burning fruit that has been thrown on, they become intoxicated by the odor, just as the Greeks do by wine; and that the more fruit that is thrown on the more intoxicated they become, until they rise up to dance and betake themselves to singing."

Herodotus, commenting on marijuana use by the Scythians, a nomadic central Asian barbarian group (McKenna, 1992)

Cannabis appears to have been used for its intoxicating effects in these parts of the world for an extended time. Not until the 19th century did the Western world begin to be exposed to cannabis, primarily through descriptions of the hashish experience in medical writings and the popular press. The use of cannabis was introduced to Great Britain primarily by William O'Shaughnessy, an Irish physician. In India, he observed the medical applications of cannabis and described them in his writings. Suggestions regarding the use of cannabis were made in France by Dr. Jacques Moreau, a physician who thought it could be used in the treatment of mental illness (Bloomquist, 1971). Subsequently, the use and effects of cannabis were described in detail in the works of other French authors. Perhaps most notable was Théophile Gautier, a famous and influential poet and essayist, who was introduced to cannabis by Moreau. Gautier graphically described his initiation into *Le Club des Hachichins* (The Hashish Club), which met in Paris in the exclusive Hotel Pimodan in the 1840s. The hashish consumed was contained in a sweetmeat called Dawamesc. Gautier's descriptions of the drug effects were graphic (some excerpts from his writings are presented in the Drugs and Culture Box 11.1). His descriptions of the hashish experiences included elements of mystery, intrigue, joy, ecstasy, fear, and terror.

Despite what appeared to some as attractive features of cannabis and hashish, the use of this drug did not immediately catch on in Europe. In fact, using cannabis for its psychoactive properties did not become widespread in Europe until the 1960s, when it was reintroduced by, among others, tourists from the United States (Bloomquist, 1971).

DRUGS AND CULTURE BOX 11.1

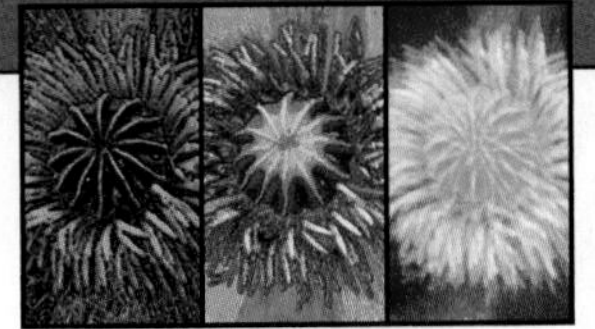

Gautier's Experiences at the Hashish Club

As noted in the text, the Frenchman Théophile Gautier wrote in graphic detail of his experiences using hashish in the 1840s. These drug-use descriptions are of interest to us today for several reasons. They provide an opportunity for us to observe the similarities in the marijuana experience then and now, at least as described by those who write of their experiences. In addition, these descriptions allow us to observe the use of drugs in different cultures. In the present case, the user is a French hashish user, the setting is a club in Paris, and the time is the mid-19th century.

The hashish Gautier and his friends used was contained in a sweetmeat (a food rich in sugar, such as candied or crystallized fruit) called Dawamesc, which they ate at the Paris hotel that housed *Le Club des Hachichins* (The Hashish Club). The drug-laced sweetmeat was eaten before dinner. After dinner, sitting in a large drawing room, Gautier (1844) described the scene:

> Solitude reigned in the drawing room, which was studded with only a few dubious gleams; all of a sudden, a red flash passed beneath my eyelids, innumerable candles burst into light and I felt bathed in a warm, clear glow. I was indeed in the same place, but it was as different as a sketch is from a painting: everything was larger, richer, more gorgeous. Reality served as a point of departure for the splendors of the hallucination. (Solomon, 1966, p. 126)

This period was followed by a state Gautier labeled "fantasia," after which *al-kief* was experienced:

> I was in that blessed state induced by hashish which the Orientals call al-kief. I could no longer feel my body; the bonds of matter and spirit were severed; I moved by sheer willpower in an unresisting medium.
>
> Thus I imagine the movement of souls in the world of fragrances to which we shall go after death. A bluish haze, an Elysian light, the reflections of an azure grotto, formed an atmosphere in the room through which I vaguely saw the tremblings of hesitant outlines; an atmosphere at once cool and warm, moist and perfumed, enveloping me like bath water in a sort of enervating sweetness. When I tried to move away, the caressing air made a thousand voluptuous waves about me; a delightful languor gripped my senses and threw me back upon the sofa, where I hung, limp as a discarded garment.
>
> Then I understood the pleasure experienced by the spirits and angels, according to their degree of perfection, when they traverse the ethers and the skies, and how eternity might occupy one in Paradise. (Solomon, 1966, pp. 130–131)

Al-kief was replaced by a nightmarish stage in which Gautier felt fear, fury, and aspects of paranoia. Then, finally, around five hours after entering The Hashish Club, the drug effects ended:

> The dream was at an end.
>
> The hashisheen went off, each in his own direction, like the officers in *Marlborough Goes to War*.
>
> With light steps, I went down the stairs that had caused me so much anguish, and a few moments later I was in my room, in full reality; the last vapors raised by the hashish had vanished. (Solomon, 1966, p. 135)

Cannabis in the New World

The presence of cannabis in the New World dates to 1545, when the Spaniards brought it to Chile. In the North American colonies, the Jamestown settlers in Virginia raised the cannabis plant for fiber in 1611. Not long after, this hemp product was firmly entrenched as a basic staple crop and was cultivated by George Washington, among many others. Cannabis was harvested in New England starting in 1629; it remained a core U.S. crop until after the Civil War. The center of hemp production was Kentucky, where it was a major crop product for decades.

Despite its widespread presence, the marijuana plant was relatively unknown as a mind-altering substance. There was some recognition of its uses beyond the fiber component, however. Following the lead of European doctors, American physicians used cannabis in the 1800s, as a general, all-purpose medication (Nahas, 1973). The most commonly used preparation was Tilden's Extract of Cannabis Indica, an Indian hemp

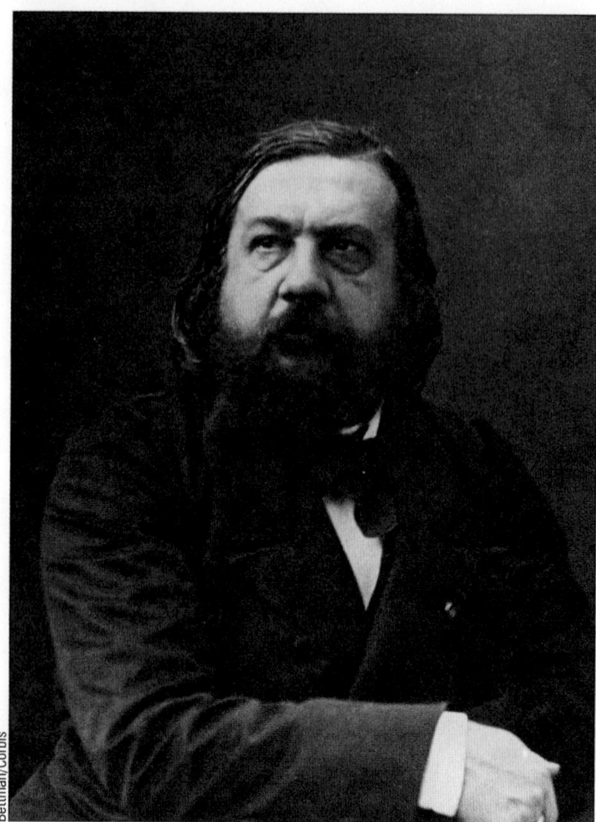
Bettman/Corbis

French writer Théophile Gautier described in detail his consumption of hashish at the *Le Club des Hachichins.*

plant produced in East Bengal. By the 1850s, marijuana was listed in the *United States Pharmacopeia,* a listing of legitimate therapeutics; it remained there until 1942. The cannabis extract also was listed in the less select *National Formulary.*

Cannabis was consumed for recreational purposes only to a limited extent during this period, and descriptions of its psychoactive effects were not common. One notable exception was the publication in 1857 of the book *The Hasheesh Eater.* Written by Fitz Hugh Ludlow, this volume details his cannabis-eating experiences over a four-year period beginning at around age 16. Ludlow lived in the town of Poughkeepsie, north of New York City in the Hudson River Valley. He spent much of his time with a friend named Anderson, an **apothecary**, and often experimented with the varied substances in Anderson's drugstore. One day, Anderson pointed out to Ludlow a new arrival: a marijuana extract from Tilden and Co. Ludlow began experimenting with the substance. At first, he experienced no immediate drug effects, but he described the onset of effects after several hours as follows:

> Ha! what means this sudden thrill? A shock, as of some unimagined vital force, shoots without warning through my entire frame, leaping to my fingers' ends, piercing my brain, startling me till I almost spring from my chair.
>
> I could not doubt it. I was in the power of the hasheesh influence. (Ludlow, 1857/1979, p. 20)

apothecary A pharmacist.

Ludlow continued his experimenting, graphically describing the varied cannabis effects. For example, in a chapter titled "The Kingdom of the Dream," he noted:

> The moment that I closed my eyes a vision of celestial glory burst upon me. I stood on the silver strand of a translucent, boundless lake, across whose bosom I seemed to have been just transported. A short way up the beach, a temple, modeled like the Parthenon, lifted its spotless and gleaming columns of alabaster sublimely into a rosy air—like the Parthenon, yet as much excelling it as the godlike ideal of architecture must transcend that ideal realized by man. (p. 34)

Ludlow also identified two "laws of the hasheesh operation." The first was that "after the completion of any one fantasia has arrived, there almost invariably succeeds a shifting of the action to some other stage entirely different in its surroundings" (pp. 36–37). The second law was that "after the full storm of a vision of intense sublimity has blown past the hasheesh-eater, his next vision is generally of a quiet, relaxing, and recreating nature" (p. 37).

The 1920s brought a wider use of cannabis. Edward M. Brecher, in The Consumers Union Report on *Licit and Illicit Drugs* (1972), attributes this increase to alcohol prohibition. He writes, "Not until the Eighteenth Amendment and the Volstead Act of 1920 raised the price of alcoholic beverages and made them less convenient to secure and inferior in quality did substantial commercial trade in marijuana for recreational use spring up" (p. 410). In New York City, for example, a number of marijuana

tea-pads (estimated at more than 500 in Harlem alone) opened in the early 1920s, generally in a room or apartment. As described by Mayor LaGuardia's Committee on Marihuana (1944),

> The "tea-pad" is furnished according to the clientele it expects to serve. Usually, each "tea-pad" has comfortable furniture, a radio, Victrola or, as in most instances, a rented nickel-odeon. The lighting is more or less uniformly dim, with blue predominating. An incense burner is considered part of the furnishings. The walls are frequently decorated with pictures of nude subjects suggestive of perverted sexual practices. The furnishings, as described, are believed to be essential as a setting for those participating in smoking marihuana. (p. 10)

tea-pads
Historically, places where people gathered to smoke marijuana. The sites could be anything from a rented room to a hotel suite.

The committee went on to note:

> The marihuana smoker derives greater satisfaction if he is smoking in the presence of others. His attitude in the "tea-pad" is that of a relaxed individual, free from the anxieties and cares of the realities of life. The "tea-pad" takes on the atmosphere of a very congenial social club. The smoker readily engages in conversation with strangers, discussing freely his pleasant reactions to the drug and philosophizing on subjects pertaining to life in a manner which, at times, appears to be out of keeping with his intellectual level. . . . A boisterous, rowdy atmosphere did not prevail and on the rare occasions when there appeared signs indicative of a belligerent attitude on the part of a smoker, he was ejected or forced to become more tolerant and quiescent. (p. 10)

The origins of the practice of smoking marijuana in this country in the early part of this century are not clear, but most agree that one of the earliest introductions was through Mexican laborers crossing the border into the United States. The greatest extent of use was in New Orleans, also in the early 1920s. In fact, New Orleans was a central dispensing arena for marijuana as late as the 1930s. The marijuana could be sent up the Mississippi River to river ports and then distributed throughout the country. According to Nahas (1973), marijuana was available in the larger cities by 1930, although its use was limited to primarily black Americans, not infrequently jazz musicians.

"Prolonged use of marihuana frequently develops a delirious rage which sometimes leads to high crimes, such as assault and murder. Hence marihuana has been called the 'killer drug.' The habitual use of this narcotic poison always causes a very marked mental deterioration and sometimes produces insanity."

Excerpt from a 1936 pamphlet entitled "Marijuana or Indian Hemp and its Preparations," distributed by the International Narcotic Education Association

There was little public concern over the use of marijuana during this period, with one notable exception. In 1926, a series of articles was printed in two New Orleans newspapers. They sensationally "exposed" the "menacing" presence of marijuana and attributed a number of crimes and heinous acts to use of the drug. Although many of these lurid reports were ridiculous and fabricated, a Louisiana law mandating a maximum penalty of a $500 fine and/or six months imprisonment for conviction of possession or sale of marijuana was passed the next year. This law had little effect on the sale or use of marijuana in New Orleans, however, except for a possible moderate increase in the price of a marijuana cigarette (Brecher, 1972).

Even though marijuana had not threatened to enter the mainstream of American life, additional government and legal action continued into the next decade. Much of this activity was promoted by Harry J. Anslinger, who became director of the Federal Bureau of Narcotics in 1932. Anslinger was convinced that marijuana represented a major threat to the safety and well-being of the country. He successfully encouraged many states to restrict the trafficking and use of marijuana. In 1930, only 16 states had statutes prohibiting the use of marijuana; by 1937, virtually all states had such statutes.

Anslinger's efforts culminated in the 1937 passage of the Marijuana Tax Act. The act did not officially ban marijuana; rather, it acknowledged the medicinal uses of marijuana and permitted the prescription of marijuana following payment of a license fee of $1 per year. Any other possession or sale of marijuana was strictly outlawed. Punishments for violation were a $2,000 fine, five years of imprisonment, or both.

Anslinger's efforts overall were successful in reducing the legal spread of marijuana; in the following year, only 38 physicians paid the $1 license fee to prescribe marijuana (Brecher, 1972). Furthermore, Anslinger's efforts set the stage for progressively stricter penalties for marijuana sale and possession in the ensuing years. Throughout the 1960s, judges often had the option of sentencing users or sellers of marijuana to life imprisonment. A second offense of selling marijuana to a minor in Georgia could be punished by death.

Since 1970, the penalties for marijuana possession and use have been moderated significantly. In addition, there has been a gradual movement toward decriminalizing the possession of small amounts of marijuana, much of this trend spurred by grass-roots movements and public referendums. Nevertheless, there continues to be a strong political emphasis on "zero tolerance" and the "war on drugs."

Committee Reports on Marijuana

Several comprehensive reports on the use of marijuana and its effects have appeared during the past century. One of the earliest was the Indian Hemp Drugs Commission Report released in 1894. The committee preparing the report included four British and three Indian commissioners. A second report was the 1933 Panama Canal Zone Military Investigations, which spanned the years between 1916 and 1929. A third, and one of the most widely known investigations, was the LaGuardia Committee Report published in 1944. Because the conclusions of these three commissions were similar, we focus on the LaGuardia findings.

"A person may be a confirmed smoker for a prolonged period, and give up the drug voluntarily without experiencing any craving for it or exhibiting withdrawal symptoms."

Excerpt from the Laguardia Commission Report (1944)

Mayor LaGuardia's Committee on Marihuana was created by the New York Academy of Medicine at the request of New York City Mayor Fiorello LaGuardia. The study, second in scope only to the Indian Hemp Drugs Commission, was a truly multidisciplinary report, including coordinated input by physicians, psychologists, pharmacologists, and sociologists. Data were gathered on marijuana use and effects in tea-pads as well as in laboratory settings. The general finding of the study was that marijuana use was not particularly harmful to users or to society at large. The report failed to find evidence for the claim that aggression, violence, and belligerence were common consequences of marijuana smoking. This was not intended to suggest, however, that marijuana did not induce psychoactive effects. A number of individual changes were noted, including in more extreme form "mental confusion and excitement of a delirious nature with periods of laughter and of anxiety" (p. 216).

These report findings were consistent with those of commission reports published earlier. Subsequent reports also have mirrored these basic conclusions. These investigations include the 1968 Baroness Wootton Report from Great Britain, the 1972 Report of the Canadian Government's LeDain Commission, and the First Report of the National Commission on Mental Health and Drug Abuse (titled *Marihuana: A Signal of Misunderstanding*) in 1972. Subsequent reports in the United States, such as *Marijuana and Health,* the Ninth Report to the U.S. Congress (NIDA, 1982) and *Drug Abuse and Drug Abuse Research* (USDHHS, 1984, the first in a series of several triennial reports to Congress), have likewise not provided markedly discrepant findings, although they were much more cautious in describing nonnegative effects of marijuana use.

Several other reports have been issued in the years since. Two influential documents recommended the approval of smoking marijuana for treating certain categories of medical disorders. The first report was prepared by Britain's House of Lords (1988) and the second by the United States National Academy of Sciences (Joy, Watson, & Benson, 1999). The latter report concluded that there was scientific foundation for studying marijuana as a treatment vehicle in such areas as pain relief, control of nausea and vomiting, and appetite stimulation. A more recent report, entitled *Cannabis: Our Position for a Canadian Public Policy* (Senate Special Committee on Illegal Drugs, 2002), provided a series of recommendations. First, they recommended amendments to existing law to allow compassionate medical access to cannabis and its derivatives. Second, they recommended a system through which licensed individuals would produce and sell cannabis. Third, the committee recommended that the government of Canada declare an amnesty for any person convicted of possession of cannabis under current or past legislation.

Epidemiology

Marijuana is the most widely used illicit drug in the Western world and the third most commonly used recreational drug after alcohol and tobacco (Iversen, 2000). According to the World Health Organization, it also is the illicit substance most widely cultivated, trafficked, and abused.

For a number of years, the United Nations has been compiling annual surveys of worldwide drug use, including cannabis. Reflecting the difficulties and uncertainties associated with developing estimates of the number of people who use drugs (such as the quality of the data gathered and the methodologies used to sample populations), the latest United Nations estimates are presented in ranges, reflecting the lower and upper estimates indicated through the array of surveys available. In their 2009 report (covering 2007), the United Nations estimated that between 142.6 and 190.3 million people between the ages of 15 and 64 had used cannabis in the past year, representing between 3.3% and 4.4% of the world's population (UN Office on Drugs and Crime, 2009b).

Looking at specific regions of the world, surveys have found that the highest per capita rate of use in the past year was in Oceania (the countries and territories in the Pacific Ocean, including Australia), where between 11.0% and 11.5% of adults reported past-year use. Past-year prevalence estimates for other regions were 7.0% to 7.1% for the Americas, 5.4% to 10.5% for Africa, 5.2% to 5.4% for Europe, and 1.6% to 2.3% for Asia. Past-year cannabis use estimates for subregions include 9.3% to 15.6% for west and central Africa, 10.5% for North America, 7.7% for western/central Europe, 4.3% to 6.7% for the Caribbean, 3.4% for South America, and 2.9% to 3.1% for eastern Europe (UN Office on Drugs and Crime, 2009b).

As in most other countries, marijuana is the most frequently used illicit drug in the United States. Its use rose dramatically throughout the 1960s and 1970s, followed by steady decreases into the early 1990s. However, the use of marijuana by high school seniors increased again in 1993, although it has been decreasing since the late 1990s.

Data gathered as part of the 2007 National Survey on Drug Use and Health (SAMHSA, 2008) revealed that just over 100 million Americans (41% of the population) have used marijuana at least once in their lives. An estimated 14.4 million Americans were current marijuana users (that is, they used marijuana in the last 30 days), representing 5.8% of the U.S. population aged 12 and older. The breakdown by age for current use of marijuana was 6.7% among those aged 12 to 17; 16.4% among those aged 18 to 25; 7.9% among those aged 26 to 34; and 3.0% among those 35 and older.

Data on lifetime, annual (that is, use in the past year), and current use over time among Americans aged 12 and older are shown in Figure 11.1. The figure shows that

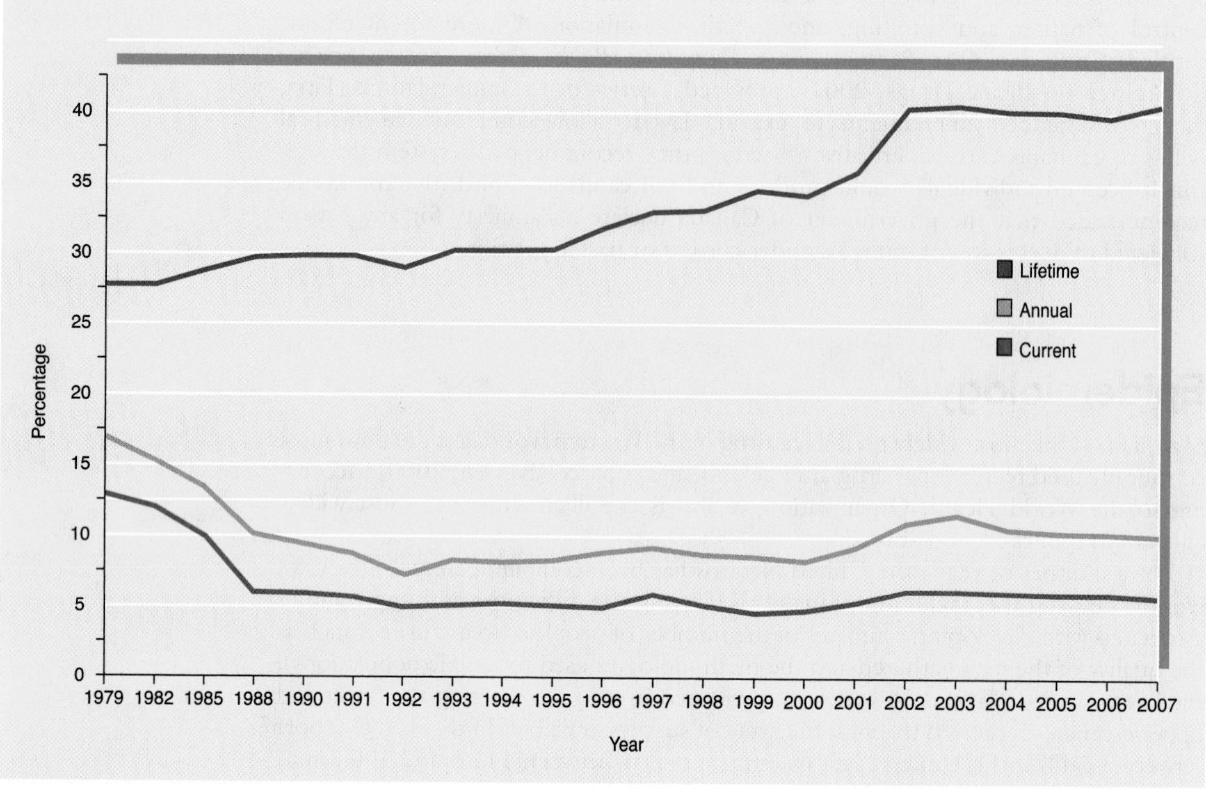

FIGURE 11.1
Trends in the prevalence of lifetime use, annual use, and current use of marijuana or hashish among Americans aged 12 and over (from SAMHSA, 2008)

annual and current rates decreased significantly from 1979 to 1988, decreased more gradually for several more years, and were generally stable from around 1993 until the increases noted in 2001 and 2002. Rates have been relatively stable through the latest survey. Prevalence rates of lifetime use have been gradually rising since the mid-1990s, with a larger increase apparent from 2000 to 2002.

Data on current use over that same period of time, broken down by age, are shown in Figure 11.2. Two patterns are evident. First, rates of current marijuana use were significantly higher in the late 1970s and early 1980s than they are now for those under the age of 35. Second, rates of current use have been consistently higher among those aged 18 to 25 and consistently lower among those over the age of 35. Third, current use among those aged 26 to 34 was consistently higher than for those aged 12 to 17 until the mid-1990s. In the late 1990s, current use was higher among those aged 12 to 17, with current use since 2000 being fairly comparable.

Three other findings from the 2007 National Survey on Drug Use and Health are noteworthy. First, men were more likely than women to be current users of marijuana (8.0% versus 3.8%). Second, current marijuana use varied by race or ethnicity. Current marijuana prevalence was 7.9% among American Indians/Alaska Natives, 7.2% among blacks, 6.0% among whites, 4.5% among Hispanics, 2.8% among Native Hawaiians or other Pacific Islanders, and 2.6% among Asians. The rate of current use among individuals describing themselves as being of two or more races was 10.4%. A third finding

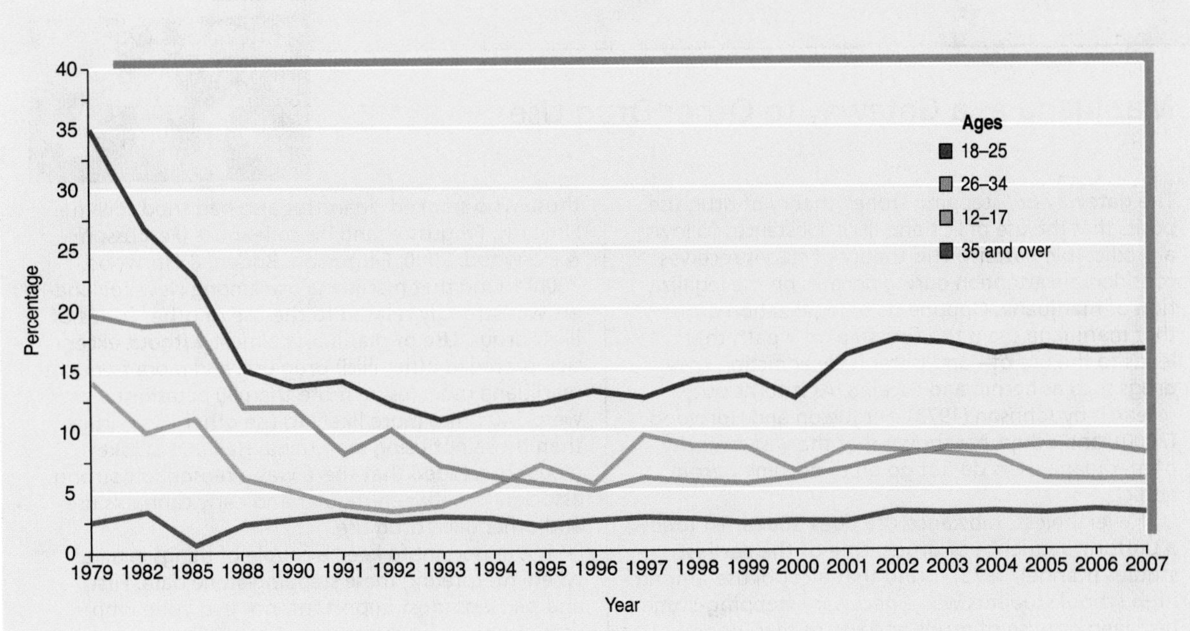

FIGURE 11.2
Trends in the current (past month) use of marijuana or hashish for different age groups (from SAMHSA, 2008)

concerned frequency of use. Among those who smoked marijuana in the past year, 34% reported using marijuana on 1 to 11 days, 19% on 12 to 49 days, 10% on 50 to 99 days, 23% on 100 to 299 days, and 14% on 300 or more days.

The reasons for the overall decline in marijuana use since the late 1970s and early 1980s in the National Survey on Drug Use and Health (even when considering the increases in the early 2000s) have not been specified. The decreases probably reflect broad cultural factors, growing concerns about health and fitness, and concerns over possible negative effects of drug use in general.

The same decreases in marijuana use in the national surveys also appeared—until 1992—in the annual surveys of high school seniors. As you can see in Figure 11.3, the percentages of seniors ever using, using in the past month or year, and using daily for the past month all dropped from around 1979 until 1992. Starting in 1993, however, the data revealed that marijuana was making a comeback, at least among high school seniors. As shown in Figure 11.3, marijuana use increased significantly in 1993, and continued to rise through 1997. It remained relatively constant for the following years. Gradual decreases have been recorded since around 2000. For example, lifetime prevalence decreased from 48.8% in 2000 to 42.6% in 2008. On other indicants of marijuana use among high school seniors, annual prevalence (use in the past year) decreased from 36.5% in 2000 to 32.4% in 2008, 30-day prevalence from 21.6% to 19.4%, and 30-day prevalence of daily use from 6.0% to 5.4%. In attempting to account for these decreases, the authors of the survey speculated they are related to increases in the proportion of students viewing marijuana use as dangerous and reporting personal disapproval of marijuana use. In addition, there has been a continuing decline in the proportion of students saying it would be easy for them to obtain marijuana if they wanted some.

CONTEMPORARY ISSUE BOX 11.2

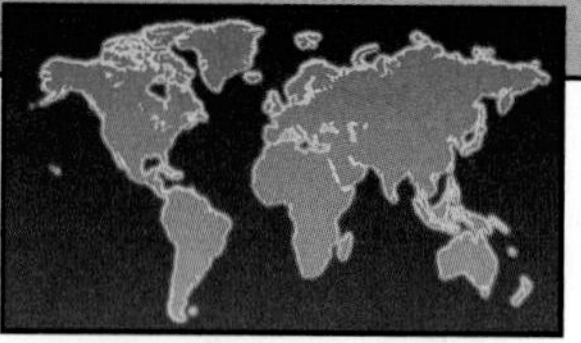

Marijuana as a Gateway to Other Drug Use

The gateway or "stepping stone" theory of drug use posits that the use of licit and illicit substances follows a predictable pattern. This theory of stages receives considerable attention during debates on the legalization of marijuana. Opponents of legalization argue that marijuana use is the first step on a path that leads to the use of—and potentially addiction to—drugs such as heroin and cocaine. As it turns out, research by Johnson (1973), Fergusson and Horwood (2000), and others has shown that the vast majority of marijuana users do not go on to become heroin addicts.

Nevertheless, substance use does appear to follow a uniform sequence of drugs. One of the earliest studies (Kandel, 1975) found that alcohol use among high school students was a necessary stepping-stone between nonuse of drugs and use of marijuana. This finding was replicated in research conducted at the New York State Research Institute on Addictions (Welte & Barnes, 1985; Windle, Barnes, & Welte, 1989). High school students (white, black, and Hispanic) tend to use drugs in the same sequence: alcohol, marijuana, and then the so-called hard drugs (such as cocaine, crack, hallucinogens, and heroin). In a later study, Kandel and Yamaguchi (1993) found that crack users almost always had used marijuana earlier. Indeed, only 10% of crack users in high school had not previously used marijuana. Adler and Kandel (1981) found similar patterns in the sequence of drug use among adolescents in Israel and France.

More recently, researchers at the Center on Addiction and Substance Abuse at Columbia University found that teenagers who experimented with alcohol, cigarettes, and marijuana were more likely than other youths to use cocaine and other "hard drugs." The report noted that 17% of children (aged 12 to 17) who had used marijuana had tried cocaine as well; 5% of those who drank alcohol and 6% of those who smoked cigarettes also had tried cocaine. Similarly, Fergusson and his colleagues (Fergusson & Horwood, 2000; Fergusson, Boden, & Horwood, 2006) found that marijuana use among New Zealanders was strongly related to the use of other forms of illicit drugs. Use of marijuana almost without exception preceded other illicit drug use, and more frequent marijuana users (using more than 50 occasions a year) were 140 times more likely to use other illicit drugs than those not using marijuana. Hall and Lynskey (2005) concluded that there was a reasonably strong association between regular and early cannabis use and other illicit drug use.

It is important to keep a couple of things in mind when interpreting these stepping-stone data. First, and perhaps most important, not everyone who uses alcohol will subsequently use marijuana, and not everyone who uses marijuana will subsequently use other illicit drugs. (Indeed, in both cases, most will not.) Second, people who start using marijuana after previously using alcohol typically do not stop using alcohol. Instead, both substances can be in the person's drug-use repertoire. Finally, consider that an alternative to the gateway theory has been proposed. Called the "correlated vulnerabilities" theory, it suggests that the so-called "stepping-stone" pattern of substance use is explained by the common characteristics (i.e., a general predisposition to use drugs) of those who use cannabis and other drugs (Hall & Lynskey, 2005; Morral, McCaffrey, & Paddock, 2002).

The studies mentioned have implications for people who work in the areas of prevention and drug policy. As an example (and you probably can imagine others), these studies suggest that people who do not use marijuana for the most part will not use "hard drugs" such as cocaine or heroin. Prevention efforts that focus on not using marijuana potentially will decrease the pool of marijuana users who will subsequently use other drugs.

Methods of Use

joint
A hand-rolled marijuana cigarette.

Marijuana and hashish have been administered in a number of ways in their use as psychoactive agents. For example, they were ingested in India centuries ago in liquid and food form. People can also experience the psychoactive effects of marijuana by chewing marijuana leaves. However, the most common procedure for ingesting cannabis in this country has been and remains smoking, typically in cigarette (**joint**) form. Inhalation through cigarettes is also the most efficient method for absorption

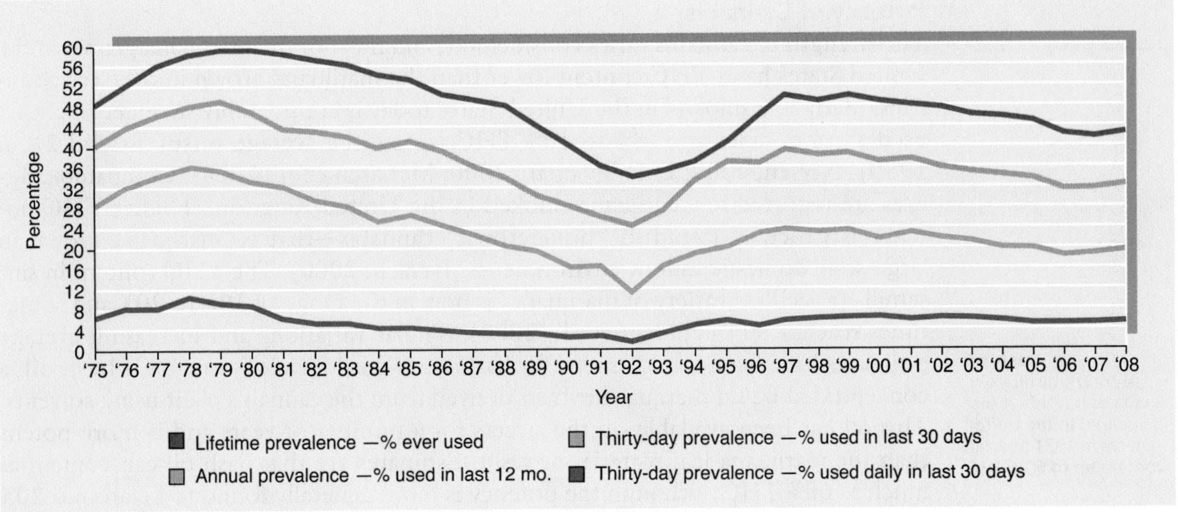

FIGURE 11.3
Trends in the prevalence of marijuana or hashish use among high school seniors (from Johnston, O'Malley, Bachman, & Schulenberg, 2009)

of cannabis. Other methods of smoking marijuana include water pipes (often called bongs) or blunts (a cigar that is emptied of tobacco and refilled with marijuana). The smoking of blunts has increased in popularity among American urban youth (Ream et al., 2008) and may present some unique health risks, given the combined intake of the marijuana and tobacco (as the cigar wrapper is a tobacco leaf). For example, smoking marijuana in a tobacco leaf appears to increase the risks of marijuana by enhancing carbon monoxide exposure and increasing heart rate, relative to smoking marijuana in joint form (Cooper & Haney, 2009).

Active Ingredients

The first chemical analysis of cannabis apparently was performed in 1821 (Mechoulam, 1973). Since then, studies have shown cannabis to be a complex plant. More than 400 individual chemical compounds have been identified in the plant. Over 60 of these chemicals, collectively called **cannabinoids**, are unique to the cannabis plant (El Sohly, 2002). Continued research will probably identify additional cannabis chemical compounds and cannabinoids.

Despite years of study, the principal psychoactive agent in cannabis was not isolated until 1964. This substance has been labeled **delta-9-tetrahydrocannabinol** but is more commonly known as Δ-9-THC, or simply THC. The THC compound was first reported by Gaoni and Mechoulam (1964), two researchers working in Israel. Research since 1964 has shown that the Δ-9-THC cannabinoid accounts for the vast majority of the known specific pharmacological actions of marijuana. Although THC is the prime psychoactive agent in cannabis, other cannabinoids, such as cannabidiol and cannabinol, can be biologically active and can modify THC effects. However, they tend not to be psychoactive in and of themselves.

cannabinoids
The more than 60 chemical compounds present in cannabis. One is delta-9-tetrahydrocannabinol (better known as THC).

delta-9-tetrahydrocannabinol
The principal active cannabinoid in marijuana responsible for the psychoactive effects.

Potency of Cannabis

The strength of cannabis varies considerably, and most of the marijuana grown in the United States has a THC content lower than the marijuana grown in overseas countries. Marijuana smoked in the United States today is considerably stronger than that used three decades ago (8% to 10% THC is now the average versus around 2% in 1980) (Iversen, 2000; El Sohly et al., 2000; McLaren et al., 2008). Comparable figures are reported for marijuana smoked in the United Kingdom. Higher THC potency is generally found in "homegrown" cannabis—that is, marijuana grown in large-scale domestic indoor environments (Iversen, 2000). The THC content in sinsemilla (a seedless variety of marijuana) is now in the range of 10% to 20% and sometimes reaches 30% (Pijlman et al., 2005). Similar variations and increasing average potencies have been found as well for hashish. A third form of cannabis is **hash oil**, a concentrated liquid marijuana extract derived from the cannabis plant using solvents. This oil has been available on the streets for a number of years and is more potent than the marijuana leaf material or resin. Estimates are that hash oil can contain as much as 60% THC, although the potency is more generally found to be around 20% (Iversen, 2000).

hash oil
A potent distillate of marijuana or hashish. It first appeared in the United States in 1971 and can contain up to 60% THC.

Pharmacokinetics

Absorption

The absorption of THC depends primarily on the mode of consumption. The most rapid and efficient absorption of marijuana occurs through smoking. Inhalation results in absorption directly through the lungs, and the onset of the THC action begins within minutes. Assessments of blood plasma reveal that peak concentrations occur 30 to 60 minutes later. The drug effects can be experienced for two to four hours.

Several factors can influence the amount of THC absorbed through smoking. One important variable, of course, is the potency of the cannabis being smoked. Only about half of the THC available in a marijuana cigarette is in the smoke, and the amount ultimately absorbed into the bloodstream is probably less. Another variable is the amount of time the inhaled smoke is held in the lungs; the longer the smoke is held, the more time for absorption of the THC. Another factor influencing intake is the number of people who share the cigarette because more smokers may decrease the amount of marijuana available to any one user. The amount of THC in a marijuana cigarette that is actually absorbed by smoking averages around 20%, with the other 80% lost primarily through combustion, sidestream smoke, and incomplete absorption in the lungs (Iversen, 2000).

Oral ingestion of marijuana is much slower and relatively inefficient. The onset of action is longer than when smoked, taking as long as an hour. The marijuana is absorbed primarily through the gastrointestinal tract, and peak plasma levels can be delayed for as long as two to three hours following ingestion. An important difference from absorption through smoking is that blood containing orally ingested marijuana goes through the liver before going to the brain. The liver processes or clears much of the THC so that lesser amounts have the opportunity to exert action in the brain. The drug effects following oral ingestion can be experienced for longer periods of time, however, generally four to six hours. The dose needed to create a comparable high when orally ingested is estimated as three times greater than that needed when smoking.

Distribution, Metabolism, and Excretion

Using peak plasma THC levels to assess cannabis effects can be misleading because the psychoactive cannabinoids are highly lipid-soluble; that is, the cannabinoids are lipids, which means they are almost entirely insoluble in water. The cannabinoids instead are a dark, viscous, oil-like substance. Plasma levels of THC decrease rapidly because the THC is deposited in the tissues of various organs, particularly those that contain fatty material. Assessments of organs following cannabis ingestion reveal marked concentrations of THC in the brain, lungs, kidneys, and liver. Thus, even when blood levels of THC are zero, the levels of THC in other organs can be substantial. Also, THC is capable of crossing the placental barrier and reaching the fetus.

As noted, THC is carried through the bloodstream and deposited within various organs. The THC is then metabolized to less active products over time. Although this process occurs primarily in the liver, it can occur in other organs as well. The THC metabolites are excreted slowly through the feces and urine. Approximately half of the THC is excreted over several days and the remainder by the end of about a week. However, some metabolites of the THC, a number of which may still be active in the system, can be detected in the body at least 30 days following ingestion of a single dose and in the urine for several weeks following chronic use.

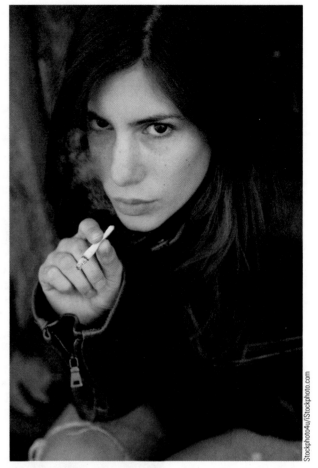

Stockphoto4u/iStockphoto.com

There has been growing concern over the use of marijuana by young people.

Mechanisms of Action

Research Findings

The psychotropic actions of marijuana occur in the brain and are a result of the drug's effect on chemical neurotransmission. Much of the early research in this area (typically performed with animals) focused on the effects of marijuana on acetylcholine, a chemical transmitter involved in memory. THC in relatively small doses has been shown to decrease the turnover in acetylcholine, particularly in the hippocampus, resulting in a decrease in neurotransmitter activity. Similar inhibitory effects of THC have been observed on a variety of neurotransmitters, including L-glutamate, GABA, noradrenaline, dopamine, and 5-HT (Iversen, 2003). In addition, THC facilitates release of the neurotransmitter serotonin and produces changes in the dopamine system, thus enhancing activation of movement.

Although specification of the drug action remains somewhat speculative, important advances are occurring. Foremost among these has been research on THC receptors in the brain (Adams & Martin, 1996; Iversen, 2003). Two types of cannabinoid receptors (called CB1 and CB2) have been identified (Devane et al., 1988; Herkenham et al., 1990; Matsuda et al., 1990; Munro, Thomas, & Abu-Shaar, 1993). These receptors are uniquely stimulated by THC. CB1 receptors are located predominantly in brain areas that control memory, cognition, the motor system, and mood. CB2 receptors are most prevalent in the immune system.

Research on cannabinoid receptors opened the door to efforts to study pathways in the brain that may be involved in cannabinoid actions and to the search for naturally occurring chemicals in the body (called endogenous chemicals) that normally would interact with the identified receptors. One research team (Devane et al., 1992) identified such a chemical (named "anandamide" from the Sanskrit word for "bliss") that binds to the same receptors on brain cells as do cannabinoids. Researchers now are using the compound anandamide to study how the cannabinoid receptors affect functions such as memory, movement, hunger, and pain, which are affected by marijuana use. Another endogenous chemical identified as interacting with cannabinoid receptors is 2-arachidonoyl-glycerol, or 2-AG (Pertwee, 2002; Sugiura et al., 2000).

Newer research methods, such as positron emission transaxial tomography (PET), which assesses cerebral blood flow, have opened new avenues for exploring marijuana effects. For example, it has been shown that THC increases blood flow in most brain regions in both the cerebral cortex and deeper brain structures (Iversen, 2000; Quickfall & Crockford, 2006). Such blood flow is greatest in the frontal cortex (Matthew et al., 1997), which is critical to "executive" brain functions. Other recent research has focused on identifying and investigating areas of the brain that have greater densities of cannabinoid receptors, such as the cerebral cortex.

Tolerance and Dependence

Tolerance to cannabis has been well documented in animal species (for example, Agurell et al., 1986; Harris, Dewey, & Razdan, 1977). The evidence for tolerance to cannabis in humans is less clear, with many studies indicating tolerance but a number

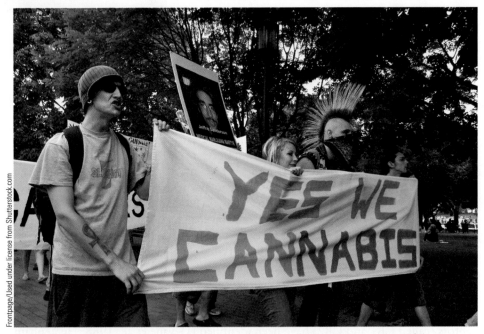

A number of public demonstrations have been organized around the country in support of the legalization of marijuana. This rally took place in front of the White House in Washington, DC, on July 4, 2009.

of others not. Some of the discrepancies in the human studies can be attributed to the dose of marijuana and the duration of use being studied. Tolerance is more likely to occur with higher doses used over longer periods of time. Research has typically been done in controlled laboratory settings, where the doses and frequencies of use studied are generally much greater than those reported by marijuana users in the general population. The mechanisms by which tolerance occurs are still unknown.

There is an ongoing debate as to whether physical dependence can occur in the context of marijuana use. Some have argued that there is no significant withdrawal syndrome identifiable (Compton et al., 1996; Smith, 2002), and certainly no clustering of withdrawal indicators as identified for other substances such as alcohol or heroin. Jones (1980), on the other hand, described several aspects of dependence associated with sustained heavy use of marijuana. These aspects entailed sleep disturbance, nausea, irritability, and restlessness following cessation of marijuana use. It has been more recently posited that these symptoms reflect a reliable and clinically significant withdrawal syndrome (Budney et al., 2004), although debate continues as to whether these symptoms are more indicative of a psychological as opposed to physical dependence on marijuana. At present, it appears that aspects of physical dependence, when they occur, are most likely to be associated with sustained heavy use of marijuana.

Medical and Psychotherapeutic Uses

History of Therapeutic Use

Cannabis has a long history of use for medical and health purposes, with the earliest documented use attributed to Shen Nung in the 28th century B.C. As we noted earlier, Shen Nung purportedly recommended that his people use cannabis for its medicinal benefits. The earliest physical evidence of marijuana used as a medicine was uncovered recently by Israeli scientists who found residue of marijuana buried with the body of a young woman who apparently died in childbirth 1,600 years ago. They suggested that the marijuana was used to speed the birth process and to ease the associated pain. Indications that cannabis had been used during childbirth had been found earlier in Egyptian papyri and Assyrian tablets (Martin et al., 1993). More systematic uses of cannabis as a therapeutic agent did not occur until the 1800s. For example, the Paris physician Jacques Moreau used cannabis in the mid-1800s to treat mental illnesses. (Recall that Moreau supplied the cannabis used by Gautier at *Le Club des Hachichins.*) Much greater legitimization of the medical use of marijuana was provided by Dr. William O'Shaughnessy, the Irish physician who, in an 1838 treatise, described the use of cannabis to treat such problems as rheumatism, pain, rabies, convulsions, and cholera.

Cannabis also was used widely in the United States for many complaints. It was recognized as a therapeutic drug well into the 1900s. At that time, cannabis extract was listed for varying periods of time in the *United States Pharmacopeia,* the *National Formulary,* and the United States *Dispensatory.* In the *Dispensatory,* for example, cannabis was recommended for treating neuralgia, gout, rheumatism, rabies, cholera, convulsions, hysteria, mental depression, delirium tremens, and insanity.

Well into the 1930s, cannabis was an ingredient in a variety of over-the-counter medicines, such as remedies for stomach pain and discomfort, restlessness, and coughs (Iversen, 2000). One company marketed cannabis cigarettes for the treatment of asthma. These medicinal uses of cannabis rapidly began to decline, however, for two reasons. The first was the advances made in medicine and specific knowledge about various diseases and their treatments. The second factor was the Marijuana Tax Act of 1937. This legislation markedly decreased prescribed medicinal uses of marijuana.

The therapeutic uses of marijuana today are much more circumscribed. For the most part, synthetic products (such as dronabinol [trade name Marinol] and nabilone [Cesamet]) that chemically resemble the cannabinoids have been used in current treatment efforts because they provide the active elements of THC in a more stable manner (see Joy, Watson, & Benson, 1999; Sussman et al., 1996). Synthetics also can provide better solubility. Unfortunately, a downside to the synthetics is the absence of the rapid effect experienced when marijuana is smoked. When synthetic THC is taken orally, it is broken down prior to entering the bloodstream and absorption thus is delayed. A recent development with promise is a cannabis oral spray (trade name Sativex), which has been approved in several countries for use as a painkiller for sufferers of multiple sclerosis. Sativex also holds promise for alleviating pain associated with rheumatoid arthritis and may even suppress the disease. Sativex has also shown some promise in animal research for improving memory loss in Alzheimer's disease.

The discovery of the cannabinoid receptor by Devane and his colleagues (described earlier) has important implications for future medical and psychotherapeutic uses of cannabis. The identification of the cannabinoid receptor also has advanced knowledge about the neurobiology of cannabis abuse. Perhaps more importantly in the context of therapeutics, it has opened wide investigation of compounds related to the endogenous cannabinoid system for potential applications with multiple disorders (de Fonseca & Schneider, 2008). For example, a medication based on the cannabinoid CB1 receptor, the antagonist rimonabant, is being used in the treatment of complicated obesity. Other medications based on the endogenous cannabinoid system are now in development or under evaluation.

"A past evaluation by several Department of Health and Human Services (DHHS) agencies . . . concluded that no sound scientific studies supported medical use of marijuana for treatment in the United States, and no animal or human data supported the safety or efficacy of marijuana for general medical use. There are alternative FDA-approved medications in existence for treatment of many of the proposed uses of smoked marijuana."

Press release issued by the United States Food and Drug Administration, April 20, 2006

Meanwhile, the past several decades have witnessed sustained efforts to legalize marijuana use for medicinal purposes. Much of this effort has been spurred by an increased use of marijuana by AIDS patients who claim that marijuana reduces the nausea and vomiting caused by the disease and that it stimulates appetite, thus helping them to regain weight lost during their illness. The passage of propositions in Arizona, California, Colorado, and Oregon, along with a handful of other states, demonstrates public sympathy for those positions. An offshoot of these efforts has been the establishment of "cannabis clubs" in several major U.S. cities. These organizations purchase marijuana in bulk and provide it (free or at cost) to patients with AIDS, cancer, and other diseases. As noted in the Contemporary Issue Box 11.3, the cannabis club in San Francisco has, on and off, operated fairly openly and was shielded for a while by a city law that made medicinal marijuana use a low priority for its police force.

The debate over legalizing marijuana for medicinal purposes is not likely to be resolved in the near future. In the meantime, there are several disorders—especially nausea and cachexia—for which cannabis is prescribed in synthetic form, and we describe these briefly in the following sections.

Nausea and Vomiting

Cannabis and THC synthetics have been used to counter the nausea and vomiting frequently associated with chemotherapies (and some radiation treatments) for cancer. These side effects, which can last for several hours or even several days, often are not ameliorated by traditional antiemetic medications (although significant advances are

CONTEMPORARY ISSUE BOX 11.3

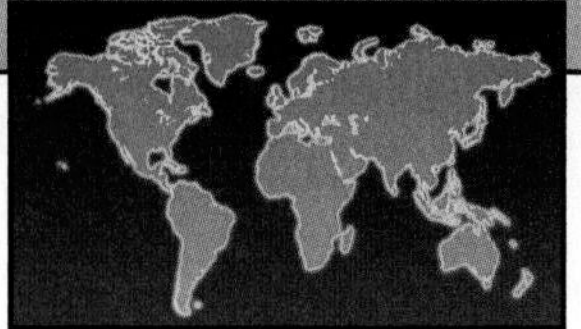

The San Francisco Cannabis Buyers Club

A coffee shop environment where you can buy and smoke marijuana for medicinal purposes? Sure, you might think—in Amsterdam. But here in the United States? Well, there are such enterprises, and the best known is the Cannabis Buyers Club in San Francisco.

The Cannabis Buyers Club was founded by Dennis Peron, following the 1990 death of a friend from AIDS. Peron was instrumental in collecting petition signatures to have a proposition to make marijuana available to sick people placed on the San Francisco citywide ballot in 1991.

The proposition was overwhelmingly approved, and the Cannabis Buyers Club opened in 1992. Although operating at that time in violation of state law, the club was able to remain in operation mainly because local government and law enforcement agencies in San Francisco relegated the enforcement of marijuana-related laws to a low priority. Consider this statement by Frank Jordan, the then-mayor of San Francisco: "I have no problem whatsoever with the use of marijuana for medical purposes. I am sensitive and compassionate to people who have legitimate needs. We should bend the law and do what's right."

The Cannabis Buyers Club was housed on several floors of a building in downtown San Francisco. The setting included couches, chairs, and coffee tables, similar to what one would find in a coffee house. Available for purchase, as identified on a "menu" placed on the wall, were such items as marijuana banana bread, marijuana "magic" brownies, "merry pills" (high-grade THC and olive oil in a capsule), vials of marijuana tincture that can be dropped into tea or coffee, and a variety of grades of loose marijuana (purchased mostly from local growers). Members could take their purchases home or consume them at the club.

The club membership at one point exceeded 8,000. To join, one needed to present a doctor's note to certify that one has AIDS, cancer, or another condition with symptoms marijuana may alleviate. The club was selling more than 40 pounds of marijuana per week.

The Cannabis Buyers Club was the best known of such establishments, but it is not alone. Similar clubs exist overtly or covertly in cities and towns throughout the United States. The extent to which these clubs remain open is uncertain. The Cannabis Buyers Club was afforded a bit more security by the 1996 passage of California Proposition 215, which permitted use of marijuana for medicinal purposes. However, federal injunctions have periodically halted—at least temporarily—distribution of marijuana at this and other such clubs. Stay tuned for future developments on the state and national levels, as this issue very much remains in a state of flux.

being made in the development of more powerful antisickness drugs). Researchers in the 1970s began more systematic study of the antinausea and antivomiting effects of THC (usually administered orally), and their results were favorable. This research, incidentally, followed anecdotal reports by chemotherapy patients that their private use of marijuana had reduced the aversive side effects of their treatments.

Positive outcomes have emerged in subsequent research. Furthermore, there are indications that children undergoing cancer chemotherapy may particularly benefit from orally administered high doses of cannabinoids (see Abrahamov, Abrahamov, & Mechoulam, 1995; Martin et al., 1993). More recent studies have included the use of THC synthetics. The main drawback to the use of cannabis and THC synthetics is the resultant mental effects, which some patients have viewed as uncomfortable and disorienting. Nevertheless, many patients undergoing chemotherapy find the THC side effects an acceptable price to pay for reduced side effects. Only limited research is being conducted, despite the classification of synthetic THC as a Schedule III drug, which means some medical value is recognized. The synthetic had once been classified as a Schedule I drug, meaning it was a prohibited substance with no recognized medical benefit. Marijuana not in synthetic form remains a Schedule I drug. Meanwhile, advances have been occurring with newer antiemetic drugs, not cannabis-based, that have been well tolerated and effective.

"If anybody needed proof that the FDA has become totally politicized, this is it. This isn't a scientific statement; it's a political statement. There is abundant evidence that marijuana can help cancer patients, multiple sclerosis patients and AIDS patients. There is no scientific doubt that marijuana relieves nausea, vomiting, certain kinds of pain and other symptoms that don't respond well to conventional drugs, and does it more safely than other drugs."

Bruce Mirken, Communications Director for the Marijuana Policy Project, in response to the April 20, 2006, FDA press release on medical uses of marijuana

Cachexia

Cachexia is a disorder in which an individual physiologically "wastes away," often due to HIV infection or cancer. Based partly on anecdotal reports that marijuana use is associated with increased frequency and amount of eating, it has been proposed that patients with cachexia use marijuana to stimulate appetite and thus weight gain. These anecdotal reports have some empirical support. Plasse et al. (1991) found a relationship between marijuana ingestion and appetite. Accordingly, some individuals who have disorders that include cachexia have been turning to marijuana to stem the tide of weight loss and to gain weight. Abrams et al. (2003), for example, found that smoked marijuana or oral THC each effectively induced weight gain among HIV-infected adults. A caution on the use of smoked marijuana is that patients with HIV, for example, might be uniquely vulnerable to any immunosuppressive effects of the drug (Joy et al., 1999). More study in this area appears justified (Robson, 2001).

Glaucoma

Glaucoma is a generic term used to denote ocular diseases that involve increases in intraocular pressure. This pressure damages the optic nerve and represents the leading cause of blindness in the United States. More than 2 million Americans over age 35 have developed glaucoma, and an estimated 300,000 new cases are diagnosed yearly. Almost 67 million people are affected by glaucoma worldwide. Although drug and surgical interventions are available, their effectiveness is variable.

Cannabis has been shown to decrease intraocular pressure (Joy et al., 1999), although patients have experienced side effects regardless of whether the cannabis was administered orally, through injection, or by smoking (Hepler & Petrus, 1976; Merritt et al., 1980). These side effects include increased heart rate and psychological effects. Some effects dissipate with extended exposure to the cannabis. Of more concern, marijuana may also reduce blood flow to the optic nerve and possibly exacerbate the loss of vision.

The mechanisms through which the cannabis reduces intraocular pressure have not been determined. Cohen and Andrysiak (1982) suggested that cannabis dilates the vessels that drain excess fluids from the eyeball. This draining is thought to prevent fluid buildup and the resultant pressure that causes optic nerve damage.

Clinical research on the potential benefits of cannabis as a treatment for glaucoma is continuing, with two emphases. The first is on developing synthetic formulas that reduce side effects, and the second emphasis is on modes of application. Particular attention is given to developing a topical preparation that could be applied directly onto the eye. Meanwhile, most experts believe that existing non-THC medications have equal or greater benefit in the treatment of glaucoma (Amar, 2006; Joy et al., 1999).

Other Uses

Cannabis and THC synthetics have been used to a lesser extent or in exploratory fashion in the treatment of several other disorders. For example, ajulemic acid, a synthetic analog of THC, is receiving attention as an analgesic that does not produce feelings of being "high" (Burstein et al., 2004; Karst et al., 2003). Other clinical areas for which THC and cannabis-based treatments are being studied include muscle spasticity, convulsant activity, epilepsy, chronic pain, insomnia, hypertension, asthma, anxiety, Tourette's syndrome, and depression. However, the data in support of these uses so far have been preliminary or mixed, and more research is needed to specify the potential utility of cannabis in these areas.

Physiological Effects

Acute Effects

Although cannabis produces physiological effects, most of these actions are different for different users, not only in strength or intensity of the effect but also in duration. In general, the acute physiological effects of marijuana in a healthy individual are not dramatic. In fact, the LeDain Commission (1972) reported the "short-term physiological effects of a typical cannabis dose on normal persons are generally quite benign, and are apparently of little clinical significance," a finding often reported in subsequent research.

The most commonly experienced effects are cardiovascular. Predominant among these is injection of the conjunctiva, or bloodshot eyes. This effect, a result of vasodilation, is most obvious about an hour after smoking, and it is generally dose-related. Although some cite a concomitant dilation of the pupil, research does not support this claim. It appears more likely that the dilation is a consequence of smoking the marijuana in a darkened room. There does, however, tend to be a cannabis-induced sluggish reaction to light.

The second most common cardiovascular effect is an increase in heart rate and pulse rate (Grotenhermen, 2007; Kelly, Foltin, & Fischman, 1993). Both of these effects last for about an hour, and each appears to be dose-related. The peak heart rate occurs around 20 minutes after smoking. In addition to these effects, blood pressure tends to become slightly elevated. No evidence indicates that these effects create any permanent damage within the normal cardiovascular system (Institute of Medicine, 1982; Workshop on the Medical Utility of Marijuana, 1997).

Another general effect following cannabis use is a generalized decrease in motor activity. The only real exception to this is the talkative behavior of many following smoking. Some users also report drowsiness. Cannabis use also can have a marked effect on sleep stages, tending in part to decrease the total REM sleep achieved. However, this effect typically occurs only with higher doses of cannabis.

Other effects have also been reported, but they tend to be minor or infrequent and often variable from person to person. These other effects include (but are not limited to) dry mouth, thirst, fluctuations in respiration and body temperature, hunger or "the munchies" (peaking two to three hours after smoking), nausea, and headache or dizziness.

Longer-Term Effects

Data on the longer-term effects of marijuana unfortunately are sparse and difficult to interpret. The research that has been conducted has focused on four central systems: respiratory, cardiovascular, immune, and reproductive.

Respiratory System

Little controlled research has been done on the long-term effects of smoking cannabis. Proper lung functioning appears to be altered as a consequence of smoking cannabis, but much of this impairment, such as airway obstruction, is reversed following abstinence from smoking. Marijuana cigarettes contain more tar than tobacco cigarettes. Additionally, cannabis tar contains greater amounts of cancerous agents than does tobacco tar (Jones, 1980). This is particularly noteworthy because marijuana smokers (in an effort to maximize the effects of the drug) inhale deeply and hold the smoke in their lungs. The long-term consequences unfortunately are not known. One difficulty in specifying these effects is that cannabis smokers frequently also smoke cigarettes, and separating the effects of the two substances is difficult. Nevertheless, the possibility of irreversible lung damage due to marijuana smoking remains.

Cardiovascular System

The vast majority of cardiovascular effects associated with cannabis smoking were described earlier in this section as short term (or acute). No evidence shows that smoking marijuana produces deleterious cardiovascular effects among healthy individuals. The acute effects produced (for example, increased heart rate) are, however, potentially dangerous among people who have existing cardiovascular problems, such as abnormal heart functioning or atherosclerosis.

Immune System

Although some of the early research on this topic was contradictory, it appears now that cannabis poses no significant long-term threat to the immune system. Thus, although cannabis can act as an immunosuppressant and decrease resistance to some viruses and bacteria, its clinical significance among otherwise healthy individuals remains questionable. The mechanism through which this immune dysfunction occurs has not yet been defined.

Reproductive System

Studies using animals and humans suggest that cannabis does disrupt the reproductive system in both males and females. For example, chronic marijuana use has been associated with decreases in the number of sperm and sperm motility among men. The potential effects of these disruptions on fertility are difficult to specify. Frequent use of cannabis by women may produce nonovulatory menstrual cycles, in which menstruation is not preceded by the release of an ovum. As in the males, the delayed effects of these disruptions on fertility are not known. In reviews, researchers (Ehrenkranz & Hembree, 1986; Budney, Moore, & Vandrey, 2004; and Zimmer & Morgan, 1997) concluded that disruptions in reproductive function are not obvious, although subtle alterations may be operative.

Of more concern are possible teratogenic effects. The active agents present when marijuana is smoked readily cross the placental barrier and expose a fetus to an array of cannabinoids. Although few data are available for humans, it does not appear that major birth malformations result. This does not mean significant effects cannot occur, however. The use of marijuana by pregnant women is associated with increased risk of premature birth, shorter body length, and lower infant birth weight (e.g., Day & Richardson, 1991; Fried, 1986). A more recent concern is that children born to mothers who used marijuana during pregnancy may be at greater risk of developing certain forms of childhood cancer (Robison et al., 1989; Grufferman et al., 1993). In addition, newborn infants whose mothers used marijuana during pregnancy have been noted to exhibit tremor, startle response, and altered visual responses (Jones, 1980), although the functional impact of these effects has not been determined. Longer-term consequences also have been reported. Children exposed to marijuana prenatally were found to show deficits on a sustained attention task at age 6 (Fried, Watkinson, & Gray, 1992), and to be more impulsive, hyperactive, and delinquent at age 10 (Goldschmidt, Day, & Richardson, 2000). The prudent advice is to not use cannabis during pregnancy.

Summary of Longer-Term Effects

It appears the majority of effects associated with marijuana use are more acute than chronic and that longer-term effects tend to be reversible with the termination of drug use. Significant exceptions may occur, however. Smoking marijuana may be found to be linked to various respiratory disorders, including cancer. Most of the negative

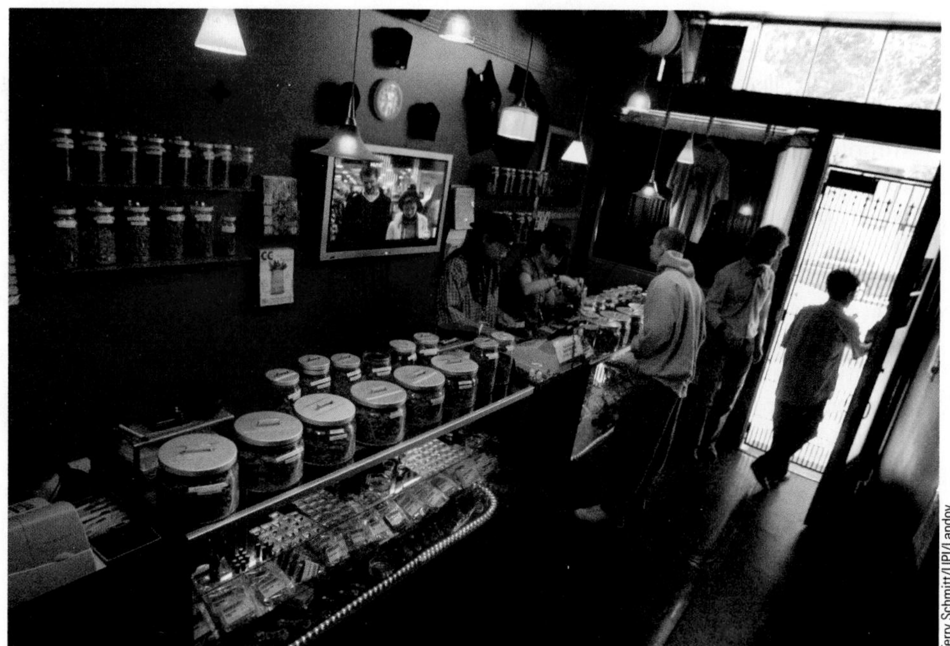
Terry Schmitt/UPI/Landov

Cannabis buyers' clubs, such as this one in San Francisco, have been established in a number of locations to provide cannabis to individuals who have medical conditions such as AIDS, cancer, or other conditions with symptoms that marijuana may alleviate. Here, a buyer looks over some of the products available for sale.

effects found are correlated with higher doses and frequency of use than those described by most cannabis smokers in this country. Nevertheless, these indications are tentative and await confirmation from more systematic and controlled research.

Psychological Effects

Although cannabis can produce the varied effects previously noted, most marijuana users use the drug to experience its psychological effects, some of which are reported consistently and others more idiosyncratically. The psychological effects that marijuana users generally experience can be divided into three domains: behavioral, cognitive, and emotional.

Some cannabis effects, especially those associated with the "marijuana high" that users describe, are learned. This learning process has been described in detail by Becker (1953; 1963). According to Becker, the first step is mechanical, when the smoker learns to inhale the smoke and hold it in the lungs to maximize intake and absorption. The second step is to learn to perceive the effects of the cannabis, which can be physical as well as psychological. The final step described by Becker is learning to label these effects as pleasant. This learning process accounts for the frequent finding that experienced users are more sensitive to cannabis effects than novice smokers are.

Behavioral Effects

The most common behavioral effect is a generalized decrease in psychomotor activity and decrements in some domains of psychomotor performance. These effects appear to be dose-related, with more pronounced changes associated with greater amounts of marijuana taken in. The general decrease in motor activity appears to be pervasive, and the state is described as associated with feelings of relaxation and tranquility. The only exception to this effect appears to be speech because marijuana use is associated with rapid or slurred speech, circumstantial talk, and loquaciousness. These speech effects often are observed more in the early smoking phase, followed by the more traditional relaxation.

Although relaxation and a sense of well-being are the usual responses to cannabis, some users first experience a stage in which they feel excited and restless. Fairly soon, however, these users virtually always experience a transition to the relaxation stage. Furthermore, despite feeling relaxed, users sometimes also feel their senses are markedly keener. Many users, for example, describe more intense perceptions of touch, vision (especially in perceiving colors), hearing, and smell. The research cited to support these reports is not strong, though. Finally, other research has shown a decreased sensitivity to pain during marijuana intoxication.

Concomitant with the feelings of relaxation and decreased motor activity is a subtle impairment in some areas of psychomotor performance. There appear to be dose-related dysfunctions in motor coordination, signal detection, and the ability to monitor a moving object. The data on reaction time are not conclusive. Taken together, these findings have implications for driving a motor vehicle after using cannabis. Laboratory studies that use a driving simulator have revealed detrimental effects of marijuana on driving skill. Some of these impairments may be cognitively mediated in that drivers under the influence of marijuana showed impaired judgment and concentration along with other general driving skills. Others have suggested that some of the detriments in driving skill may be due to decreased vigilance and thus less awareness of peripheral stimuli. Therefore, it appears that cannabis can cause psychomotor impairment and that this impairment becomes more apparent in tasks that require thinking and concentration.

The influence of marijuana on sexual behavior and functioning is not fully understood, but its effects vary considerably from user to user. Some report that sexual pleasures are more intense and enjoyable when using marijuana, whereas others describe a disinterest in sex. Those who report increased sexual pleasure when smoking probably are responding to the enhanced sensory sensitivity that frequently accompanies marijuana use. The drug itself produces no known specific physiological response that stimulates sexual drive or performance. Long-term or heavy use of marijuana has been associated with temporary impotence among men and temporary decreases in sex drive among women.

Cognitive Effects

Two primary cognitive consequences of cannabis intoxication have been documented. The first is impaired short-term memory and the second is the perception that time passes more slowly.

The impairment in short-term memory seen following cannabis use can occur with intake of a fairly low dose (Deahl, 1991). The degree of impairment increases rapidly with the complexity of the memory task. This effect has been observed with various types of stimuli, such as word lists and conversational materials. More generally, the evidence indicates that cannabis intake impairs multiple aspects of memory, including the encoding, consolidation, and retrieval of information (Grotenhermen, 2007; Ranganathan & D'Souza, 2006).

The mechanisms of marijuana's effects on memory have not been specified, but Paton and Pertwee (1973) have identified several possibilities. The first cause simply may be that the user is not motivated to attend to or to retrieve the material presented. Although this hypothesis is plausible, indications suggest participants in these experiments perceive the tasks administered as a challenge and respond actively to the task demands. A second possibility is that the perceptual changes created by cannabis produce a "curtain of interference" that blocks or hinders intake or retrieval of material. The third hypothesis proposed by Paton and Pertwee (1973) is that marijuana causes a decreased ability to concentrate and attend to the material presented. This mechanism was advocated by Abel (1971) and by DeLong and Levy (1974). These latter researchers have proposed a model of attentional processes as a central key in understanding the cognitive effects of cannabis. Finally, cannabis drug action may interfere with the neurochemical processes that operate in memory and retrieval operations. The exact factor, or set of factors, remains unknown, but it is likely that they operate in concert to affect short-term memory. However, likely mechanisms include cannabis effects on long-term potentiation and long-term depression and the inhibition of neurotransmitter (GABA, glutamate, acetylcholine, dopamine) release.

Altered perception of the passage of time is the second common cognitive effect of cannabis (Chait & Pierri, 1992). This is perhaps best described in statements like "a few minutes seemed to pass like hours." The effect has been noted in both surveys and the experimental literature. However, the time distortion is not as pronounced in the research reports as it is in more subjective self-reports that marijuana users provided.

Other cognitive effects of marijuana have been reported but not as consistently as those already described. One effect is decreased ability to attend and concentrate so that the user is easily distracted. Many users report that cannabis produces racing thoughts and "flight of ideas," in which various (and sometimes seemingly random) ideas "fly" in and out of the mind. Another perception sometimes reported is enhanced creativity. Writers and painters have especially noted this. Finally, some cannabis users describe occasional feelings of "unreality" (see Hollister, Richards, & Gillespie, 1968) and the attachment of increased meaning to events or objects not previously perceived as important. Most of the effects noted are short-term.

The effects of long-term cannabis use on cognitive functioning have received much less attention. Research in this area has been increasing, although providing a mixed picture so far. Solowij (1998), for example, reported that a longer history of use was associated with greater cognitive impairment, even after stopping marijuana use. Messinis et al. (2006) found that frequent marijuana users (smoking four or more joints per week) performed worse than nonusers on several measures of cognitive functioning, including divided attention (paying attention to more than one task at a time) and verbal fluency. Among the marijuana users, those who had used marijuana for 10 or more years had more difficulties with their thinking abilities than those who had used marijuana for 5 to 10 years. Other recent studies comparing the cognitive functioning of current heavy users, former heavy users, light users, and nonusers have not found such a relationship (Lyketsos et al., 1999; Pope et al., 2001). Pope et al. (2001) found that intellectual impairment associated with heavy marijuana use is apparently reversible with abstinence. More generally, the available research on persistent cognitive effects from long-term marijuana use is at best equivocal (Grant et al., 2003; Van Amsterdam, van der Laan, & Slangen, 1996).

Emotional Effects

Positive emotional changes following cannabis intake are cited frequently as key motivators to smoke marijuana. Alterations in mood can occur, but there is uncertainty regarding the extent to which these are direct drug effects. A host of nonpharmacological factors can contribute to the drug effects experienced (Adesso, 1985; Zinberg, 1984). Chief among these nondrug influences are past experiences with cannabis, attitudes about the drug, expectancies regarding the drug-use consequences, and the situational context of drug use. These factors must be considered in conjunction with the dose of THC absorbed to understand the emotional changes attributed to the drug.

The typical emotional response to cannabis is a carefree and relaxed state. This feeling has been described in various ways: euphoric, content, happy, and excited. It frequently includes laughter and loquaciousness and may take on the character of a dreamlike state. Most generally, the response is viewed as pleasant and positive. It appears the intensity of the response is positively correlated with the dose.

It is noteworthy that negative emotional feelings, such as anxiety or dysphoria, are more common than might be expected. Additionally, a variety of somatic consequences have been experienced, including headache, nausea, and muscle tension; less frequently reported are suspiciousness and paranoid ideation. About a third of marijuana users at least occasionally experience some negative effects; however, the effects can be transitory. A user may fluctuate between experiencing these negative feelings and the more positive states described earlier. Also, the negative effects often are reported more by inexperienced cannabis users.

In recent years, there has been an increased focus on the relationship between cannabis use and various mental health outcomes, such as schizophrenia, anxiety disorders, and depression. A review of the literature on this issue concluded that cannabis use increases one's risk for psychotic behavior outcomes (including schizophrenia), and not just among heavy users (Moore et al., 2007). In this regard, they found that marijuana users had around a 40% higher chance of developing a psychotic condition later in life, relative to nonusers (although the risk is fairly low overall). Although the data used to address this issue do not prove that marijuana use increases the risk for psychosis (instead, it could be something else about cannabis users, such as their use of other drugs or particular personality traits), the association is still noteworthy. A comparable relationship between cannabis use and anxiety disorders and depressive disorders was not found in the Moore et al. (2007) study. In another report, however, a modest link between cannabis use and the risk for a later episode of depression was found (van Laar et al., 2007). The mechanisms underlying these relationships are not known, although they do not appear to be related to cannabis-induced changes in brain anatomy (DeLisi, 2008; Linszen & van Amelsvoort, 2007). Instead, the positive relationship may reflect the impact of cannabis on the dopaminergic pathway, perhaps especially among genetically vulnerable individuals (Di Forti et al., 2007).

Social and Environmental Effects

Three hypothesized social and environmental consequences of cannabis use have received attention: the role of marijuana in enhancing interpersonal skills, the effect of cannabis on aggression and violence, and the role of marijuana use in what has been called the **amotivational syndrome**.

amotivational syndrome Loss of effectiveness and reduced capacity to accomplish conventional goals as a result of chronic marijuana use.

Many young users of marijuana have said they use the drug because it enhances their social skills and allows them to be more competent in social situations. Although insufficient data are available to evaluate it fully, this claim has not been supported by the available research. Rather, what seems to occur is that users either are more relaxed in the situation and thus perceive less anxiety or interpret their behavior differently while under the influence of marijuana. In any event, marijuana does not seem to significantly enhance competence in social situations.

A long-standing claim regarding cannabis use, dating in this country to 1920s newspaper articles in New Orleans cited previously, is that marijuana causes users to be aggressive and violent. The overwhelming conclusion drawn from data, including surveys, laboratory investigations, and field studies, however, is that cannabis use is not causally related to increased aggression (Institute of Medicine, 1982). When aggression is observed, it probably is more a function of the beliefs and characteristics of the individual drug users (Cherek et al., 1993). In fact, levels of aggression actually decrease following cannabis use.

Perhaps the most controversial social/environmental consequence of cannabis use is the amotivational syndrome. The term was used independently in the late 1960s by McGlothlin and West (1968) and Smith (1968) to describe the clinical observation "that regular marijuana use may contribute to the development of more passive, inward turning, amotivational personality characteristics" (McGlothlin & West, 1968). Based on case reports, the phenomenon was most likely to be seen among younger users who were using marijuana daily or heavily. The list of behaviors proposed as part of the syndrome includes apathy, decreased effectiveness, lost ambition, decreased sense of goals, and difficulty in attending and concentrating.

Although there does not seem to be much question that these characteristics cluster in some marijuana users, the causal influence of cannabis is not clear (Brick, 1990). Also, there is some debate about just how commonly the syndrome occurs, with some citing it as fairly infrequent (Duncan, 1987). In addition, anthropological investigations of heavy cannabis users in other countries generally have not found the presence of the amotivational syndrome (for example, Carter, 1980; Carter & Doughty, 1976; Comitas, 1976; Duncan, 1987; Page, 1983), and laboratory studies on cannabis use in humans have not supported the hypothesized syndrome (Foltin et al., 1989; Foltin et al., 1990). Furthermore, survey studies do not always find the differences between

CONTEMPORARY ISSUE BOX 11.4

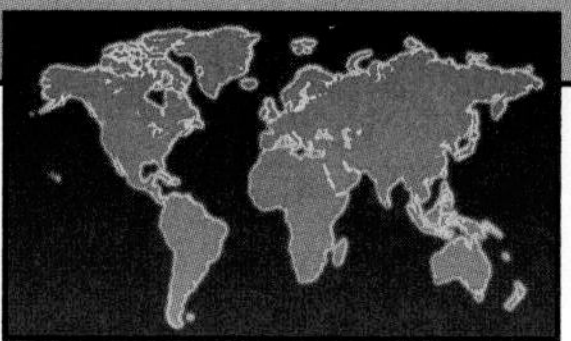

AMP: Combining Embalming Fluid and Marijuana

There is seemingly no end to the number of ways in which a drug can be used or abused. Sometimes the effects of a drug are much more pronounced when the drug is taken, for example, intravenously versus orally. Sometimes the way a substance is prepared has an effect on how and what effects are experienced. One dramatic example of changing the preparation of a psychoactive substance is the drug known as AMP in the 1980s and now also called "dank." AMP/dank is marijuana soaked in embalming fluid or formaldehyde (the fluid's main ingredient) and dried before being smoked. Ivan Spector, a physician at Baylor College of Medicine in Texas, first described this in the clinical literature in 1985.

According to Spector, who provided case examples of patients seeking treatment after they smoked AMP, these users showed some profound psychiatric effects and impairments. Several of them reported they "immediately felt as if a transparent field has been placed between them and their surroundings." Among the symptoms associated with AMP intoxication are a slowed sense of time, memory impairment, disorientation, paranoid thoughts, anxiety, confusion, disordered thought and difficulties in reality testing, and tremor. Physiological components in the response to AMP intake include elevated blood pressure, hypersalivation, tachycardia, and psychomotor excitement.

It may be instructive to describe one of the cases seen by Spector. A 35-year-old woman, called Ms. D., was presented for treatment three days after smoking AMP. She felt anxious, was tremulous, was salivating excessively and sweating, and had a racing heartbeat. All of this followed closely the actual AMP smoking. Several hours later, she exhibited psychomotor retardation, secluded herself, reported she could not think well, lost all motivation, and described paranoid thoughts. Ms. D. also described hallucinations in which she saw blood on the walls. After three days, many of these complaints disappeared, with the exception of the anxiety and tremulousness. She was treated with an antianxiety medication, and the discomfort cleared within several days.

Ms. D's scenario was similar to those of the other AMP users described in the report, and we can offer two conclusions. One is that any given drug can be prepared in ways that markedly influence its effect on the user. For example, in some areas, the formaldehyde is combined with the drug PCP before soaking the marijuana so as to increase the high. This form of preparation has been referred to as "fry." A second conclusion is that drug users may be in a situation in which the drug they are using is not quite what they thought it was. Some AMP users reported they were given AMP by friends who told them it was only marijuana.

marijuana users and nonusers that would be expected if marijuana caused this clustering of effects. And, the amotivational syndrome has been seen in youths who do not use marijuana and is often not seen in other daily users of marijuana. Thus, both preexisting personality characteristics and some drug effects together probably account for the clustering labeled the amotivational syndrome, when it occurs.

Summary

- The plant *Cannabis sativa* is more commonly known as marijuana. It once was harvested primarily for its fiber but now is most often grown for its psychoactive effects.
- Marijuana is the leafy top portion of the plant, and hashish is made from the resin the plant produces for protection from the sun.
- The use of cannabis for its intoxicating effects appears to have been centered in Asia, the Middle East, and North Africa for an extended period of time before Europe was exposed to these effects in the 19th century.
- Cannabis in the New World dates to 1543, when the Spaniards brought it to Chile. The cannabis plant was raised in the American colonies for its fiber.
- Several influential reports have appeared on the use of marijuana and its effects, including the 1894 Indian Hemp Drugs Commission Report and the 1944 LaGuardia Commission Report. Such reports have tended to find that marijuana use overall is not particularly harmful to society at large.
- Marijuana is the most frequently used illicit drug in the United States, although its use has decreased over the last decade.
- The most common and efficient procedure for ingesting cannabis is smoking.
- The principal psychoactive agent in cannabis, isolated in 1964, is delta-9-tetrahydrocannabinol, more commonly known as Δ-9-THC or simply THC.
- The potency of cannabis varies widely. Most of the marijuana grown in the United States has a lower THC content than that imported from overseas. The THC potency of marijuana smoked in the United States typically is 8% to 10% (10% to 20% for sinsemilla, a seedless variety of marijuana). Values for hashish and hash oil are higher, with hash oil containing up to 60% THC.
- The onset of THC action occurs within minutes of inhalation, and peak concentrations occur 30 to 60 minutes later. The effects usually are experienced for two to four hours. Most of the THC metabolites are excreted slowly, approximately half within several days and the remainder by the end of about a week. Some metabolites can be detected in the body for up to and beyond 30 days.
- The main actions of marijuana occur in the brain and result from the drug's effect on neurotransmitters. Although specification of the drug action remains speculative, recent advances include work on THC receptors in the brain.
- Tolerance, when it occurs, is most likely when high doses of cannabis are used over extended periods of time. Dependence on cannabis has been documented, although there is debate as to whether this dependence is more psychological than physical.
- Cannabis has long been used for medicinal and psychotherapeutic purposes. Today, it is used mostly to reduce nausea and vomiting associated with cancer chemotherapies and as an appetite stimulant among patients with cachexia.
- The acute effects of marijuana generally are benign. They include bloodshot eyes, increased heart rate and pulse rate, and decreased motor activity.
- Research on the long-term effects of marijuana is sparse. Some effects associated with long-term marijuana use appear to be reversible with termination of its use. There may be significant exceptions, such as the possible association between marijuana and lung cancer.
- Psychological effects of cannabis include decreased psychomotor activity, happy feelings and relaxation, impaired short-term memory, and altered time perception.
- Marijuana has not been shown to enhance social skills or to induce aggression or violence. The data on cannabis causing an amotivational syndrome are mixed. Both preexisting personality characteristics and drug effects probably account for what has been labeled the amotivational syndrome.

Answers to *"What Do You Think?"*

1. The cannabis plant was raised for its psychoactive properties by the settlers at Jamestown and later by George Washington.
   F *Although they did cultivate the cannabis plant, it was for the use of its fiber and not for its psychoactive properties.*
2. The Eighteenth Amendment prohibiting the use of alcohol had the paradoxical effect of increasing the prevalence of marijuana use in the United States.
   T *As the price of alcoholic beverages rose and the quality of these products declined during the Prohibition era, commercial trade in marijuana "sprang up."*
3. Criminal penalties in the United States for the possession and use of marijuana have increased steadily since the 1960s.
   F *The penalties have been moderated significantly over this period, including the gradual decriminalization for possession of small amounts of marijuana. Throughout the 1960s, judges had the option of sentencing users or sellers to life in prison.*
4. Data recently gathered both in national household surveys and in annual surveys of high school seniors demonstrate a lower prevalence of marijuana use relative to the 1970s.
   T *The prevalence of annual and current marijuana use is markedly lower than the rates observed in the 1970s.*
5. The marijuana smoked in the United States today is more potent than that smoked 20 years ago.
   T *The potency is approximately two to three times greater today.*
6. Drug effects following oral ingestion of marijuana last longer than after the drug is smoked.
   T *Although the onset of action is slower and up to three times as much marijuana is needed to create a comparable high, the drug effects following oral ingestion last four to six hours compared to two to four hours when smoked.*
7. Tolerance to cannabis has been well-documented in animal studies.
   T *Tolerance to cannabis has been well-documented in animals. The evidence for tolerance in humans is less clear, with some studies indicating tolerance but others not.*
8. Marijuana has been used effectively to treat the nausea and vomiting often associated with chemotherapy in the treatment of cancer.
   T *Cannabis and THC synthetics have often been used for this purpose.*
9. Marijuana cigarettes contain more tar than tobacco cigarettes.
   T *There is more tar in a marijuana cigarette than in a tobacco cigarette. In addition, cannabis tar contains a greater amount of cancerous agents than does tobacco tar.*
10. Marijuana use often causes long-term damage to the cardiovascular system.
    F *Although marijuana use does cause short-term increases in heart rate and pulse rate, no evidence shows that marijuana smoking produces deleterious cardiovascular effects in healthy individuals. The acute effects may be dangerous to individuals who have preexisting cardiovascular problems.*
11. One consequence of cannabis intoxication is the impairment of short-term memory.
    T *This impairment is a common consequence of marijuana use and can occur with intake of a fairly low dose. The degree of impairment increases rapidly with the complexity of the task.*
12. The most commonly reported emotional effects of cannabis use are suspiciousness and paranoid ideation.
    F *The typical emotional response to cannabis is a carefree and relaxed state. Paranoia and suspiciousness are reported less frequently and more often by inexperienced cannabis users.*
13. An area of concern regarding marijuana use is that it often causes users to be aggressive and violent.
    F *The overwhelming conclusion drawn from available data is that cannabis use is not causally related to increased aggression. In fact, levels of aggression decrease following cannabis use.*

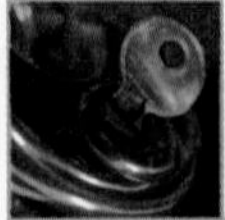

Key Terms

amotivational syndrome
apothecary
cannabinoids
delta-9-tetrahydrocannabinol
hash oil
joint
tea-pads

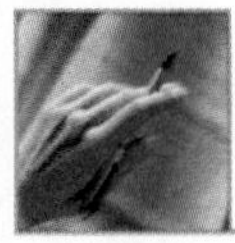

Essays/Thought Questions

1. Should marijuana be legalized, or at least markedly decriminalized? Would the use of marijuana increase? What would be the advantages and disadvantages to society as a whole?
2. What do you think might be the critical determinants of a person's decision to use marijuana?
3. If under a doctor's supervision, should one be able to purchase and use marijuana for medicinal purposes?

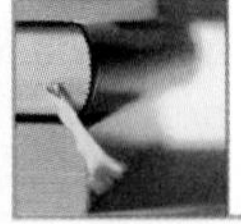

Suggested Readings

Becker, H. S. (1953). Becoming a marihuana user. *American Journal of Sociology, 59*, 235–242.

Booth, M. (2003). *Cannabis: A history.* New York: St. Martin's Press.

Earleywine, M. (2002). *Understanding marijuana: A new look at the scientific evidence*. New York: Oxford University Press.

Hall, W., & Pacula, R. L. (2003). *Cannabis use and dependence*. Cambridge: Cambridge University Press.

Iversen, L. L. (2000). *The science of marijuana.* New York: Oxford University Press.

Joy, J. E., Watson, S. J., & Benson, J. A. (1999). *Marijuana and medicine: Assessing the science base.* Washington, DC: National Academy Press.

Ludlow, F. H. (1857/1979). *The hasheesh eater, being passages from the life of a Pythagorean.* San Francisco: City Lights Books.

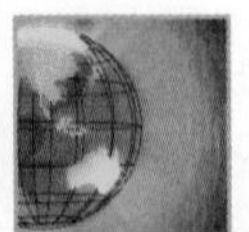

Web Resources

Visit the Book Companion Website at www.cengage.com/psychology/maisto to access study tools including a glossary, flashcards, and web quizzing. You will also find links to the following resources:

- United States National Institute on Drug Abuse
- National Organization for the Reform of Marijuana Laws
- *Cannabis Culture* online magazine
- Marijuana and Medicine: Assessing the Science Base (National Academy of Sciences Report)

CHAPTER 12

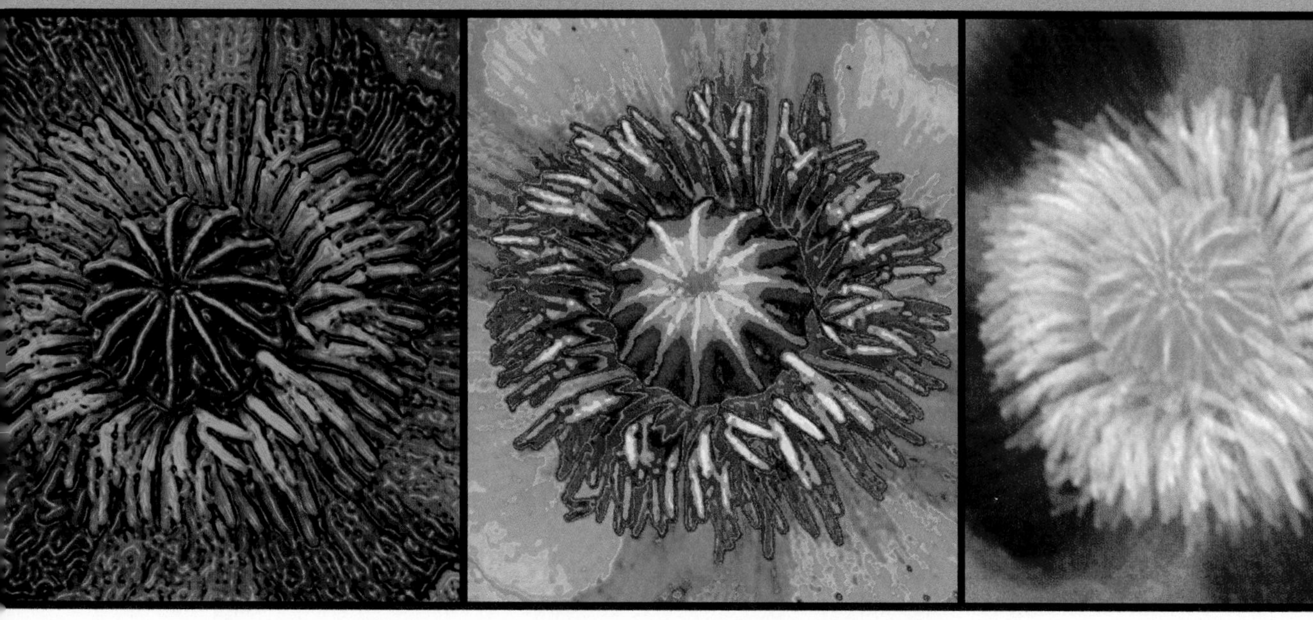

Hallucinogens

What Do You Think? True or False?

Answers are given at the end of the chapter.

___ 1. Unlike other classes of drugs, most hallucinogens are derived from synthetic compounds.

___ 2. Hallucinogenic compounds were commonly used in the early 1900s throughout Europe and America.

___ 3. The hallucinogenic properties of LSD were discovered by accident.

___ 4. LSD and Ecstasy were once used in psychotherapy.

___ 5. Federal law mandates that anyone using LSD more than five times be declared legally insane.

___ 6. Use of LSD, even once, is likely to cause permanent chromosome damage and subsequent birth defects.

___ 7. Ecstasy (MDMA) produces vivid visual hallucinations.

___ 8. Ecstasy has been linked to long-term changes in brain chemistry.

___ 9. Hallucinations experienced under the influence of drugs such as LSD are very similar to those experienced by schizophrenics.

___ 10. Dependence develops easily to hallucinogens such as LSD.

___ 11. Reports of LSD flashbacks are now considered urban myth.

___ 12. Phencyclidine (PCP or angel dust) was originally used as an animal tranquilizer.

Overview

Among the most fascinating, but also confusing, classes of drugs is the group called hallucinogens. These drugs are fascinating because they can alter consciousness in profound and bizarre ways. They are at the same time confusing because so many different drugs act in a variety of ways as hallucinogens and because these drugs have been named and classified in many different ways over the years. Called "phantastica" by Lewin (1964), hallucinogens have gone through dozens of name changes. Some researchers have used the term *psychotomimetics* because of the belief that these drugs mimic the symptoms of functional psychoses such as schizophrenia. This usage is rare today; it is now clear that, although intriguing similarities exist, the effects of hallucinogens differ in many respects (to be considered later) from natural psychosis. During the 1960s, advocates of hallucinogen use referred to them as *psychedelics*, a term coined by one of the early LSD experimenters, Humphrey Osmond. Osmond defined psychedelic as "mind-expanding or mind-revealing" (Stevens, 1987), but whether LSD or other hallucinogens actually possess such properties is controversial at best, and we avoid the term for that reason.

We are left with the term *hallucinogen,* but even this term is misleading. It does focus attention on hallucinations and other alterations in perception, and indeed most of the drugs in this category generally do produce sensory disturbances or alterations that can be considered hallucinogenic. However, that is certainly not the only effect these drugs produce. Hallucinogens exert profound effects on mood, thinking processes, and physiological processes as well. Hallucinogens alter nearly all aspects of psychological functioning, and the phrase "altered state of consciousness" describes these drugs better than any we have considered.

An additional complexity is that more than 90 different species of plants and many more synthetic agents can produce these kinds of effects (Siegel, 1984). To simplify this complex group of drugs, we divide them on the basis of their effects and mechanisms of action into four different subgroups to be treated separately.

The first and historically most important group is referred to as the **serotonergic hallucinogens**. This category includes the synthetic compound lysergic acid diethylamide (LSD) and related drugs, such as **mescaline** (from the peyote cactus) and **psilocybin** (from certain mushrooms), along with many other less well-known compounds. These drugs all produce vivid visual hallucinations and a variety of other effects on consciousness. Numerous experiments suggest that, despite differing chemical structures, these drugs also have in common the action of influencing serotonergic transmission in the brain (Meyer & Quenzer, 2005).

serotonergic hallucinogens
A class of drugs that includes LSD and drugs with similar effects and mechanisms of actions.

mescaline
An LSD-like hallucinogen found in the peyote cactus.

psilocybin ('sī-ə-'sī-bən)
An LSD-like hallucinogen found in mushrooms.

methylated amphetamines
A class of drugs including MDA and MDMA (ecstasy).

The second class of hallucinogens includes MDA and MDMA (ecstasy), referred to as the **methylated amphetamines**. As the name suggests, these drugs are structurally related to amphetamine (as is mescaline). MDA and MDMA produce alterations in mood and consciousness with little or no sensory change. Like amphetamine and cocaine, these drugs act on dopamine, norepinephrine, and serotonin synapses, but their effects are most potent on the serotonergic system (Iversen, 2008).

A third class of hallucinogens, called the **anticholinergic hallucinogens**, is less familiar to most people and includes drugs such as atropine and scopolamine found in plants such as mandrake, henbane, belladonna, and jimsonweed. These drugs produce a dreamlike trance in users from which they awaken with little or no memory of the experience. The drugs in this class act on cholinergic synapses of the brain (Meyer & Quenzer, 2005).

anticholinergic hallucinogens
A class of drugs including atropine and scopolamine.

A fourth class of hallucinogens includes phencyclidine (PCP or angel dust) and the related compound ketamine. These are often referred to as the **dissociative anesthetics** because of their ability to produce surgical anesthesia while an individual remains at least semiconscious. Dissociative anesthetics are thought to act through a receptor that influences activity of the excitatory amino acid neurotransmitter, glutamate (Balazs, Bridges, & Cotman, 2006).

dissociative anesthetic
A class of drugs including PCP and ketamine.

Finally, one of the most widely used hallucinogens in recent years is salvinorin A, a chemical found in a plant in the sage family (*Salvia divinorum*) and often referred to as diviner's sage or just salvia. Almost completely unknown a decade ago, salvia is not currently a federal controlled substance, although some states have banned it. Although relatively little is known about salvinorin A, it appears to act differently on the brain from any of the previously known hallucinogens by affecting specialized opiate receptors known as kappa receptors, and thus we classify it as a kappa hallucinogen.

Serotonergic Hallucinogens: LSD and Related Compounds

Early History

Table 12.1 lists some of the major drugs that are thought to obtain their hallucinogenic properties by altering serotonin function in the brain. LSD is the prototype hallucinogen of this class, but drugs with effects similar to those of LSD were used long before LSD was synthesized. As you can see in Table 12.1, LSD-like hallucinogens are found in a wide variety of plants. The hallucinogenic properties of these plants were primarily discovered and used by the Indian peoples of Central and South America (an exception is ibogaine, which was discovered and used by tribal peoples of Africa). Historians and anthropologists have reconstructed the uses to which these hallucinogenic plants were put and these are worth some consideration here.

When the Spanish *conquistadores* began to explore and colonize Mexico and other parts of Central and South America, they encountered new civilizations with customs and religious practices unfamiliar to Europeans. Among these practices was the use of

TABLE 12.1 Serotonergic Hallucinogens

Drug	Botanical Source	Area Found	Other Names
Lysergic acid diethylamide (LSD)	Synthetic, but derived from the ergot fungus	Ergot native to Europe	Acid, many others
Ibogaine	Iboga plant: *Tabernanthe iboga*	Africa	—
Psilocybin	Mushrooms of genus *Psilocybe, Conocybe, Panaeolus,* and *Stropharia*	Throughout the world	Teonanacatl
Dimethyltryptamine (DMT)	Virola tree: *Virola calophylla* and other species	South America	Yakee, yopo
Mescaline	Peyote cactus: *Lophophora williamsii*	Mexico and Southwest U.S.	Peyote
Harmaline, Harmine	Ayahuasca vine: *Banisteriopsis caapi, Banisteriopsis inebrians*	South America	Yagé
Lysergic acid amide	Morning glory seeds: *Rivea corymbosa, Ipomoea violacea*	Throughout the world	Ololuiqui

hallucinogenic plants in religious ceremonies. One of the earliest documentations was by Fernando Hernandez, the royal physician to the king of Spain (Stewart, 1987). In 1577, he studied the plants the Aztecs used and noted the use of peyote cactus (referred to as peyotl), psilocybe mushrooms (called teonanacatl), and morning glory seeds (called ololuiqui). Although each of these plants contains a different drug, all produce vivid visual hallucinations, and the Indians took the visions as oracles that could reveal the future and solve other mysteries, help in decision making, and aid the medicine man or shaman in healing the sick (see the Drugs and Culture Box 12.1).

The Aztec and Mayan peoples called the psilocybe mushrooms *teonanacatl,* which means "flesh of the gods," and as one might guess from that name, the mushrooms were viewed as sacred. Mushroom icons found in Mayan ruins dating back to before 1000 B.C. suggest that the use of the sacred mushroom was an ancient practice (Schultes, 1976). One Spanish writer, de Sahagun in the 1500s, described the use of mushrooms by Aztecs as follows:

"Rotating kaleidoscopes . . . kaleidoscopes moving horizontally . . . weeds, lots of yellow weeds multiplying, embellished with colors . . ."

Description of a peyote vision (Siegel, 1992)

> These mushrooms caused them to become intoxicated, to see visions and also to be provoked to lust. . . . They ate the mushrooms with honey and when they began to feel excited due to the effect of the mushrooms, the Indians started dancing, while some were singing and others weeping. . . . Some Indians who did not care to sing, sat down in their rooms, remaining there as if to think. Others, however, saw in a vision that they died and thus cried; others saw themselves eaten by a wild beast; others imagined that they were capturing prisoners of war; others that they were rich or that they possessed many slaves; others that they had committed adultery and had their heads crushed for this offense. . . . (Schlieffer, 1973, p. 19)

This may be the first description of hallucinogenic drug effects that captures the range of experiences different individuals may have after taking the drug. The use of sacred mushrooms persists in parts of Mexico in rituals for healing and divination (Schultes, 1976).

DRUGS AND CULTURE BOX 12.1

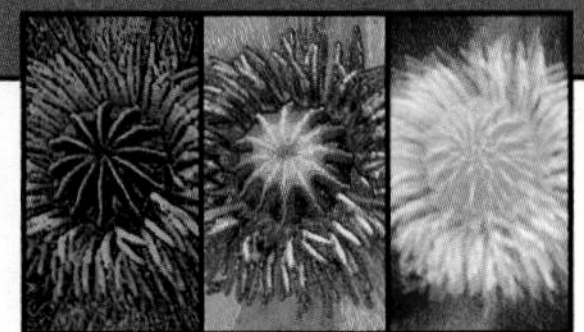

Peyote

Peyote may have been the most widespread hallucinogenic drug in the New World, which is surprising given that the range of the peyote cactus is limited to a relatively small area of northern Mexico and southwestern Texas. The Aztecs used peyote in their rituals, and de Sahagun noted, "Those who eat or drink it see visions either frightful or laughable . . ." (Stewart, 1987, p. 19). Peyote, like ololiuqui and sacred mushrooms, was forbidden to the Indians by the Spaniards, who regarded its use for religious purposes as blasphemous. Thus, the use of all these agents persisted only "underground," and little is known of them before the 20th century. The peyote religion spread widely during the 18th and 19th centuries, however, to unite most Indian tribes in western Mexico and the United States.

The southwestern tribes gathered peyote by cutting the cactus at the soil line, leaving the root intact. The cactus was sliced and dried into hard "buttons." These buttons could be transported great distances without losing their potency, and indeed they found their way to Native American tribes living throughout the West and as far north as Minnesota and Wisconsin. The ritual itself is almost identical regardless of the tribe studied. The all-night ceremony takes place in a large tepee where the participants sit in a circle around a fire, eating peyote buttons and drinking peyote tea. They smoke tobacco in cigarettes or a pipe. The night is spent chanting, singing, praying, and later on discussing and interpreting the peyote-induced visions. These ceremonies are still conducted today by some Native American people, much as they were many centuries ago (Stewart, 1987).

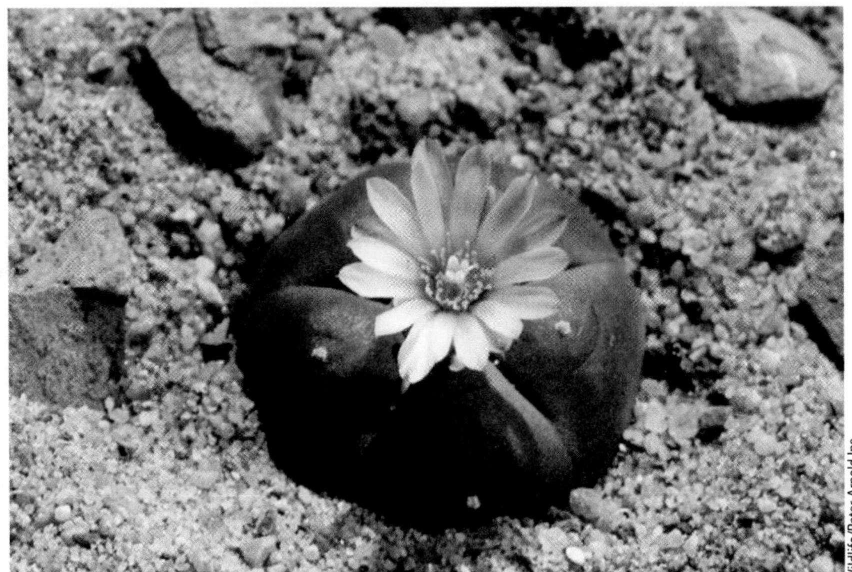

Mescaline comes from the peyote cactus, *Lophophora williamsii*.

In South America, a number of different hallucinogenic plants traditionally have been used in much the same way as peyote and psilocybin were used farther north. Two hallucinogens, harmine and harmaline, are found in the bark of the vines *Banisteriopsis caapi* and *B. inebrians*. These plants are known as *ayahuasca* and *caapi* by indigenous people of the western Amazon area of Brazil, Colombia, Peru, Ecuador, and Bolivia. Local names for the drink made from the bark of these vines are *yagé*, *pinde*, and *dapa*. These plants are used in healing ceremonies, initiation rites, and

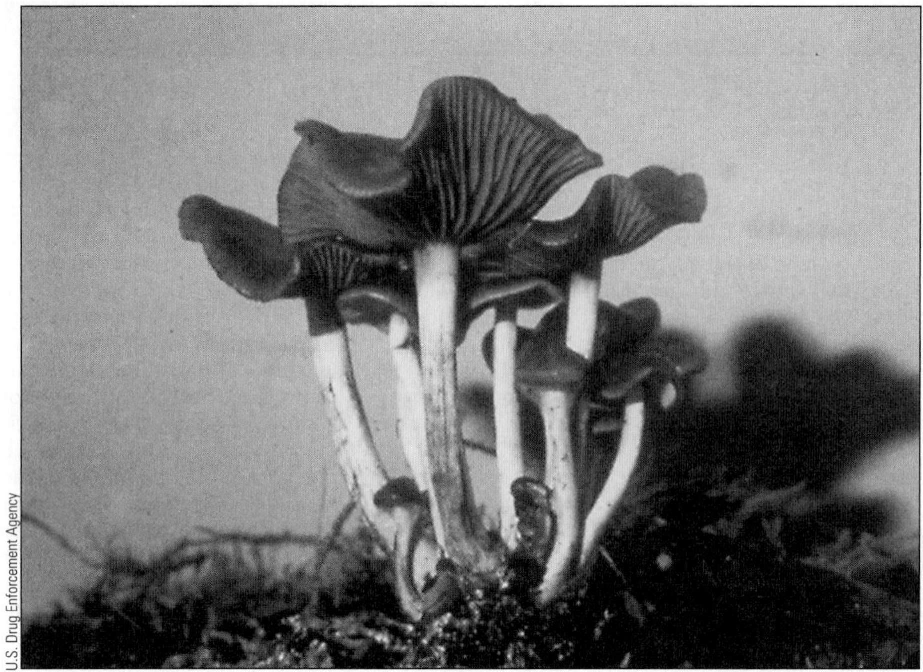

Psilocybin comes from mushrooms such as this *Psilocybe cubensis.*

other rituals. It is said that the plants provide users with telepathic powers, but this claim has no scientific support (Schultes, 1976), and in fact, the effects are similar to those of the other serotonergic hallucinogens. Another group of South American plants used for their hallucinogenic properties includes the various species of the Virola tree (*Virola calophylla, V. calophylloidea,* and *V. theiodora*) of Brazil, Colombia, and Venezuela. The bark of these trees is taken as a snuff called yopo that contains the hallucinogen dimethyltryptamine (DMT), and DMT is also one of the active compounds in yagé preparations. The effects of DMT are consistent with those noted previously except that DMT has a shorter duration of action (Riba et al., 2001). Virola snuff is taken by some Amazon tribes in a funeral ritual in which the powdered bones of the deceased are consumed along with the snuff (Schultes, 1976).

Recent History

Despite the long history of hallucinogenic drug use, these drugs had virtually no impact on mainstream European or American culture until the 1960s, when hallucinogen use exploded. The history of the "psychedelic movement" began in Basel, Switzerland, where Albert Hofmann, a chemist working in Sandoz Laboratories, discovered LSD in 1938. Hofmann was studying derivatives of ergot, a fungus that infests grain and occasionally caused outbreaks of disease (St. Anthony's Fire) in medieval Europe when infected bread was eaten. Ergot derivatives have medical use in the treatment of migraine headache and to induce uterine contractions during pregnancy, and this accounted for Sandoz's interest. Hofmann eventually synthesized compounds involving lysergic acid, the 25th of which was lysergic acid diethylamide —abbreviated LSD-25 on the bottle. LSD underwent several preliminary animal tests, but it showed no commercially interesting properties and was shelved. It stayed unknown until 1943, when Hofmann decided to reexamine its properties. During a laboratory experiment, Hofmann apparently spilled a small amount of LSD on his hand, where it was absorbed. Thus, Hofmann became the first person to experience the effects of LSD. He described his reaction as follows:

> I was forced to interrupt my work in the laboratory in the middle of the afternoon and proceed home, being affected by a remarkable restlessness, combined with a slight dizziness. At home I lay down and sank into a not unpleasant intoxicated-like condition, characterized by an extremely stimulated imagination. In a dreamlike state, with eyes closed . . . I perceived an uninterrupted stream of fantastic pictures, extraordinary shapes with intense, kaleidoscopic play of colors. (Hofmann, 1980, p. 15)

Hofmann decided the bizarre experience must have been due to contact with LSD, so he decided to test that hypothesis with an experiment. He reasoned that LSD must be very potent to have produced such effects through an accidental exposure, and he measured out for oral administration 250 micrograms—a minute amount by the standards of drugs known at that time. What Hofmann could not have known is that LSD is *so* potent that this dose was at least twice as potent as the normal effective dose (25 to 125 micrograms).

After taking the drug, Hofmann (1980) noted in his journal: "Beginning dizziness, feeling of anxiety, visual distortions, symptoms of paralysis, desire to laugh" (p. 16). At this point, Hofmann was overcome by the drug and could no longer write. He asked his assistant to escort him home, and he later wrote about his LSD trip:

> On the way home, my condition began to assume threatening forms. Everything in my field of vision wavered and was distorted as if seen in a curved mirror. . . . Finally we arrived at home safe and sound, and I was just barely capable of asking my companion to summon our family doctor and request milk from the neighbors . . . as a nonspecific antidote for poisoning.
>
> My surroundings had now transformed themselves in more terrifying ways. Everything in the room spun around, and assumed grotesque, threatening forms. They were in continuous motion, animated, as if driven by an inner restlessness. The lady next door, whom I scarcely recognized, brought me milk. . . . She was no longer Mrs. R., but rather a malevolent, insidious witch with a colored mask. . . . (pp. 16–17)

Later, as the intensity of the drug effects began to subside, Hofmann reported enjoying the hallucinations and altered thought processes. After he recovered and made his report to Sandoz, many other experiments followed.

Sandoz began to distribute LSD to psychologists and psychiatrists for use as an adjunct to psychotherapy. The theory was that the drug would break down the patient's normal ego defenses and thus facilitate the psychotherapy process. Psychiatrists were encouraged to try LSD themselves so they would better understand the subjective experience of schizophrenia. The idea was that LSD was psychotomimetic—that is, it mimicked psychosis.

By the early 1960s, many people had tried LSD, and it was beginning to generate some publicity. One user was movie star Cary Grant, who said in an interview that his LSD psychotherapy changed his whole life and brought him true peace of mind. Another famous user, Henry Luce, head of Time Inc., said he talked to God under LSD's influence. The British author Aldous Huxley, who earlier had tried peyote and written a book about his experiences (Huxley, 1954), promoted LSD and other hallucinogenic drugs as leading to the next step in human evolution! But the most influential of the early LSD users were Harvard psychologist Timothy Leary and writer Ken Kesey.

Leary and his Harvard associate Richard Alpert (who later became known as religious writer Baba Ram Das) had taken LSD and other hallucinogens and become convinced of their psychological and spiritual value. What began as legitimate experiments, including work on the possible beneficial effects of hallucinogens on prison inmates, began to look suspiciously like LSD parties involving Harvard faculty, students, and an assortment of celebrities and intellectuals. At some point, Leary had stepped out of his role as a scientist and had become the leader of a social and religious movement. Calling himself "High Priest," Leary claimed LSD was a ticket for a trip to spiritual enlightenment. He exhorted an entire generation to "Turn on. Tune in. Drop out" (Stevens, 1987). Leary left Harvard under duress in 1963, but continued to proselytize for LSD and in fact became a media celebrity. Harassment by law enforcement officials continued to increase Leary's eminence, and he became viewed as something of a martyr, winning new converts as a curious nation heard more and more about the wonders of LSD.

On the West Coast, LSD was popularized by Ken Kesey, celebrated author, and his "merry pranksters." Kesey is the author of *One Flew over the Cuckoo's Nest.* As recounted by Wolfe (1969), Kesey's "acid tests" were large parties where hundreds of people were "turned on to LSD" in a single night. LSD began to make an impact on the emerging hippie subculture, particularly through the music of groups like the Grateful Dead, Jefferson Airplane, Jimi Hendrix, and others whose music became known as "acid rock." Eventually, the Beatles became part of the movement, and the surreal images of songs such as "Lucy in the Sky with Diamonds" had the entire Western world talking about, if not using, LSD.

By the late 1960s, LSD had become the most controversial drug in the world. As many as 2 million people in the United States had tried LSD, but the positive statements about LSD were counterbalanced by increasing negative publicity. LSD was claimed to cause chromosome damage; users were said to be likely to have mutant children. It was said to cause insanity, suicide, acts of violence, and homicidal behavior (Stevens, 1987). All of this controversy led to a decline in LSD use in the 1970s and 1980s, but perhaps equally important was a loss of faith in the LSD mystique, the recognition that spiritual enlightenment produced by LSD was a false hope. As Hunter S. Thompson (1971) put it in his chronicle of the era:

> This was the fatal flaw in Tim Leary's trip. He crashed around America selling consciousness expansion without ever giving a thought to the grim meat-hook realities that were lying in wait for all the people who took him too seriously. . . . Not that they didn't deserve it: No doubt they all Got What Was Coming To Them. All those pathetically eager acid freaks thought they could buy Peace and Understanding for three bucks a hit. But their loss and failure is ours, too. What Leary took down with him was the central illusion of a whole lifestyle that he helped to create . . . a generation of permanent cripples, failed seekers, who never understood the essential old-mystic fallacy of the Acid Culture: the desperate assumption that somebody—or at least some force—is tending that Light at the end of the tunnel. (pp. 178–179)

The use of LSD did not vanish, but it did decline throughout the 1980s. Then LSD use, along with other hallucinogens, increased once again in the 1990s. For example, a national survey of high school seniors showed increases in reported LSD use through the early part of that decade, reaching a peak in 1996, when 8.8% reported having used LSD during the past year. LSD use has declined substantially since then with only 2.7% of America's high school seniors reporting use of LSD during 2008 (Johnston et al., 2009a).

However, hallucinogens, including LSD, became associated with the "club" scene in recent years, and the protracted parties or concerts that are sometimes referred to as "raves" are often occasions for hallucinogen drug use. Although MDMA or Ecstasy is generally considered the prototypical "club drug," LSD is used as well. For example, in one study of clients in treatment for substance abuse (Hopfer et al., 2006),

LSD use was reported by nearly half (48.6%) of those under 18 years old, as compared to 32.3% reporting MDMA use. Among older clients (18 to 32 years), the pattern was similar, with 42.9% reporting LSD use compared with 37.0% using MDMA (Ibid.). So, LSD remains a significant issue in the United States today.

Mechanisms of Action of LSD-Like Drugs

The mechanisms by which LSD and related drugs are capable of producing—in such small doses—such dramatic effects as visual hallucinations and alterations of consciousness remain enigmatic, but there is increasing consensus that an important feature is the alteration of activity of brain systems mediated by the neurotransmitter serotonin. The first bit of evidence was suggested by the chemical structures of some of the major hallucinogens. LSD, psilocybin, and many of the other drugs listed in Table 12.1 have similar chemical structures that resemble that of the naturally occurring transmitter serotonin. The structural similarity led to the notion that LSD and related compounds might act by mimicking serotonin and thus activate serotonin receptors in the brain. This hypothesis has now received considerable support. For example, it has been shown that LSD and the related hallucinogens bind to certain subtypes of serotonin receptors (5-HT2A receptors) and that this effect correlates strongly with the potency of the drug as a hallucinogen (Iversen et al., 2009; Nichols, 2004).

One problem with this analysis that has puzzled researchers is the structure of mescaline. Mescaline's chemical structure is different from the others; in fact, mescaline is far more similar to amphetamine than to LSD. For this reason, it has often been classified as having a different mechanism from LSD. Unlike amphetamine (and the methylated amphetamines like MDA, discussed later), however, mescaline produces vivid visual hallucinations virtually identical in form to those of LSD. Further evidence for a common mechanism of action between LSD and mescaline comes from studies on tolerance. Tolerance to all the effects of LSD develops fairly rapidly, and the same is true for mescaline. In addition, there is cross-tolerance between LSD, mescaline, and other drugs of this class (Abraham, Aldridge, & Gogia, 1996), suggesting a common mechanism of action. Finally, mescaline, like LSD, is an agonist at the specialized group of serotonin receptor subtypes called 5-HT2A receptors, providing further support that these receptors play an important role in mediating the visual hallucinations common to all the drugs in this class (Meyer & Quenzer, 2005).

As we noted in Chapter 3, serotonin is distributed widely in the brain. This may account for the enormously varied effects of LSD-like hallucinogens. Serotonin is thought to play an important role in mood, which is consistent with the powerful emotional effects of these drugs. The precise areas of the brain responsible for the hallucinogenic actions of these drugs remain open to debate. Interestingly, many drugs that affect serotonin do *not* produce hallucinations (e.g., MDMA, SSRI antidepressants), and thus many questions remain regarding just how serotonergic hallucinogens produce their remarkable effects on visual experience (Iversen et al., 2009).

Pharmacokinetics of LSD-Like Drugs

As we have noted, all the hallucinogens that act on serotonin receptors have similar effects. However, these drugs differ widely in potency, duration of action, and other pharmacokinetic variables. LSD is the most potent of the class, with oral doses as small as 25 micrograms producing effects. Street doses range from about 12 to 350 micrograms and are prepared by placing a small amount of LSD solution in a gel (windowpane), in a tablet, or, most commonly, on paper (blotter) with colorful cartoon designs (Dal Cason & Franzosa, 2003). LSD is rapidly absorbed, and subjective effects are usually noted within 20 to 60 minutes after consumption. The drug is distributed throughout the body and readily penetrates the blood-brain barrier. The effects of LSD persist for 8 to 12 hours, and the drug is rapidly metabolized and eliminated from the body. Even the most sensitive techniques can detect LSD or its metabolites in urine for no longer than 72 hours after use (Hawks & Chiang, 1986). Although the hallucinogen found in morning glory seeds (lysergic acid amide) is similar to LSD, it is far less potent—perhaps 10% as strong as LSD (Julien, Advokat, & Comaty, 2008).

People normally take psilocybin orally by either eating the mushrooms or drinking a brew containing them. It is difficult to specify doses because the amount of psilocybin varies depending on the species of mushroom, among other things. Typically, 5 to 10 grams of mushrooms are taken, which contain 10 to 20 milligrams of psilocybin. Thus, psilocybin is about 1% as potent as LSD. The duration of action is about four to six hours. As is true of virtually all the serotonergic hallucinogens, tolerance develops to both LSD and psilocybin, and both show cross-tolerance with each other as well as with other members of the class (Grinspoon & Bakalar, 1979).

Mescaline is normally taken by consuming peyote buttons, as described. Usually 5 to 20 buttons are eaten, delivering 200 to 800 milligrams of mescaline. Mescaline is about 1/3000 as potent as LSD, with 200 milligrams considered an effective dose. Duration of action is about 10 to 14 hours (Strassman, 2005).

Less information is available about the other serotonergic hallucinogens, but most are similar. One noteworthy exception is dimethyltryptamine (DMT), which is usually taken by using the bark of the Virola as a snuff or by smoking. Its effects begin within minutes of use but persist for only about 60 minutes (Dal Cason & Franzosa, 2003).

Psychotherapeutic Uses

LSD and the related hallucinogens historically have been thought to have two applications in psychotherapy but neither is well accepted today. One notion was that LSD produced a model psychosis and that psychotherapists would benefit from having experiences similar to those of their patients. It is true that hallucinations, unusual affective reactions, and loss of reality contact are characteristics of both schizophrenia and hallucinogenic experiences, but there also are important differences. For example, the hallucinations experienced under the influence of LSD are primarily visual, whereas those of schizophrenics are usually auditory (Strassman, 2005), so the subjective experiences of the psychotic are certainly not identical to those of the hallucinogen user. An intriguing similarity is that chlorpromazine and the other antipsychotics used in the treatment of schizophrenia are effective antagonists of LSD effects. Thus, hallucinogens may yet provide clues about the biochemistry of mental disorders (e.g., Marona-Lewicka, Thisted, & Nichols, 2005).

Paradoxically, the other major application of hallucinogens has been its use as an adjunct to psychotherapy. The general idea was that therapists would be able to learn important information when their patients were using LSD and that the patients would be better able to gain insight into their condition because LSD could break down ego defenses. Many extravagant claims have been made about the benefits of LSD for mental health and spiritual development, but the use of LSD in psychotherapy gradually has declined. Although one important reason for this was the political climate, another was that most therapists thought the potential risks of LSD outweighed the benefits. In fact, it never has been demonstrated scientifically that the use of LSD is superior to placebo as an adjunct to psychotherapy. Some therapists think these drugs deserve further evaluation as possible psychotherapeutic agents (Grinspoon & Bakalar, 1983; Strassman, 2005), but the current controversy has shifted to the related drug MDMA or Ecstasy (see a later discussion in this chapter).

Effects of Serotonergic Hallucinogens

The physiological effects of LSD and related hallucinogens are generally similar to those of amphetamine and cocaine; that is, they are sympathomimetic. Thus, the effects include pupil dilation, increased heart rate and blood pressure, increased body temperature, and increased sweating (Grinspoon & Bakalar, 1979).

The psychological effects are more difficult to characterize. Experiences with hallucinogens are tremendously variable among individuals and may vary from one experience to the next for a single individual. Common to all the serotonergic hallucinogens are profound changes in visual perception, although there is some consistency in the types of visual changes that occur. Many were summarized by Albert Hofmann (1980) in his account of his first LSD trip described earlier:

> Kaleidoscopic fantastic images surged in on me, alternating, variegated, opening, and then closing themselves in circles and spirals, exploding in colored fountains, rearranging and hybridizing themselves in constant flux. It was particularly remarkable how every acoustic perception, such as the sound of a door handle or a passing automobile, became transformed into optical perceptions. Every sound generated a vividly changing image, with its own consistent form and color. (p. 19)

The spiral explosions and vortex patterns Hofmann described have been noted by Siegel (1992) to be among the most common forms in hallucinogenic experiences. Siegel calls them form constants because they are reported so frequently, not only in drug-induced states but also in hallucinations experienced by people with medical conditions such as migraine headache and high fever. Siegel noted another form constant, the lattice pattern: a checkerboard pattern that appears in an otherwise plain surface. The experience of sensing a sound stimulus as a visual one that Hofmann described is called **synesthesia**, and others have reported it as well. Other visual effects are flashing lights, increased brightness and saturation of colors, trails or plumes around objects, and the sense of movement in stable objects (for example, the wall breathes or moves rhythmically). Visual patterns may be come to be seen as familiar or unfamiliar images that may be perceived as in motion (see Strassman, 2005, for a review).

synesthesia
An effect sometimes produced by hallucinogens that is characterized by the perception of a stimulus in a modality other than the one in which it was presented (for example, a subject may report "seeing" music).

There is a good bit more to the "trip" than just a light show, however. Other perceptions may be altered. Mood is extremely labile, and bizarre cognitive experiences occur (Stevens, 1987). Some examples of such experiences are described in the Contemporary Issue Box 12.2. Although the descriptions recounted are quite different, they do reveal some similarities. All are characterized by strong affect, although the nature of the emotional state varies. All involve "magical" thinking and, particularly in the last two, events are fraught with cosmic significance. If the visions are terrifying (as in the second quote), the subject may behave in a psychotic manner; this is usually referred to as a bad or bum trip. The insights, enlightenments, and beliefs that occur and seem so significant during the trip often turn out to be trivial or false afterward. For example, users are often convinced they possess telepathic or clairvoyant abilities under the influence of the drug, but when tested, these abilities are not present. Nonetheless, it is easy to see how such experiences must have led prescientific cultures to attach mystical and religious significance to hallucinogens.

Adverse Effects of Serotonergic Hallucinogens

The LSD controversy revolves around the adverse effects of its use. One major concern about LSD use involved the claim that it produced chromosome damage—that those who used the drug, male or female, would stand a high risk of having deformed children. This concern was based on a study that found that LSD produced chromosome breaks in white blood cells artificially cultured in the laboratory. The study

CONTEMPORARY ISSUE BOX 12.2

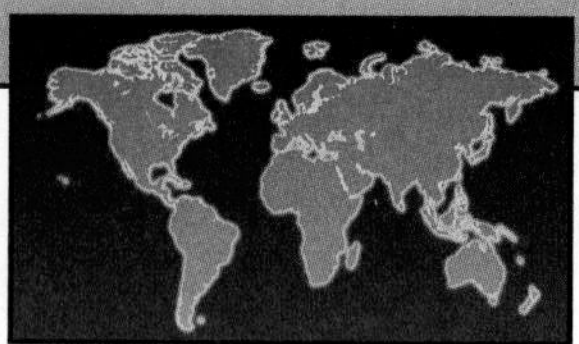

Descriptions of the Subjective Effects of LSD

Many attempts have been made to describe the effects and experiences produced by LSD. Such accounts are remarkably diverse, often confusing, and sometimes contradictory, yet some features are common. The following are vivid recollections given by well-known LSD users, illustrating the variety of the experience.

> I looked into the glass of water. In its swirling depths was a vortex which went down the center of the world and the heart of time. . . . A dog barked and its piercing howl might have been all the wolves in Tartary. . . . At one moment I would be a giant in a tiny cupboard, and the next, a dwarf in a huge hall. (Humphrey Osmond on mescaline, in Grinspoon & Bakalar, 1979, p. 100)
>
> I was lying on my back on the floor. Then the room itself vanished and I was sinking, sinking, sinking. From far away I heard very faintly the word "death." I sank faster, turning and falling a million light years from the earth. The word got louder and more insistent. It took shape around me, closing me in. "DEATH . . . DEATH . . . DEATH." I thought of the dread in my father's eyes in his final hours. At the last instant before my own death I shouted, "No." Absolute terror, total horror. ([Richard] Lingeman on LSD, in Grinspoon & Bakalar, 1979, p. 112)
>
> Now a series of visions began. The imagery appeared to synchronize with the phonograph music. . . . I envisioned myself at the court of Kubla Khan . . . at a concert being held in an immense auditorium . . . in some futuristic Utopia . . . at Versailles . . . at a statue of Lincoln. . . . I felt myself engulfed in a chaotic, turbulent sea. . . . There were a number of small boats tossing on the raging sea . . . [I was] in one of these vessels . . . we came upon a gigantic figure standing waist-deep in the churning waters. . . . His facial features were graced by an unforgettable look of compassion, love, and concern. We knew that this was the image of God. We realized that God, too, was caught in the storm. ([Stanley] Krippner on psilocybin, in Grinspoon & Bakalar, 1979, pp. 100–101)

raised fears that LSD also might damage human gametes (Cohen & Marmillo, 1967). However, breaking chromosomes in white cells in a test tube under high doses of LSD has not been shown to generalize to in vivo conditions. After considerable research into this question, there is no convincing evidence that LSD (or any other serotonergic hallucinogen) increases birth defects in offspring when taken in normal doses (Wiegand, Thai, & Benowitz, 2008). As with most drugs, however, there is risk of fetal damage if taken by pregnant women (Grinspoon & Bakalar, 1979).

Other adverse effects of LSD and related hallucinogens are more cause for concern. An important problem has been acute panic or paranoid reactions to the drug. These bad trips can leave individuals in an acute psychotic state during which they may harm themselves or others. The frequency of bad trips is difficult to estimate, but it was high enough in the 1960s to lead to the widespread development of walk-in crisis centers where victims could be brought for reassurance (talking the subject down) and, if necessary, hospital referral. Bad trips appear to be less frequent today, perhaps because more is known about how to prevent them. The psychological state of the user and the environmental setting are important. For example, one of the few documented LSD suicides took place after a man was administered LSD without his knowledge in an experiment conducted by the CIA in the 1950s (Grinspoon & Bakalar, 1979). Being exposed to the drug without foreknowledge is apparently frightening and disturbing. Individuals seem to be less likely to have bad trips if they are aware and frequently reminded that they are under the influence of a drug. A calm and comfortable setting and low doses of LSD are thought to reduce the frequency of bad trips as well, although bad trips may occur even under the best of circumstances (Abraham, Aldridge, & Gogia, 1996).

DRUGS AND CULTURE BOX 12.3

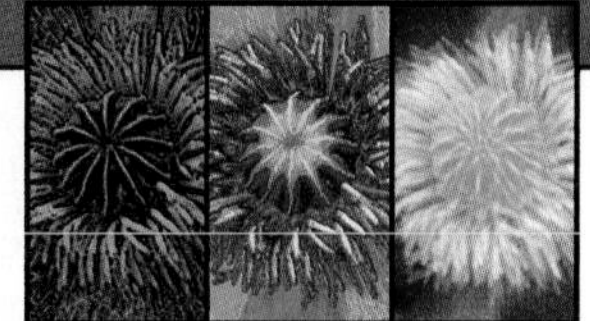

Hallucinogenic Ibogaine: New Rx for Addiction?

Tabernathe iboga is a shrub native to West Africa. Several tribal groups in the region made up of Cameroon, Congo, and Gabon have used this plant for many centuries for its hallucinogenic properties. The bark of the iboga root is eaten in ceremonies by members of the Bwiti religion who believe that the plant produces divine visions and permits them to commune with their ancestors. Iboga contains a number of psychoactive chemicals, but the critical component isolated from the bark preparation seems to be the chemical ibogaine. Although ibogaine is generally classified as a serotonergic hallucinogen (see previous discussion), recent studies have suggested that its neurochemical actions may be more complex, including effects on glutamate, endorphin, and dopamine pathways (Vastag, 2005). In recent years, ibogaine has become quite controversial because of claims that it may be of value in the treatment of addiction. Anecdotes from ex-addicts who believe that ibogaine visions helped in their recovery from dependency on alcohol, cocaine, and heroin have circulated since the 1960s, and although interest in this possibility has increased in recent years, there has been very little research on it. Most treatment experts are skeptical of these claims, but certainly studies are needed. As Frank Vocci, director of antiaddiction drug development for the National Institute on Drug Abuse (NIDA), put it: "There's basically a vast uncontrolled experiment going on out there" (Vastag, 2005, p. 345). Some data show that ibogaine can reduce alcohol consumption in rats (Rezvani et al., 2003), but until controlled clinical outcome studies are available, ibogaine treatment will remain controversial.

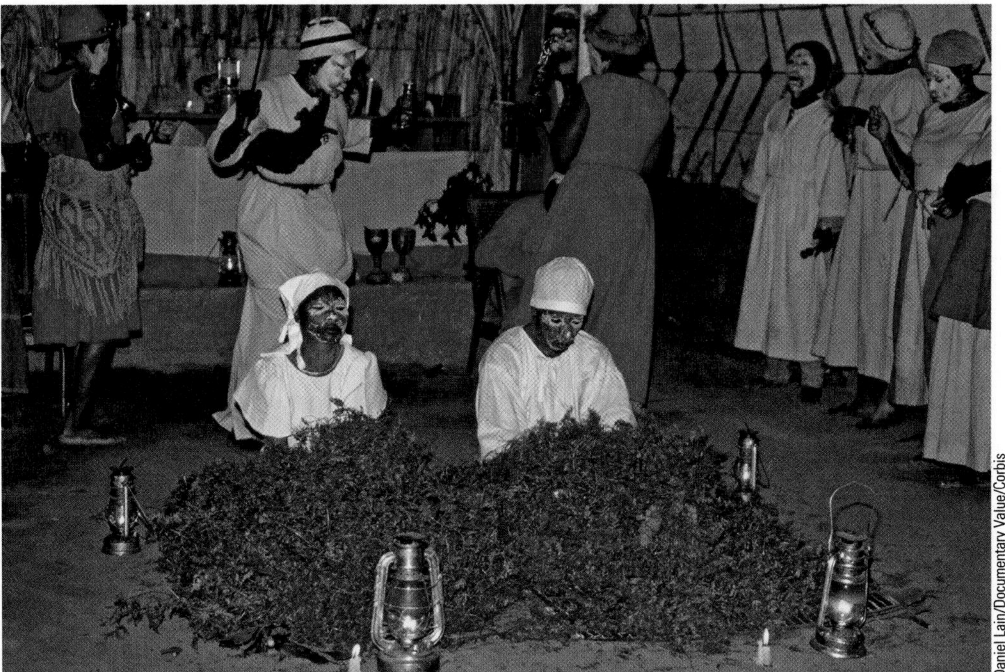

Daniel Lain/Documentary Value/Corbis

Hallucinogenic iboga root is eaten by West Africans who follow the Bwiti religion.

Another problem associated with LSD use is a phenomenon known as the **flashback**. Flashbacks are a reexperience of some aspect of a hallucinogenic trip that may have occurred months or even years before. The nature of the experience usually involves visual disturbances such as flashes of color, trails in the visual field, or fleeting perceptions in the peripheral field of view. Flashbacks are often brought on by stress, fatigue, entering

flashback
A sudden recurrence of an LSD-like experience.

a dark environment, or marijuana use (Abraham, Aldridge, & Gogia, 1996). In a review, Halpern and Pope (2003) noted that it is difficult to estimate the frequency of flashbacks. In most cases, it appears that users do not find their flashbacks to be problematic, and so, no doubt, many go unreported. In unusual cases, flashbacks can be frequent and severe and may disrupt the individual's life. The DSM-IV diagnosis of hallucinogen persisting perception disorder is applied to such cases. Very rarely, the visual distortions are nearly constant and may reflect permanent loss of serotonergic neurons. Treatment with antipsychotics or benzodiazepines may relieve the symptoms of such cases (Halpern & Pope, 2003; Young, 1997).

LSD also has been linked to long-term psychiatric disorders. Perhaps the most publicized and horrifying example is Charles Manson and his "family." The Manson family used LSD heavily, but it is unclear what role, if any, the drug played in the development of their psychopathology and subsequent mass murders. When one is confronted with a psychotic individual who has used LSD, it is difficult to determine whether LSD caused the psychosis or the person was psychotic to begin with and LSD made the symptoms more flagrant. To complicate matters further, most users of LSD who are diagnosed as psychotic have extensive histories with other drugs as well, and the role these other drugs may have played is rarely certain. It generally is agreed that hallucinogens may precipitate or exacerbate psychosis or emotional disturbance in certain vulnerable individuals. LSD has also been linked to chronic psychiatric disorders in rare cases. Then, the controversy focuses on the precise role of LSD and related hallucinogens. Some have argued that LSD may be capable of producing psychosis even in the absence of other predisposing conditions, but the general consensus seems to be that, when chronic psychiatric problems occur following serotonergic hallucinogen use, it generally involves individuals who had already been diagnosed with or have manifested psychotic or prepsychotic symptoms before the drug use (Halpern & Pope, 1999; Wiegand, Thai & Benowitz, 2008).

Methylated Amphetamines

Overview

MDMA (Ecstasy) has become perhaps the most controversial illegal drug in our society today. One reason was its rapid increase in popularity in the late 1990s. Prior to 1996, the annual high school senior survey did not even have a specific category for MDMA; in that year, 4.6% of America's high school seniors reported having used it during the past year. That number rose explosively, doubling by 2001, when 9.2% reported using it; after that peak, however, use declined and has leveled off in recent years (see Figure 12.1; Johnston et al., 2009a). One important reason for this decline is the publicity about the many adverse effects of MDMA, including claims that it may produce brain damage and death. These claims, in turn, have generated considerable controversy and a tremendous amount of research on MDMA in the past few years. We discuss this in some detail because of the importance of this drug on college campuses today.

MDMA is one of a group of drugs known as methylated amphetamines because of their chemical structures. Dozens of drugs fall into this category, and the more well-known variations are listed in Table 12.2. These drugs are often categorized with the serotonergic hallucinogens, and indeed their chemical structures resemble that of mescaline. In addition, they influence serotonin transmission, and also dopamine and norepinephrine (Morton, 2005). DOM (2,5-dimethoxy-4 methylamphetamine) not only resembles mescaline in structure but also produces similar effects, including visual hallucinations.

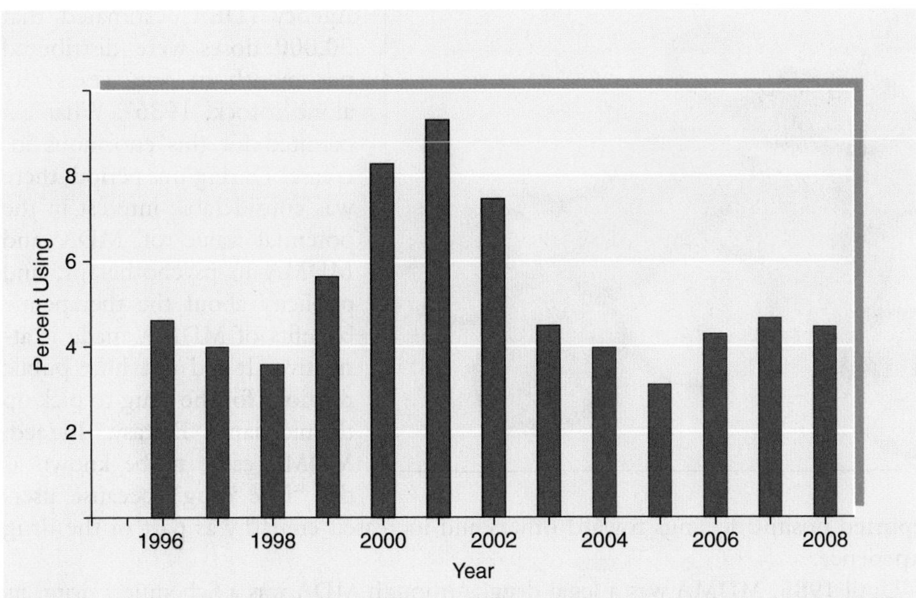

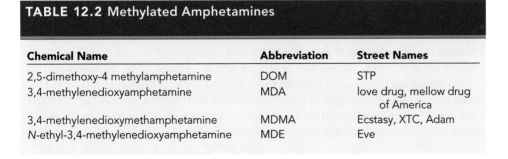

FIGURE 12.1
Percent high school seniors reporting MDMA use during their senior year (Johnston et al. 2009a)

The others (MDA, MDMA, MDE) are more similar to amphetamine in effects (see Chapter 6) and differ from the serotonergic hallucinogens in that they produce few or no visual hallucinations. The effects of MDA and MDMA seem to be primarily a mild euphoria accompanied by openness, feelings of warmth and empathy, and lack of defensiveness. These properties led some psychotherapists to advocate the use of these drugs, particularly MDMA, as an adjunct to therapy. Some scientists classify MDMA with the hallucinogens, others with the amphetamines, and still others consider these drugs as belonging to a unique category (Cohen, 1998).

History and Epidemiology

Methylated amphetamines were developed in the early 1900s, but attracted little attention until relatively recently. For example, MDMA was patented in 1914, by Merck Pharmaceuticals in Germany, but the drug was not marketed or even much studied until many years later (Iversen, 2008). DOM was first reported on the street in the late 1960s, when its potent hallucinogenic effects and very long duration of action (as long as 24 hours) led to many bad trips. MDA also surfaced on the street about this time, but it had a better reception. It was called "mellow drug of America" because it has fewer perceptual effects than LSD. The use of MDA declined along with LSD in the 1970s, whereas MDMA began to increase in popularity. In 1976, an estimated 10,000 doses of MDMA were used in the United States. In 1985, the Drug Enforcement

TABLE 12.2 Methylated Amphetamines

Chemical Name	Abbreviation	Street Names
2,5-dimethoxy-4 methylamphetamine	DOM	STP
3,4-methylenedioxyamphetamine	MDA	love drug, mellow drug of America
3,4-methylenedioxymethamphetamine	MDMA	Ecstasy, XTC, Adam
N-ethyl-3,4-methylenedioxyamphetamine	MDE	Eve

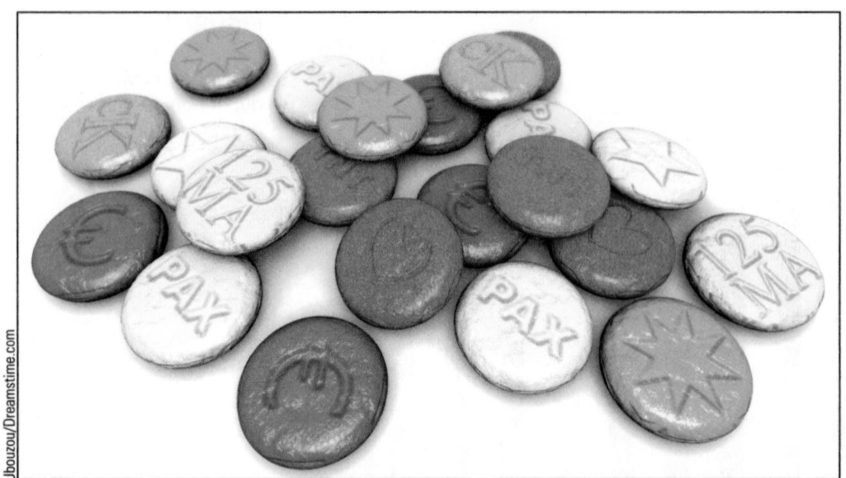

Jbouzou/Dreamstime.com

Ecstasy tablets

Agency (DEA) estimated that 30,000 doses were distributed per month in one Texas city alone (Stock, 1986). What accounted for this enormous increase? During this period, there was considerable interest in the potential value of MDA and MDMA in psychotherapy, and publicity about the therapeutic benefits of MDMA made it attractive. It did not hurt public relations for the drug to pick up the nickname "Ecstasy." Indeed, MDMA came to be known as the "love drug" because users reported positive feelings toward others and increased empathy as part of the drug experience.

Until 1985, MDMA was a legal drug. Although MDA was a Schedule I drug, its close relative MDMA had not yet been classified. Thus, dealers preferred the low risks associated with the designer drug Ecstasy. In the face of the explosive rise in MDMA use, coupled with animal research implicating the drug in brain damage, however, the DEA classified MDMA as Schedule I in 1985, on an emergency basis. Amid considerable controversy over whether MDMA had legitimate medical uses, this decision was affirmed in 1986, and MDMA was permanently placed in Schedule I (Holland, 2001).

MDMA grew in popularity as it became associated with the "club" or "rave" subcultures. Originating in Europe in the late 1980s, the rave movement swept rapidly through the United States, and indeed much of the world, in the 1990s (Holland, 2001). Raves were usually large-scale, all-night dance parties featuring "techno," "house," or "trance" musical styles often accompanied by light shows. Alcohol was rarely associated with raves; rather, the "club drugs" tended to be drugs like MDMA, methamphetamine, Ritalin (see Chapter 6), LSD, and GHB (see Chapter 14). Bright fluorescent clothing and jewelry along with paraphernalia such as pacifiers (to avoid teeth grinding or bruxism, a side effect of MDMA) were common, and the settings varied from empty warehouses, airplane hangers, and open fields to smaller venues such as clubs. The popularity of raves declined in the late 1990s, but by the early 2000s, MDMA was the fastest-growing illicit drug across the United States, western Europe, and Australia (Inciardi, 2002), and had become known as the prototype of club drugs. Even considering the recent decline in use noted among U.S. high school seniors (see Figure 12.1), MDMA remains one of the most world's most popular recreational drugs. After marijuana, it is the most widely used illegal drug in Europe, and more than 8 million people are thought to have used MDMA at least once (Morton, 2005).

"The rave scene is crazy, fun, dangerous—yet exciting. It's deadly. It's happening. It's all about how you dress and how you dance. It's about standing out and meeting people and just being able to live your youth."

Rave attendee (Cohen, 1998)

Effects of Methylated Amphetamines

The effects of MDMA, MDA, and MDE are similar enough to be discussed together (DOM effects are like those of mescaline or LSD and are not considered further). These drugs are usually taken orally but can be injected or absorbed intranasally (snorted). They are absorbed rapidly, and their duration of action is about six to eight hours. The neural mechanisms of action involve increased release of monoamines, particularly serotonin. MDMA also blocks the reuptake of serotonin and, to a lesser extent, dopamine.

Thus, there is an initial overall increase in serotonin and dopamine activity after taking the drug, but this is followed after several hours by a marked decrease in serotonin activity (Iversen, 2008). At effective doses (75 to 150 mg for MDMA, 50 to 150 mg for MDA, 1 to 2 mg for MDE), these drugs produce clear sympathomimetic effects, including increased heart rate, blood pressure, and pupil dilation. Additional physical effects include muscle tension, teeth grinding (bruxism), increased body temperature, appetite suppression, and insomnia—effects remarkably similar to those of amphetamine (Freedman, Johanson, & Tancer, 2005). The psychological effects claimed for these drugs are euphoria, increased emotional warmth and empathy, lowered defensiveness, and increases in verbal behavior (Bravo, 2001). Hallucinations are uncommon or absent at ordinary doses. Few experiments have directly compared the psychological effects of MDMA to amphetamine, but Tancer and Johanson (2003) studied young adults under various doses of both drugs. Participants reported stronger reinforcing effects for MDMA than amphetamine at all doses tested, and they also consistently reported that they liked MDMA better. The profile of MDMA effects were generally quite similar to those of amphetamine, so in the Tancer and Johanson (2003) study, the main difference was a preference for the MDMA drug effect over amphetamine.

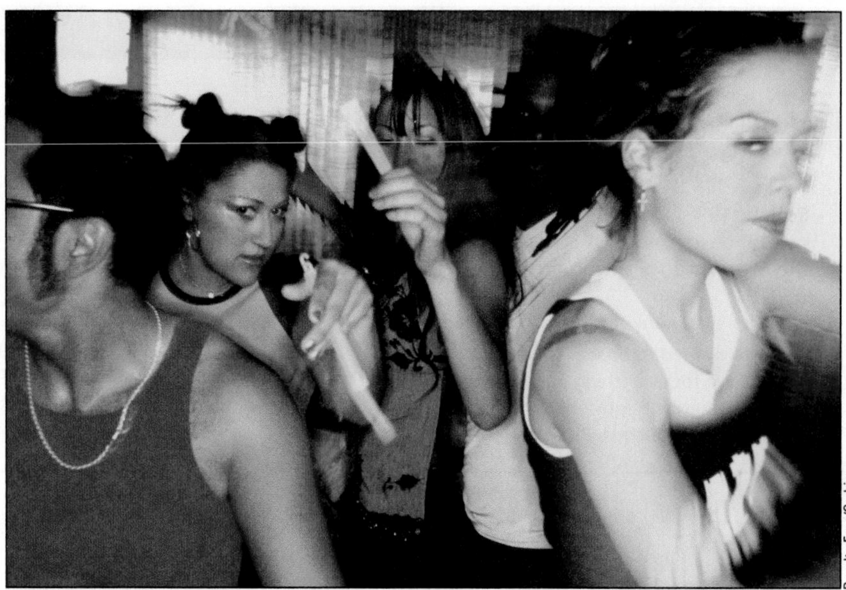

Royalty-Free/Corbis

The club scene is associated with LSD and ecstasy.

A clinical description of this sort does not capture the allure of MDMA. Remember that both the user and the setting determine the effects of any drug. For MDMA, the setting often includes the pulsing rhythm of techno music, strobe lights, dancing, and bonding with other individuals. The combination of drug and setting produces effects that users sometimes describe as a trancelike state with feelings of peace and unity. Researchers have interviewed hundreds of MDMA users about their experiences, and some excerpts from their descriptions are given in the Drugs and Culture Box 12.4. Because of these desirable effects, some users develop a pattern of heavy, binge use. Although MDMA is not associated with dramatic physical withdrawal symptoms, commonly reported aftereffects include drowsiness, muscle pain, depression, paranoia, and anxiety (Hegadoren, Baker, & Bourin, 1999). These effects typically dissipate within a few days but can be more persistent in some cases.

The belief that MDMA might enhance communicative ability and empathy and decrease defensiveness led some therapists to advocate the use of these drugs as an adjunct to psychotherapy. The logic was much the same as that described for LSD therapy, but because MDMA does not produce hallucinations or the dissociation of LSD, it was seen as less likely to produce adverse reactions. Although some therapists involved in this work reported that MDMA was beneficial (Naranjo, 2001; Riedlinger & Montagne, 2001), controlled studies are lacking, so little experimental evidence supports the value of MDMA (or any other drugs of this class) in psychotherapy. Recent

DRUGS AND CULTURE BOX 12.4

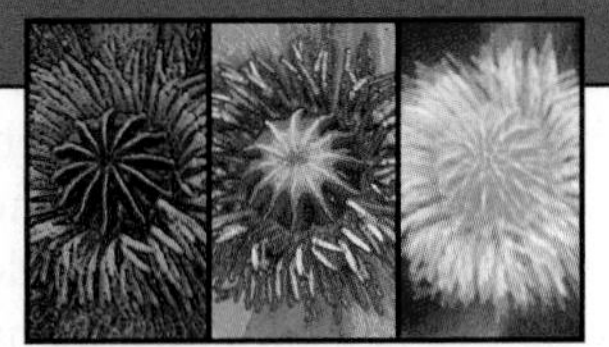

Voices of Ecstasy

Cohen (1998) and Iversen (2008) have published several descriptions of MDMA users' experiences on the drug. The following are some brief excerpts:

> "Ecstasy is more or less a happy speed."
> "All I wanted to do was smile. I was so wide awake, and I felt love for everything and everyone."
> "Pure energy. Happy energy. I felt tingly all over. It felt good to be touched. Being touched was so intense."
> "It made me able to let my guard down and reveal my true self. I did experience mood fluctuations (ups and downs)."
> "Everyone was my friend. I don't think that anything could have brought me down. I loved it."
> "I had a bad experience. I felt like I was surrounded by water and drowning. It must have been panic."
> "Floating, flying, highly sexual. I felt like I was on this really high mountain and I just wanted to stay there."
> "It was the most euphoric experience of my life."

years have seen a renewed interest in the possibility of MDMA therapy, and controlled trials are underway to determine whether MDMA is of value in the treatment of post-traumatic stress syndrome and other psychological disorders (c.f., Bouso et al., 2008).

Toxicity

The increased use of MDMA in the late 1990s was associated with reports of toxic reactions and deaths. Toxic reactions include dehydration, heatstroke and heat exhaustion, muscle breakdown, kidney failure, stroke, seizures, and heart attacks (Eede et al., 2009; Ghatol & Kazory, 2009). Most toxic reactions to MDMA occur after high doses or multiple doses (stacking) have been ingested, but in some cases, serious reactions and even deaths have occurred after relatively low doses (Hegadoren, Baker, & Bourin, 1999; Schifano, 2004). The toxic effects of MDMA are often related to elevated body temperature, and the pharmacological effects of the drug may be compounded by intense physical activity of users and by the high temperatures of many clubs. Users are often advised to drink fluids to avoid dehydration and overheating, but some MDMA emergency cases have involved collapse due to low sodium levels, possibly caused by excessive fluid intake altering the salt balance (Schifano, 2004). Complicating our ability to evaluate toxic reactions to MDMA is the fact that tablets sold on the street as MDMA often contain other drugs that may also be toxic in some cases. Adulterants are so common in street MDMA that one organization (DanceSafe) maintains a website with pictures of commonly sold MDMA tablets along with the results of their chemical analysis. Many different compounds have been revealed in these analyses; among the more common adulterants in samples posted in the first half of 2009 were benzodiazepines, methamphetamine, caffeine, ketamine, and dextromethorphan. Interestingly, many of the samples contained no active chemical at all (see Parrott, 2004)!

Residual Effects of MDMA

One of the major controversies about MDMA and other methylated amphetamines concerns the possibility that they may produce long-term damage of certain brain structures. The report sounding the alarm (Ricaurte et al., 1985) showed that, after several administrations of high doses of MDA, rats had a depletion of serotonin apparently caused by the degeneration of serotonergic neuron terminals. Similar results have now been reported for MDMA in several species, including primates, and it appears that the neurotoxic effects can be produced after a single high dose (20 mg/kg) is administered or after several lower doses (5 mg/kg) are administered over consecutive days (Bauman, Wang, & Rothman, 2007). One criticism of this work is that even the doses considered moderate in these animal studies are higher than doses generally used on the street. This point is somewhat difficult to evaluate in that MDMA tablets vary enormously in the dose contained. In a worldwide survey, Parrott (2004) found that most pills sold as MDMA contained an average of 70 to 100 mg MDMA, which would deliver between 1 to 2 mg/kg to an adult human depending on body weight. This is below the dose range shown to be neurotoxic in nonhumans. However, some tablets have contained up to 300 mg (according to information on www.dancesafe.org), and many users take multiple tablets during the course of an evening; two or three tablets could certainly deliver a dose capable of producing neurotoxic effects. Indeed, some users report commonly taking 15 or more tablets in a night, and this would likely produce doses well above those shown to produce long-term serotonin deficits in nonhumans (Schifano, 2004). Of course, human users may take lower doses of MDMA but take them many times, intermittently, over many years, and we do not yet know what neural consequences may occur following this pattern of use. How rapidly neurons recover from the toxic effects of the drugs is also open to debate, but one study showed effects that persisted for as long as seven years after drug administration in primates (Hatzidimitriou, McCann, & Ricaurte, 1999). As noted in Chapter 3, serotonin is a neurotransmitter that modulates sleep, mood, and many other functions, so depletion of serotonin could lead to serious problems. Thus, whether MDMA produces these neurotoxic effects in humans is a critical issue.

As you might imagine, in recent years, many researchers have attempted to determine whether MDMA users show evidence of brain damage or other residual effects. Numerous studies have used brain imaging technology such as PET and SPECT techniques (see Chapter 3) and consistently have found reductions in serotonergic functioning between heavy MDMA users and controls; however, there is also evidence that the serotonin system recovers from these effects after a period of abstinence (McCann et al., 2005; Selvaraj et al, 2009).

Although ecstasy users do show evidence of serotonin neurotoxicity, the functional significance of these neural changes has been controversial. Dozens of studies have compared MDMA users and controls on tests of mood, psychopathology, memory, and attention. In many of these studies, heavy users of MDMA showed more evidence of sleep problems, depressed mood, and memory as well as related cognitive deficits when compared to nonusers (see Morton, 2005, for a review). Of course, these studies have many interpretive problems. For example, the accuracy of the drug histories used to form the groups is open to question. As noted, many different drugs are sold as MDMA, and some of these may produce more toxicity than MDMA alone.

It is also difficult to determine from study results whether the differences between users and nonusers are actually caused by MDMA. MDMA users may differ in many respects from the nonusing control sample, and these other differences may influence the measured variables. For example, most MDMA users also use other drugs, and in many studies, the MDMA user group differs from the control group with respect to overall drug use—not just MDMA. The potential importance of such a confound has been demonstrated in some recent studies. Parrott et al. (2001) studied 618 polydrug users and 150 nonusers in England and Italy. In keeping with the studies reviewed here, they found that heavy MDMA users showed more evidence of psychopathology than nonusers. However, drug users who did not report using MDMA did not differ from MDMA users in psychopathology, so the role of MDMA use was unclear. These findings have been replicated by Daumann et al. (2004) and by a study that focused on depressive symptoms (Roiser & Sahakian, 2004). In summary, frequent MDMA users generally show more psychopathology (particularly depression) than controls who do not report use of illegal drugs, but when compared to polydrug users or marijuana users who do not use MDMA, these differences tend to disappear.

Similar results have been obtained with respect to cognitive impairments associated with MDMA use. For example, several studies (Croft et al., 2001; Dafters, Hoshi, & Talbot, 2004; de Sola et al., 2008) have compared groups of MDMA users (who also reported marijuana use) with groups of participants who reported only marijuana use and with control groups who did not use drugs on various neuropsychological tests. MDMA users performed more poorly than controls on tests of attention and memory, but the participants who used marijuana only were equally impaired. These studies suggest that the memory deficits often reported in MDMA users might have been caused by their coincident use of marijuana. However, other researchers have found that MDMA users showed more severe deficits on memory and other cognitive tasks than control participants matched for drug use other than MDMA (Dafters, 2006; Daumann et al., 2005; Halpern et al., 2004), so it remains possible that MDMA use may play a role.

In sum, the jury is still out on what long-term effects are associated with MDMA use. Although scientific opinion does not support the "horror scenarios of our kids' brains rotting out by the time they were 30" touted by the media in the 1990s (Iversen, 2008), neither does it support the notion that MDMA is a safe drug. On the contrary, MDMA and related drugs pose risks of acute toxic effects and possible deficits in neuropsychological functioning, particularly among heavy users.

Anticholinergic Hallucinogens

atropine An anticholinergic hallucinogen found in certain plants.

scopolamine An anticholinergic hallucinogen found in certain plants.

Atropine and **scopolamine** are drugs that block acetylcholine receptors in the brain. In low doses these drugs are used for a variety of medical purposes, and atropine in particular has been in the news recently because it is standard issue to troops in the Middle East where there is risk of nerve gas attack. Deadly nerve gases (sarin and soman) are toxic because they inhibit the enzyme that breaks down acetylcholine, and as an acetylcholine antagonist, atropine is an antidote if administered rapidly after exposure. However, drugs like atropine and scopolamine also can produce hallucinogenic effects. They are found in a number of plants known throughout the world and have a long history of use. Hundreds of years before the birth of Christ, the ancient Greeks at the oracle of Delphi used plants containing scopolamine and atropine. In the Middle Ages, such plants were included in the infamous witches' brews. Plants such as belladonna, also called deadly nightshade (*Atropa belladonna*); mandrake (*Mandragora officinarum*); henbane (*Hyoscyamus niger*) of Europe; jimsonweed (*Datura stramonium*); and other plants of the *Datura* genus from the New World have been eaten for their hallucinogenic properties (Schultes, 1976). Although these drugs are not widely used for witchcraft today, *Datura* is allegedly one of the ingredients in zombie powder in Haiti (Davis, 1988).

Anticholinergic hallucinogens produce a variety of physiological effects, including dry mouth, blurred vision, loss of motor control, and increased heart rate and body temperature. These drugs can be fatal as they cause respiratory failure at doses only slightly higher than the effective dose (Grinspoon & Bakalar, 1979). The psychological experience appears to be a dreamlike trance or stupor. Users seem delirious and confused but may be able to describe visions if asked. A unique feature of the drugs of this class is that memory of the drug experience is poor, and users may be unable to recall any details of the experience. These drugs are rarely seen on the street today.

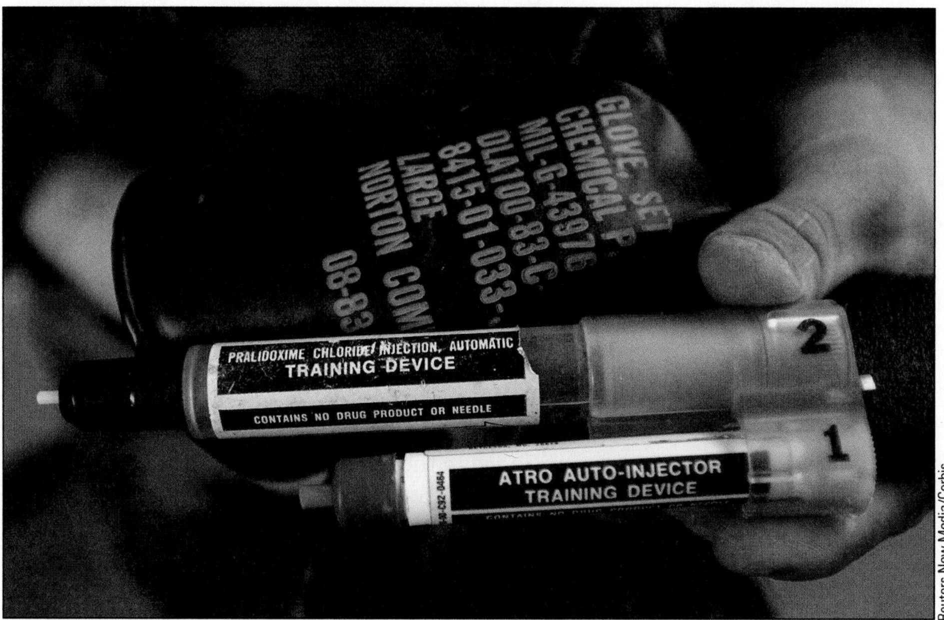

Reuters New Media/Corbis

Atropine auto-injections are provided to soldiers who are at risk of nerve gas attacks.

One additional plant to be discussed in this section is the fly agaric mushroom (*Amanita muscaria*). Fly agaric contains several different hallucinogenic chemicals, including muscarine, which is a cholinergic agonist, and muscimole, a hallucinogen that may be similar to the LSD-like drugs. Although rarely used today, the mushroom represents one of the earliest forms of hallucinogen use. Fly agaric grows throughout much of Europe and Asia, and it may have been the mysterious "Soma" described in the Hindu *Rig-Veda* more than 2,000 years ago. The *Rig-Veda* describes the rather bizarre practice of recycling the drug effect by drinking the urine of the intoxicated individual. Muscimole is the only hallucinogen known that passes unchanged through the system into the urine (Wasson, 1979). The effects of the mushroom are unique among hallucinogens. Users of the fly agaric typically fall into a stupor for several hours during which they experience visions, and later they experience intense euphoria and energy accompanied by visual hallucinations (Ibid.).

Dissociative Anesthetic Hallucinogens

History

The final class of hallucinogens to be considered is a large group, but only two of its members, **phencyclidine** (PCP, angel dust) and its close analogue **ketamine** (special K, vitamin K), have been used enough to warrant discussion here. PCP was synthesized in 1956, and was tested as an anesthetic because it had pronounced tranquilizing effects. With animals, it produced a general anesthesia that left the animal conscious but not feeling pain, even during surgery. In clinical trials of PCP and ketamine with humans, however, some patients experienced hyperexcitability, delirium, and visual disturbances. Thus, these drugs were largely abandoned for human use, although both were marketed for use as anesthetics and tranquilizers in veterinary medicine (Dal Cason & Franzosa, 2003; Linder, Lerner, & Burns, 1981).

phencyclidine
A dissociative anesthetic.

ketamine
A dissociative anesthetic.

PCP emerged in the 1970s as a street drug of preference. Sold under a variety of names, including "angel dust," "hog," "horse tranquilizer," and "lovely," it was often taken as sprinkled powder on a cigarette or joint. Although PCP also is effective taken orally and can be injected, smoking remains the most popular route of administration. By the early 1980s, some surveys were finding that more than 20% of America's high school students had tried PCP. Because of the high incidence of dangerous side effects, PCP became a notorious drug and its use declined. The high school senior surveys indicated that the number of high school seniors who used PCP through the 1990s was near 3%, and by the 2008 survey, this was down to 1.8% reporting they had tried the drug (Johnston et al., 2009a).

Although PCP is no longer extensively used in veterinary medicine, ketamine remains quite popular in this regard, and ketamine abuse appears to be increasing as it is often included among the "club" drugs. Most of the ketamine or "special K" that appears on the street today is diverted from veterinary supplies and is seen as a crystalline powder or in solution. It can be snorted, injected, taken orally, or smoked (Jansen, 2004). Ketamine has not yet been included in the senior survey, so less is known about current levels of use. In one study, Hopfer et al. (2006) reported that over 18% of young clients (18 to 32 years old) in treatment for substance abuse had used ketamine, making it one of the popular club drugs used in this population.

Pharmacokinetics

The mechanism of PCP and ketamine action involves antagonism of a subset of receptors for the excitatory amino acid glutamate (Balazs, Bridges, & Cotman, 2006). PCP is absorbed rapidly after smoking or injection, with peak blood concentrations noted 5 to 15 minutes after smoking. In contrast, peak concentrations are reached two hours after oral administration. The drug remains in the system unmetabolized for more than two days, and PCP is detectable in urine for several weeks after a single use (Hawks & Chiang, 1986).

Effects of PCP and Ketamine

A moderate dose (1 to 10 mg) of the dissociative anesthetics produces feelings of euphoria and numbness resembling alcohol intoxication. Speech may be slurred, and generally there is motor discoordination. Users may be catatonic and rigid with a blank stare or may be aggressive and hyperactive. Effects include profuse sweating, increased heart rate and blood pressure, and rapid jerky eye movements called nystagmus (Linder, Lerner, & Burns, 1981; Young, Lawson, & Gacono, 1987). Subjects often report blurred vision or double vision but rarely visual hallucinations. Rather, there are changes in perception of body image, distortions of the tactile senses, and sometimes dreamlike visions. Consider these descriptions from PCP users:

> It's weirdly hallucinogenic. It makes you go, boy that's steep stairs I have to climb there, that you realized you climb in five minutes you know, and stuff, and it actually feels like you're going to float off the couch and stuff, you know. Your arm is over somewhere. I can remember like crawling down the stairs because the only thing that I trusted was my fingers and my knees. . . .
>
> The most frequent hallucination is that parts of your body are extremely large or extremely small. You can imagine yourself small enough to walk through a keyhole, or you can be lying there and all of a sudden you just hallucinate that your arm is twice the length of your body. (Feldman, Agar, & Beschner, 1979, p. 133)

> My body image was distorted beyond recognition—fantastically elongated pipe-cleaner legs and arms, spindly E.T.-like fingers, and morphing alien-insect head in the mirror. . . . (Jansen, 2004, p. 75)

"In Donna's ketamine eyes the hallway leading to the restroom looked like a tunnel stretching for miles. To make matters more difficult, Donna felt that she was only two feet tall. . . ."

(Siegel, 1992)

These effects, described as being in the "K-hole," normally last four to six hours but are variable and, particularly after high doses, may persist for days or weeks. Overdoses (more than 20 mg) may result in seizures, prolonged coma, and sometimes death from respiratory failure (Carroll, 1990). Like LSD, anesthetic hallucinogens may produce transient psychotic states or "bad trips." Toxic psychosis produced by PCP and ketamine is often characterized by paranoia and sometimes violence and may persist for several days (Young, Lawson, & Gacono, 1987). Long-term cognitive impairments have also been reported for PCP and ketamine (Morgan et al., 2004). Talking the subject down from a bad trip with these drugs generally is difficult. Physical restraint and intensive medical care are often necessary. Dissociative anesthetics are far more likely than other hallucinogens to produce medical or psychiatric complications (Boutros & Bowers, 1996; Morgan et al., 2004; Young, Lawson, & Gacono, 1987).

Salvinorin A (Salvia)

Salvia divinorum is a plant in the sage family that has been cultivated by the Mazatec people of southern Mexico and used in religious ceremonies for many centuries. Traditionally, salvia was ingested by chewing the leaves or drinking a tea brewed from them. Today, the leaves are often dried and smoked, and concentrated extracts are also available for oral use or smoking. Use of salvia was virtually unheard of 10 years ago in the United States, but use has grown rapidly in recent years. Because it is not a scheduled drug in the United States, salvia can be sold legally in many states (it is illegal in Delaware, Florida, Illinois, Kansas, Louisiana, Mississippi, Missouri, North Carolina, North Dakota, Ohio, Oklahoma, South Dakota, Tennessee, and Virginia and several other states are reviewing salvia's status). A recent national survey indicated that 1.8 million people had tried the drug (SAMHSA, 2008). Literally thousands of YouTube videos document salvia trips, and the publicity this generated has made salvia the focus of considerable attention.

The hallucinogenic effects of salvia are relatively short-lived (generally less than 30 minutes in duration), but are often intense and produce a trancelike state. The effects include visual hallucinations and other sensory disturbances and impaired motor control. Although this is often reported as pleasant, frightening experiences that resemble the bad trips associated with some of the types of hallucinogens reviewed previously can also occur. The active chemical in salvia is a compound called salvinorin A. Effective in doses of 100 to 500 micrograms, it is considered to be the most potent of any naturally occurring hallucinogen (Julien, Advokat, & Comaty, 2008). The mechanism of salvinorin A action is also quite unlike any of the hallucinogens reviewed previously, but rather appears to act as an agonist of a subset of opioid receptors called kappa receptors (Butelman et al., 2009). Little is known about the functions of these kappa receptors. They are not the same receptors that produce the pleasurable effects of opiate drugs reviewed in Chapter 10, but they are thought to be involved in regulating pain.

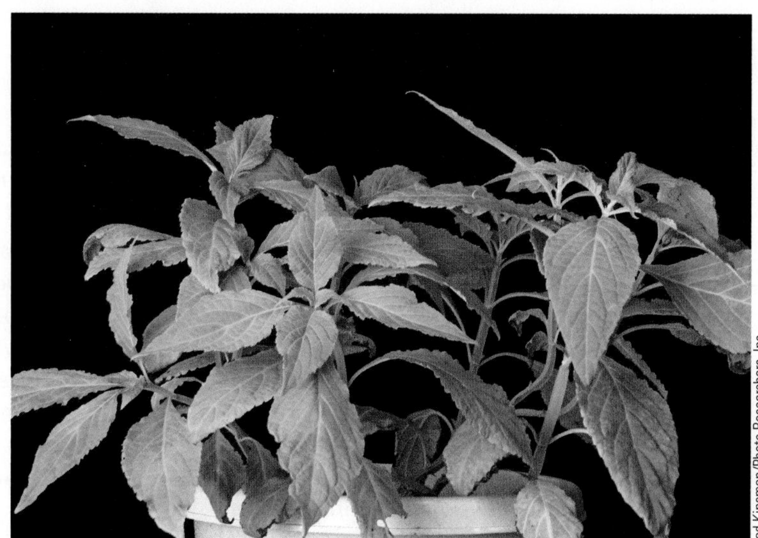

Salvia divinorum

There is considerable scientific interest in salvinorin A as it may open the door to learning more about the functions of the kappa receptor system in the brain. In the meantime, very little is known about the possible adverse or long-term effects of salvia use. Given the increasing popularity of the drug, it is currently under review by the DEA, and it would not be surprising to see salvia become a federally scheduled drug in the near future.

Summary

- Hallucinogens are a group of drugs that have the capacity to alter perceptual, cognitive, and emotional states.
- Hallucinogens may be divided into four classes: serotonergic hallucinogens, methylated amphetamines, anticholinergic hallucinogens, and dissociative anesthetics.
- Serotonergic hallucinogens include drugs such as LSD, psilocybin, and mescaline. Psilocybin comes from mushrooms of the *Psilocybe* genus, and mescaline from the peyote cactus. These drugs have a long history of use by early Indian peoples for religious purposes.
- LSD is a synthetic compound. Its hallucinogenic properties were discovered by the Swiss chemist Albert Hofmann, but it was made popular by counterculture figures such as Timothy Leary and Ken Kesey.
- LSD and the other drugs in this class affect serotonergic neurons. They are sympathomimetic drugs as well.
- The psychological effects of these drugs are diverse but include visual hallucinations, alterations of mood and thought, and dreamlike visions.
- Many adverse effects have been linked to LSD and other drugs in this class, including acute psychotic reactions (bad trips), flashbacks, and long-term psychological deficits.
- Methylated amphetamines include drugs such as MDA and MDMA (ecstasy). These drugs are sympathomimetic and produce many other effects similar to LSD but generally do not produce visual hallucinations.
- Anticholinergic hallucinogens include atropine and scopolamine, which are chemicals found in plants such as the deadly nightshade, mandrake, jimsonweed, and henbane. These drugs produce a semi-sleep state characterized by vivid visions and poor memory of the experience later.
- Phencyclidine (PCP) and ketamine are classified as dissociative anesthetic hallucinogens. They produce a potent intoxication at moderate doses and complete surgical anesthesia at higher doses.
- Salvinorin A is a hallucinogenic chemical found in a species of plant in the sage family (*Salvia divinorum*) and is often referred to as diviner's sage. It is unique among hallucinogens in acting on kappa receptors in the brain.

Answers to "What Do You Think?"

1. Unlike other classes of drugs, most hallucinogens are derived from synthetic compounds.
   F *There are more than 90 different species of plants, in addition to many more synthetic agents, that can be used to produce hallucinogenic effects.*
2. Hallucinogenic compounds were commonly used in the early 1900s throughout Europe and America.
   F *Although hallucinogens were used for centuries by Indians of South and Central America, these drugs had virtually no impact on mainstream European or American culture until the 1960s.*
3. The hallucinogenic properties of LSD were discovered by accident.
   T *Albert Hofmann of Sandoz Laboratories in Switzerland accidentally discovered the effects of LSD when he spilled some on himself and it was absorbed through his skin.*
4. LSD and Ecstasy were once used in psychotherapy.
   T *Both LSD and Ecstasy were used in psychotherapy, but their benefits were never successfully defended.*

5. Federal law mandates that anyone using LSD more than five times be declared legally insane.
   F *Although there is concern about long-term psychiatric effects of chronic LSD use, no such law exists.*
6. Use of LSD, even once, is likely to cause permanent chromosome damage and subsequent birth defects.
   F *LSD should be avoided by pregnant women but otherwise has not been shown to cause birth defects.*
7. Ecstasy (MDMA) produces vivid visual hallucinations.
   F *Ecstasy rarely produces true hallucinations.*
8. Ecstasy has been linked to long-term changes in brain chemistry.
   T *Long-term destruction of serotonergic terminals has been associated with Ecstasy, and problems consistent with such damage have been reported in controversial human studies.*
9. Hallucinations experienced under the influence of drugs such as LSD are very similar to those experienced by schizophrenics.
   F *The hallucinations experienced under the influence of LSD are primarily visual in nature, whereas those of schizophrenics are usually auditory.*
10. Dependence develops easily to hallucinogens such as LSD.
    F *The problems associated with LSD do not include drug dependence, but it is nonetheless a potentially dangerous drug.*
11. Reports of LSD flashbacks are now considered urban myth.
    F *Heavy users of LSD sometimes report vivid flashbacks.*
12. Phencyclidine (PCP or angel dust) was originally used as an animal tranquilizer.
    T *Phencyclidine and the related compound ketamine are still widely used for nonhuman anesthesia.*

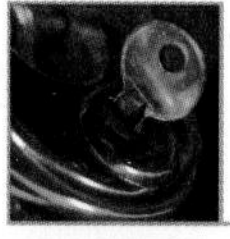

Key Terms

anticholinergic hallucinogens
atropine
dissociative anesthetic
flashback
ketamine
mescaline
methylated amphetamines
phencyclidine
psilocybin ('sī-ə-'sī-bən)
scopolamine
serotonergic hallucinogens
synesthesia

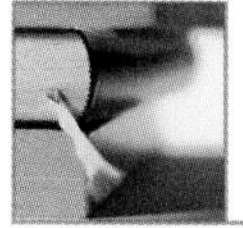

Suggested Readings

Iversen, L. (2008). *Speed, ecstasy, Ritalin: The science of amphetamines.* Oxford: Oxford University Press.

Laing, R. (2003). *Hallucinogens: A forensic drug handbook.* London: Academic Press.

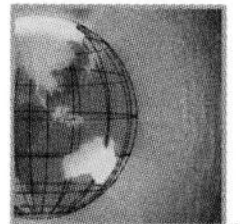

Web Resources

Visit the Book Companion Website at www.cengage.com/psychology/maisto to access study tools including a glossary, flashcards, and web quizzing. You will also find links to the following resources:

- NIDA on club drugs
- Erowid site on psychedelic drugs
- Site on salvia
- DanceSafe on club drugs
- NIDA Ecstasy research

CHAPTER 13

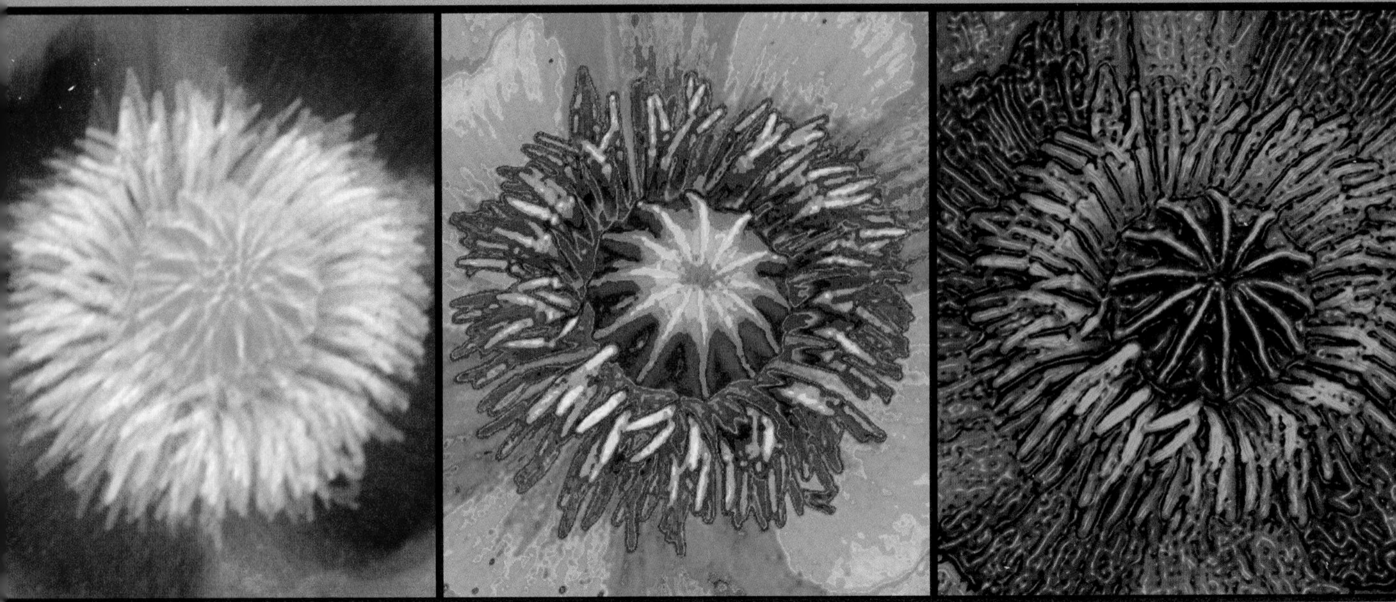

Psychotherapeutic Medications

What Do You Think? True or False?

Answers are given at the end of the chapter.

___ 1. One of the first successful attempts to treat the symptoms of mental illness with psychotherapeutic drugs occurred in the 1840s, when Moreau used cannabis to treat patients with both depressive and manic symptoms.

___ 2. Since the 1950s, the number of patients hospitalized for psychiatric conditions has decreased significantly.

___ 3. Almost half of the adults in the United States will meet the criteria for a mental illness at some point in their lives.

___ 4. The prevalence of psychotherapeutic medication is twice as high among men as among women.

___ 5. Psychotherapeutic drugs are rarely abused.

___ 6. As with most drugs, the age group least likely to misuse psychotherapeutic drugs is the elderly.

___ 7. Most psychotherapeutic medications are administered intravenously, with direct transport in the bloodstream.

___ 8. Schizophrenia is one of the most common psychiatric disorders in the United States.

___ 9. Stimulants are often used to treat chronic depression.

___10. Because antidepressants are absorbed rapidly, their effects are often immediate.

___11. Nitrous oxide (laughing gas) is no longer used by the medical profession.

___12. The effects of a moderate dose of a barbiturate drug resemble the effects of alcohol.

___13. Withdrawal from depressant sleeping pills can trigger rebound insomnia.

___14. Withdrawal from barbiturates is similar to alcohol withdrawal.

___15. Benzodiazepines (Valium) are one of the most commonly prescribed drugs in America.

___16. Benzodiazepines are a common street drug known as "bennies."

___17. Overdose of benzodiazepines was the cause of the suicide death of Marilyn Monroe.

___18. The main depressant drugs (barbiturates, benzodiazepines, and alcohol) all act by vastly different physiological mechanisms and affect different areas of the body.

___19. Depressant drugs may show cross-tolerance with cocaine.

___20. Alcohol in combination with other depressant drugs is the leading cause of drug overdose deaths in the United States.

___21. Lithium, a natural alkaline metal, is often used to treat manic attacks.

___22. Psychotherapeutic drugs pose little or no threat to the fetus and may be used safely during pregnancy.

Psychoactive substances have been used to treat mental illnesses for centuries. In fact, many of the substances described in this text, such as alcohol, cannabis, and opium, have been used as treatments for mental illness at one time or another. In some cases, the motivation to administer psychopharmacological agents to the mentally ill has been simply to subdue them. More typically today, medications are intended to provide people with some relief and ideally with the opportunity to function better in their environments.

The development, testing, and distribution of psychotherapeutic drugs, as described in Chapter 5, are a major worldwide industry. Fewer than a dozen countries (predominantly the United States, Italy, Japan, Germany, France, the United Kingdom, Brazil, Spain, and Canada) account for approximately 75% of the world's pharmaceutical sales. In the United States alone, over 250 million prescriptions are processed yearly for the lawful use of psychotherapeutics, including, for example, antidepressants, stimulants, and sedative hypnotics.

psychotherapeutic Exerting a special or unique action on psychological functioning.

We open this chapter with an overview of the use of psychotherapeutic drugs. Following a brief historical overview, we discuss some epidemiological features of what are called **psychotherapeutic** drugs. The term *psychotherapeutic* describes those drugs that have a special or unique effect on the mind or mental functioning. (In the field of psychiatry, these psychotherapeutic drugs are often called psychotropics.) We discuss mechanisms of drug action, and provide an overview of four major classes of psychotherapeutic drugs: antipsychotics, antidepressants, antianxiety agents, and antimanic or mood-stabilizing drugs. We supplement this material with case examples to give you a feeling for the problems or disorders these drugs are intended to relieve.

Historical Overview

The roots of psychopharmacology are based in the 19th century, when a science of chemistry was developing, and the field grew rapidly during the 20th century. The actual coining of the term *psychopharmacology* in 1920 is attributed to David Macht, an American pharmacist (Caldwell, 1970).

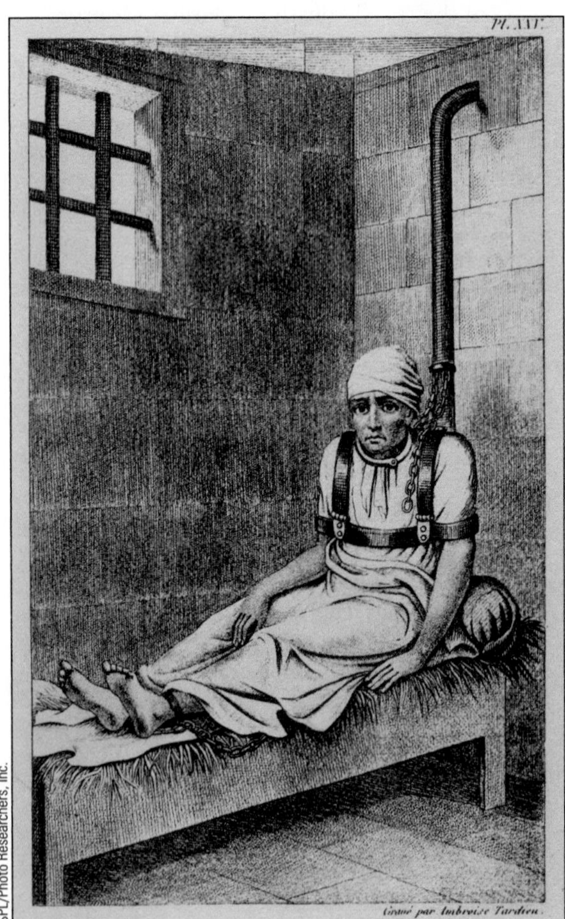

SPL/Photo Researchers, Inc.

Early psychiatric hospitals did not have the advantages of psychotherapeutic drugs to treat mentally ill patients. This drawing depicts a mentally ill patient during the early 1800s.

The Pre-Chlorpromazine Era

Nineteenth-century society had very little understanding of mental illness. Although there were several compendia of treatments and psychopharmacological agents for mental illnesses (especially in England, France, and Germany), the proposed remedies were mostly speculative and without scientific support. Many of the approaches used were actually cruel, including bloodletting, hot irons, flogging, revolving chairs, starvation, and sneezing powder (Spiegel & Aebi, 1983). Nevertheless, attempts were made to understand and treat, or in some cases, "cleanse" those with mental illness. The efforts of Emil Kraepelin, Phillip Pinel, and J. E. Esquirol were particularly noteworthy. These scientists were involved in the development of a classification system of mental illnesses. They believed that a scientific understanding and categorizing of mental illnesses were prerequisites to the identification of effective treatments.

One of the more systematically studied drugs in this period was cannabis. In the 1840s, the French physician Jacques-Joseph Moreau de Tours was working at a mental hospital in Paris. He theorized that treatment should "substitute symptoms of mental illness with similar but controllable drug-induced symptoms" (Caldwell, 1978, p. 16). Moreau used cannabis and found gaiety and euphoria to be among its effects. He decided to give cannabis to two hospital patients with depression to see whether it would produce similar results in them. These patients did indeed respond to the cannabis, appearing happy and becoming talkative. Moreau also found that

manic patients given cannabis subsequently calmed down and relaxed. Unfortunately, the effects of the cannabis tended to be temporary.

The first half of the 20th century brought further attempts to use drugs and other therapies to treat mental illness. For example, tests were conducted on the effectiveness of giving amphetamines to depressed and **narcoleptic** patients, and carbon dioxide inhalation procedures were used in the treatment of illnesses referred to as psychoses and **neuroses**. Also used in the treatment of psychoses were antihistamines, insulin shock, and **psychosurgery**. Electroshock therapy was used to treat severe depression (a procedure still used today). Finally, in 1949, an Australian physician named John Cade discovered that the alkali metal lithium successfully moderated manic conditions, although concerns about toxic reactions to it prevented its approval for use in the United States until 1970. Lithium remains a mainstay in the treatment of bipolar illnesses today.

Despite many efforts, the collective impact of these advances in the treatment of mental illness was modest at best. In fact, the total positive impact of this progress pales in comparison to the successes experienced in the later use of another drug, chlorpromazine. To the extent that psychopharmacology is defined as the use of psychotherapeutic medications to restore and maintain some degree of mental health, its true coming of age was in Paris in 1951.

manic
Relating to mania, a mood disturbance that typically includes hyperactivity, agitation, excessive elation, and pressured speech.

narcoleptic
A state characterized by brief but uncontrollable episodes of sleep.

neuroses
Nonpsychotic emotional disturbance, pain, or discomfort beyond what is appropriate in the conditions of one's life.

psychosurgery
Surgery that entails the cutting of fibers connecting particular parts of the brain or the removal or destruction of areas of brain tissue with the goal of modifying severe behavioral or emotional disturbances.

The Age of Chlorpromazine

Chlorpromazine was synthesized by Paul Charpentier in 1950. Its first use was as a psychotherapeutic medication in general surgery. Chlorpromazine was used as an anesthetic; it decreased patients' anxiety about surgical preparations and prevented shock during surgery. Henri Laborit primarily conducted this work in surgery, and his observation of chlorpromazine's calming effects led him to suggest its potential use in psychiatry. This application was initially tried at Val-de-Grace, a military hospital in Paris. Agitated psychotic patients appeared calm following administration of chlorpromazine. In addition, the patients' thoughts appeared to become less chaotic and the patients were less excitable. Notably, the patients did not exhibit any loss of consciousness. Instead, they showed a disinterested and detached demeanor, or what Deniker (1983) has called "the syndrome of psychomotor indifference" (p. 166).

Chlorpromazine has had a profound effect on the field of psychiatry. As described by Caldwell (1978):

> By May 1953, the atmosphere in the disturbed wards of mental hospitals in Paris was transformed: straightjackets [sic], psychohydraulic packs and noise were things of the past! Once more, Paris psychiatrists who long ago unchained the chained, became pioneers in liberating their patients, this time from inner torments too, and with a drug: (chlorpromazine). It accomplished the pharmacologic revolution of psychiatry—then and there. (p. 30)

Word of the successful use of chlorpromazine spread rapidly, and it was adopted throughout Europe, then in the United States and the rest of the world. The effects following introduction of chlorpromazine in the United States were just as dramatic. Since 1955, the number of hospitalized psychiatric patients in the United States has decreased significantly. In 1955, the figure was 600,000, and today, there are approximately 150,000 hospitalized psychiatric patients, despite an increase in the general population. Of course, other factors have contributed to today's lower figure (for example, the development of other psychotherapeutic drugs and the movement toward deinstitutionalizing psychiatric patients), but the starting point was chlorpromazine.

The decades following the introduction of chlorpromazine witnessed much growth in the field of psychopharmacology. The next major event was the appearance of reserpine in 1954. This drug, similar to chlorpromazine, was originally used in the treatment of another medical disorder (arterial hypertension), and the physicians using the drug noted symptoms of indifference in their patients. Because of this effect, reserpine was given to psychiatric patients. The drug had positive effects overall, but its action often took several weeks to be apparent (see Deniker, 1983), and patients who took the medication often appeared depressed. Thus, reserpine never achieved the popularity of chlorpromazine.

Other advances in the field were antianxiety (or anxiolytic) medications, such as meprobamate (which also was used as a muscle relaxant), and antidepressant medications, such as monoamine oxidase inhibitors (MAOIs) and tricyclic antidepressants. Another drug that received renewed attention was LSD. Because of the psychotic-like effects produced by LSD, researchers used it to create a "model psychosis" to study (with limited success, to date) possible etiological factors contributing to mental illness. They could also treat the LSD-created symptoms with psychotherapeutic drugs.

In retrospect, the 1950s were a frontier period for psychopharmacology. Much growth was experienced, and advances in the field continue to be made (although none with quite the impact and significance of chlorpromazine, which is widely used today). These advances have had a profound effect on the current treatment of mental illness. As noted, psychopharmacology contributed to decreases in the numbers of hospitalized psychiatric patients. Unfortunately, there have been downsides to this deinstitutionalization. Although psychotherapeutic medications often ameliorate the primary symptoms associated with a disorder, this does not necessarily mean that social coping skills or general "life skills" simultaneously materialize or reappear. Thus, some form of continuing care is often warranted. It had been expected that a variety of outpatient psychiatric services would be available to serve the needs of those discharged with chronic mental illness. Because that has not been the case, many patients once under psychiatric care are now without such services. It also has been argued that this lack of ongoing care contributes to the increased incidence of homeless people, many of whom suffer from psychiatric illnesses.

Epidemiology

Approximately one-quarter of the U.S. adult population experiences some form of mental disorder in any given year. Most of these people are experiencing symptoms associated with one of three problems: anxiety states, depression and affective disorder, or substance abuse. However, only a minority seeks clinical services for their disorders. These mental health problems exact an enormous toll for individuals, employers, and society as a whole (e.g., Langlieb & Kahn, 2005).

A picture of the nature and extent of mental illness in the United States was provided in the recent National Comorbidity Survey Replication (NCS-R) (Kessler, Berglund, Demler, et al., 2005; Kessler, Chiu, et al., 2005; Wang, Berglund, et al., 2005; Wang, Lane, et al., 2005), a national household survey of over 9,000 adults (age 18 and older). The survey focused on four major categories of mental illness: anxiety disorders (such as panic and posttraumatic stress disorders), mood disorders (such as major depression and bipolar disease), impulse-control disorders (such as attention deficit/hyperactivity disorders), and substance abuse. Among the findings were the following:

- One in every four adults in the United States (26.2%) suffers from a diagnosable mental disorder in a given year. This figure roughly translates to nearly 58 million individuals. A quarter of these individuals were classified as having had a "serious" disorder, in that it significantly disrupted their ability to function day to day.
- The most prevalent "past-year" mental disease classes are anxiety disorders (18%), mood disorders (10%), impulse-control disorders (9%), and substance abuse (15%).
- Almost half of U.S. adults had met the criteria for a mental illness at some point in their lives. Most of these cases were mild, not severe, and typically did not require treatment.
- Comorbidity, which refers to the simultaneous occurrence of two or more mental illnesses, was common. In fact, almost half (45%) of the adults with one mental disorder met the criteria for at least one other disorder.
- Fewer than half of those in need get treatment, and those who do often wait many years before doing so.
- The signs of mental illness appear to be evident early on. Half of those who were diagnosed with a mental disorder showed signs of the disease by age 14, and three-quarters showed signs by age 24. Unfortunately, few sought help.

It should be noted that these prevalence rates may be underestimates of mental illness in the United States. First, the sample drawn was household listings and thus did not include individuals who were homeless or institutionalized (such as in nursing homes or psychiatric hospitals). Second, the study did not assess some less common psychiatric disorders, such as schizophrenia and autism.

The symptoms associated with mental health disorders frequently are treated with prescription medications, most commonly prescriptions for an antidepressant or anti-anxiety agent. In 2005, antidepressant agents became the most commonly prescribed class of medications in outpatient offices and clinics, surpassing antihypertensive agents (Olfson & Marcus, 2009). (Antipsychotic medications account for a small fraction of the total number of prescriptions provided.) And considerable relief is reported: National surveys suggest that approximately three-fourths of patients who receive these medications report some degree of symptomatic relief.

There are important trends among people who use psychotherapeutic medications. First, the prevalence of psychotherapeutic medication use is about twice as high among women as among men. Second, psychotherapeutic drug use increases with age, a trend seen more dramatically among men. Third, greater use of psychotherapeutics is found among those who live alone, those with more education, and those with higher incomes.

Although most psychotherapeutic medications are used as prescribed, the nonprescribed use and abuse of psychotherapeutic drugs are a significant problem. Abuse of prescription drugs can take many forms, ranging from patients who exceed recommended dosages to the street sale of pharmaceuticals (Weiss & Greenfield, 1986). People who abuse prescription drugs divert them from legal distribution by stealing from drugstores or pharmaceutical companies, pilfering supplies of hospitals or clinics, and altering or forging prescriptions. Estimates indicate that several hundred million of the drug dosage units prescribed each year in the United States for psychiatric disorders are diverted to street or other illicit use. The consequences of prescription drug abuse are immense. For example, prescription drug abuse is implicated in significant numbers of injuries and deaths, drug-related emergency room cases, and drug-related deaths.

The drugs most often abused or misused in Western cultures are depressants and stimulants. People of all ages have been known to misuse prescription drugs, but it is an especially notable problem among the elderly. The elderly use approximately one-third of the drugs taken yearly in the United States, while accounting for a much smaller proportion of the population. It is not uncommon to see the elderly misuse prescribed medications in combination with each other, with over-the-counter drugs (see Chapter 14), or with alcohol. (The use of multiple prescription drugs is not always intentional because doctors sometimes provide prescriptions to the elderly without being aware of other prescription medications they already are using.)

Over the years, both legislative and medical association groups have made efforts to monitor and control the availability of and access to prescribed medications. Most legal guidelines are consolidated in the Comprehensive Drug Abuse Prevention and Control Act of 1970 (better known as the Controlled Substances Act; see Chapter 2). In particular, this act mandates explicit procedures for distributing and dispensing prescription medications. Most psychotherapeutic medications are under federal control and require a prescription for use.

Several information-gathering networks have been established to monitor the distribution and use (legal and otherwise) of drugs overall, including psychotherapeutic drugs. The largest of these is the Drug Abuse Warning Network (DAWN), which uses reports from emergency rooms and medical examiners' offices to produce yearly statistics on morbidity and mortality associated with drug use. DAWN, along with other monitoring programs, provides an ongoing tracking of trends in drug use and consequences. The usefulness of this information, of course, is a direct function of the accuracy with which the original data are gathered.

Before leaving the discussion on prescription drug misuse and abuse, we should note that a variety of over-the-counter substances with psychoactive properties are also subject to abuse. Examples are nonprescription hypnotics that contain antihistamines, nonprescription cold and allergy products, laxatives, nonprescription stimulants, and diet pills. These are described in more detail in Chapter 14.

Classes of Drugs and Their Actions

Psychotherapeutic drugs, like other drugs, can be classified along a variety of dimensions, such as chemical structure, clinical actions, and sites of action (see Chapter 1). However, the most common classification used in psychiatry, and the one we use, is by therapeutic usage. This classification yields four basic categories: antipsychotics, antidepressants, antianxiety agents, and antimanic medications. In the following sections, we describe representative psychotherapeutics in each of these classifications.

Antipsychotics

As you will recall, the introduction of antipsychotic medications in the 1950s was a major turning point in the treatment of severe psychiatric disorders, especially schizophrenia. *Schizophrenia* is a term that encompasses an array of thought disorders, including disturbances in areas of functioning such as language, affect, perception, and behavior. These disturbances, depending on the type of schizophrenia, may include distortions of reality (such as delusions and hallucinations), profoundly blunted mood, and withdrawn or bizarre behavior. The symptoms that are most likely to respond to antipsychotic medications are agitation, mania, hallucinations, delusions, fury, and accelerated and disorganized thinking processes (Magliozzi & Schaffer, 1988). It is estimated that schizophrenia affects approximately 1% of people over a lifetime, and the rate appears to be slightly higher among men than women (APA, 2000b; Lewine, 1988).

Sometimes an individual has previously or concurrently experienced a significant depressive or manic episode, in which case a diagnosis of schizoaffective disorder might be given to reflect the presence of symptoms of both schizophrenia and a major affective disorder.

To a lesser extent, antipsychotics also have been used in the treatment of mania, **agitated depression**, toxic (such as drug-induced) psychoses, emotionally unstable personalities, and psychoses associated with old age. Antipsychotic medications are also known as **neuroleptics** or major tranquilizers (the latter term is used much less frequently now). The term *neuroleptic* is derived from the Greek word that means "to clamp the neuron" (Snyder & Largent, 1989). *Antipsychotics* is the term more commonly used in the United States, with *neuroleptics* used more often in Europe. The terms are used interchangeably in this discussion. Representative antipsychotic medications are listed in Table 13.1.

The basic—but oversimplified—notion regarding antipsychotic medications is that they primarily affect the reticular activating system, the limbic system, and the hypothalamus. The effects on the reticular activating system generally moderate spontaneous activity and decrease the patient's reactivity to stimuli. The action within the limbic system serves to moderate or blunt emotional arousal. These actions are thought to produce the drug's dramatic effects on schizophrenic or agitated behavioral patterns. The effects on the hypothalamus help modulate metabolism, alertness, and muscle tone. Because of these effects, antipsychotics are

agitated depression
Depressed mood accompanied by a state of tension or restlessness. People with agitated depression show excessive motor activity, as they may, for example, be unable to sit still or may pace, wring the hands, or pull at their clothes.

neuroleptics
Tranquilizing drugs used to treat psychoses; a synonym is *major tranquilizer*.

"Sometimes people are taking away parts of my body and putting them back. Sometimes I think they are going to kill me."

22-year-old schizophrenic describing his thoughts and feelings (*Time Magazine*, July 6, 1992)

TABLE 13.1 Representative Antipsychotic Medications

Generic Name	Trade Name
Phenothiazines	
Chlorpromazine	Thorazine
Prochlorperazine	Compazine
Trifluoperazine	Stelazine
Fluphenazine	Prolixin
Thioridazine	Mellaril
Pimozide	Orap
Perphenazine	Trilafon
Promazine	Prazine
Mesoridazine	Serentil
Trifluopromazine	Psyquil
Nonphenothiazines	
Haloperidol	Haldol
Thiothixene	Navane
Loxapine	Loxitane
Clozapine	Clozaril
Molindone	Moban
Quetiapine	Seroquel
Risperidone	Risperdal
Olanzapine	Zyprexa
Ziprasidone	Zeldox
Sertindole	Serlect
Quetiapine	Seroquel
Aripiprazole	Abilify
Amisulpride	Solian
Paliperidone	Invega
Zotepine	Nipolept

paranoid schizophrenia A type of schizophrenia distinguished by systematic delusions or auditory hallucinations related to one theme.

the major approach to the drug treatment of schizophrenia. The following is a case example of clinical **paranoid schizophrenia:**

Mr. Simpson is a 44-year-old, single, unemployed, white man brought into the emergency room by the police for striking an elderly woman in his apartment building. Mr. Simpson had been continuously ill since the age of 22. During his first year of law school, he gradually became more and more convinced that his classmates were making fun of him. He noticed that they would snort and sneeze whenever he entered the classroom. When a girl he was dating broke off the relationship with him, he believed that she had been "replaced" by a look-alike. He called the police and asked for their help to solve the "kidnapping." His academic performance in school declined dramatically, and he was asked to leave and seek psychiatric care.

Mr. Simpson got a job as an investment counselor at a bank, which he held for seven months. However, he was getting an increasing number of distracting "signals" from co-workers, and he became more suspicious and withdrawn. It was at this time that he first reported hearing voices. He was eventually fired, and soon thereafter was hospitalized for the first time, at age 24. He has not worked since.

Mr. Simpson has been hospitalized 12 times, the longest stay being eight months. However, in the past five years he has been hospitalized only once, for three weeks. During the hospitalizations he has received various antipsychotic drugs. Although medication has been prescribed on an outpatient basis, he usually stops taking it shortly after leaving the hospital. Aside from twice-yearly lunch meetings with his uncle and his contacts with mental health workers, he is isolated socially. He lives on his own and manages his own financial affairs, including a modest inheritance. He reads the *Wall Street Journal* daily. He cooks and cleans for himself.

Mr. Simpson maintains that his apartment is the center of a large communication system that involves all three major television networks, his neighbors, and apparently hundreds of "actors" in his neighborhood. There are secret cameras in his apartment that carefully monitor all his activities. When he is watching TV, many of his minor actions, such as getting up to go to the bathroom, are soon directly commented on by the announcer. Whenever he goes outside, the "actors" have all been warned to keep him under surveillance. Everyone on the street watches him. His neighbors operate two different "machines"; one is responsible for all of his voices, except the "joker." He is not certain who controls this voice, which "visits" him only occasionally and is very funny. The other voices, which he hears many times each day, are generated by this machine, which he sometimes thinks is directly run by the neighbor whom he attacked. For example, when he is going over his investments, these "harassing" voices constantly tell him which stocks to buy. The other machine he calls "the dream machine." This machine puts erotic dreams into his head, usually of "black women."

Mr. Simpson describes other unusual experiences. For example, he recently went to a shoe store 30 miles from his house in the hope of getting some shoes that wouldn't be "altered." However, he soon found out that, like the rest of the shoes he buys, special nails had been put into the bottom of the shoes to annoy him. He was amazed that his decision concerning which shoe store to go to must have been known to his "harassers" before he himself knew it, so that they had time to get the altered shoes made up especially for him. He realizes that great effort and "millions of dollars" are involved in keeping him under surveillance. He sometimes thinks this is all part of a large experiment to discover the secret of his "superior intelligence." (Spitzer et al., 1989; Reprinted with permission from the *Diagnostic and Statistical Manual of Mental Disorders.* Copyright 1981 & 1989 American Psychiatric Association.)

Although several theories address the action of antipsychotics, the dopamine hypothesis is generally accepted. This theory is based on the observation of amphetamine-induced psychosis, which serves as a pharmacological model of schizophrenic behavior. The symptoms evidenced in this model of psychosis are readily ameliorated through the use of neuroleptic drugs. Furthermore, it appears that most amphetamine-induced psychotic behavior is mediated through increased release of dopamine in the brain. Thus, the dopamine theory has two core components: (1) Psychosis is induced by increased levels of dopaminergic activity, and (2) most antipsychotic drugs block postsynaptic dopamine receptors (Baldessarini, 1985; Bishara & Taylor, 2008; Gardner, Baldessarini, & Waraich, 2005). Unfortunately, it is not certain what leads to this dopaminergic overactivity in the first place.

It is believed that although antipsychotic medications block norepinephrine, serotonin, and acetylcholine, their primary action is as central dopamine antagonists (Galenberg, 1991; Meyer & Quenzer, 2005). That is, these drugs block central dopamine receptors, particularly the D_2 subtype, and thus inhibit dopaminergic neurotransmission in the brain. The postsynaptic receptor blockade in the limbic system is thought to reduce the schizophrenic symptoms.

The preceding discussion presents the predominant beliefs about the general actions of antipsychotic medications. Much research is ongoing, however, to identify the precise mechanisms of action that account for their effects. Although the precise mechanisms underlying the actions of neuroleptics remain to be isolated, current knowledge does point to at least some role for dopamine in the modulation of psychotic behaviors.

Although the antipsychotics have produced many positive effects in the treatment of mental disorders, their use comes with significant side effects. Antipsychotics also affect the **extrapyramidal** tract by blocking postsynaptic receptors in the basal ganglia, and these actions produce some of the most profound side effects associated with antipsychotics. Chief among the acute side effects are motor disturbances, which, taken together, give the appearance of a Parkinsonian syndrome. People who have Parkinson's disease are characterized by tremor, blank rigidity, gait and posture changes, and excessive salivation. Extrapyramidal symptoms are the most apparent motor disturbances, primarily **dyskinesia** (disordered movements) and **akinesia** (slowness of movement and underactivity). These are experienced acutely by at least 50% of patients who take antipsychotics (Bhana et al., 2001; Chakos et al., 1992; Mackay, 1982). The side effects of antipsychotics tend to be dose related: Stronger side effects are associated with higher doses of the antipsychotic medication.

extrapyramidal
Outside the pyramidal tracts, with origin in the basal ganglia. These cell bodies are involved with starting, stopping, and smoothing out movements.

dyskinesia
Disordered movements.

akinesia
Slowness of movement and underactivity.

The most common side effect associated with the long-term use of antipsychotics is another extrapyramidal complication known as **tardive dyskinesia**. Tardive dyskinesia, which typically can be seen after two years or more of antipsychotic drug use, is characterized most often by repetitive involuntary movements of the mouth and tongue (often in the form of lip smacking), trunk, and extremities. Most cases of tardive dyskinesia are preceded by the Parkinson-like symptoms described earlier. The current estimates are that tardive dyskinesia occurs among about one-third of treated patients (Fait et al., 2002; Gitlin, 1990), and many if not most of the tardive dyskinesia symptoms are permanent. The effects are seen more among women than men. Efforts to control or eliminate these effects include reducing the dose of the drug, which sometimes reduces the side effect and still provides some relief from the psychotic symptoms; administering medications designed to treat the side effects symptomatically (for example, benztropine [trade name Cogentin] or trihexyphenidyl [Artane]); and instituting what are called "drug holidays," during which the patient is off medication to have a physiological break from the use of the drug.

tardive dyskinesia
An extrapyramidal complication characterized by involuntary movements of the mouth and tongue, trunk, and extremities; a side effect of long-term (two or more years) use of antipsychotic drugs.

Although great strides have been made in the pharmacological treatment of psychotic disorders, concerted efforts in this area are continuing. One focus is on developing neuroleptics that provide symptom relief but act through different mechanisms. The hope is to avoid or minimize the side effects (especially tardive dyskinesia) of current antipsychotic medications. A second emphasis is on developing neuroleptics that not only diminish the obvious symptoms such as hallucinations but also alleviate some less visible symptoms, such as emotional withdrawal. One excellent example in this regard is clozapine (trade name Clozaril), used in the treatment of psychotic and schizophrenic disorders. Clozapine was the first of a new class of antipsychotics collectively referred to as atypical or second-generation antipsychotics (Bonham & Abbott, 2008). Most of the subsequent antipsychotics in this class seek to emulate the pharmacological properties believed to be responsible for clozapine's particular clinical profile (Grunder, Hippius, & Carlsson, 2009). The major attractive feature of clozapine is that it has yielded antipsychotic efficacy among patients who have not responded to other antipsychotics, such as haloperidol. In addition, clozapine appears to produce a minimum of acute extrapyramidal side effects and is a rare antipsychotic that does not appear to produce tardive dyskinesia. Like all medications, however, clozapine has side effects. The most significant concern with clozapine is the occasional side effect of agranulocytosis, a destructive condition in which the bone marrow stops producing white blood cells, thus opening the door to infection. If undetected, agranulocytosis results in death, so close monitoring of the patient is required. Close monitoring of heart functioning also is needed, especially early in the course of treatment, based on recent reports of fatal myocarditis, an inflammation of the heart lining. Though initially not available to large numbers of clients because of the high costs of the drug and the associated blood-test monitoring, the

DRUGS AND CULTURE BOX 13.1

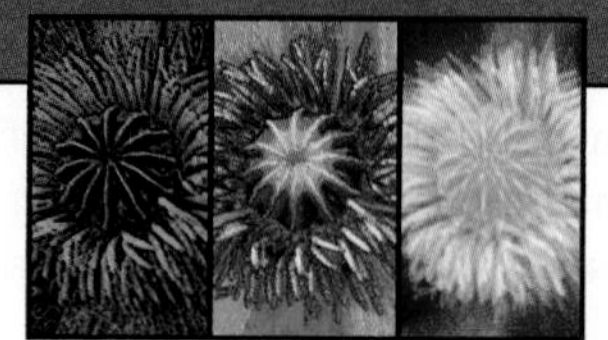

The Right to Refuse Psychotherapeutic Medications

As you are aware, countries and cultures vary considerably in the extent to which they tolerate freedom of speech and other forms of behavioral expression. Not surprisingly, this often predicts the extent to which patients with mental illness (however defined) have any say in how they are treated. In some cultures, the response to behaviors viewed as "different" or "mentally ill" is to subdue people through incarceration, restraints, drugs, or some combination of these interventions. In other cultures, treatment might include a more collaborative approach in which patients discuss their problems with a counselor or work with a psychiatrist in trying different drugs to see how they work.

The United States has a long constitutional history of endorsing the rights of the individual. But how far should this privilege extend? For example, should a person who is voluntarily or involuntarily admitted to a psychiatric facility have the opportunity to refuse psychotherapeutic drugs? For many years, people hospitalized for psychiatric treatment had little if any say in whether drugs would be administered, based in part on the assumption that they had no expertise in the area of psychotherapeutic medications and that being hospitalized to begin with suggested impaired functioning and thus the inability to make decisions.

This issue has been addressed in court cases over the years. In one case, seven Boston State Hospital patients filed suit to stop the (nonemergency) administration of medications without their informed consent. Relatedly, the patients claimed the right to refuse medication. The psychiatrists faced a dilemma. On the one hand, they knew by experience that certain drugs were able to significantly relieve emotional distress. On the other hand, some of these drugs had unpleasant side effects and patients understandably might want to avoid these. The court decided in favor of the patients. It ruled that patients (whether voluntarily or involuntarily admitted to the hospital) should be presumed competent to accept or refuse psychotherapeutic medications. The court added that when a patient was not deemed competent, a court-appointed guardian needed to make the decision whether to use medications.

Is this the final word? No, probably not. New cases arise and can yield different rulings. However, the practical implication of the Boston State Hospital case may not arise very often for the simple reason that hospitalized psychiatric patients do not frequently raise the issue of refusing their medications.

subsequent availability of generics of clozapine is allowing more patients to benefit from the use of this medication.

Another area of recent attention has been evaluation of the relative effectiveness of antipsychotic medications. The general clinical experience is that no one antipsychotic medication is the "magic pill" for all patients with schizophrenia. Instead, treatment providers have sometimes needed to shift patients from one medication to another until finding the medication with the best individual effect. In one study, for example, five medications (olanzapine [trade name Zyprexa], perphenazine [Trilafon], quetiapine [Seroquel], risperidone [Risperdal], and ziprasidone [Zeldox]) used to treat schizophrenia were compared (Lieberman et al., 2005). It was found that all five medications blunted the symptoms of schizophrenia, but that nearly 75% of the patients stopped taking the drugs they were on because of discomfort or specific side effects. One of the drugs—olanzapine (Zyprexa)—appeared to help more patients control symptoms for a longer period of time, although with a higher risk of side effects that in turn increased risk of diabetes.

Finally, it should be noted before closing that other pharmacological treatments for schizophrenic or psychotic disorders continue to be evaluated and distributed for use in clinical settings. Among the latest is risperidone (trade name Risperdal), which provides many of the benefits associated with clozapine without the agranulocytosis risk. Unfortunately, risperidone appears to present an increased risk of diabetes (as indicated in the aforementioned Lieberman et al. 2005 study). Further, patients taking risperidone (along with quetiapine, olanzapine, and clozapine) may have an increased risk of sudden death from cardiac arrhythmias and other cardiac causes than patients not taking these medications (Ray et al., 2009). A second promising treatment is aripiprazole (Abilify), which seeks to stabilize the dopamine system. Both medications have shown very positive outcomes and many fewer and less severe side effects. Finally, another opening frontier in the advance of antipsychotics medications revolves around glutamate (as opposed to the more traditional focus on dopamine). Glutamate is central to brain processes involving perception, memory, and learning. Experimental work is underway with a drug called ketamine (often used in pediatric anesthesia) that targets glutamate receptors, with some preliminary positive indications.

Antidepressants

Depression is among the most common psychiatric disorders in the United States. Approximately 20% of the U.S. population will experience a depressive episode in their lifetimes (Kessler, Berglund, et al., 2005). Depressions vary in severity, duration, and frequency of occurrence; the most common symptoms that contribute to what has been characterized as a depressive syndrome (as opposed to cases where a person might feel sad or blue) include dysphoric mood, loss of interest, disturbances in appetite

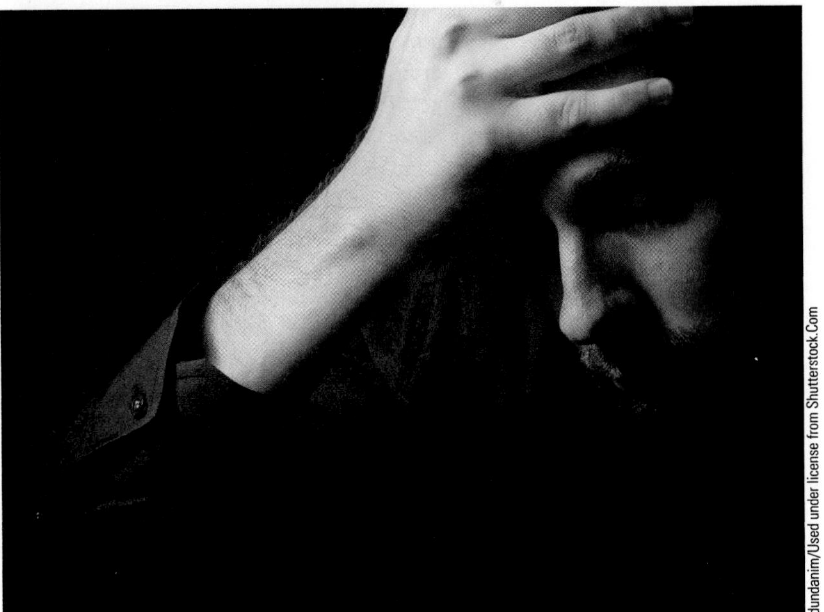

Common symptoms of depression are dysphoric mood, loss of interest, sleep disturbance, withdrawal, and difficulties in concentration.

endogenous
Developed from within. When applied to depression, the term means that depressive symptoms seem to be due to genetic factors.

exogenous
Developed from without. When applied to depression, the term means that depressive symptoms seem to be in reaction to a particular situation or event.

and weight, sleep disturbance, fatigue, withdrawal, thoughts of suicide, and difficulties in concentration. Depressions frequently are classified as either **endogenous**, in which symptoms tend to be chronic and associated with genetic constitutional factors, or **exogenous**, in which symptoms are thought to be in response to some situation or event (Cooperrider, 1988). The average age for onset of a first depressive episode traditionally has been in the late 30s or early 40s, although depressions are being seen more frequently among younger people and even among preschool children under the age of 6 (Luby et al., 2009). The length of a depressive episode is also variable, although periods of six months are common. Depression is diagnosed much more frequently among women than among men (Ebmeier, Donaghey, & Steele, 2006). Around 50% of the people who experience a major depressive episode do not have a recurrence of the illness (Coryell & Winokur, 1982).

The following case, excerpted from Spitzer et al. (1989), is an example of major depression rated as moderately severe.

> Connie is a 33-year-old homemaker who separated from her husband three months previously. She has a 4-year-old son, Robert.
>
> Connie left her husband, Donald, after a five-year marriage. Violent arguments between them, during which Connie was beaten by her husband, had occurred for the last four years of their marriage, beginning when she became pregnant with Robert. During their final argument, about Connie's buying an expensive tricycle for Robert, her husband had held a loaded gun to Robert's head and threatened to shoot him if she didn't agree to return the tricycle to the store. Connie obtained a court order of protection that prevented Donald from having any contact with her or their son. She took Robert to her parents' apartment, where they are still living.
>
> Connie is an only child, and a high school and secretarial school graduate. She worked as an executive secretary for six years before her marriage and for the first two years after, until Robert's birth. Before her marriage Connie had her own apartment. She was close to her parents, visiting them weekly and speaking to them a couple of times a week. Connie had many friends whom she also saw regularly. She still had several friends from her high school years. In high school she had been a popular cheerleader and a good student. In the office where she had worked as a secretary, she was in charge of organizing office holiday parties and money collections for employee gifts.
>
> During their first year of marriage, Donald became increasingly irritable and critical of Connie. He began to request that Connie stop calling and seeing her friends after work, and refused to allow them or his in-laws to visit their apartment. Connie convinced Donald to try marital therapy, but he refused to continue after the initial two sessions.
>
> Despite her misgivings about Donald's behavior toward her, Connie decided to become pregnant. During the seventh month of the pregnancy, she developed thrombophlebitis and had to stay home in bed. Donald began complaining that their apartment was not clean enough and that Connie was not able to shop for groceries. He never helped Connie with the housework. He refused to allow his mother-in-law to come to the apartment to help. One morning when he couldn't find a clean shirt, he became angry and yelled at Connie. When she suggested that he pick some up from the laundry, he began hitting her with his fists. She left him and went to live with her parents for a week. He expressed remorse for hitting her and agreed to resume marital therapy.
>
> At her parents' and Donald's urging, Connie returned to her apartment. No further violence occurred until after Robert's birth. At that time, Donald began using cocaine every weekend and often became violent when he was high.
>
> In the three months since she left Donald, Connie has become increasingly depressed. Her appetite has been poor, and she has lost ten pounds. She cries a lot and often wakes up at five in the morning, unable to get back to sleep. Ever since she left Donald, he has been

calling her at her parents' home and begging her to return to him. One week before her psychiatric evaluation, Connie's parents took her to their general practitioner. Her physical examination was normal, and he referred her for psychiatric treatment.

When seen by a psychiatrist in the outpatient clinic, Connie is pale and thin, dressed in worn-out jeans and dark blue sweater. Her haircut is unstylish, and she appears older than she is. She speaks slowly, describing her depressed mood and lack of energy. She says that her only pleasure is in being with her son. She is able to take care of him physically, but feels guilty because her preoccupation with her own bad feelings prevents her from being able to play with him. She now has no social contacts other than with her parents and her son. She feels worthless and blames herself for her marital problems, saying that if she had been a better wife, maybe Donald would have been able to give up the cocaine. When asked why she stayed with him so long, she explains that her family disapproved of divorce and kept telling her that she should try harder to make her marriage a success. She also thought about what her life would be like trying to take care of her son while working full-time and didn't think she could make it. (Reprinted with permission from the *Diagnostic and Statistical Manual of Mental Disorders*. Copyright 1981 & 1989 American Psychiatric Association.)

Although stimulants once were used as a treatment for depression, their effectiveness was limited, especially among people with severe depressions. Today, stimulants are rarely used for depression. Instead, several classes of antidepressant medications are prescribed, each acting in a manner different from stimulants, which produce a euphoria that does not generally occur with the antidepressants (Cooperrider, 1988). The first class includes the cyclic antidepressants. Historically, these were referred to as tricyclic antidepressants because of their three-ring chemical structure nucleus. Some more recent antidepressants have more varied chemical structures, however, and have been identified as heterocyclic antidepressants. Included among these are antidepressant medications called selective serotonin reuptake inhibitors (SSRIs), which often treat the symptoms of depression more effectively than the tricyclics and are associated with fewer side effects for many users. The most common SSRIs are fluvoxamine (trade name Luvox), paroxetine (Paxil), fluoxetine (Prozac), and sertraline (Zoloft). We use the term cyclic when referring to these antidepressants generally and the term tricyclics when referring to that specific group of antidepressants. The second class of antidepressants includes MAOIs (recall that this acronym refers to the monoamine oxidase inhibitors), which are used less frequently than the cyclic antidepressants. Finally, in the third class are newer antidepressant medications that either have mechanisms of action that are not yet well understood or have specific therapeutic effects that mirror those of both the tricyclics and the SSRIs. Representative antidepressant medications in these three categories are listed in Table 13.2.

Both the tricyclics and MAOIs were available in the late 1950s. As with other psychotherapeutic medications, their potential antidepressant effects were discovered serendipitously. The tricyclics initially were being investigated as antipsychotic agents, whereas the MAOIs initially were used in the treatment of tuberculosis. In both cases, investigators noted antidepressant effects—for example, some tuberculosis patients treated with an MAOI showed an energized state.

Before discussing the cyclics and MAOIs in more detail, we need to present the postulated biochemical hypotheses for depression. It is believed that depression results from a deficiency in biogenic amines, specifically catecholamines and serotonin, which act as central nervous system neurotransmitters (see Chapter 3). According to the catecholamine hypothesis, depression results from a deficiency in catecholamines (particularly norepinephrine) at varied neuron receptor sites in the brain. The cyclics are believed to block the reuptake of norepinephrine from the synaptic cleft. Thus, the

"After a few weeks on Prozac, I realized my outlook on life was brighter. Since taking it, my friendships have blossomed, I've developed a couple of friendships at work that I never had before. I didn't know that I could look at life without seeing all the bad."

33-year-old professional woman describing the effects of Prozac (*Washington Post Health*, August 28, 1990)

TABLE 13.2 Representative Antidepressant Medications

Generic Name	Trade Name
Cyclic antidepressants	
Fluoxetine	Prozac
Imipramine	Tofranil, Imavate, Antipress
Amitriptyline	Amitril, Elavil
Desipramine	Norpramine
Doxepin	Sinequan
Nortriptyline	Aventyl, Pamelor
Protriptyline	Vivactil
Amoxapine	Asendin
Clomipramine	Anafranil
Maprotiline	Ludiomil
Sertraline	Zoloft
Paroxetine	Paxil
Fluvoxamine	Luvox
MAOIs	
Tranylcypromine	Parnate
Isocaroxazid	Marplan
Phenelzine	Nardil
Newer medications	
Trazodone	Desyrel
Venlafaxine	Effexor
Mirtazapine	Remeron
Nefazodone	Serzone
Bupropion	Wellbutrin
Reboxetine	Edronax
Citalopram	Celexa
Escitalopram	Lexapro
Duloxetine	Cynbalta
Milnacipran	Pristiq
Desvenlafaxine	Ixel, Savella

Note: The most frequently prescribed antidepressant drugs include sertraline (Zoloft), escitalopram (Lexapro), fluoxetine (Prozac), and bupropion (Wellbutrin).

result is a greater concentration of norepinephrine in the synaptic cleft, alleviating the hypothesized neurotransmitter deficiency. This cyclic-mediated process is thought to occur in the amygdala and reticular formation areas of the brain.

The catecholamine theory is derived in large part from observations of the effects of the antipsychotic agent reserpine, discussed earlier in the historical overview. Patients given reserpine often exhibit a depressed appearance. Furthermore, reserpine was found to deplete brain concentrations of norepinephrine. Thus, there was the suggestion that such depletions were causally related to depression.

The serotonin hypothesis, the other central theory of antidepressant action, postulates that depression is the result of a deficiency of the neurotransmitter serotonin in the brain stem (Galenberg & Schoonover, 1991; Kalus, Asnis, & van Praag, 1989). People who are depressed have reduced levels of serotonin and chemicals involved in its metabolism in their cerebrospinal fluid. Like the catecholamine norepinephrine, the cyclics have been found to prevent the uptake of serotonin (Cooperrider, 1988).

Although the cyclics block the uptake of amines, MAOIs prevent the breakdown of the neurotransmitters (Cohen, 1997; Cooperrider, 1988; Meyer & Quenzer, 2005). The enzyme monoamine oxidase metabolizes a variety of neurotransmitters, including norepinephrine and serotonin. MAOIs inhibit this degradation process and thus enhance the availability of the transmitter within the neuron. Thus, the actions of the cyclics and MAOIs each are consistent with the hypothesis that decreased brain catecholamine activity causes depression and that these antidepressants (using different mechanisms) reverse this process by increasing catecholamine activity in the brain.

Taken together, the cyclics and MAOIs each appear to enhance the functional activity of one or more neurotransmitters, but our understanding of the mechanisms remains clouded. One finding that contributes to our lack of understanding is that the effects noted occur within hours, although the therapeutic antidepressant action can take days or weeks for the patient to experience.

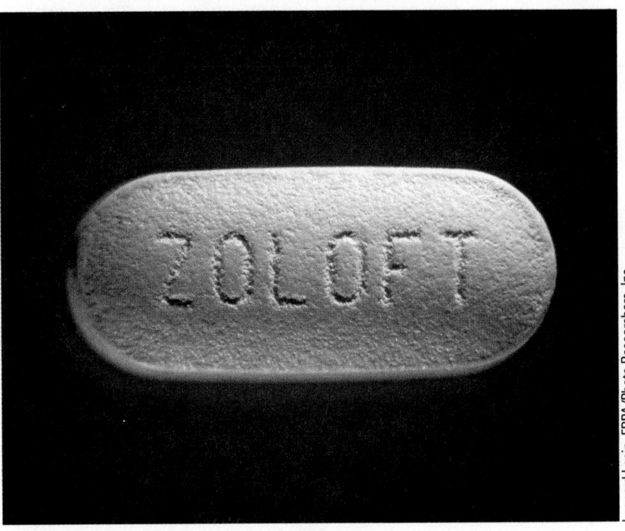

Leonard Lesin, FBPA/Photo Researchers, Inc.

Zoloft is among the most commonly prescribed antidepressant medications.

Although current theories about the actions of antidepressants are best viewed as tentative, recent work on the neurobiology of depression has provided some exciting new insights. A link has been known to exist between depression (and also chronic stress and anxiety) and atrophy and cell loss in the hippocampus. Research by several researchers (e.g., Duman, 2004; Duman, Nakagawa, & Malberg, 2001; Malberg et al., 2000; Santarelli et al., 2003) has demonstrated that antidepressant treatment increases neurogenesis, or new cell growth, in the hippocampus. This neurogenesis may block or reverse the effects of depression on hippocampal neurons. Further, the new cell growth appears to take several weeks to occur, and this may account for the fact that antidepressant medications typically take several weeks to exert their action. The findings suggest that increased cell proliferation and increased neuronal numbers may be mechanisms by which antidepressant treatment overcomes the atrophy and loss of hippocampal neurons associated with depression.

The cyclics and MAOIs are absorbed readily through the gastrointestinal tract (Fait et al., 2002). The cyclics are administered only rarely through injection, and MAOIs always are taken orally. Following absorption, relatively high concentrations of the drugs develop in the brain especially but also in other organs. Then the antidepressant pharmacokinetics resemble those of the antipsychotics, especially chlorpromazine (Baldessarini, 1985). More is known of the absorption and distribution of the cyclics than of the MAOIs, in part because of the difficulty in isolating MAOI metabolites (Tyrer, 1982b). Metabolism for each occurs primarily in the liver, with most excreted through the urine.

Despite the rapid absorption of antidepressant medications, one disadvantage in their use (noted previously) is that clinical action frequently takes two to three weeks to be apparent in the patient's functioning. Unfortunately, patients experience most of the undesired side effects of antidepressants during this initial period of use, and many patients terminate their use because they experience the side effects in the absence of rapid symptom relief. The most common side effects of the cyclics are drowsiness; a variety of anticholinergic effects such as dry mouth, constipation, and difficulty in urinating; blurred vision; orthostasis (dizziness upon standing up); decreased libido; weight gain; and tachycardia (Andrews & Nemeroff, 1994). In addition, use of some of the newer SSRI antidepressant medications may be associated with a greater risk of bone breaks (Richards et al., 2007) and, among older women, an increased rate of bone loss at the hip (Diem et al., 2007). The most common side effects of the

"What we're going to find out about the brain is mind-boggling. Every time a new drug is found another disease disappears, and makes one very curious about what other diseases have a biological basis."

Drug therapist Dr. Paul Wender (*Newsweek*, March 26, 1990)

MAOIs are drowsiness, dry mouth, dizziness, weight gain, insomnia, constipation, and fatigue. In addition, MAOI use is associated with two other unwanted effects. The first is temporary low blood pressure when changing position (such as from sitting to standing), and the second is impaired sexual functioning. Men may experience impotence and difficulty in ejaculating, and women may report orgasmic inhibition. The use of MAOIs also requires dietary restrictions. Most significant among these is avoiding substances that contain tyramine, such as most cheeses and some alcoholic beverages (especially Chianti wine). MAOIs and tyramine interact to cause potentially severe hypertensive reactions. Finally, a concern in the use of antidepressants is their potential for lethal use. Overdosing on cyclics can result in coma, respiratory difficulties, and a variety of cardiac problems. Accordingly, the patient's potential for suicide has to be assessed before most of the cyclics are prescribed. MAOIs do not produce intoxicating effects, and overdosing on them is not common.

An area of recent concern regarding some antidepressants, primarily SSRIs, is the possibility of suicide, especially among children. This concern prompted the U.S. Food and Drug Administration (FDA) to issue a warning that people taking antidepressants can become suicidal and should be closely monitored, especially when patients start using an antidepressant or when the dose is increased or decreased. The FDA urged the manufacturers of 10 popular antidepressants (trade names Prozac, Zoloft, Wellbutrin, Zyban, Paxil, Celexa, Effexor, Serzone, Luvox, and Remeron) to issue revised warning labels for the medications identifying these concerns. These concerns also led Great Britain to markedly increase restrictions on the prescribing of

CONTEMPORARY ISSUE BOX 13.2

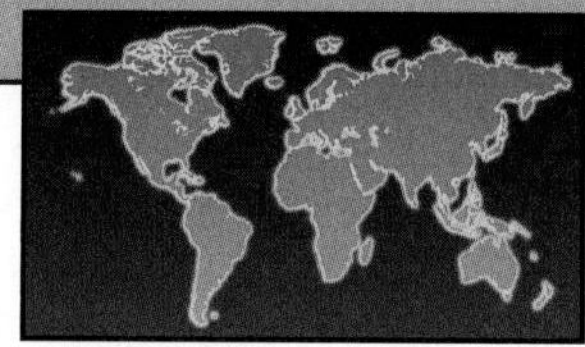

Antidepressant Medications: Drug versus Placebo Effects

An issue often discussed in the context of psychotherapeutic medications is whether receiving a medication provides more relief than receiving a placebo (a patient receives an inactive pill but believes it is an active medication). Part of the reason for comparing those who receive the active medication with those who receive a placebo is to account for the therapeutic effects associated with receiving a medication, such as the expectation of improvement, independent of the medication's active ingredients.

In a review of many studies comparing the effects of antidepressant medications with placebo, Kirsch and Sapirstein (1999) concluded that only about 25% of the "response" to medication treatment was due to the pharmacological effect of the medication. Fully 50% of the effect was due to the psychological impact of administering the medication (the placebo effect). The remaining 25% of the treatment response was attributed to "nonspecific factors," such as the therapeutic relationship between the doctor and the patient. According to Dr. Sapirstein, "People benefiting from drugs are benefiting because they think that taking the antidepressant medicine is working. If we take these results and say that improvement is due to what the patients think, then how people think and its effect on how they feel are more powerful than the chemical substance."

More recently, Dr. Andrew Leuchter and his colleagues (Leuchter et al., 2002) have demonstrated that placebo medications can actually induce changes in brain functioning for individuals with major depression. These alterations are different from the brain changes caused by antidepressant medications. Patients who responded to the placebo showed increased activity in the prefrontal cortex of the brain, whereas those who responded to the medication showed suppressed activity in that area. According to the authors of this study, the finding raises questions about two commonly held beliefs. The first is that administration of an inert pill appears to be an active treatment rather than no treatment, as previously thought. And second, the placebo response is not equivalent to an active drug response because the two groups' brain physiology was altered differently. They caution, though, that their data do not indicate a causal link between brain changes and the effects of a placebo or medication. Further research is needed to assess causal links and longer-term outcomes for these two groups of patients.

antidepressants for children. In 2003, the British Medicines and Healthcare Products Regulatory Agency declared Celexa, Effexor, Lexapro, Luvox, Paxil (called Seroxat in Britain), and Zoloft as too risky for children under age 18. Physicians, and also patients and parents, will need to incorporate these considerations into decisions on whether and which antidepressants to use, and on balancing the risks of using antidepressants against leaving the illness untreated pharmacologically.

The therapeutic effects of antidepressants for many patients are impressive once the lag time has passed. The cyclics in particular markedly alleviate depressive symptoms. MAOIs also have strong supportive treatment effectiveness rates when compared with placebos, although the positive outcomes are not as dramatic as with the cyclics. Also, MAOIs, when compared directly with cyclics, tend to be less effective. This has led to a tendency, in the United States at least, for the cyclics along with the newer medications identified in Table 13.2 to be the treatment of choice for most depressions, with MAOIs used when these do not produce desired results. Nevertheless, they do not provide relief for all (Moncrieff & Kirsch, 2005), and research continues on the development of more effective medications as well as alternatives to medication (including the use of electroconvulsive therapy, or ECT, in the most severe cases of depression that do not respond to medication). Nondrug therapies, aside from psychotherapy, include herbs (such as St. John's wort, see Contemporary Issue Box 13.3), dietary supplements,

CONTEMPORARY ISSUE BOX 13.3

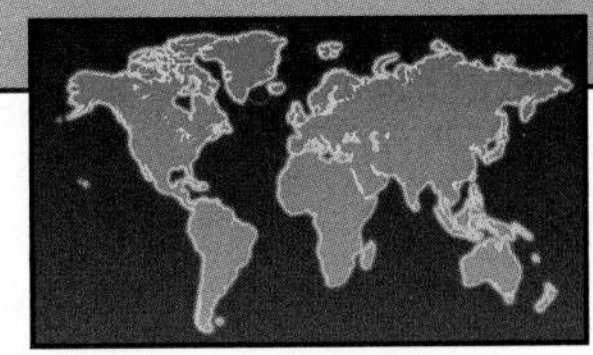

Herb Treatment for Depression?

This chapter deals overall with psychotherapeutic medications for mental illnesses, but that does not mean alternative interventions do not exist. One example is the herb St. John's wort (sometimes spelled St. Johnswort). The word *wort* means plant, and this particular yellow-flowered plant carries the Latin name *Hypericum perforatum*. Also called goatweed, hypericum, and Klamath weed, St. John's wort grows wild in the western United States and throughout Europe. Its peak blooming period is late June, around the time of the traditional birthday of John the Baptist (June 24), thus the name of the plant.

St. John's wort is thought to have been used many centuries ago as protection from evil spirits and later for colds, tuberculosis, and worms, among other ailments. Much more recently—over the past two decades—it has been used extensively throughout Europe as an herbal treatment for mild to moderate depression. It has its greatest popularity in Germany, where it is a leading treatment for depression and is prescribed by doctors more frequently than Prozac—by a ratio estimated at 15–20:1. The medication is available in liquid, capsule, and dried form. The plant extracts contain a variety of chemical compounds, and it is not clear just which active agents are contributing to the observed effects of the herb.

A number of studies have suggested St. John's wort as a viable treatment for depression. In one study of more than 3,000 patients with mild to moderate depression, over three-quarters showed improvement after four weeks of using the herb. In another study, patients who received St. John's wort showed significantly more improvement than patients who received a placebo. Taken together, the research in support of St. John's wort in the treatment of mild to moderate forms of depression is reasonably strong (Lawvere & Mahoney, 2005); research on its effectiveness in the treatment of major depression is less consistent (Hypericum Depression Trial Study Group, 2002; Linde, Berner, & Kriston, 2008; Shelton et al., 2001).

Clinical researchers are continuing their efforts to understand better how St. John's wort works and how it will fare in more direct tests comparing it with more traditional psychotherapeutic treatments for depression. In the meantime, users of St. John's wort need to be aware of recent research showing that the herb can cause decreases in the blood levels of a variety of prescription drugs. It is believed that St. John's wort influences drug metabolism by increasing the production of a liver enzyme that speeds elimination of many common drugs, including oral contraceptives and medications for elevated levels of cholesterol. More recently, Smith (2004) found that St. John's wort may compromise the effectiveness of an anticancer drug (imatinib mesylate [trade name Gleevec]) used in the treatment of chronic leukemia.

light therapy (daily exposure to a box providing artificial light), and exercise. Another recent development is transcranial magnetic stimulation (TMS), a noninvasive procedure that activates the brain's emotive centers. This may be especially helpful for patients with depression who have not responded to other treatment interventions and have been classified as having "treatment-resistant depression" (Matthew, 2008).

Antianxiety Agents

barbiturates Depressant drugs formerly used as sleeping pills; currently used in anesthesia and treatment for epilepsy.

anxiolytic Anxiety-reducing.

sedative-hypnotic effects The calming and sleep-inducing effects of some drugs.

general anesthesia The reduction of pain by rendering the subject unconscious.

Before describing anxiety and today's approaches to its treatment, we provide some background and historical perspective on depressant drugs more generally. We should note, first of all, that although alcohol is the prototype depressant drug (see Chapter 9), many other drugs can depress the CNS and behavior. These include a variety of different chemical agents but especially the **barbiturates**, the benzodiazepines, nonbarbiturate sedatives, and the general anesthetics (see Tables 13.3 and 13.4). These drugs are often classified according to their most common medical uses, but such a classification can be misleading. On the one hand, benzodiazepines such as diazepam (trade name Valium) and chlordiazepoxide (Librium) are often labeled as **anxiolytic** (antianxiety) drugs. Although moderate doses of these compounds do indeed relieve anxiety and are widely used for this purpose, in larger doses, benzodiazepines produce **sedative-hypnotic effects** (that is, they induce sleep) and are now prescribed widely as sleeping pills. Barbiturates, on the other hand, often are called sleeping pills and can certainly be effective in this regard. In lower doses, barbiturates are also anxiolytic, and if the dose is high enough, these and other depressants can produce surgical anesthesia. All depressant drugs (including alcohol) can relieve anxiety at low-dose levels, produce intoxication at moderate levels, induce sedation and sleep at still higher levels, produce **general anesthesia** at very high-dose levels, and eventually lead to coma and death (see Figure 13.1). Due to differing potency, duration of action, and safety, some depressants are used for specific purposes more often than others (for example, nitrous

TABLE 13.3 Representative Depressant Drugs

Generic Name	Brand Name	Slang Name
Hypnotics		
Barbiturates		
Pentobarbital	Nembutal	yellow jackets, nembies
Secobarbital	Seconal	reds
Amobarbital	Amytal	blues, Amys, blue Angels
Phenobarbital	Luminal	
Methohexital	Brevital	
Thiopental	Pentothal	
Aprobarbital	Alurate	
Mephobarbital	Mebaral	
Chloral hydrate		
Methaqualone	Quaaludes	ludes
Ethchlorvynol	Placidyl	
Zolpidem	Ambien	
General anesthetics		
Halothane	Fluothene	
Propofol	Diprivan	
Nitrous oxide		

TABLE 13.4 Representative Antianxiety Agents

Generic Name	Trade Name
Benzodiazepines	
Chlordiazepoxide	Librium
Diazepam	Valium
Flurazepam	Dalmane
Alprazolam	Xanax
Lorazepam	Ativan
Oxazepam	Serax
Temazepam	Restoril
Clorazepate	Tranxene
Triazolam	Halcion
Flunitrazepam	Rohypnol
Midazolam	Versed
Estazolam	ProSom
Clonazepam	Klonopin
Prazepam	Centrax
Halazepam	Paxipam
Nonbarbiturates, nonbenzodiazepines	
Meprobamate	Equanil
Hydroxyzine	Vistaril, Atarax
Ethinamate	Valmid
Buspirone	BuSpar

Note: The most frequently prescribed antianxiety drugs incude alprazolam (Xanax), lorazepam (Ativan), clonazepam (Klonopin), and diazepam (Valium).

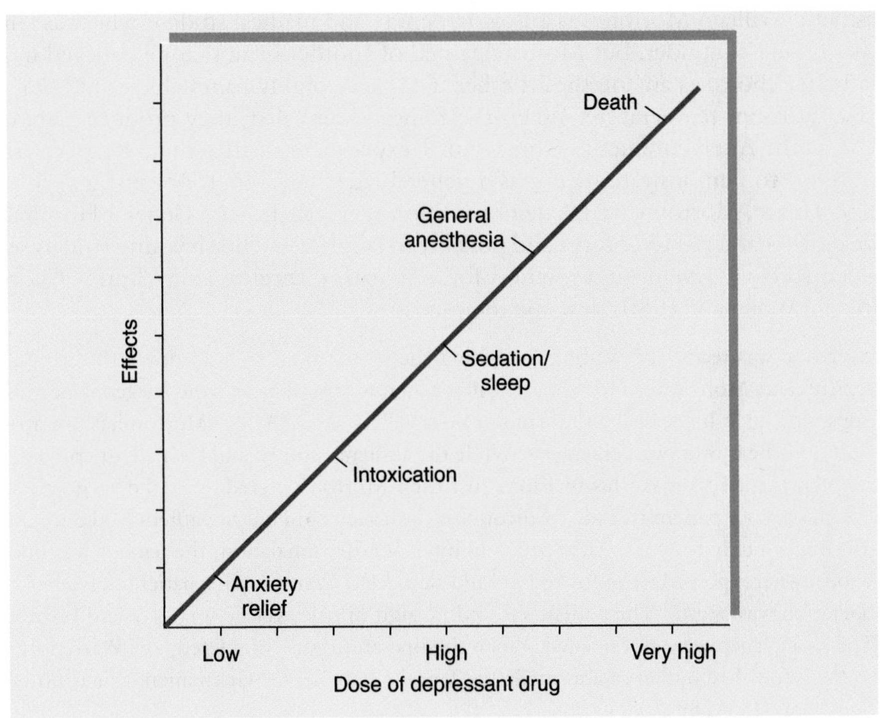

FIGURE 13.1
Effects Per Dose of a Depressant Drug

oxide is used almost exclusively for anesthesia). The benzodiazepines are currently the most important class of drugs for treating anxiety and sleeping disorders.

Early History

Perhaps the first depressant compound other than alcohol to be used was the gas nitrous oxide, discovered by Joseph Priestley and synthesized by Humphry Davy in 1776. These English scientists were the first to note that inhalation of nitrous oxide produced a short period of intoxication similar to drunkenness. Because the euphoric state that nitrous oxide produces often results in laughter and giggling, it came to be known as laughing gas (Brecher, 1972). Although Davy and others experimented with the gas for recreational purposes, its use in medicine was long delayed by one of the most famous stories in the history of medicine.

The story begins in 1845, in Hartford, Connecticut, where a young dentist named Horace Wells attended an exhibition of the effects of laughing gas. People paid admission to sniff nitrous oxide or just to watch others. One of the users apparently tripped and was badly cut during the exhibition, and Wells noticed that he seemed to feel no pain despite the severe injury. As a dentist, Wells immediately realized the possible uses of such a drug. Dentistry and other surgeries were immensely painful during this era that lacked anesthetic agents. Wells then experimented with nitrous oxide and discovered that teeth could be pulled without pain. After proclaiming his discovery, Wells was invited to demonstrate his procedure at the Massachusetts General Hospital in Boston. There, before a prestigious group of physicians, Wells placed a patient under anesthesia. Wells had not studied the drug well enough to establish dosages reliably, however, and the patient awakened during surgery screaming in pain. Wells was laughed out of the amphitheater by the skeptical scientists, and the use of nitrous oxide as an anesthesia was set back many years. Today, nitrous oxide is widely used in dentistry and some types of surgery.

The next era in the history of depressants also involved the search for an effective anesthetic. William Morton was a Boston dentist and medical student who was familiar with Wells's blunder, but Morton learned of another drug that he believed might be a better choice as an anesthetic: ether. Ether is a highly flammable liquid that vaporizes at room temperature. When the fumes are inhaled, they produce a state of intoxication. After conducting some initial experiments with ether, Morton asked permission to demonstrate its use as a general anesthetic. In 1846, just a year after Wells's failure, Morton gave his demonstration at Massachusetts General Hospital. A large crowd gathered to observe and possibly to laugh at the brash young student who claimed to have developed a method for eliminating surgical pain. Smith, Cooperman, and Wollman (1980) describe the events:

> Everyone was ready and waiting, including the strong men to hold down the struggling patient, but Morton did not appear. Fifteen minutes passed, and the surgeon, becoming impatient, took his scalpel and turning to the gallery said, "As Dr. Morton has not arrived I presume he is otherwise engaged." While the audience smiled and the patient cringed, the surgeon turned to make his incision. Just then Morton entered . . . [the surgeon] said, "Well, sir, your patient is ready." Surrounded by a silent and unsympathetic audience, Morton went quietly to work. After a few minutes of ether inhalation, the patient was unconscious, whereupon Morton looked up and said, "Dr. Warren, your patient is ready." The operation was begun. The patient showed no sign of pain, yet he was alive and breathing. The strong men were not needed. When the operation was completed, Dr. Warren turned to the astonished audience and made the famous statement, "Gentlemen, this is no humbug." (pp. 258–259)

Morton had just given the first public demonstration of surgical anesthesia and had revolutionized the practice of surgery. The use of ether as an anesthetic quickly became widespread, and it is still used today occasionally along with newer anesthetics such as halothane, related gases, and barbiturates.

Barbiturates

A number of depressant drugs were introduced in the 19th century, including chloroform, chloral hydrate, and paraldehyde, but the next truly significant development was the introduction of the barbiturates in 1862. The first barbiturate was developed in that year in the Bayer laboratories in Munich, Germany. Barbiturate compounds are synthesized using, among other things, chemicals found in urine, and some say Bayer gave the drugs their name to honor a woman named Barbara who provided the urine samples (Barbara's urates?). Others claim the name was to honor St. Barbara, and there are other stories as well (Perrine, 1996). We may never know, but regardless of how they were named, the class of depressant drugs called barbiturates now includes more than 2,000 different compounds (although only about 50 are currently available in the United States). Because so many barbiturates have been developed, custom dictates that both generic and brand names of these drugs end with the suffix "-al." A few representative barbiturates are listed in Table 13.3.

The effects of these various barbiturates are generally similar, differing primarily in potency and duration of action. Thus, pentobarbital and secobarbital are considered potent and short acting (duration of action 2 to 4 hours), amobarbital is intermediate (6 to 8 hours), and phenobarbital longer acting (8 to 10 hours). Barbiturates, like benzodiazepines, are thought to act by influencing inhibitory neurotransmission, a mechanism of action we discuss later in this chapter. In general, barbiturates that have a rapid onset and short duration of action are used as anesthetics today (for example, pentobarbital), whereas those with slower onset and longer duration of action are

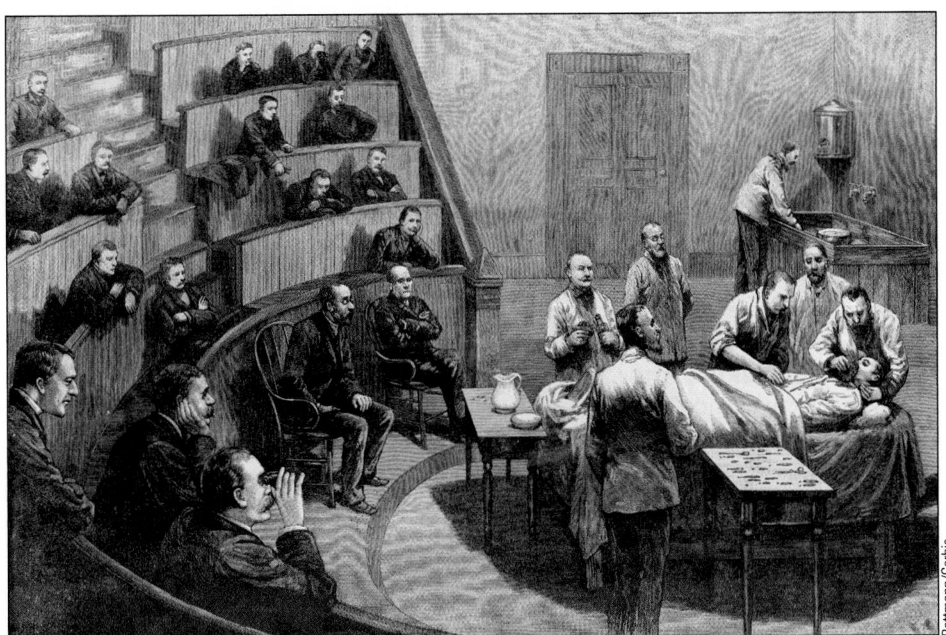

Bettmann/Corbis

William Morton successfully used ether inhalation to render a patient unconscious in the first public demonstration of surgical anesthesia.

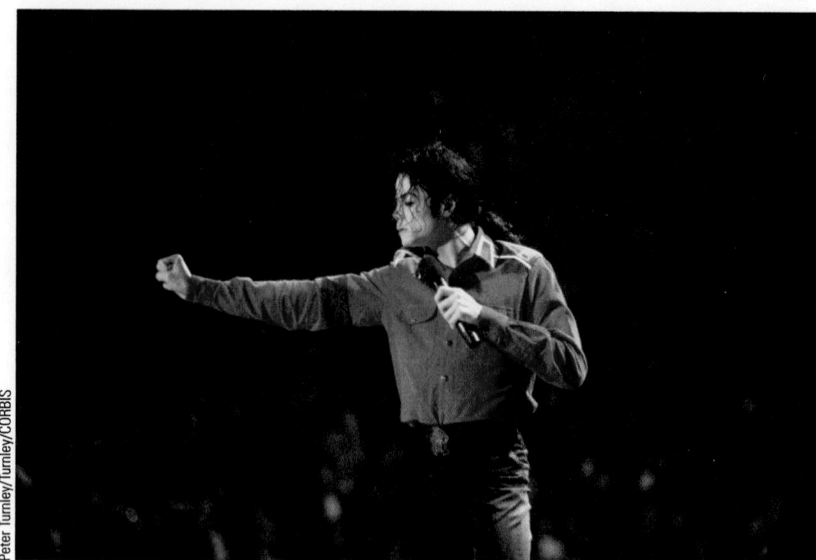
Peter Turnley/Turnley/CORBIS

The toxicology results carried out on the blood of singer Michael Jackson showed that he died of an overdose of propofol (trade name Diprivan), a powerful sedative/anesthetic sometimes prescribed for insomnia. On the day Jackson died, his doctor had also given Jackson diazepam (Valium), lorazepam (Ativan), and midazolam (Versed).

preferred for the treatment of epilepsy (phenobarbital).

Barbiturates were introduced into general medical practice in 1903, when barbital was marketed under the brand name Veronal. They soon became popular as a treatment for anxiety and as the first "sleeping pills" (Brecher, 1972). Use of barbiturates continued to increase until the 1960s, but has declined markedly in the years since. Several reasons account for the rise and fall of barbiturate use. Of the various afflictions people experienced in the 20th century and currently, sleeping disorders and anxiety problems are among the most common. Thus, any drug that offers relief from anxiety or promises sleep to insomniacs has potential for tremendous popularity and commercial success. The barbiturates do have the capacity to induce sleep and to relieve anxiety, and this accounts for their ascendance. However, consumers and physicians did not at first know a number of the problems associated with barbiturate use (discussed next). These led to the decline of barbiturate use in the past 25 years.

All the barbiturates possess the properties of CNS depressants. Thus, in moderate doses, they produce a drunken euphoric state. Similar to alcohol, barbiturates may produce a loss of motor coordination, a staggering gait, and slurred speech. Loss of emotional control and behavioral disinhibition are also characteristic effects. Sedation and sleep are produced by increased doses, and higher doses produce surgical anesthesia. Physiological effects include respiratory depression, which is responsible for most of the overdose deaths associated with barbiturates. In addition, some depression of heart rate, blood pressure, and gastrointestinal activity is noted at higher doses.

As noted, the barbiturates once were used extensively as sedative-hypnotic drugs, but except for certain specialized uses, they now have been replaced by the safer benzodiazepines. Short-acting barbiturates still are used to produce anesthesia. Other current uses include emergency treatment of convulsions and prevention of seizures in people with certain types of epilepsy (Perrine, 1996).

One major reason for the movement away from the medical use of barbiturates involves tolerance and dependence. Tolerance develops fairly rapidly to many effects of the barbiturates. Whereas a given dose may be effective at inducing sleep for a while, the patient soon may require a higher dose to sleep if the drug is used regularly. If doses escalate too much and regular use persists, patients will experience an abstinence syndrome when they attempt to withdraw from barbiturates. The symptoms of the barbiturate withdrawal syndrome are similar to those of alcohol—shakes, perspiration, confusion, and full-blown delirium tremens (DTs) in some cases (see Chapter 9)—but convulsions and seizures are more likely to occur in barbiturate withdrawal; they are seen in 5% to 20% of the cases (Schuckit, 1995). As with alcohol, the severity of barbiturate withdrawal depends upon the extent of use. Mild symptoms such as

rebound insomnia (discussed next) and anxiety may occur after a brief use of barbiturates, whereas life-threatening convulsions occur only after heavier use.

rebound insomnia
Inability to sleep produced as a withdrawal symptom associated with some depressant drugs.

Many people became dependent on barbiturates even though the drugs were used only under medical supervision. Suppose someone is in crisis—say, after the death of a spouse or other loved one. A physician may prescribe a sleeping pill to help the person rest during the crisis. After a few weeks, the patient may feel emotionally ready to sleep without the drug—and indeed may be. But the first night the patient attempts to sleep without the barbiturate, the person may have a great deal of trouble because of rebound insomnia, one of the features of barbiturate withdrawal (Mendelson, 1980). That is, after the chronic use of barbiturates, abstinence produces insomnia even in someone who was untroubled with insomnia previously.

A related problem involves the type of sleep experienced while under the influence of barbiturates and after heavy use of sleeping pills. Barbiturates do induce sleep, but like alcohol, they reduce the amount of time spent in the rapid eye movement or REM stage of sleep. This may account in part for the "hungover" feeling some people report after sleeping with the aid of a drug. Although they get enough hours of sleep, it may not be "high-quality" sleep. Further, when subjects try to sleep without a pill after taking drugs for several nights, they may experience **REM rebound**; that is, they spend more time than normal in REM. Often accompanying REM rebound are vivid dreams and nightmares with nocturnal awakening.

REM rebound
An increase in the rapid eye movement or REM stage of sleep when withdrawing from drugs that suppress REM time.

So even if the tired patients are able to sleep without drugs during barbiturate withdrawal, they may awaken early in the morning and not be able to get back to sleep. Other factors may be involved, but it is clear that once dependence on sleeping pills has developed, considerable time must pass before normal sleep patterns return (Mendelson, 1980). All of these factors make it easy to understand why dependence on drugs such as barbiturates for sleeping so often develops. Dependence certainly limits the usefulness of these and other depressants as a treatment of sleep disorders.

"You can get drunk on them [benzodiazepines and other minor tranquilizers]; you can become addicted to them; and you can suffer delirium tremens when they are withdrawn."

(Brecher, 1972)

An additional problem with the barbiturates is the risk of fatal drug overdose. The lethal dose of many barbiturates is fairly low compared to the effective dose in inducing sleep, and accidental overdoses have been a problem. This is particularly evident when barbiturates are taken in combination with alcohol or other depressant drugs, because these drugs potentiate one another (Schuckit, 1995). Barbiturates often were prescribed to people suffering from depression because sleeping disorders are a common symptom of clinical depression. Because there is a risk that severely depressed patients may attempt suicide, having a prescription for barbiturates could make them more likely to succeed in their attempt. Barbiturates have been the lethal drug in many suicides, including celebrated cases such as that of Marilyn Monroe.

Barbiturates (particularly the short-acting barbiturates) produce a euphoric state similar to alcohol intoxication. In fact, a recent laboratory study compared the behavioral and subjective effects of alcohol with those of the barbiturate pentobarbital and concluded that they were virtually identical, with the exception that the barbiturate was somewhat more sedating and more likely to be abused than alcohol (Mintzer et al., 1997). As a result, barbiturates became significant recreational drugs on the street during the 1950s and 1960s. An estimated 5 billion doses of barbiturates entered the illicit market in 1969 alone (Brecher, 1972). Clearly, barbiturates were causing some major societal problems, and the quest was on for safer drugs to relieve anxiety and induce sleep.

Quaaludes and Other Nonbarbiturate Sedatives

Several nonbarbiturate sedatives were introduced in the 1950s and 1960s, as possible alternatives in the treatment of anxiety and sleep disorders. Meprobamate (trade name Equanil), ethchlorvynol (Placidyl), and glutethimide (Doriden) have all been used in this way, but each seemed to possess the same undesirable properties as the barbiturates. One important candidate as an alternative to barbiturates was methaqualone, first marketed under the brand names Quaalude and Sopor in 1965. Although some thought methaqualone would be much safer because it was not a barbiturate, this did not prove to be true. It quickly became evident that methaqualone was toxic at high doses, especially when taken in combination with alcohol. In addition, dependence develops rapidly to methaqualone, with abstinence symptoms similar to those produced by alcohol and barbiturates. Thus, medical enthusiasm for methaqualone was quickly dampened. Because it produces a pronounced state of "drunkenness" and developed a reputation as a sexual enhancer, however, methaqualone became a major street drug in the 1970s, and was sometimes known as "disco biscuits" or "ludes." Very little research is available about the true effects of methaqualone on sexuality. Anecdotal data are mixed: Some users report a disinhibition they find enhances sexual experience, but others report it interferes with sexual behavior (Abel, 1985). Actually, given the similarity in pharmacology between methaqualone and other depressants such as alcohol, it would be surprising if there were any major differences in the way these drugs affect sexual behavior (see Chapter 9).

The problems of abuse with methaqualone and other nonbarbiturate sedatives far outweigh their medical benefits, and currently these drugs are rarely used for the management of sleep problems or anxiety. In fact, methaqualone has become a Schedule I drug and is no longer produced for medical use. A major reason these drugs and the barbiturates have lost favor is the widespread acceptance of the benzodiazepines as the treatment of choice in these disorders.

The Problem of Anxiety

At this point, it makes sense to define anxiety and to provide some background and perspective on its treatment today. (A list of the most commonly prescribed antianxiety drugs is provided in Table 13.4.) Anxiety is frequently experienced as some or all of four categories of symptoms: (1) motor tension (for example, shakiness, muscle tension, restlessness); (2) autonomic hyperactivity (sweating, pounding heart, stomach tightness, flushing); (3) apprehensive expectation (anxiety, fear, rumination); and (4) vigilance (impatience, hyperattentiveness, insomnia) (APA, 2000a). Approximately 29% of adults in the United States will meet the criteria for an anxiety disorder at some point in their lives, and 18% will meet the criteria in any given year. Clinicians frequently speak of two types of anxiety. The first is a trait or characterological anxiety, in that people seem to experience their anxiety practically all the time. The second is a more transient state, called situational anxiety, wherein the anxiety is much greater at some times than at others, when the person may not even feel anxious at all. A related type of anxiety is panic attacks, which are recurrent and unpredictable periods of intense fear and impending doom (Ibid.). These attacks frequently include sweating, palpitations, dizziness, and difficulty in breathing. A case illustration of panic attacks from Spitzer et al. (1989) follows:

> Mindy is a stylishly dressed, 25-year-old art director who is seeking treatment for "panic attacks" that have occurred with increasing frequency over the past year, often two or three times a day. These attacks begin with a sudden intense wave of "horrible fear" that seems to come out of nowhere, sometimes during the day, sometimes waking her from sleep. She begins to tremble, is nauseated, sweats profusely, feels as though she is gagging, and fears that she will lose control and do something crazy, like run screaming into the street.
>
> Mindy remembers first having attacks like this when she was in high school. She was dating a boy her parents disapproved of, and had to do a lot of "sneaking around" to avoid confrontations with them. At the same time, she was under a lot of pressure as the principal

CONTEMPORARY ISSUE BOX 13.4

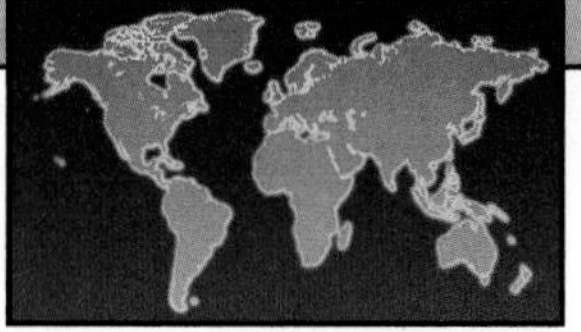

Internet Pharmacies: Rx for Disaster?

Prescription drugs have become easier than ever to obtain, thanks to the proliferation of Internet-based pharmacies. Literally thousands of such sites, both foreign and domestic, have appeared in recent years. In many cases, people may obtain drugs without speaking to a doctor and/or without having a prescription.

Many view the marketing of prescription drugs over the Internet as a dangerous trend. They cite concerns about three different types of online providers. First, and of greatest concern, are sites that sell products like GHB, a "date rape" drug. Second are sites, predominantly foreign, that sell misbranded, counterfeit, or out-of-date drugs. And third are sites that sell drugs to individuals who do not hold a prescription obtained through a qualified health professional.

The near boundary-less nature of the Internet has made it difficult for regulators trying to get a handle on Internet drug sales. At minimum, the sheer number of online pharmacies in operation overwhelms regulators. They are hoping that ongoing efforts to craft Internet licensing criteria will provide much-needed relief. In addition, a host of legislative efforts are underway. One example is the Ryan Haight Online Pharmacy Consumer Protection Act of 2008, which addresses the purchase or dispensing of controlled substances via the Internet. The act is named for a teenager whose death resulted in part from the ease with which he obtained a narcotic drug over the Internet without a valid prescription. The act amends the Controlled Substances Act to prohibit the delivery, distribution, or dispensing of a controlled substance over the Internet without a valid prescription. The act also requires that a face-to-face physician contact occur prior to the issuance of a prescription for a controlled substance.

designer of her high school yearbook, and was applying to Ivy League colleges. She remembers that her first panic attack occurred just after the yearbook went to press and she was accepted by Harvard, Yale, and Brown. The attacks lasted only a few minutes, and she would just "sit through them." She was worried enough to mention them to her mother; but because she was otherwise perfectly healthy, she did not seek treatment.

Over the eight years since her first attack, Mindy has had them intermittently, sometimes not for many months, sometimes, as now, several times a day. There have also been extreme variations in the intensity of the attacks, some being so severe and debilitating that she had to take a day off from work.

Apart from her panic attacks and a brief period of depression at 19, when she broke up with a boyfriend, Mindy has always functioned extremely well, in school, at work, and in her social life. She is a lively, friendly person who is respected by her friends and colleagues both for her intelligence and creativity and for her ability to mediate disputes.

Even during the times that she was having frequent, severe attacks, Mindy never limited her activities. She might stay home from work for a day because she was exhausted from multiple attacks, but she never associated the attacks with particular places. (Reprinted with permission from the *Diagnostic and Statistical Manual of Mental Disorders.* Copyright 1981 & 1989 American Psychiatric Association.)

Before the 20th century, the common palliative for anxiety symptoms was drinking alcohol, perhaps the oldest known means of sedation. For much of this century, into the 1950s, anxiety was treated primarily with bromide salts (which were available without prescription) and barbiturates. By the 1930s, scientists were discovering that the use of the bromides had many dangerous side effects (Feldman, Meyer, & Quenzer, 1997). Barbiturates, such as phenobarbital, were used then more frequently as an anxiolytic agent. As noted earlier, however, it gradually became clear that these drugs were physically addictive because users developed tolerance and exhibited a severe withdrawal reaction when drug use ceased. As a result, efforts were directed at developing an anxiolytic medication that would effectively treat the anxiety but not be physically addicting. The first in the desired group of nonbarbiturate sedatives was meprobamate, but again, it was found that a severe withdrawal syndrome was associated with discontinuing its use after some period of time on the drug. The world was still looking for a safer anxiolytic.

Benzodiazepines

benzodiazepines Currently the most widely prescribed anxiolytic drugs.

In the late 1950s, scientists at Roche Laboratories synthesized a new group of compounds known as the **benzodiazepines**. Animal tests with these drugs showed sedative, anticonvulsant, and muscle-relaxant effects similar to those of the barbiturates. An additional feature was that they produced a "taming" effect in monkeys. Even more intriguing, these drugs showed very low toxicity: The lethal dose is sufficiently high that it is difficult to attain. The first of the benzodiazepines, chlordiazepoxide (trade name Librium), was first marketed in 1960, closely followed by the introduction of its more potent cousin, diazepam (Valium) in 1963 (Sternbach, 1983). These two drugs quickly came to dominate the market as treatments for anxiety and insomnia. By the 1970s, they were among the best-selling drugs in America, with 100 million prescriptions written for benzodiazepines in 1975 alone (Harvey, 1980). More recently, because of widespread concern about dependence and other side effects, the use of these drugs is down, but they are still frequently prescribed.

"Valium is . . . a leveler. It evens things out silently, quietly. No rush. No thrill. No charge."

(Gordon, 1979)

Depressant drugs share many traits. Alcohol, barbiturates, nonbarbiturate sedatives, and of course benzodiazepines all have similar effects when equated for dose. In addition, cross-tolerance occurs between these drugs, and they potentiate one another. Cross-dependence also occurs because an appropriate dose of any depressant can be used to reduce the withdrawal symptoms produced by any other. In fact, benzodiazepines are commonly used to withdraw alcoholics from alcohol. Thus, substantial evidence indicates a common mechanism of action for depressant drugs (Julien, 2001).

By the 1970s, evidence had begun to accumulate that GABA, the brain's major inhibitory neurotransmitter, might provide the common link (Costa, Guidotti, & Mao, 1975; Ticku, Burch, & Davis, 1983). The problem was that no direct evidence was found that any of the depressant drugs bound to the GABA receptor site. Then, in 1977, two independent laboratories reported the discovery of binding sites for benzodiazepines (Möhler & Okada, 1977; Squires & Braestrup, 1977), and it was subsequently shown that, although specific to benzodiazepines, these receptors are part of what is now called the GABA/benzodiazepine receptor complex (Feldman, Meyer, & Quenzer, 1997). Apparently the normal neural inhibition produced by GABA is greatly enhanced when there is activity at the benzodiazepine receptor. Benzodiazepines act by enhancing neural inhibition in the GABA system.

When taken orally, benzodiazepines generally are absorbed slowly and have a long duration of action. Considerable variability exists in duration of action, however, which accounts for the different uses for and effects of the different benzodiazepines. Table 13.5 shows the half-lives for some of the widely used benzodiazepines (the time required for half of the drug to be metabolized). The longer-acting benzodiazepines such as Valium are considered most useful when it is desirable to maintain the patient at a constant level of drug over an extended period—for example, when an individual is suffering from an anxiety reaction. The short- and intermediate-duration benzodiazepines are more useful for treating insomnia when it is desirable to have the drug effects wear off by morning.

TABLE 13.5 Kinetic Classification of Representative Benzodiazepines

Type	Half-life (hours)
Long half-life	
Flurazepam (Dalmane)	75
Diazepam (Valium)	50
Intermediate half-life	
Alprazolam (Xanax)	15
Lorazepam (Ativan)	15
Short half-life	
Triazolam (Halcion)	4
Midazolam (Versed)	1

A number of reasons exist for the commercial success of the benzodiazepines. First, they are effective at relieving anxiety and inducing sleep. In fact, benzodiazepines are sometimes claimed to be uniquely effective as anxiolytic agents. It is true they relieve anxiety in animal studies and in humans at doses that do not produce motor impairment (ataxia) or pronounced sedation. In animals, anxiolytic action is tested by determining the ability of a drug to increase rates of a punishment response (see Chapter 5). Animals, typically rats, are trained to press a lever to produce food or water reinforcement. Then, during some periods, lever pressing is punished by electric shock; during other periods, no shock is delivered. Normally, rats will show decreased rates of lever pressing in the punishment component. When benzodiazepines are given to animals trained with such procedures, the rates of lever pressing in the punishment component go up almost to baseline levels at doses that do not affect the unpunished component. The clinical efficacy of various benzodiazepines measured in humans is correlated closely with these antipunishment actions, and for this reason, the facilitation of a punishment response is viewed as an excellent animal model of human anxiety. In fact, novel anxiolytic drugs have been discovered on the basis of antipunishment effects on this animal model. Although other depressant drugs also show antipunishment effects, none is as selective in this regard as benzodiazepines. This is one reason for considering benzodiazepines as possessing some unique anxiolytic actions.

The potent anxiolytic actions of benzodiazepines occur at doses that produce fewer serious side effects than barbiturates. Although drowsiness may occur when taking benzodiazepines, it is less of a problem than with other depressant drugs. Because the lethal dose is so high, suicide and accidental overdose are far less of a risk with benzodiazepines than with other depressant drugs. Benzodiazepines do interact to potentiate alcohol and other depressant drugs, however, and fatal overdoses are not uncommon with such drug combinations. So benzodiazepines, though not nearly so toxic as depressants such as barbiturates or methaqualone, are not without overdose risk.

"You can get roaring drunk on 'barbs.'"

(Brecher, 1972)

In addition to use in anxiety disorders, benzodiazepines are often prescribed for insomnia. These drugs are effective at reducing both the amount of time required to fall asleep and the amount of awake time in cases where the person wakes up after the initial sleep onset. As we noted for the barbiturates, though, benzodiazepines also change the pattern of sleep. Benzodiazepines suppress the amount of REM sleep and change the EEG patterns observed during non-REM sleep. Unlike barbiturates, the short- or intermediate-duration benzodiazepines—sleeping pills such as the popular and controversial triazolam (trade name Halcion) or temazepam (Restoril)—do not often produce "hangover" or day-after effects. Rebound insomnia is a problem with all of the benzodiazepines but to a lesser extent than it was with the barbiturates (Parrino & Terzano, 1996). Finally, other side effects have been reported, particularly depression and paranoia with Halcion.

Benzodiazepines also are used for purposes other than anxiety and insomnia management. For example, benzodiazepines have muscle-relaxant and anticonvulsant actions and are often used as a treatment for muscle spasms and seizures. Short-acting benzodiazepines such as midazolam (trade name Versed) are used as anesthetics in some surgical procedures.

Finally, benzodiazepines are frequently used to medically manage withdrawal from alcohol. Because alcohol shows cross-dependence with benzodiazepines and other depressants, tapering off from alcohol use is made easier through the use of benzodiazepines. The general practice, often referred to as *detoxification*, involves providing an initial dose of the benzodiazepine that is sufficient to suppress potentially dangerous alcohol withdrawal symptoms. Then, over a period of weeks, the dose is gradually reduced. There is great concern that an individual with a history of alcohol problems may simply substitute benzodiazepine abuse for alcohol, so the goal of most detoxification programs is to taper the client off benzodiazepines as rapidly as possible.

Tolerance develops to benzodiazepines, and there is cross-tolerance between them and other depressants. Tolerance to benzodiazepines develops slowly, however, and fairly high doses are needed for tolerance to develop. There is some controversy about the frequency of withdrawal symptoms following benzodiazepine use. It has been argued that withdrawal occurs only at very high doses, but more recent studies find withdrawal affects between 5% and 35% of patients who have taken benzodiazepines for one month or longer (Miller & Greenblatt, 1996). When withdrawal syndromes do occur, they are similar to those associated with alcohol and barbiturates but generally not so severe. Abstinence symptoms may not appear for several days or even more than a week and may persist for up to four weeks. The main symptoms are rebound insomnia, anxiety, tremors, sweating, and occasionally more serious problems such as seizures (Schuckit, 1995). One of the problems in interpreting benzodiazepine withdrawal is differentiating abstinence symptoms from the symptoms the drug was suppressing. For example, a great deal of controversy about Valium was stirred by the autobiographical book and movie *I'm Dancing as Fast as I Can* by Barbara Gordon (1979). Gordon was a successful professional whose psychiatrist was maintaining her on very high doses of Valium. When she decided to quit Valium, her physician told her to simply stop taking the drug rather than tapering off. This was certainly a poor decision. Gordon describes her withdrawal symptoms vividly:

> By early afternoon I began to feel a creeping sense of anxiety. But it was different from my usual bouts of terror. It felt like little jolts of electricity, as if charged pins and needles were shooting through my body. My breathing became rapid and I began to perspire. . . .
>
> My scalp started to burn as if I had hot coals under my hair. Then I began to experience funny little twitches, spasms, a jerk of a leg, a flying arm, tiny tremors that soon turned into convulsions. (p. 51)

Gordon was unable to leave her own house, much less work. Her relationships with her lover and other friends deteriorated, and eventually she required hospitalization for several months. Nevertheless, her symptoms persisted even beyond this time. The book is a moving description of anxiety disorder, though perhaps not a very typical description of Valium withdrawal. As we noted, although some withdrawal symptoms are very persistent (Modell, 1997), it is difficult to differentiate long-lasting withdrawal from the reemergence of previous anxiety symptoms. Thus, Barbara Gordon's experience may illustrate a case where the severity of her symptoms was revealed only when the drug, which had masked them, was removed.

The issues of abuse of and dependence on benzodiazepines have been controversial. Benzodiazepines do turn up on the street but far less frequently than barbiturates or Quaaludes did in their day. In general, the potential for abuse of benzodiazepines is considered to be fairly moderate in comparison with most other depressants (Cappell, Sellers, & Busto, 1986). There are still reports of abuse and dependence, and they appear to be most common in individuals who abuse other drugs (King, 1994). The risk of abuse is higher for people who have a history of drug or alcohol problems than for those without such a history. For example, one laboratory study compared the effects of alprazolam (trade name Xanax) in a group of men with alcoholism who had abstained from alcohol for up to 72 hours with a group of men without alcoholism. The pharmacokinetics (absorption and metabolism) of the drug did not differ in the two groups, but those with alcoholism reported that they "liked" the effects of the drug more. "Liking" the drug was measured on a questionnaire that correlates with drug-abuse liability (Ciraulo et al., 1988). Griffiths et al. (1980) also have investigated benzodiazepine self-administration in human volunteers who have histories of sedative abuse. In double-blind laboratory studies, these researchers have shown that humans will self-administer benzodiazepines and prefer them to placebo but, like nonhumans, prefer barbiturates (Griffiths et al., 1980). When different benzodiazepines were compared, the more potent drugs with a rapid onset of action, such as Valium and Xanax, were preferred to the less potent compounds with slower onset of action, such as oxazepam (Griffiths, McLeod, Bigelow, Liebson, Roache, & Nowowieski, 1984; Griffiths, McLeod, Bigelow, Liebson, & Roache, 1984; Mumford, Rush, & Griffiths, 1995). This observation may explain the recent rash of reports of abuse of the potent benzodiazepine Rohypnol (flunitrazepam), or "roofies" as they are referred to on the street (see Contemporary Issue Box 13.5).

CONTEMPORARY ISSUE BOX 13.5

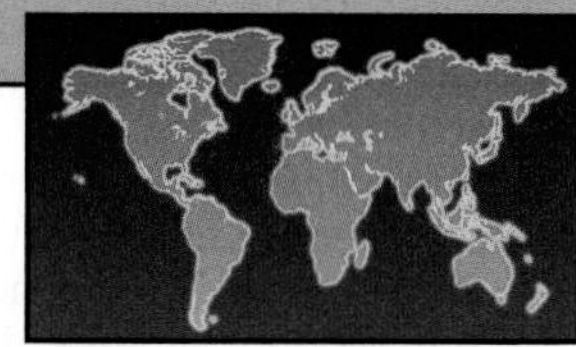

Roofies: A New Wave of Sedative Abuse

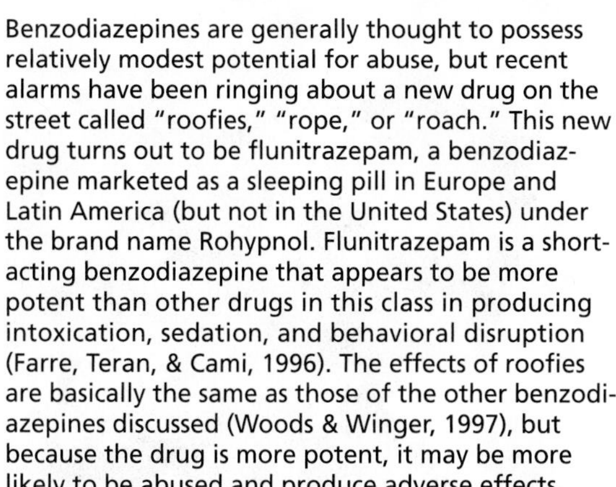

Benzodiazepines are generally thought to possess relatively modest potential for abuse, but recent alarms have been ringing about a new drug on the street called "roofies," "rope," or "roach." This new drug turns out to be flunitrazepam, a benzodiazepine marketed as a sleeping pill in Europe and Latin America (but not in the United States) under the brand name Rohypnol. Flunitrazepam is a short-acting benzodiazepine that appears to be more potent than other drugs in this class in producing intoxication, sedation, and behavioral disruption (Farre, Teran, & Cami, 1996). The effects of roofies are basically the same as those of the other benzodiazepines discussed (Woods & Winger, 1997), but because the drug is more potent, it may be more likely to be abused and produce adverse effects.

Of particular concern is the link between roofies and memory loss or blackouts. This effect has resulted in roofies' apparent association with date rape. Cases have surfaced that involved men slipping the drug into a woman's drink without her knowledge and, after the drug "knocked her out," raping her (Seligman & King, 1996). Prosecution of these cases can be difficult because the women are often unable to remember much about the crime. In addition, there is concern about the potential of roofies to produce dependence and dangerous drug interactions. A synergistic combination of flunitrazepam and alcohol put rock star Kurt Cobain into a coma just a month before his suicide. At this writing, flunitrazepam remains a Schedule IV drug, like most other benzodiazepines, but its status is under review and stiffer penalties seem likely in the future. In the meantime, keep your eyes on your drink!

Tolerance, dependence, and abuse are associated with the benzodiazepines, but the problems produced are far milder than those connected with other depressant drugs. Over the years, however, a number of other problems associated with benzodiazepine use have emerged. As with other depressants, the significant side effects of benzodiazepines are drowsiness and motor impairment. Although even these side effects are rare with benzodiazepines alone (see Cappell, Sellers, & Busto, 1986, for a review), they may become particularly problematic when benzodiazepines are taken, as they often are, in combination with alcohol or other depressant drugs (see Contemporary Issue Box 13.6).

anterograde amnesia Loss or limitation of the ability to form new memories.

A more recently recognized problem is that benzodiazepines may interfere with the storage of memories, a phenomenon called **anterograde amnesia**. Thus, when individuals are awakened by a phone call from sleep induced by benzodiazepines, they may fail to remember the phone conversation. The drug may be present in sufficient dose the next morning so that the patients forget what they had for breakfast or what was read in the morning paper. These are examples of benzodiazepine-induced amnesia, and evidence is mounting that it is a common problem, particularly with some of the popular

CONTEMPORARY ISSUE BOX 13.6

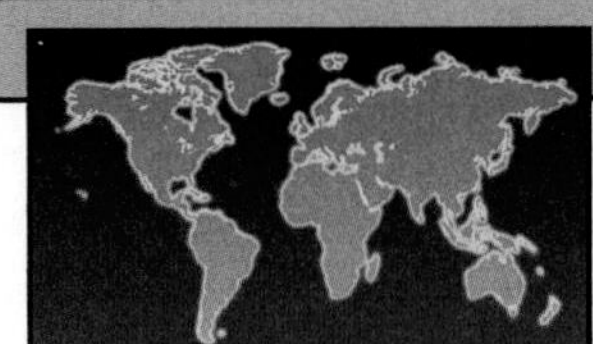

Depressant Drugs and Potentiation

All the depressant drugs reviewed to this point tend to potentiate one another; that is, the effects of the drugs when combined are greater than would be expected from the individual doses considered alone. Potentiation is among the most dangerous aspects of drug use. The vast majority of deaths from drug overdose are due not to overdose of a single drug but rather to smaller doses of more than one drug taken in lethal combination. Alcohol, barbiturates, nonbarbiturate sedatives (Quaaludes, meprobamate), and benzodiazepines all interact to produce additive effects. They interact with heroin and other opiate drugs to produce additive effects as well. Many deaths attributed to heroin overdose actually involve heroin taken in combination with alcohol or other depressant drugs, and the largest number of deaths from drug overdose in America every year involve alcohol taken in combination with other depressants, according to the National Institute on Drug Abuse. Such a combination of depressants killed Elvis Presley, and it kills thousands of others every year.

Another problem with additive effects involves cases in which lower doses are consumed. Consider a young woman who is given a prescription for Valium to help her weather a family crisis. Suppose after taking her Valium, she goes out with some friends for dinner and has a couple of beers. Perhaps she could tolerate this much alcohol without impairment under normal conditions, but by drinking in combination with the Valium, she may find herself quite intoxicated. If she attempts to drive home after such a drug combination, the loss of motor coordination may prove fatal. Combinations of alcohol with another depressant are thought to be responsible for many highway deaths above and beyond those caused by alcohol alone (O'Hanlon & De Gier, 1986). Never combine depressant drugs with alcohol or one another.

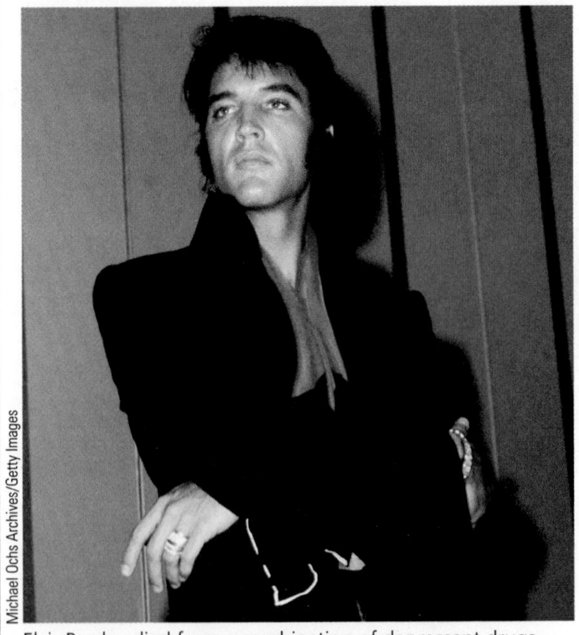

Michael Ochs Archives/Getty Images

Elvis Presley died from a combination of depressant drugs.

benzodiazepines such as triazolam (trade name Halcion) and alprazolam (Xanax) (Perrine, 1996; Salzman, 1992). This type of effect is not unique to benzodiazepines. After all, alcohol is known to produce the more dramatic memory loss of the blackout (see Chapter 9). Barbiturates and methaqualone also produce blackouts, which suggests that some type of memory deficit may be characteristic of any depressant drug.

Nonbenzodiazepine Treatment

Because of the problems reviewed in the preceding sections, considerable interest has focused on the development of new drugs for the treatment of anxiety problems and sleep disorders. One example is a drug called zolpidem (trade name Ambien). Zolpidem's chemical structure is different from the benzodiazepine drugs, but it is still thought to act as an agonist of the same "benzodiazepine" receptors. Thus, zolpidem produces more or less the same array of depressant drug effects that are associated with the benzodiazepines. However, zolpidem is effective at inducing sleep at doses that interfere very little with the "natural" sleep structure. That is, zolpidem induces sleep with less suppression of the REM stage than benzodiazepines, and it appears less likely to produce "hangover" effects or rebound insomnia (Parrino & Terzano, 1996). As a result, Ambien has become one of the most widely prescribed drugs for the treatment of insomnia. However, it should be noted that, depending on the dose, zolpidem can produce the same side effects as the benzodiazepines (Rush & Griffiths, 1996).

Another nonbenzodiazepine anxiolytic drug is buspirone (trade name BuSpar). Buspirone's chemical structure and activities are very different from any of the traditional depressant drugs. It appears to affect the serotonin neurotransmitter system, not the GABA/benzodiazepine receptor complex. Perhaps because of its different mechanism of action, buspirone has been shown to be effective in the treatment of anxiety with fewer side effects than the alternatives. For example, no withdrawal symptoms have been reported following chronic use of buspirone, and it is considered to have no significant abuse potential. Animals will not self-administer buspirone, and humans report no intoxication or euphoria after using it (Rush & Griffiths, 1997; Tunnicliff, Eison, & Taylor, 1991). Little sedation or motor impairment is seen during buspirone treatment, and it interacts less with alcohol than other depressant drugs (Rush & Griffiths, 1997). Simply put, buspirone seems to relieve anxiety without producing many of the undesirable effects of the other anxiolytic drugs. One difference is that buspirone's anxiolytic effects are delayed: It often requires three to four weeks of treatment before benefits appear. In contrast, the benzodiazepines are immediate. Also, buspirone appears less effective in the treatment of panic disorder and does not relieve insomnia (Coplan, Wolk, & Klein, 1995). Despite these limitations, buspirone is a valuable alternative for the treatment of anxiety and raises the hope that developments in psychopharmacology may lead to safer treatments for psychological problems.

Beyond these issues, it should be noted that antidepressant medications also are used in the treatment of anxiety disorders. Tricyclic antidepressants and SSRIs both have been used in the treatment of such anxiety disorders as panic disorder, obsessive-compulsive disorder, and posttraumatic stress disorder.

Mood-Stabilizing Drugs

The most specific treatment for the mood disorders of mania and bipolar disorder is lithium. Mania is a state with pronounced elevations in mood and increased activity. Symptoms of a manic episode typically include increased talkativeness, flights of ideas or racing thoughts, grandiosity, decreased need for sleep, and excessive involvement in behaviors that can produce negative consequences (such as buying sprees or sexual indiscretions) (APA, 2000a). Although these symptoms seem to describe someone who is "happy-go-lucky" or "pleasantly high," their occurrence and severity generally are profound and significantly disrupt the person's functioning. For people with this disorder, the first manic episode generally occurs in the 20s or 30s, although there are exceptions in both directions. The natural course of an untreated manic episode is generally a couple of months.

Manic attacks are usually a component of what is called bipolar, or manic-depressive, disorder; these individuals often experience periodic episodes of depression as well. The following case (Spitzer et al., 1989) illustrates the manic component of bipolar disorder. It is an example of the development of manic symptoms late in life:

> A wealthy, 72-year-old widow is referred by her children, against her will, as they think she has become "senile" since the death of her husband six months previously. After the initial bereavement, which was not severe, the patient had resumed an active social life and become a volunteer at local hospitals. The family encouraged this, but over the past three months, has become concerned about her going to local bars with some of the hospital staff. The referral was precipitated by her announcing her engagement to a 25-year-old male nurse, to whom she planned to turn over her house and a large amount of money. The patient's three sons, by threat and intimidation, have made her accompany them to this psychiatric evaluation.
>
> Initially in the interview the patient is extremely angry at her sons and the psychiatrist, insisting that they don't understand that for the first time in her life she is doing something for herself. She then suddenly drapes herself over the couch and asks the psychiatrist if she is attractive enough to capture a 25-year-old man. She proceeds to elaborate on her fiancé's physique and sexual abilities and describes her life as exciting and fulfilling for the first time. She is overtalkative and repeatedly refuses to allow the psychiatrist to interrupt her with questions. She says that she goes out nightly with her fiancé to clubs and bars and that although she does not drink, she thoroughly enjoys the atmosphere. They often go on to an after-hours place and end up breakfasting, going to bed, and making love. After only three or four hours' sleep, she gets up, feeling refreshed, and then goes shopping. She spends about $700 a week on herself and gives her fiancé about $500 a week, all of which she can easily afford. (Reprinted with permission from the *Diagnostic and Statistical Manual of Mental Disorders.* Copyright 1981 & 1989 American Psychiatric Association.)

"At this point in my existence I cannot imagine leading a normal life without both taking Lithium and having had the benefits of psychotherapy. Lithium prevents my seductive but disastrous highs, diminishes my depressions, clears out the wool and webbing from my disordered thinking, slows me down, gentles me out, keeps me from ruining my career and relationships, keeps me out of a hospital, alive, and makes psychotherapy possible."

Kay Redfield Jamison, *An Unquiet Mind* (1995, p. 88–89)

Lithium is an alkaline metal readily available throughout nature and is found in the form of silicate in such rocks as petalite, lepidolite, and spodumene (Tyrer & Shaw, 1982). Most of the lithium used in the United States is mined in North Carolina. Lithium's mood-stabilizing properties were discovered in the 1940s. An Australian physician, John Cade, was giving research animals lithium in an attempt to decrease uric acid–induced kidney damage. In the course of his work, he observed a calming effect on the animals and speculated that lithium might be useful in humans as a mood attenuator (Baldessarini, 1985; Sack & DeFraites, 1977). Cade administered lithium to a sample of manic patients and observed positive responses. Subsequent research eventually led to the approval of lithium for clinical use in the United States in 1970, although it was in clinical use in Europe several years earlier. Although lithium may have some value in treating other psychiatric disorders (such as depression, some schizophrenias, alcoholism, impulsive-aggressive behaviors, and movement disorders), it is approved in the United States only for the treatment of manic episodes and prophylactically to prevent the recurrence of manic episodes. There is strong evidence that lithium is effective with these two indications. Lithium probably is, incidentally, the only drug in psychiatry for which there is effective prophylaxis against disease recurrence (Fieve, 1976; Sack & DeFraites, 1977).

As with the antidepressants discussed earlier, the major biological theory regarding mania concerns the monoamine neurotransmitters. In depression, underactivity of neurotransmitters is hypothesized, and the hypothesis for mania is increased functional activity of the neurotransmitters. Within these hypotheses, the central focus is on catecholamines and serotonin. At the presynaptic level, lithium appears to enhance reuptake of serotonin and norepinephrine. Lithium also appears to decrease dopamine and norepinephrine effects at the postsynaptic receptors (Gitlin, 1990). Importantly, lithium serves to normalize the mood of manic patients, not just offset mania through sedation.

The most common preparations of lithium salts are carbonates (lithium carbonate, or Li_2CO_3), which are prepared in tablet form. In terms of pharmacokinetics, lithium, which is taken orally, is absorbed completely from the gastrointestinal tract (primarily the small intestine) and distributed throughout the system. The lithium is distributed in the body water and is not metabolized. Excretion occurs almost entirely by the kidneys, with between 90% and 95% eliminated through urine.

Despite its success in the treatment of mania, cautions must be taken into account prior to and during lithium use. Several of these considerations pertain to lithium's therapeutic index, or safety margin. In this regard, the difference between the therapeutic and toxic levels is small. When the therapeutic range is exceeded, at least several of the following symptoms might be observed: drowsiness, blurred vision, ataxia, confusion, cardiac irregularities, and even seizures and coma. Some deaths have been reported. Thus, lithium use requires close medical supervision. Also, pretreatment medical work-ups are specifically geared toward ruling out cardiovascular problems or renal disease. Cardiac problems are a concern because toxic effects can cause cardiac irregularities, which could then exacerbate preexisting cardiovascular problems. Renal functioning must be satisfactory so that the lithium is efficiently excreted. If it is not, lithium will accumulate in the body. Finally, several side effects are associated with lithium use, including gastrointestinal problems such as nausea, diarrhea, fine hand tremor, urinary frequency, and dry mouth. These side effects often decrease within a period of weeks, however.

Although lithium remains the major drug used in the treatment of mania, other drugs are available when the patient does not tolerate lithium or when the patient does not respond to the lithium. The most frequently used alternative is carbamazepine (trade name Tegretol), better recognized as an antiepileptic drug. Chemically related to the tricyclic antidepressants, carbamazepine has been shown to be effective with patients who have rapid-cycling manic-depressive episodes. Other alternatives to lithium that are available are clonazepam (trade name Klonopin), topiramate (Topamax), tiagabine (Gabitril), and valproic acid (Depakote), another anticonvulsant drug. There also has been recent interest in the use of several of the atypical antipsychotic medications because of their mood-stabilizing properties (in particular olanzapine [Zyprexa], aripiprazole [Abilify], and quetiapine [Seroquel]) (Alda et al., 2009).

Psychotherapeutic Drugs and Pregnancy

No psychotherapeutic medication is totally safe for use during pregnancy, and all carry FDA warnings regarding use when a patient is pregnant. As a result, a judgment needs to be made between the health of the mother on the one hand and the risks to the unborn child on the other. The approach most recommended is that psychotherapeutics not be used during pregnancy unless absolutely necessary and then only after nondrug interventions, such as counseling, have been tried first.

Psychotherapeutic drug use during pregnancy is potentially unsafe for several reasons. Certainly, on one level, the risks to the mother are at least the same as when she is not pregnant. However, the risks are increased when one considers the variety of physical changes that occur during pregnancy, including alterations in metabolism and endocrine, renal, and cardiac changes (Kerns & Davis, 1986). These and other changes create an environment in which absorption, distribution, and excretion of the drug can occur. One effect of antipsychotic medication on the mother is lowered blood pressure, which can compromise the placental blood flow to the fetus.

teratogenic Producing abnormalities in the fetus.

The fetus also faces risks, particularly **teratogenic** effects, long-term effects on neurobehavioral functioning, and direct toxic effects of the drug. This is especially the case during the first trimester of pregnancy, when particularly critical fetal development (including organ and limb development) occurs (Howland, 2009). Three points should be kept in mind (Kerns & Davis, 1986). First, all classes of psychotherapeutic drugs cross the placenta. Second, drug effects can change the blood flow within the placenta and thus influence the transport and nutritive functions of the placenta. Third, the fetus, compared to an adult, has greater cardiac output and a greater proportion of blood flow to the brain. This results in a greater exposure of the drug to the brain. Comparable considerations, to a lesser extent, come into play in the context of breast-feeding. Concentrations of some psychotherapeutic medications are detectable in the breast milk of mothers taking such medications (Field, 2008).

The effects of psychotherapeutic drugs on the fetus are not well established. Most of the research has been conducted, for obvious reasons, on animals rather than humans. And the work involving humans, usually follow-up studies on women who used these drugs during pregnancy and their offspring, is hard to interpret. For example, many of the pregnant women who use psychotherapeutic medications have used more than one drug, and many have used other substances as well, such as alcohol or cigarettes. Nevertheless, there are indications, with varying levels of risk, that various teratogenic, neurobehavioral, and toxic consequences can occur when psychotherapeutics are used during pregnancy. Perhaps the most widely recognized effect is the association of lithium used during the first trimester of pregnancy with a significant teratogenic risk of cardiovascular system impairment (Fait et al., 2002).

Summary

- Psychotherapeutic medications are prescribed in hopes of providing mentally ill people some relief and ideally the opportunity to function better in their environments.
- Early efforts to deal with mental illness included a variety of speculative approaches, many of which were cruel. These included bloodletting, hot irons, flogging, and starvation.
- Later on, in the mid-1800s, cannabis was studied as a treatment for depression and mania.
- During the first half of the 1900s, amphetamines were used in the treatment of depression and narcolepsy, and carbon dioxide in the treatment of various psychotic and neurotic conditions.
- In 1949, the Australian physician John Cade discovered the benefits of lithium in the treatment of mania, and lithium remains a mainstay in the treatment of that disorder today.
- The greatest advance in psychopharmacology was the use, starting around 1950, of the drug chlorpromazine as an antipsychotic medication. A host of other drugs were introduced in the years following, including antianxiety medications (including meprobamate, a muscle relaxant) and antidepressant medications (including the cyclic antidepressants and monoamine oxidase inhibitors).
- About one-quarter of the U.S. population experience some form of mental disorder in any

given year. Most have symptoms associated with anxiety, depression, or alcohol abuse.

- Psychotherapeutic drug use is more likely among women, older people, people living alone, the more educated, and those with higher incomes.
- The illicit use of prescription medications is a serious problem. Prescription drugs are a factor in a large number of drug-related emergency room cases and drug-related deaths. Information-gathering networks, such as the Drug Abuse Warning Network (DAWN), have been established to monitor the distribution and use (legal and otherwise) of drugs overall, including psychotherapeutic drugs.
- Psychotherapeutic drugs can affect the neurotransmitter/receptor system. The prominent processes are binding directly to the receptor site, serving as a receptor agonist or antagonist; causing the release of more neurotransmitters; blocking the reuptake of neurotransmitters back into the presynaptic neuron; changing the number of receptor sites or the sensitivity of the receptors; altering the metabolism of the neurotransmitter; and altering the enzymatic degradation of the neurotransmitter.
- Like other drugs, psychotherapeutic drugs can be classified in different ways. The most common way is by therapeutic use, and the four major categories are antipsychotics, antidepressants, antianxiety agents, and mood-stabilizing drugs.
- Antipsychotic medications, also known as neuroleptics or major tranquilizers, are used to treat schizophrenia and other disorders, such as mania, agitated depression, toxic psychoses, emotionally unstable personalities, and psychoses associated with old age. These medications affect primarily the reticular activating system, the limbic system, and the hypothalamus.
- The dopamine hypothesis is the most accepted explanation of the action of antipsychotic medications. Two core elements of the dopamine hypothesis are that increased levels of dopaminergic activity induce psychoses, and most antipsychotic drugs block postsynaptic dopamine receptors.
- Tardive dyskinesia is a major side effect of long-term use of antipsychotic drugs. It is characterized by repetitive, involuntary movements of the mouth and tongue, trunk, and extremities.
- Depression is one of the most common psychiatric disorders in the United States. Depression often is classified as one of two major types: endogenous or exogenous.
- Two major classes—cyclic antidepressants and monoamine oxidase inhibitors (MAOIs)—of antidepressant medications now are prescribed. In the United States, cyclics are prescribed more frequently than MAOIs.
- Antidepressant-medication treatment of depression follows from the biochemical hypothesis of the disorder. The hypothesis is that depression results from a deficiency in two biogenic amines —catecholamines and serotonin—that act as CNS neurotransmitters.
- All depressant drugs (including alcohol) produce similar effects. At low doses, they relieve anxiety; at moderate doses, they induce sleep; and at higher doses, they produce general anesthesia and eventually coma and death.
- The first depressants discovered were drugs used for general anesthesia, such as nitrous oxide and ether. Modern surgery would not be possible without this development.
- The development of the barbiturate drugs led to the use of depressants as sleeping pills and as treatment of anxiety symptoms and epilepsy.
- The use of barbiturates was limited when adverse effects were discovered. These include rapid development of tolerance, severe withdrawal symptoms, high risk of overdose, and high abuse potential.
- A number of barbiturate-like compounds have been developed (such as methaqualone, or Quaaludes), but they have the same undesirable effects as the barbiturates.
- The discovery of benzodiazepines revolutionized the medical use of depressant drugs because they relieve anxiety with fewer side effects than previous depressants.
- Benzodiazepines and other depressant drugs are believed to act at the GABA receptor site in the central nervous system.
- The anxiolytic effects of benzodiazepines are more selective than those of other depressants because they relieve anxiety at doses that produce minimal sedation and motor impairment.

- Although less problematic than barbiturates, benzodiazepines may produce tolerance and dependence, and withdrawal symptoms may occur.
- Lithium is the major drug used to treat the mood disorders of mania and manic-depressive illness. Lithium is the only psychotherapeutic drug that is an effective prophylaxis against disease recurrence.
- Use of lithium is based in the biological theory that bipolar disorder results from an overactivity of the neurotransmitters in the brain. Lithium appears to enhance reuptake of serotonin and norepinephrine at the presynaptic level and to decrease dopamine and norepinephrine effects at the postsynaptic receptors.
- No psychotherapeutic drug is totally safe for use during pregnancy. The best approach is that psychotherapeutic drugs be given to a pregnant woman only when necessary and when nondrug therapies, such as counseling, have been tried and have failed.
- Psychotherapeutic drug use during pregnancy can pose a health risk to both the mother and the fetus. Although the experimental evidence is not solid, the fetus may face various teratogenic, neurobehavioral, and toxic consequences of its mother's use of psychotherapeutic medications during pregnancy.

Answers to "What Do You Think?"

1. One of the first successful attempts to treat the symptoms of mental illness with psychotherapeutic drugs occurred in the 1840s, when Moreau used cannabis to treat patients with both depressive and manic symptoms.
   T *Patients with depression who were treated with cannabis became more talkative and happy, whereas patients with manic symptoms calmed down and relaxed. Unfortunately, these effects were temporary.*
2. Since the 1950s, the number of patients hospitalized for psychiatric conditions has decreased significantly.
   T *The introduction of chlorpromazine was the starting point of this trend. Other contributing factors include the development of other psychotherapeutic drugs and the movement toward deinstitutionalization.*
3. Almost half of the adults in the United States will meet the criteria for a mental illness at some point in their lives.
   T *Most of these cases, though, are mild, not severe, and typically do not require treatment.*
4. The prevalence of psychotherapeutic medication is twice as high among men as among women.
   F *The use of psychotherapeutic medication is twice as high among women as among men.*
5. Psychotherapeutic drugs are rarely abused.
   F *The nonprescribed use and abuse of psychotherapeutic drugs are a significant problem.*
6. As with most drugs, the age group least likely to misuse psychotherapeutic drugs is the elderly.
   F *The elderly are the age group most likely to misuse psychotherapeutic drugs.*
7. Most psychotherapeutic medications are administered intravenously, with direct transport in the bloodstream.
   F *Most psychotherapeutic medications are taken orally, absorbed in the gastrointestinal tract, and modified in the liver before being transported in the bloodstream.*
8. Schizophrenia is one of the most common psychiatric disorders in the United States.
   F *Schizophrenia affects only about 1% of the population.*
9. Stimulants are often used to treat chronic depression.
   F *Although stimulants were once used as a treatment for depression, their effectiveness is limited. Antidepressant medications are generally used to treat depression.*
10. Because antidepressants are absorbed rapidly, their effects are often immediate.
    F *Despite the rapid absorption, the effects of antidepressant medications take two to three weeks to become apparent.*
11. Nitrous oxide (laughing gas) is no longer used by the medical profession.
    F *Nitrous oxide is still widely used in dentistry and some types of surgery.*

12. The effects of a moderate dose of a barbiturate drug resemble the effects of alcohol.
    T *Barbiturate effects closely resemble those of alcohol, as do most depressant drugs.*
13. Withdrawal from depressant sleeping pills can trigger rebound insomnia.
    T *Insomnia and REM sleep rebound occur after barbiturates or benzodiazepines are used to induce sleep.*
14. Withdrawal from barbiturates is similar to alcohol withdrawal.
    T *Delirium tremens–like effects characterize withdrawal from all depressants.*
15. Benzodiazepines (Valium) are one of the most commonly prescribed drugs in America.
    T *A recent survey revealed that four different benzodiazepines (Valium, Dalmane, Ativan, and Tranxene) are among the most commonly prescribed drugs in America.*
16. Benzodiazepines are a common street drug known as "bennies."
    F *"Bennies" are a type of amphetamine, whereas benzodiazepines are considered a depressant. Also, although benzodiazepines do turn up on the street, their prevalence is less widespread than other depressant drugs.*
17. Overdose of benzodiazepines was the cause of the suicide death of Marilyn Monroe.
    F *Benzodiazepines have a very high LD 50. Highly toxic barbiturates were the fatal drugs for Marilyn Monroe.*
18. The main depressant drugs (barbiturates, benzodiazepines, and alcohol) all act by vastly different physiological mechanisms and affect different areas of the body.
    F *Substantial evidence indicates a common mechanism of action for depressant drugs. GABA is one of the primary inhibitory neurotransmitters of the brain, and many depressants are thought to act through this system.*
19. Depressant drugs may show cross-tolerance with cocaine.
    F *Depressant drugs show cross-tolerance with other depressant drugs, such as barbiturates or alcohol.*
20. Alcohol in combination with other depressant drugs is the leading cause of drug overdose deaths in the United States.
    T *Alcohol and other depressant drugs produce strong potentiation.*
21. Lithium, a natural alkaline metal, is often used to treat manic attacks.
    T *Although lithium may have some value in treating other disorders, its use in the United States is approved only for treatment of manic episodes.*
22. Psychotherapeutic drugs pose little or no threat to the fetus and may be used safely during pregnancy.
    F *When psychotherapeutic drugs are taken during pregnancy, the fetus faces the risk of teratogenic effects, long-term effects on neurobehavioral functioning, and the direct toxic effects of the drug. Therefore, it is most often recommended that psychotherapeutic drugs not be used during pregnancy unless absolutely necessary.*

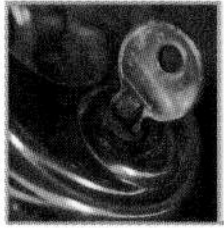

Key Terms

agitated depression
akinesia
anterograde amnesia
anxiolytic
barbiturates
benzodiazepines
dyskinesia
endogenous
exogenous
extrapyramidal
general anesthesia
manic
narcoleptic
neuroleptics
neuroses
paranoid schizophrenia
psychosurgery
psychotherapeutic
rebound insomnia
REM rebound
sedative-hypnotic effects
tardive dyskinesia
teratogenic

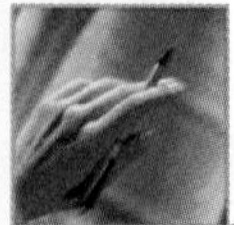

Essays/Thought Questions

1. Should herbal remedies such as St. John's wort be available to consumers without a prescription? What guidelines, if any, should be in place to ensure the safe use of such remedies and to establish that the remedy acts as advertised?
2. What are the advantages and disadvantages of a pregnant woman's use of psychotherapeutic medications?

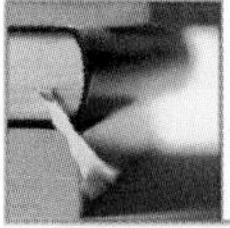

Suggested Readings

Gordon, B. (1979). *I'm dancing as fast as I can*. New York: Bantam Books Inc.

Russo, E. (2001). *Handbook of psychotropic herbs: A scientific analysis of herbal remedies for psychiatric conditions*. Binghamton, NY: Haworth Herbal Press.

Silverman, H. M. (2008). *The pill book* (13th ed.). New York: Bantam Books Inc.

Spitzer, R. L., Gibbon, M., Skodol, A. E., Williams, J. B. W., & First, M. B. (1989). *DSM-III-R casebook*. Washington, DC: American Psychiatric Press Inc.

Styron, W. (1992). *Darkness visible: A memoir of madness*. New York: Vintage Books.

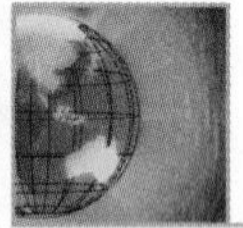

Web Resources

Visit the Book Companion Website at www.cengage.com/psychology/maisto to access study tools including a glossary, flashcards, and web quizzing. You will also find links to the following resources:

- National Institute of Mental Health
- National Alliance on Mental Illness
- Internet Mental Health
- RxList: The Internet Drug Index for Prescription Drugs and Medication
- Drug Abuse Warning Network

CHAPTER 14

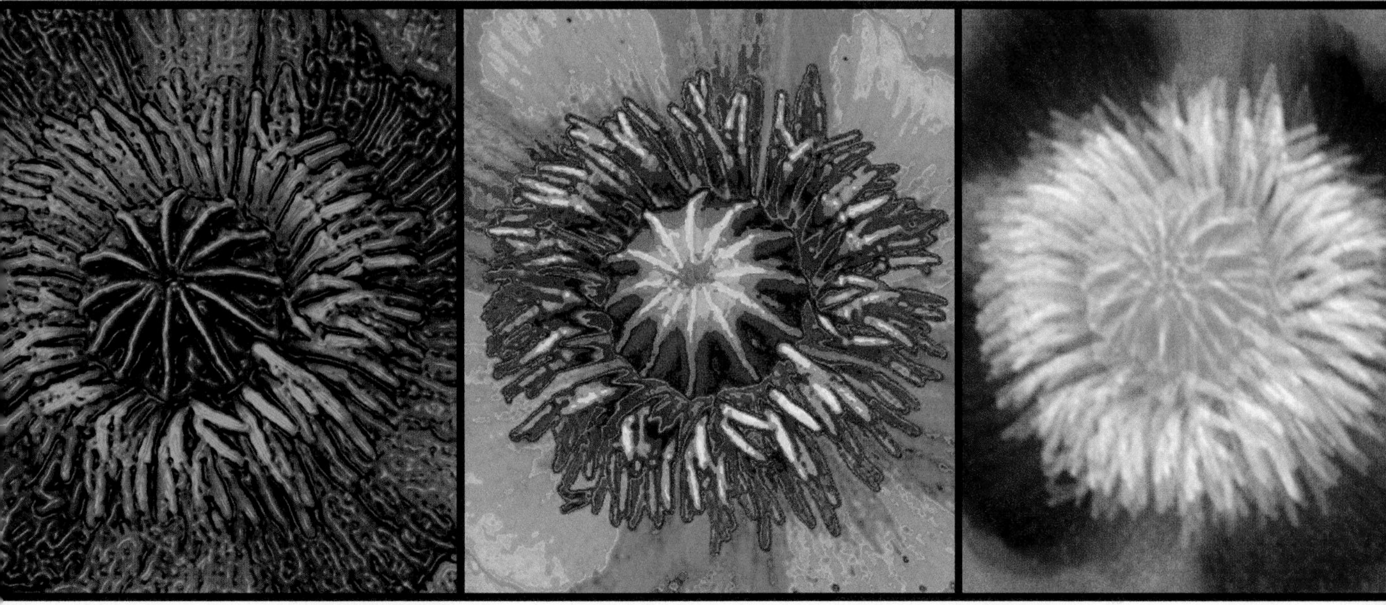

Other Prescription and Over-the-Counter Drugs

What Do You Think? True or False?

Answers are given at the end of the chapter.

___ 1. Birth control pills contain synthetic forms of one or both of the female sex hormones.

___ 2. One of the risks associated with the use of birth control pills is an increased chance of lung cancer.

___ 3. Anabolic steroids are synthetic forms of testosterone.

___ 4. Anabolic steroids are generally taken because of the high they produce.

___ 5. Acne, baldness, and liver damage are all side effects associated with steroid use.

___ 6. GRAS is a common street name for marijuana.

___ 7. Aspirin relieves pain through action on the endorphins, in much the same way that the pain-relieving effects of opiates are produced.

___ 8. Many over-the-counter diet pills contain low doses of amphetamines.

___ 9. Antitussive agents are used to suppress coughing.

___10. Antihistamines are common ingredients in over-the-counter cold remedies.

___11. GHB is a naturally occurring brain chemical.

___12. Caffeine is a common ingredient in over-the-counter stimulant preparations.

Overview

We have discussed the major traditional classes of psychoactive drugs. Other drugs of importance did not fit neatly into the earlier chapters, however. Now we review some of them. We first discuss some significant prescription drugs, including birth control pills and anabolic steroids. Next we consider psychoactive drugs that, although regulated by the Food and Drug Administration (FDA), can be legally purchased without a prescription: the over-the-counter drugs. These include primarily analgesics (such as aspirin), antihistamines and other cold and allergy medications, diet pills, and sleeping aids. Then we review an array of herbal remedies, hormones, and dietary supplements that have psychoactive properties. These products are legally available but are not regulated by the FDA. We also consider the strange case of gamma hydroxybutyrate (GHB), a drug that was originally classed as a supplement but became a major abuse problem and is now regulated as a Schedule I drug. Finally, we discuss a group of legal chemicals that produce volatile fumes with psychoactive effects: the inhalants.

combination pill Birth control pill that contains synthetic forms of both female sex hormones: progesterone and estrogen.

progesterone (prō-'jes-tə-'rō–n) One of the female sex hormones involved in the regulation of ovulation and the menstrual cycle.

estrogen ('es-trə-jən) One of the female sex hormones involved in the regulation of ovulation and the menstrual cycle.

Prescription Drugs

Birth Control Drugs

The first birth control pill became available in the early 1960s, and since that time, "the pill" has had a profound impact on our culture. It is no accident that the so-called sexual revolution of the late 1960s coincided with the widespread availability of the pill. About 11.5 million women in the United States use the birth control pill, making it the most widely used form of contraception (Center for Disease Control and Prevention, 2006).

The most common form of the birth control pill is the **combination pill**, which consists of synthetic forms of two female sex hormones: **progesterone** and **estrogen**. In some forms of the combination pill (multiphasic), the amount of synthetic progesterone or estrogen varies depending on where the woman is in the menstrual cycle. The combination birth control pill works by suppressing ovulation (release of a mature egg from the ovary). It is taken daily for 21 days and then removed for 7 days, during which a period of menstruation should occur. Most birth control pill packages contain placebo or vitamin pills to be taken during the 7 off-days to help the woman stay in the habit of taking a pill each day.

Basically, the pill works by "tricking" a woman's brain into responding as if she were already pregnant. When a woman is pregnant, she no longer ovulates. The hypothalamus and pituitary gland are responsible for regulating ovulation. When circulating levels of estrogen and progesterone are high (as in the case of pregnancy or use of the birth control pill), these structures do not release the hormones that are necessary to prepare the ovaries to release an egg, and thus ovulation is prevented.

To keep circulating levels of estrogen and progesterone continually high enough to inhibit ovulation, the woman must faithfully remember to take a birth control pill every day at approximately the same time of day. If she misses a pill, she must take it as soon as possible. If she misses more than one pill, her levels of circulating estrogen and progesterone may have dropped sufficiently low to allow ovulation to occur. Used properly, the combination pill is one of the most reliable forms of birth control available, with a failure rate of 0.5% to 8%, much lower than most alternatives (Hyde & DeLamater, 2006) (see Table 14.1 and Contemporary Issue Box 14.1). The pill has other advantages over other contraception methods as well. Because it does not require taking precautions just before or after intercourse, it permits more spontaneity in sexual activity than other approaches. A disadvantage of the pill compared to condoms, of course, is that the pill does not prevent the spread of sexually transmitted disease. In addition, the pill has a number of side effects.

One of the more serious concerns is the increased risk of blood clots in users of the combination pill. Blood clots can produce strokes or heart attacks, and indeed women older than 40 show an increased risk of heart attack when they take the combination pill. This risk is greatly increased if the woman is also a cigarette smoker. Mood changes, including severe depression, are often reported by women on the pill (Ibid.).

In an effort to minimize the side effects of estrogen, an alternative form of birth control pill has been developed that contains only small amounts of synthetic progesterone (progestin). The **progestin pill** is sometimes called the minipill. It is thought to work somewhat differently from the combination pill in that it may not always block ovulation. Rather, the major effect of progestin is to alter the cervical mucus

progestin pill
Birth control pill (sometimes called the minipill) that contains only progestin, a synthetic progesterone.

TABLE 14.1 Comparison of Contraceptive Methods

Method	Failure Rate in Typical Users (%)
Vasectomy	<0.2
Patch	<1
Ring	<1
Combination birth control pill	3
IUD	6
Condom	15
Diaphragm plus spermicide	16
Withdrawal	25
Rhythm, body temperature	25
Chance	90
Abstinence	?

CONTEMPORARY ISSUE BOX 14.1

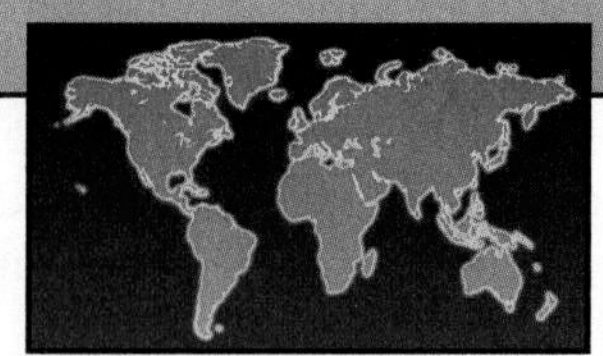

What Kind of Birth Control Is Best?

Perhaps the question most college women have when reading about the pill is whether it is the best method of contraception. It is impossible to evaluate the pill without considering the other available methods. Table 14.1 lists the failure rates for various methods of birth control in typical users. The difference between these techniques often amounts to error in their proper use. Failure is minimized with surgical procedures such as vasectomy, but in addition to the possible complications of surgery, the procedure may be irreversible. Thus, surgical procedures are uncommon among young people. Notice that the hormonal treatments (the pill, the ring, the patch) are the most effective techniques not requiring surgery. Their main drawbacks are the side effects noted in the text. The intrauterine device (IUD) is also highly effective and is a very popular technique, but the IUD also can produce side effects. The most common are irregular bleeding and pelvic pain. More serious complications are less common but may include greater risk of pelvic inflammatory disease, uterine perforation, and complications if pregnancy should occur when the IUD is in place. Women also use a variety of "barrier" techniques, including the diaphragm and the contraceptive sponge. These devices block the cervical opening and, when used with a spermicide, produce acceptable failure rates. A disadvantage of these methods is the repeated insertion and removal of the device, which some women find problematic.

The condom has gained favor as a method of birth control because it may protect users from sexually transmitted disease. With the current concern about AIDS, condoms should be recommended to most couples. Unless used properly (and reliably), however, condoms have a high failure rate, as Table 14.1 shows. As you will also note in Table 14.1, techniques such as withdrawal and rhythm have a common side effect: pregnancy! Then, of course, there is abstinence. . . .

medium in such a way as to block sperm entry. A limitation of the progestin pill is that it is less effective than the combination pill, although it is still more reliable than other reversible methods (see Table 14.1).

Another new twist is the development of the continuous birth control pill (e.g., Seasonale). These are combination estrogen/progestin pills like those discussed previously, but they differ in formulation. With the standard combination pill regimen, a woman takes estrogen/progestin pills for three weeks, followed by inactive pills for one week accompanied by a menstrual period. With continuous birth control pills, a woman takes hormonally active pills for three consecutive months followed by inactive pills for one week so that she has only four, one-week menstrual periods each year.

As we noted, a major limitation in the effectiveness of the pill is that users must remember to take it every day. Newer developments in birth control provide longer-lasting methods of delivering estrogen and progestin that require less frequent administration by users. One example is the vaginal ring, a doughnut-shaped device that is placed in the vagina where it slowly releases progestin, estrogen, or both. The vaginal ring functions much like the pill in preventing ovulation. The ring is kept in place for three weeks and is then removed for the fourth week to permit menstrual flow. A more recent development is the contraceptive patch. This is a thin strip of plastic material that attaches to the skin like a bandage. The side that makes contact with the skin releases the same hormones as the pill and the ring, in appropriate doses over a one-week period. The woman replaces a patch every seven days for three weeks and then goes for seven days without a patch. The obvious advantage of both the ring and the patch is that a woman does not need to remember to take daily pills throughout the month. Methods like the vaginal ring and patch thus have lower failure rates than the pill (estimated at 1%) and may eventually replace the birth control pill as the most popular means of contraception (Hyde & DeLamater, 2006).

An option for women who have had unprotected intercourse is to take emergency contraception (e.g., Plan B). Generally, emergency contraceptives deliver high doses of progestin and are most effective if taken within 12 to 24 hours after intercourse, with some effectiveness continuing for up to five days after intercourse. Emergency contraception may work by preventing ovulation, fertilization, or implantation—it is not thought to cause abortion. In 2005, a FDA panel judged the use of Plan B emergency contraception pills to be safe and effective and recommended Plan B be made available over the counter. The rationale behind this recommendation was that the drug is most effective when taken within a day of unprotected intercourse; thus, the delay required in arranging an appointment with a physician to receive a prescription for Plan B is problematic. However, this is a politically charged issue because some fear making the drug available over the counter sends a permissive message about sexuality. In late 2005, FDA chief Lester Crawford denied the over-the-counter request for Plan B, on the grounds that it would create regulatory difficulties. After Crawford's decision, Susan Wood, director of the Office of Women's Health, resigned her position in protest, claiming that Crawford was permitting political issues to interfere with agency decision making. Wood's resignation triggered a review of political tampering with the FDA process, which Crawford refused to cooperate with, and in October 2005, he resigned as FDA commissioner. In August 2006, the FDA announced a compromise decision. Plan B was approved as an over-the-counter option for women aged 18 and older but will remain available only by prescription for young women aged 17 and younger.

Even more controversial is the progesterone antagonist mifepristone (RU-486). If this drug is taken during the first 49 days of pregnancy, it causes the embryo to be aborted. Because it induces abortion, mifepristone has generated considerable protest, but it is in widespread use in Europe and has now been approved for use in the United States (Hyde & DeLamater, 2006).

When considering contraception controversies and in particular the potential side effects of birth control pills and other methods of contraception, one must keep things in perspective. Although risks are associated with use of the pill, they are lower than the risks involved in pregnancy and delivery.

Anabolic Steroids

Background

On a sunny day in September 1988 in Seoul, Korea, the world of sports was changed forever. Ben Johnson ran the 100-meter dash in 9.79 seconds to win the Olympic gold medal and break the world record. Johnson had become the world's fastest human—of all time. Then, just two days later, after traces of the **anabolic steroid** stanozolol were found in Johnson's urine sample, he was stripped of his record and his medal and left the games in disgrace. The reverberations in the sports world are still being felt; perhaps more significantly, Johnson's scandal opened the eyes of the public to the problem of steroid abuse.

anabolic steroids
Tissue-building drugs that produce masculinizing effects as well.

Anabolic steroids are synthetic drugs that resemble the male sex hormone **testosterone**. In addition to its role in determining male sexual characteristics such as facial and chest hair (androgenic or masculinizing effects), testosterone helps build body tissues and repair damaged tissue. Such bodily construction processes are called anabolic effects. People can also obtain anabolic effects by taking synthetic testosterone for certain medical problems or for improved athletic performance or bodybuilding. The clinical uses of anabolic steroids include treatments for testosterone deficiency, some types of anemia, breast cancer, osteoporosis, and arthritis. Anabolic steroids are

testosterone
The male sex hormone. Anabolic steroids are basically synthetic versions of testosterone.

often obtained illicitly, however, and are used for bodybuilding or otherwise enhancing athletic performance.

Anabolic steroids were first developed in Nazi Germany in the 1930s, allegedly to help create an army of supermen (Marshall, 1988). The first known use of anabolic steroids in athletics is reported to have been by Russian weight lifters and some female athletes in the early 1950s. By the 1968 Olympics, steroids were in widespread use. Consider this testimony given by Harold Connolly, Olympic gold medalist in the hammer throw, before a Senate committee:

> It was not unusual in 1968 to see athletes with their own medical kits, practically a doctor's bag in which they would have syringes and all their various drugs. . . . I know any number of athletes on the 1968 Olympic team who had so much scar tissue and so many puncture holes on their backsides that it was difficult to find a fresh spot to give them a new shot. (Hecht, 1985, p. 270)

Not until 1976 did the International Olympic Committee rule that athletes could not use steroids. Urine testing was used to enforce this policy. Since that time, a great many athletes have tested positive and have been banned from the games, but the Ben Johnson case was certainly the most notorious. At the 2008 Beijing Olympic Games, numerous athletes were disqualified or sent home due to drug violations, and many more were dropped from their teams before the games. Steroid use by athletes, particularly major league baseball players, has made regular headlines, largely stemming from repercussions from the BALCO scandal and leaks of positive steroid results from supposedly confidential urine tests conducted years ago (see Contemporary Issue Box 14.2).

"So I can't say, 'Don't do it,' not when the guy next to you is as big as a house and he's going to take your job and make the money."

—Former major league baseball player Ken Caminiti on steroids

Concern about steroids has also increased as it became evident that their use had become widespread not just among elite athletes but also for cosmetic purposes by men (and to a lesser extent, women) who simply wanted to enhance their physical appearance. Apparently "getting big" has become so important that many young people are willing to risk using steroids to achieve the larger muscles and better definition they believe are associated with these drugs.

Possession of steroids without a prescription has been illegal since 1990, when the Anabolic Steroid Control Act was passed, making these drugs Schedule III controlled substances. There was some evidence of decline in the use of steroids after the act passed. The reported use of steroids by high school seniors was 3% in 1989, dropped to 2.9% in 1990, and was less than 2.5% throughout the decade of the 1990s, with a low of 1.9% in 1996. Usage was back up to 4% in 2002, but has steadily declined since then to a rate of 2.2% in 2008 (Johnston, O'Malley, Bachman, & Schulenberg, 2009a).

Rates of steroid use may be substantially higher than this among older adults, particularly those who are weight lifters or bodybuilders, but as with any illicit drug, it is difficult to assess the actual prevalence. Rates obtained through mandatory drug testing by the NCAA, NFL, and Olympic committees have generally found less than 3% positive tests, but these data appear at odds with the reports of journalistic and governmental investigations as well as survey data (McCloskey & Bailes, 2005; Yesalis et al., 2000). The problem is that users can circumvent the drug tests. When testing occurs only at particular competitive events, like the Olympics, users can avoid a positive test by discontinuing use for a time prior to testing. Random testing is more difficult to beat, but low doses, designer steroids, use of natural compounds like testosterone and human growth hormone (HGH), and use of masking drugs are all strategies that may be effective.

So, actual use of anabolic steroids may be higher than our estimates indicate. But how high? The BALCO investigations and the claims of two former baseball stars (Ken Caminiti and Jose Canseco) that 50% to 85% of all major league baseball players

CONTEMPORARY ISSUE BOX 14.2

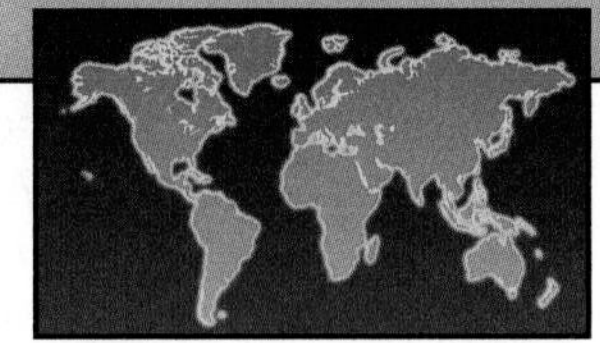

BALCO, Bonds, and Baseball

In June 2003, a track coach named Trevor Graham came into possession of an unknown drug that was being distributed by BALCO, a San Francisco outfit that provided training programs and "supplements" to many of the country's elite athletes. Graham gave the U.S. Anti-Doping Agency a syringe of the drug, which turned out to be a designer steroid, tetrahydrogestrinone (THG), that was undetectable by any of the standard drug testing screens at the time. Federal grand jury and Senate investigations in 2003 and 2004 of BALCO and its chief executive, Victor Conte, then launched what some have called "the biggest doping scandal in sports history" (McCloskey & Bailes, 2005, p. 61). Many of the nation's top athletes were named as BALCO clients and linked with use of THG, other steroids, and a host of other performance-enhancing drugs. These included many track and field athletes, among them gold medalist Marion Jones and football players like Bill Romanowski, but the sport most affected by the BALCO investigations was major league baseball. Top stars like Mark McGwire, Rafael Palmeiro, and Jason Giambi were all linked to steroid use, but the spotlight really focused on Barry Bonds.

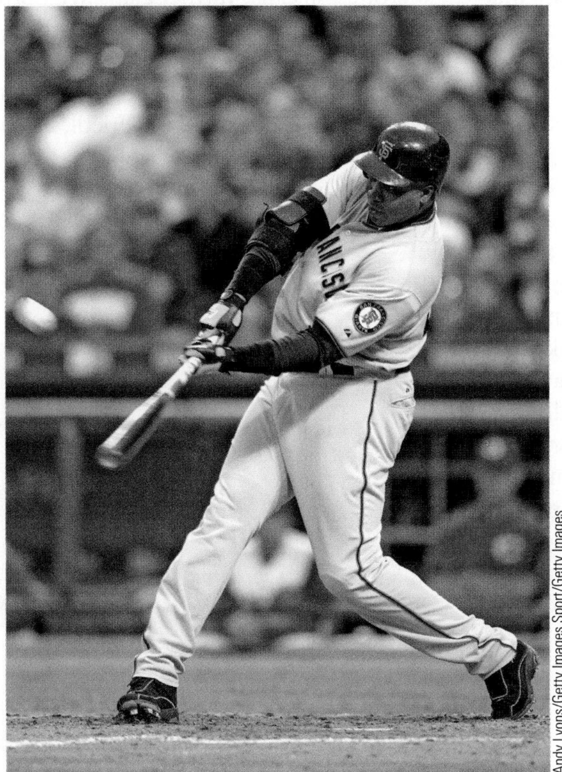

Andy Lyons/Getty Images Sport/Getty Images

Bonds shattered baseball's record for most home runs in a season (previously held by McGwire) with 73 in 2001, and in 2007 broke Hank Aaron's career record of 755. Faced with unassailable evidence that he received steroids from BALCO, Bonds admitted taking both the "clear," a liquid absorbed under the tongue, and the "cream," which was applied directly to the muscles. Both the cream and the clear were undetectable designer steroids, but Bonds denied knowing they were steroids. However, two journalists (Fainaru-Wada & Williams, 2006) provided evidence that Bonds had full knowledge of his program for use of steroids and other performing-enhancing drugs, and in 2007 Bonds was indicted for perjury on the basis of his grand jury testimony. In 2008, major league baseball implemented a new steroid-testing policy with escalating penalties for positive tests. But many say it is too little, too late. Some of the most cherished records in the sport are held by Bonds (or soon will be). Will major league baseball place a "steroid asterisk" by Bonds' home-run records?

use steroids launched a major scandal, but the accuracy of such allegations cannot be verified. In any case, the focused attention on steroid use in the past decade has led to considerable research, and we are beginning to get a better idea of just how steroids work and what side effects may follow their use.

Actions of Anabolic Steroids

The anabolic steroids include danazol, methyltestosterone, ethylestrenol, methandrostenolone, nandrolone, oxandrolone, oxymetholone, stanozolol, and tetrahydrogestrinone (brand names include Anadrol, Anavar, Danocrine, Dianabol, Metandren, and Winstrol). Although some may be taken orally or topically, others must be injected to be effective (see Table 14.2). The metabolism and elimination of steroids are variable. Steroids can be detected reliably in urine for 4 to 14 days after use, but there are reports of positive urine tests as long as 13 months after the use of nandrolone (Marshall, 1988).

A related compound, androstenedione is a precursor to testosterone and was marketed over the counter as an alternative to the illegal steroids to enhance strength and performance. Mark McGwire made "Andro" famous when he admitted to using it during his record-breaking home run streak in 1998. Because androstenedione was associated with many of the side effects of anabolic steroids, the FDA made it an illegal substance in 2004.

One ironic feature of the widespread use of steroids by athletes is that medical researchers have had great difficulty determining whether they really enhance performance. It is clear that at puberty, male testes increase testosterone output to result in the increased muscle mass and strength characteristic of males at that age. This does not necessarily mean that supplemental testosterone will cause further gains in a normal man, however. Many studies of the effects of anabolic steroids on weight gain, strength, and performance have been conducted. Although most of these have shown improvement in subjects who took steroids, some have not. Overall, the consensus in the scientific community is that steroids do produce gains in size and strength (Friedl, 2000a).

Side Effects of Anabolic Steroids

Physical side effects are associated with anabolic steroid use. Perhaps the most commonly reported are acne, balding, and reduced sexual desire. Men often experience atrophy of the testes and a related decline in sperm count and enlargement of the breasts. It seems ironic that many male steroid users have to take special drugs to prevent breast growth! These effects are usually reversible. Women may experience pronounced masculinizing effects from steroid use, and many of these effects are irreversible. They include growth of facial and chest hair, baldness, deepening of

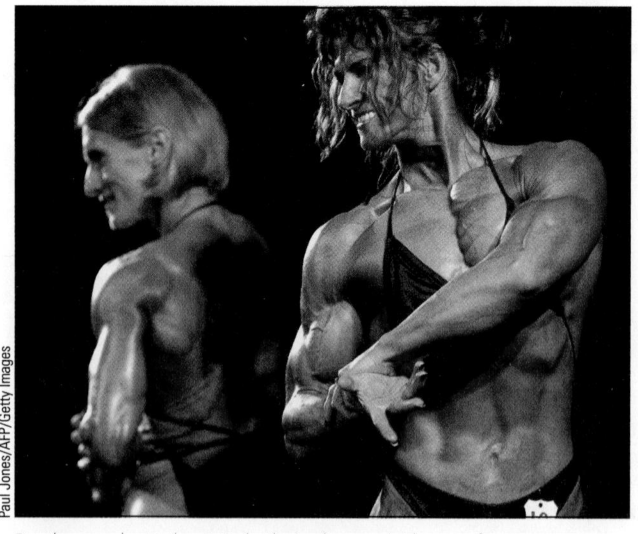

Paul Jones/AFP/Getty Images

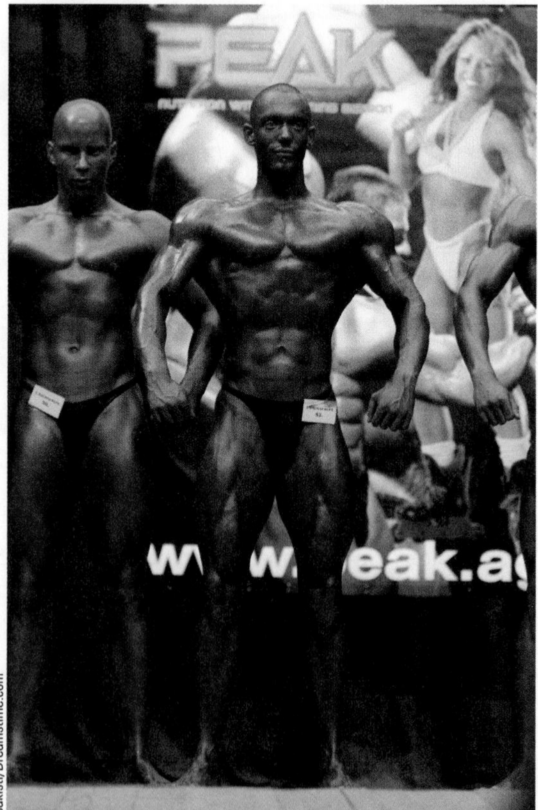

Csakisti/Dreamstime.com

Do they or don't they? Only their pharmacist knows for sure.

TABLE 14.2 Anabolic Steroids

Drug	Trade Name	Route of Administration
Danazol	Danocrine	Oral
Ethylestrenol	Maxibolin	Oral
Methandrostenolone	Dianabol	Oral
Methyltestosterone	Metandren	Oral
Oxandrolone	Anavar	Oral
Stanozolol	Winstrol	Oral
Nandrolone	Androlone, Durabolin, Nandrolin	Injection
Methandriol	Anabol, Durabolic, Methabolic, Steribolic	Injection

the voice, breast shrinkage, clitoral enlargement, and menstrual irregularities. Another cause for concern is that steroid use often changes cholesterol levels that may increase the risk of heart disease. Damage to liver function is also common and can include an increased risk of liver cancer (Langenbucher, Hildebrandt, & Carr, 2008). The late NFL All-Pro Lyle Alzado attributed his inoperable brain cancer to heavy steroid use. Whether steroids play a causal role in this and other types of cancer is controversial, however (Friedl, 2000b). Additional problems, such as premature bone fusion causing stunted growth, can occur when children and adolescents use steroids. Alteration of normal pubertal development is also a risk in young people.

In addition to the physical side effects of steroids, there are psychological effects. Most users report a mild euphoria when they use steroids, and increased energy levels also are noted. Less desirable are reports of increased irritability and aggressiveness, sometimes leading to violent behavior. Mood swings and even psychotic reactions

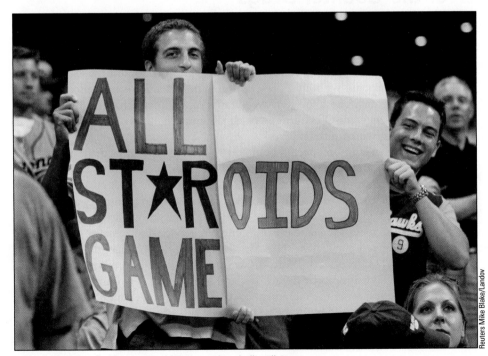

Reuters Mike Blake/Landov

Major league fans hold up a steroid poster at baseball's All-Star game.

have been reported. Pope and Katz (1988) reported on a study of 41 bodybuilders and football players who had used steroids. Nine of the subjects (22%) experienced emotional disturbance, and five (12%) developed psychotic reactions during their steroid regimens. One of the subjects deliberately drove a car into a tree at 40 mph. Another described becoming irritated at a driver in front of him who had left his blinker on. At the first stoplight, he jumped out of his car and punched out the other car's windshield! Of course, these case studies do not establish that steroids alone were responsible for these effects, but several double-blind studies have also reported increased aggression and mood swings in subjects who received steroids, albeit with less dramatic outcomes than those described here (see Kanayama, Hudson & Pope, 2008 for a review). Users of anabolic steroids also had higher-than-expected rates of violent death (Petersson et al., 2006). As well, steroid use has also been associated with withdrawal symptoms and dependence in as many as 30% of overall users in some studies (Kanayama, Hudson & Pope, 2009).

Athletes will continue to use steroids as long as they believe their competition is using them. Better testing methods are needed, but perhaps more important would be *regular* tests. Many current procedures allow athletes to discontinue the drugs prior to an important event to avoid a positive urine test. Regular random tests are more likely to reduce cheating. But what of the thousands of young men (and women) who are not Olympic-caliber athletes who are taking steroids to improve their performance at the high school or college level or just to "get big"?

"Steroids make the athlete more aggressive and in some sports that is seen as an advantage."

Al Oerter, four-time Olympic gold medalist in discus

Steroids can cause major problems, and many drug education programs do not even discuss them. Clearly there is a need to make the public aware of the potential dangers of steroid abuse.

Over-the-Counter Drugs

FDA Classification

The FDA divides drugs into two categories: those that require a prescription from a physician to purchase (such as the psychiatric drugs discussed in Chapter 13 and the birth control pills and anabolic steroids described previously) and those considered safe enough to dispense without a prescription. The latter are often called over-the-counter (OTC) drugs. The 1962 Kefauver-Harris Amendment charged the FDA with regulating and reviewing OTC drugs—no small task when you consider more than 300,000 products were on the market!

Rather than focusing on specific brands, the FDA has organized the ingredients found in these products and divided them into the categories listed in Table 14.3. As you can see, OTC drugs treat a wide range of ailments. The FDA created panels to study the ingredients and to evaluate them on two major criteria: safety and efficacy. The panel's final reports were presented in 1985. Then, those drugs authorized as OTC drugs must meet the standard of "generally recognized as safe" (GRAS) and "generally recognized as effective" (GRAE). Drugs that do not meet these criteria are removed from OTC products. Note, however, that *safety* and *efficacy* are relative terms. Some OTC drugs can be hazardous, and some are of very limited efficacy.

In addition to reviewing the ingredients of OTC drugs, FDA panels review prescription drugs and, if they are found to be relatively safe and effective, may recommend that they be made available without prescription. The pain reliever ibuprofen and some antihistamines, such as diphenhydramine and loratadine (Claritin), are examples of drugs previously available only by prescription that have now been approved as OTC drugs.

TABLE 14.3 FDA Classification of OTC Drugs

1. Antacids	13. Analgesics
2. Antidiarrheal products	14. Antitussives
3. Sunscreens	15. Eye products
4. Dandruff products	16. Dental products
5. Bronchodilators	17. Emetics
6. Stimulants	18. Antiperspirants
7. Cold remedies	19. Antimicrobials
8. Skin preparations	20. Hemorrhoidal products
9. Laxatives	21. Sedatives and sleep aids
10. Antiemetics	22. Allergy drugs
11. Vitamin and mineral products	23. Contraceptive products
12. Oral hygiene products	24. Weight-control products

Of the 24 categories of drugs listed in Table 14.3, we focus on those that have psychoactive properties: analgesics, cold and allergy medications, stimulants, and sedatives.

Analgesics

In Chapter 10, we discussed the use of opiate drugs in the treatment of pain. But the use of opiates for pain relief is usually reserved for severe cases. Many effective painkillers are available over the counter, and aspirin is the most widely known and used. **Acetylsalicylic acid** (aspirin) is closely related to a chemical found in the bark of the willow and other trees (salicylic acid). Willow bark was used in the treatment of painful conditions and fever by the ancient Greeks and by Native Americans. Salicylic acid was isolated and used as a pain reliever in Europe, but it causes severe stomach distress. Not until the late 19th century was acetylsalicylic acid synthesized and named *aspirin* by the Bayer Company of Germany. Aspirin has come to be one of the most

acetylsalicylic acid (ə-'sē-tᵊl-'sa-lə-'si-lik)
Chemical name for aspirin.

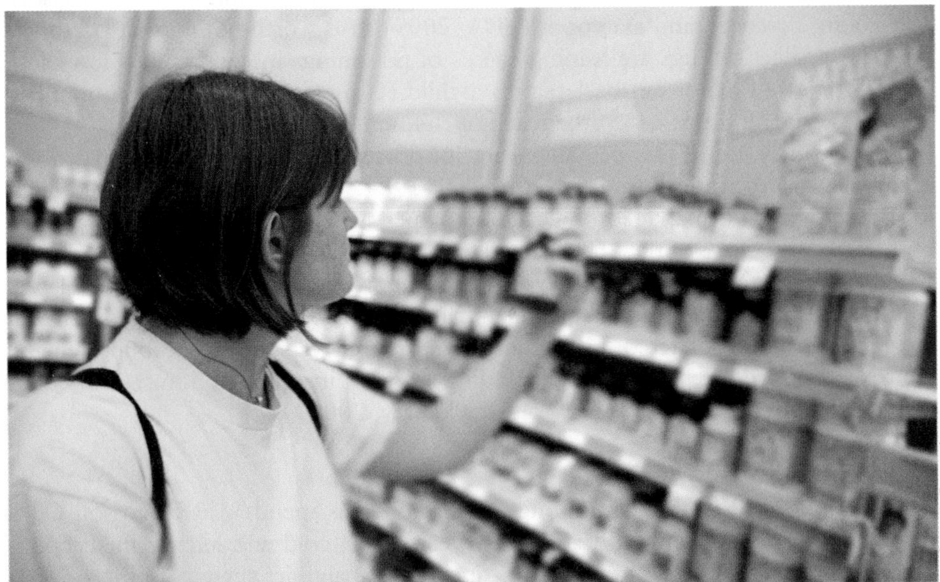

Fred Goldstein/Dreamstime.com

Over-the-counter drugs are considered safe enough to dispense without prescription.

important drugs in medicine. It is marketed under the brand names Anacin, Bufferin, and Excedrin, to name just a few, and between 10,000 and 20,000 tons of aspirin are consumed in the United States every year (Julien, Advokat & Comaty, 2008).

Aspirin is analgesic (produces pain relief without unconsciousness), antipyretic (reduces fever), and anti-inflammatory (reduces swelling). It is thought to work by means of a mechanism quite different from opiate analgesia. Aspirin (and other OTC painkillers) act by blocking the production and release of **prostaglandins**, chemicals released by the body at sites of pain. These chemicals are thought to enhance certain kinds of pain—dull pain and aches, such as headache—and to produce inflammation. Indeed aspirin is not very effective at treating sharp pains or stomach pain. It is, however, very effective with muscle aches, headaches, and soreness due to inflammation such as arthritis (Grogan, 1987).

prostaglandins ('präs-t-'glan-dən) Naturally occurring chemicals blocked by aspirin and related analgesics.

Aspirin has some adverse effects. It frequently causes stomach irritation and bleeding and is contraindicated in people who have stomach problems. Aspirin may be related to a rare and dangerous disease called Reye's syndrome. Reye's syndrome occurs only in children treated with aspirin for flu or chicken pox and involves severe vomiting, disorientation, and sometimes coma, brain damage, or death. Thus, aspirin should be avoided by children who have these diseases. Aspirin is also an anticoagulant and may prolong bleeding under certain circumstances. However, this same mechanism may be useful in the prevention of strokes and heart attacks (Julien, Advokat, & Comaty, 2008)

An effective analgesic drug useful for people with stomach problems is **acetaminophen**. This drug, marketed under brand names such as Datril and Tylenol, reduces fever and produces analgesic effects but does not cause stomach irritation. Acetaminophen is not a potent anti-inflammatory drug, however, and may cause liver problems in high doses. Acetaminophen-related overdoses are fairly common and account for over 56,000 emergency room visits and nearly 500 deaths every year. A recent FDA advisory committee noted that many of these occur because people take multiple products containing acetaminophen without knowing it, often in products that combine acetaminophen with another painkiller. The advisory committee report suggests that the recommended adult dose should be lowered (from 1,000 mg to 650 mg) and that the maximum daily dose be decreased as well. The committee also voted to eliminate products that combine acetaminophen with prescription opiate drugs, such as Vicodin, Percocet, and Darvocet, (FDA, 2009). It is worth noting that overdoses on OTC analgesic drugs are leading causes of poisonings in children. As few as 10 Extra-Strength Tylenol can be lethal to a child (Grogan, 1987). It is important to keep these and all drugs out of the reach of children.

acetaminophen (ə-'sē-tə-'mi-nə-fən) Aspirin-like analgesic.

Other widely used OTC painkillers are **ibuprofen** and **naproxen**. Ibuprofen was exclusively a prescription drug (Motrin) until 1984, when the FDA approved it for OTC use. Now it is marketed under brand names such as Advil and Nuprin and has captured a large share of the OTC painkiller market. Naproxen is marketed under the brand names of Naprosyn and Aleve and was approved as an OTC drug in 1994. These drugs have analgesic and anti-inflammatory effects that are similar to aspirin but are generally better tolerated. Like other OTC pain relievers, however, ibuprofen and naproxen can produce side effects, including stomach irritation and liver and kidney damage in high doses (Julien, Advokat, & Comaty, 2008).

ibuprofen ('ī-by ü-'prō-fən) Aspirin-like analgesic.

naproxen (nə-'prok-sən) Aspirin-like analgesic.

Cold and Allergy Medications

The common cold is common enough that its victims spend $1.3 billion on OTC cold remedies in the United States every year. OTC cold and allergy medications contain a variety of different ingredients, including analgesics such as aspirin or acetaminophen, which are of value in reducing aches, pain, and fever. In addition, many

OTC cold preparations contain a decongestant such as **pseudoephedrine** (Sudafed). Because pseudoephedrine is one ingredient used to produce illicit methamphetamine, such products are now sold behind the counter (see Chapter 6). Cold remedies also may include expectorants, which help to break up phlegm so that it may be coughed up. **Guaifenesin** is the most common expectorant. **Antitussive** agents actually suppress coughing and are often included in cold and cough formulations (dextromethorphan is an example).

Other common ingredients in OTC cold and allergy preparations are **antihistamines**. These compounds actually are more effective in the treatment of hay fever and related allergic reactions. Many allergic symptoms are caused by the release of a naturally occurring chemical called histamine. As the name suggests, antihistamines act by blocking histamine. Commonly used antihistamines include diphenhydramine, chlorpheniramine maleate, and loratadine (Claritin). Several side effects limit the usefulness of antihistamines, however. Drowsiness and fatigue are probably the most significant. It can be hard to stay awake after taking antihistamines, and in fact, diphenhydramine is the major ingredient in most OTC sleeping aids. Other side effects include thickening of mucus secretions, blurred vision, dizziness, dry mouth and nose, and sweating (Grogan, 1987).

pseudoephedrine ('sü-dō-i-'fed-rən)
An over-the-counter decongestant.

guaifenesin (gwī-'fen-ə-sin)
An over-the-counter expectorant.

antitussives
Cough-suppressant drugs.

antihistamines
Common over-the-counter drugs with decongestant effects.

Over-the-Counter Stimulants and Sedatives

The main ingredient in OTC stimulants is caffeine. Phenylpropanolamine (PPA) was a common ingredient in such preparations until 2000, when the FDA withdrew OTC approval because it was found to increase the risk of stroke. Popular brands of OTC stimulants are No-Doz and Vivarin. They certainly will induce mild central nervous system stimulation, but No-Doz, for example, contains about as much caffeine as one or two cups of coffee, so users should expect about that effect. Information on the side effects of caffeine was presented in Chapter 8.

As noted previously, the major ingredient in OTC sleeping aids is an antihistamine, diphenhydramine. Because fatigue is a common side effect of antihistamines, they sometimes can help people who are suffering from insomnia. However, other side effects associated with antihistamines (for instance, dry mouth, dizziness, and nausea) may limit their use as sleeping aids. In addition, the problems associated with using prescription sleeping pills may apply to these drugs, too, as discussed in Chapter 13.

Herbal Products, Hormones, and Dietary Supplements

In 1994, the Dietary Supplement Health and Education Act was passed. This act reduced the authority of the FDA to regulate herbal and other biological products that often contain psychoactive drugs. The change has opened up a Pandora's box of herbal remedies and products that are marketed quite freely in health food shops, grocery stores, and even drug stores. The new law changed the definition of a dietary supplement to extend beyond vitamins and to include herbs, amino acid preparations, and even some hormones. As such, herbal and other chemical preparations labeled as dietary supplements are exempt from regulations that require testing for safety and efficacy. Now, as long as the packaging for the supplement makes no specific claims with respect to treating a disease, the supplement is not considered a drug, and a company may market it freely (Spinella, 2001). So the label on a dietary supplement

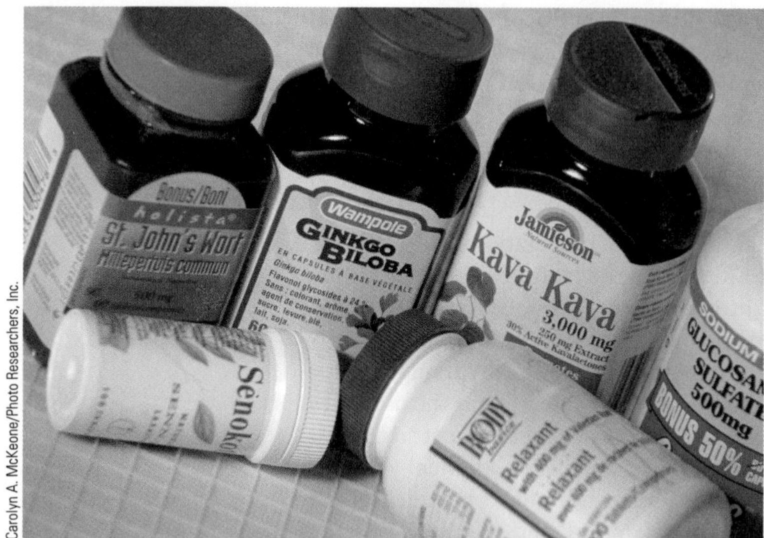

Carolyn A. McKeone/Photo Researchers, Inc.

Herbal/natural health supplements

may read "improves mood" or "calms the spirit" but not "relieves depression" or "treats anxiety."

The "health supplement" industry has burgeoned, and several controversies are now brewing. One view is that because such products are obtained directly from natural sources, they are somehow safer and more in harmony with nature than other medicines (Tyler, 2000). Many of the drugs we have already considered are also obtained directly from plants, however, including the likes of cocaine, mescaline, morphine, nicotine, and scopolamine. Clearly, a chemical found in natural plant material is not guaranteed to be risk-free. Supporters of the 1994 act argue that valuable remedies are now more readily available to people at low prices. They point, in particular, to success stories like St. John's wort (hypericum), an herbal therapy for depression. Hypericum extract from St. John's wort has been demonstrated in some studies to be effective in the treatment of depression, with few side effects. But most herbal preparations have not been well studied, so in many cases, there is little evidence of effectiveness. Even more problematic, in many cases, little is known about possible dangers that might be associated with the herb. Consumers should recognize that the FDA has not evaluated herbal preparations with respect to the GRAS and GRAE standards that are required for OTC drugs. An herbal preparation that produces serious side effects may remain on the market until enough evidence accumulates to remove it. As a case in point, consider the story of gamma hydroxybutyrate (GHB), which was marketed legally as a supplement until medical complications and abuse led to Schedule I status (see later discussion). Literally hundreds of supplements are available in the United States today. We review a few of the more important psychoactive preparations here.

Areca (Betel)

Areca catechu is a palm tree cultivated in Southeast Asia, India, and Africa. The nuts of this palm, often referred to as betel nuts, are chewed by more than 200 million people to produce a mildly stimulating effect. So, though not often seen in the United States, areca is one of the world's most popular drugs. Chewing areca or betel is a practice similar to chewing tobacco in the United States, and, like nicotine, the active chemical in areca, arecoline, affects the neurotransmitter acetylcholine. Users appear to develop a nicotine-like dependence on areca. Heavy use stains the mouth and lips red and damages the mouth and teeth, but users are often unable to quit chewing despite these problems (Spinella, 2001).

DHEA

Dehydroepiandrosterone (DHEA) is a hormone naturally secreted by the adrenal glands. It is offered as a miracle drug in health food stores with claims that it prevents heart disease, cancer, obesity, and diabetes. It is said to be an "antiaging" hormone as well. The bad news is that virtually no evidence supports any of these claims, although the hormone may have some mood-enhancing effects. DHEA is a precursor of testosterone in the body, and many DHEA effects may be related to the androgenic effects noted earlier in this chapter. So, although DHEA may not prevent aging, it may produce acne, premature baldness, and other side effects noted earlier for anabolic steroids (Julien, Advokat & Comaty, 2008).

Ephedra/Ma Huang

A number of plant species from the genus *Ephedra* have been used for many years for their stimulant effects. *Ephedra sinica* is native to Asia and is frequently sold under its Chinese name, *ma huang*. Another species, *E. nevadensis*, grows in the American West and is known as Mormon tea. The main psychoactive compound in ephedra is ephedrine. Ephedrine is a potent stimulant with effects much like those reviewed in Chapter 6. It is sympathomimetic and produces behavioral effects similar to those of other stimulants (Karch, 2000). Until 2004, ephedrine products were marketed through stores or by mail order to increase energy, prevent drowsiness, suppress appetite, and in high-dose formulations, as an "herbal" alternative to ecstasy (see Chapter 12). These products contained a wide variety of plant products and drugs, including caffeine, theophylline, pseudoephedrine, and ephedrine. Many side effects and some deaths due to heart attack and stroke were associated with ephedra products, particularly those with high doses of ephedrine (Spinella, 2001). The February 2003 death of Baltimore Orioles pitcher Steve Bechler—which was linked to his use of ephedra—prompted an expedited FDA review of ephedra preparations, and in April 2004, the FDA banned products containing ephedrine from over-the-counter sales.

Ginkgo Biloba

Extracts from the leaves of the ginkgo tree have been touted as a "smart drug," a drug that enhances memory and concentration. In fact, a number of studies have provided evidence that ginkgo extract improved memory and information processing in patients who have Alzheimer's disease, perhaps by improving blood flow to the brain (Spinella, 2001). However, these improvements are small, at best, and results from different studies have been mixed (Julien, Advokat & Comaty, 2008). Ginkgo extract contains many different chemicals, and it is unclear which are responsible for the benefits seen in Alzheimer's patients, so more research is clearly indicated on this interesting plant.

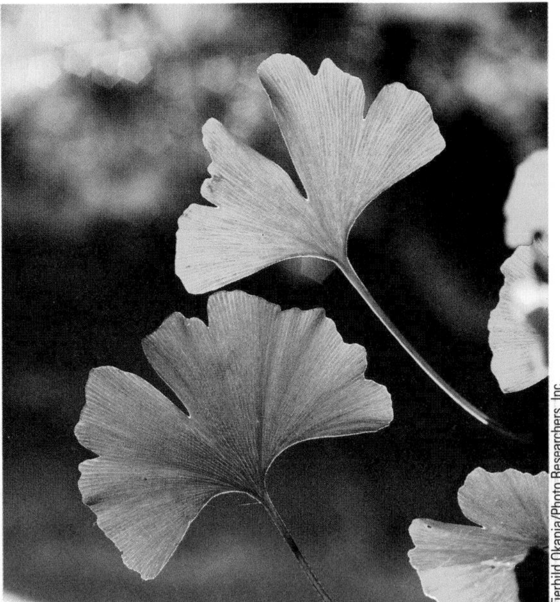

Tierbild Okapia/Photo Researchers, Inc.

Close-up shot of the leaves of a Gingko tree *(Gingko biloba)*.

Kava

The kava plant (*Piper methysticum*) is cultivated on South Pacific islands, where it has been used for religious and cultural ceremonies for hundreds of years. The roots of the plant are crushed and generally prepared in a tea. Kava appears to produce a sedating or relaxing effect similar to alcohol or other depressant drugs, and the supplement preparations sold in the United States imply that it can relieve stress and anxiety. Kava is becoming increasingly popular in the United States. Kava bars have sprung up around the country, and kava is frequently advertised and sold on the Internet as a legal high (Dennehy, Tsourounis, & Miller, 2005). Like the

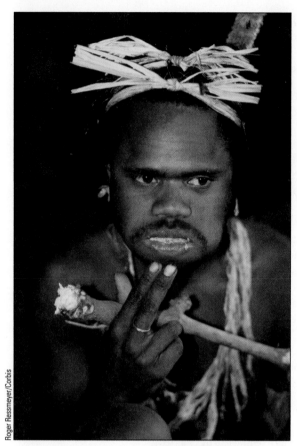
Roger Ressmeyer/Corbis

A man in Yakel village chews a mouthful of kava root.

depressant drugs, the active compounds in kava, a group of chemicals called kavalactones, appear to enhance the actions of the neurotransmitter GABA. Several controlled studies of kava preparations or kavalactones have supported the claims that kava produces relaxing or anxiolytic effects (Malsch & Kieser, 2001). Few side effects have been documented, but kava can produce an alcohol-like intoxication in higher doses, and abuse problems have been reported in the South Pacific. Side effects from kava may include drowsiness and blurred vision, and there have also been reports of liver toxicity. These have been problematic enough that kava has been banned in some countries (e.g., Canada, France, Germany), although it remains legal in the United States (Julien, Advokat, & Comaty, 2008).

Melatonin

Melatonin is a naturally occurring hormone produced by the pineal gland. It is thought to regulate biological rhythms and sleep. Numerous brands of synthetic and natural melatonin (from animal pineal gland) are available in stores, and they are recommended to consumers to treat everything from heart disease to cancer. A number of controlled studies suggest that melatonin is superior to placebo as a sleeping pill and in preventing "jet lag." Melatonin can reduce the time it takes for people to fall asleep and can lengthen sleep time (Zhdanova & Friedman, 2002). Other claims associated with melatonin have not been confirmed, however. In addition, some side effects are irritability, altered menstrual cycles, and vasoconstriction that may reduce blood flow to the brain and heart.

S-Adenosy-Methionine

S-Adenosy-methionine (SAM or SAMe) is a compound found naturally in the body that is marketed as a supplement with the formal claim that it promotes "emotional well-being." It is hyped as a treatment for depression, but these claims lack empirical support, at least with respect to the dosage forms available in the United States (Julien, Advokat, & Comaty, 2008).

St. John's Wort

St. John's wort (*Hypericum performatum*) is often held up as the poster child of the herbal alternatives movement because of its antidepressant effects. It is a perennial plant that has been cultivated in Europe for centuries. Extracts of hypericum contain a wide variety of active chemicals, including hypericin and pseudohypericin. Whether St. John's wort is really a significant antidepressant remains controversial. Some studies have found hypericum to be superior to placebo, but others have found no effects or even that patients treated with St. John's wort showed less improvement than those on placebo. Hypericum may produce side effects as well, including photosensitivity and lethargy, and it may alter the metabolization of numerous other drugs with potential for dangerous interactions, thus making St. John's wort of dubious safety (see Julien Advokat, & Comaty, 2008 for a review).

Valerian

Valerian originated in Europe and Asia, where it has been used for more than 1,000 years for a variety of purposes but primarily to treat insomnia and anxiety. Valerian preparations, derived from the root of the plant, contain active chemicals that collectively appear to enhance inhibitory neurotransmission through the GABA system. Valerian is not well studied, but several reports support the claim that it reduces sleep latency and improves sleep quality, albeit with many of the same side effects associated with benzodiazepines (Spinella, 2001).

Gamma Hydroxybutyrate

Gamma hydroxybutyrate (GHB) is a substance found in the brain that is thought to be a natural neurotransmitter or neurohormone. Its effects are generally those of depressant drugs. It is structurally related to GABA and, like many depressant drugs discussed already, influences GABA transmission. There are also specific brain receptors for GHB that may confer unique properties to GHB, but little is known about their function (Maitre et al., 2000).

GHB has an odd and interesting history. It was originally used as an anesthetic in Europe, but in the United States, it was marketed as a supplement for an odd combination of claimed benefits: to enhance athletic performance and sexual activity, and to induce sleep. GHB became a widely abused drug in the 1990s, and was linked with so many problems that it was declared a Schedule I drug in 2000. Although GHB is no longer legally available in the United States, it is still widely used. It is frequently smuggled into the country, and because it is easy to synthesize, much GHB is "home brewed."

Often considered among the "club drugs," GHB is usually taken orally in a salty-tasting liquid solution. Users report that the drug produces a euphoric intoxication; however, GHB is a potent depressant, and unconsciousness and coma have been frequently reported. Generally, these symptoms resolve within a few hours, but a number of deaths have been linked to GHB (Galloway et al., 2000). GHB toxicity and coma appears more likely when it is taken in combination with alcohol or other drugs (Liechti et al., 2006). This is consistent with findings from animal research that GHB is synergistic with alcohol and other depressants (Beardsley, Balster, & Harris, 1996). Also in keeping with the pattern of effects of most depressant drugs, tolerance and dependence to GHB have been reported. GHB is one of several drugs (for example, Rohypnol or roofies) that have been used to commit "date rape" by rendering a target unconscious (Galloway et al., 2000).

Oddly enough, GHB has been approved for medical use in the treatment of a form of narcolepsy. Narcolepsy is a rare condition (it affects about 120,000 people in the United States) in which patients suddenly and uncontrollably fall asleep. Perhaps one-third of narcoleptics also have cataplexy, a sudden loss of muscular control. Cataplexy results in collapse and, because it occurs without warning, is a very debilitating condition. GHB taken in the evening before sleep appears to markedly reduce these symptoms. In July 2002, FDA approval was given to a form of GHB to be marketed for this purpose under the brand name Xyrem. Xyrem is designated as a Schedule III controlled substance for medical use, but in another odd twist, the FDA announced that it would continue to consider the illicit use of GHB to be subject to Schedule I

TABLE 14.4 Common Inhalants and the Chemicals They Contain

Inhalant Class	Product	Chemicals
Adhesives	Airplane glue	toluene, ethyl acetate
Aerosols	Spray paint	butane, propane, fluorocarbons
	Hair spray	butane, propane
	Fabric spray	butane, trichloroethane
Anesthetics	Nitrous oxide	
	Halothane	
Cleaning agents	Spot remover	xylene, chlorohydrocarbons
	Degreaser	tetrachloroethylene
Solvents	Nail polish remover	acetone
	Paint thinner	petroleum distillates
	Correction fluid	trichloroethylene
	Gasoline	
Gases	Fuel gas	butane, isopropane
	Lighter fluid	butane
Food products	Whipped cream	nitrous oxide
	Whippets	nitrous oxide
Nitrites	Locker Room	isoamyl, butyl, or isopropyl
	Rush, poppers	nitrite

Source: Based on Sharp (1992).

penalties (FDA, 2002). This unusual move is designed to keep GHB tightly regulated, yet allow it to be available to the very small population of narcolepsy patients who need it.

So the strange story of GHB continues. The neurotransmitter was first used as an anesthetic, then moved on to become an unregulated dietary supplement, then was placed under the most stringent possible regulation as a Schedule I drug, and at present seems to be both a Schedule I drug and an approved Schedule III medical drug.

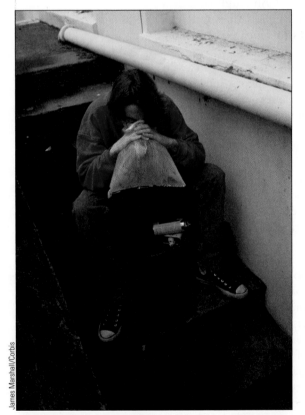

James Marshall/Corbis

A teenager uses inhalant drugs.

Inhalants

Inhalants include many different compounds related more by their method of administration than by their pharmacology. Some categories of inhalants, such as the medical anesthetics (halothane and nitrous oxide), are true depressant drugs, but inhalants also include a variety of products with widely varying pharmacologies, including glue, paint, butane gas, correction fluid, and many others (see Table 14.4 for a more detailed list). Perhaps the only thing all these products really have in common is the ability to produce a dizzy euphoria upon inhalation.

Inhalants are among the most widely abused drugs, particularly among the young. For example, in a 2008 survey, 15.7% of 8th graders reported that they used inhalants. Although fewer 12th graders reported inhalant use (9.9%), the use of inhalants, called "huffing" or "bagging," is clearly one of the major forms of dangerous drug use among young people today (Johnston, O'Malley, Bachman, & Schulenberg, 2009a).

Because of the bewildering variety of substances associated with inhalant abuse, it is difficult to characterize the hazards completely. A number of deaths have been due to cardiovascular collapse or suffocation related to the inhalation of butane, toluene, and gasoline (Cairney et. al., 2002). Chronic use of inhalants has been linked to a variety of medical problems, including psychotic behavior, movement disorders, liver and kidney toxicity, and damage to the brain's cortex and cerebellum (Cairney et al., 2005; Ridenour, Ray & Cottler, 2007).

The nitrite inhalants—amyl, butyl, and isopropyl nitrite (see Table 14.4)—are a group of inhalant drugs that deserve special mention. Amyl nitrite dilates coronary arteries when inhaled and was once prescribed to patients suffering from angina in the form of ampules that were crushed or popped before inhalation—hence the slang names "poppers" and "snappers." Nitrites also dilate cerebral blood vessels to produce a brief period of euphoria and dizziness. Nitrites have been widely used for recreational purposes, particularly in the gay community. Both gay and heterosexual users report that "poppers" inhaled during sexual activity prolong and intensify orgasm. A number of side effects have been noted from these drugs, including headache, tachycardia, eye problems, and rare sudden deaths (Rosenberg & Sharp, 1992).

The effects of inhaling nitrous oxide (laughing gas) involve a short-lived state of intoxication described by most users as a pleasant euphoria that is, as the drug's nickname implies, often accompanied by giggling and giddy laughter. However, in controlled studies, not all subjects enjoyed the effects of nitrous oxide, which they reported as confusion, feeling high, and stimulation but paradoxically also depression (Walker & Zacny, 2005).

Adverse effects reported from nitrous oxide use have included nausea, vomiting, and headache. In addition, heavy chronic use has occasionally been reported to resemble the sort of dependence that develops with other depressant drugs. With heavy use come more severe problems, including numbness of the extremities and permanent peripheral nerve damage. There have also been some reports of death by asphyxiation after using large amounts in a poorly ventilated space (Ibid.).

Summary

- The combination birth control pill contains synthetic versions of the two female sex hormones: estrogen and progesterone.
- Though highly effective at reducing the risk of pregnancy, the birth control pill has been linked to such side effects as increased risk of heart attack and stroke.
- Anabolic steroids are generally synthetic versions of the male sex hormone testosterone and are used to promote the development of muscle mass and to enhance athletic performance.
- Side effects associated with anabolic steroids include masculinizing effects in women, liver damage, acne, hair loss, and emotional disturbance.
- Three major analgesic drugs are available without prescription: aspirin, acetaminophen, and ibuprofen.
- Aspirin relieves pain, reduces fever, and is anti-inflammatory. Its side effects include stomach irritation and bleeding. The effects of ibuprofen are similar.
- Acetaminophen is a potent analgesic drug, but it lacks the anti-inflammatory effects of aspirin. It also is less likely to cause stomach irritation.

- Other ingredients of nonprescription cold and allergy medications include pseudoephedrine, guaifenesin, dextromethorphan, and antihistamines.
- The antihistamine compound diphenhydramine is the major ingredient in nonprescription sleeping pills.
- Many herbal drugs, amino acids, and hormones are marketed as dietary supplements. They include areca, DHEA, ephedra, ginkgo biloba, kava, melatonin, SAMe, St. John's wort, and valerian.
- GHB is a naturally occurring neurotransmitter that has the properties of a depressant drug. It began as a supplement but is now tightly regulated due to abuse problems.
- Inhalants are a large group of volatile compounds that can alter consciousness when taken into the lungs. Many of them are organic solvents that can damage the brain.

Answers to *"What Do You Think?"*

1. Birth control pills contain synthetic forms of one or both of the female sex hormones.
   T *Combination birth control pills contain synthetic estrogen and progesterone; the progestin pill contains only synthetic progesterone.*
2. One of the risks associated with the use of birth control pills is an increased chance of lung cancer.
   F *An increased risk of blood clots is associated with the use of birth control pills.*
3. Anabolic steroids are synthetic forms of testosterone.
   T *Anabolic steroids mimic the action of the male sex hormone.*
4. Anabolic steroids are generally taken because of the high they produce.
   F *Although steroids may produce a high, they are generally taken to increase muscle mass.*
5. Acne, baldness, and liver damage are all side effects associated with steroid use.
   T *There are other potential side effects as well.*
6. GRAS is a common street name for marijuana.
   F *GRAS stands for "generally recognized as safe."*
7. Aspirin relieves pain through action on the endorphins, in much the same way that the pain-relieving effects of opiates are produced.
   F *The pain-relieving effects of aspirin are produced by blocking prostaglandin release.*
8. Many over-the-counter diet pills contain low doses of amphetamines.
   F *Many diet pills contain ephedrine or caffeine. Amphetamines are Schedule II drugs and may not be sold without a prescription.*
9. Antitussive agents are used to suppress coughing.
   T *Antitussives are used to suppress coughing.*
10. Antihistamines are common ingredients in over-the-counter cold remedies.
    T *Antihistamines relieve nasal congestion and related symptoms.*
11. GHB is a naturally occurring brain chemical.
    T *GHB is found in the brain, where it is thought to be a neurotransmitter.*
12. Caffeine is a common ingredient in over-the-counter stimulant preparations.
    T *Caffeine and ephedrine are both commonly used.*

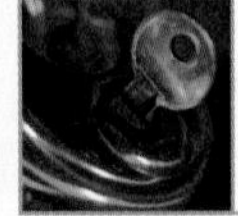

Key Terms

acetaminophen (ə-'sē-tə-'mi-nə-fən)
acetylsalicylic acid (ə-'sə-tᵊl-'sa-lə-'si-lik)
anabolic steroids
antihistamines
antitussives
combination pill
estrogen ('es-trə-jən)
guaifenesin (gwī-'fen-ə-sin)
ibuprofen ('ī-byu̇-'prō-fən)
naproxen (nə-'prok-sən)
progesterone (prō-'jes-tə-'rōn)
progestin pill
prostaglandins ('präs-tə-'glan-dən)
pseudoephedrine ('sü-dō-i-'fed-rən)
testosterone

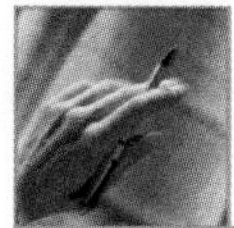

Essays/Thought Questions

1. How should athletic competitions deal with the problem of anabolic steroid use?
2. The 1994 Dietary Supplement Health and Education Act made it possible for herbal medications to be advertised and sold without FDA regulation as long as the product is not specifically represented as a treatment for a disease. What are the pros and cons of this decision?

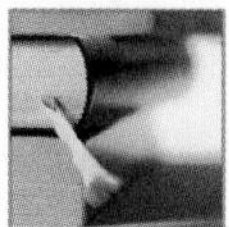

Suggested Readings

Julien, R. M., Advokat, C. D., & Comaty, J. E. (2008). *A primer of drug action* (11th ed.). New York: W. H. Freeman & Company.

Spinella, M. (2001). *The psychopharmacology of herbal medicine*. Cambridge, MA: MIT Press.

Yesalis, C. E. (2000). *Anabolic steroids in sport and exercise* (2nd ed.). Champaign, IL: Human Kinetics Press.

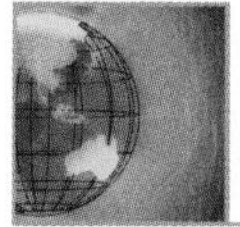

Web Resources

Visit the Book Companion Website at www.cengage.com/psychology/maisto to access study tools including a glossary, flashcards, and web quizzing. You will also find links to the following resources:

- Information on anabolic steroids
- Office of Dietary Supplements on herbal medicine and supplements
- FDA on OTC drugs
- NIH site on OTC drugs
- Project GHB

CHAPTER 15

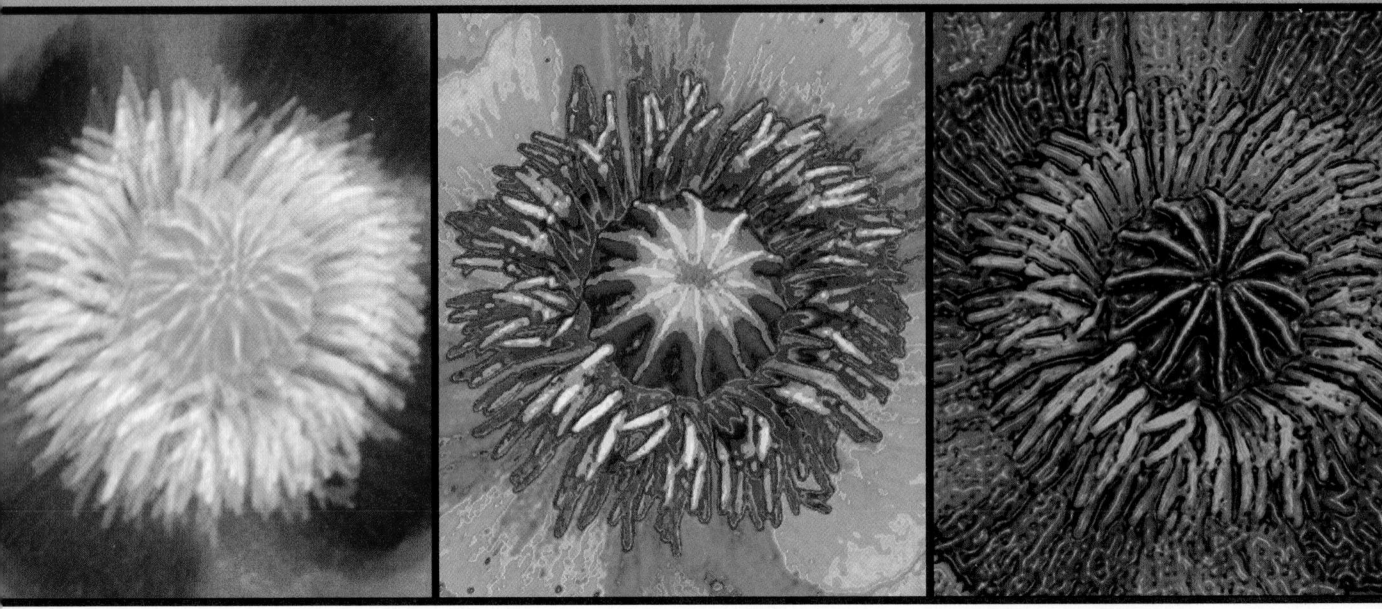

Treatment of Substance-Use Disorders

What Do You Think? True or False?

Answers are given at the end of the chapter.

___ 1. The process of changing a problem behavior seems to be different for everyone.

___ 2. Treatment is needed to change patterns of alcohol and drug abuse or dependence.

___ 3. Alcoholics Anonymous was created more than 100 years ago, and its influence is predominantly in the United States.

___ 4. It is generally agreed that substance-use disorders are caused by psychological problems.

___ 5. Assessment typically is thought to be essential to good treatment.

___ 6. The only goal of any importance in alcohol and drug treatment is the reduction of substance use.

___ 7. Abstinence from alcohol is a mandatory goal of alcohol treatment.

___ 8. Methadone maintenance seems to be an effective treatment for heroin dependence.

___ 9. Today, there are good reasons for rigid boundaries between what we call alcohol treatment and drug treatment.

___10. People who have major psychiatric problems are rarely seen in settings where alcohol and drug treatment are provided.

___11. Relapse is such a long-standing problem in alcohol and drug treatment that we can do little about it.

___12. Professional treatment for substance-use disorders is freely available to anyone who wants it.

Now that we have covered the most commonly used psychoactive substances, we are ready to address the question: What is done for people whose use becomes abuse or dependence? The question pertains to **treatment**, or planned activities designed to change some pattern of behavior(s) of individuals or their families. In this chapter, we are concerned with patterns of substance use. Both psychological and behavioral treatments and pharmacological treatments are discussed.

treatment
Planned activities designed to change some pattern of behavior(s) of individuals or their families.

Because the information about treatment is large in both volume and variety, it is useful to have a model to guide us through this chapter. Figure 15.1 is a model of what might occur during the course of treatment, from the time an alcohol or drug problem is recognized to the outcome, or the result that is attributed to treatment. In this case, the essential outcome of interest is change in alcohol or other drug use patterns.

"I always wanted to have a life. In treatment, I discovered that drug use had cost me my life."

Anonymous

You should read Figure 15.1 from left to right. For any treatment to happen, a problem must first be recognized. That recognition may come from the individual, or it may come first from other sources (family, friends, legal system, employer) in the individual's environment. Even with external feedback about a problem, individuals still may not be convinced that they actually do have a problem and need to change. This complex decision point typically is described by terms such as a person's *motivation* to change or *commitment* to change. With problem recognition, if change is initiated, it typically happens in one of three ways. People may decide to change their substance use without any kind of help. In Chapter 7, you saw that many ex-smokers stopped without help. The same applies to people with alcohol or other drug problems, though as with smoking, it may take a few tries to do so (Sobell et al., 1993). This phenomenon has been called **spontaneous remission**. Another option that individuals may choose is self-help groups, such as Alcoholics Anonymous. And a third possibility is that individuals go into some kind of professional treatment. Frequently, individuals may combine self-help group attendance with professional treatment activities.

spontaneous remission
Resolution of a problem without the help of formal treatment.

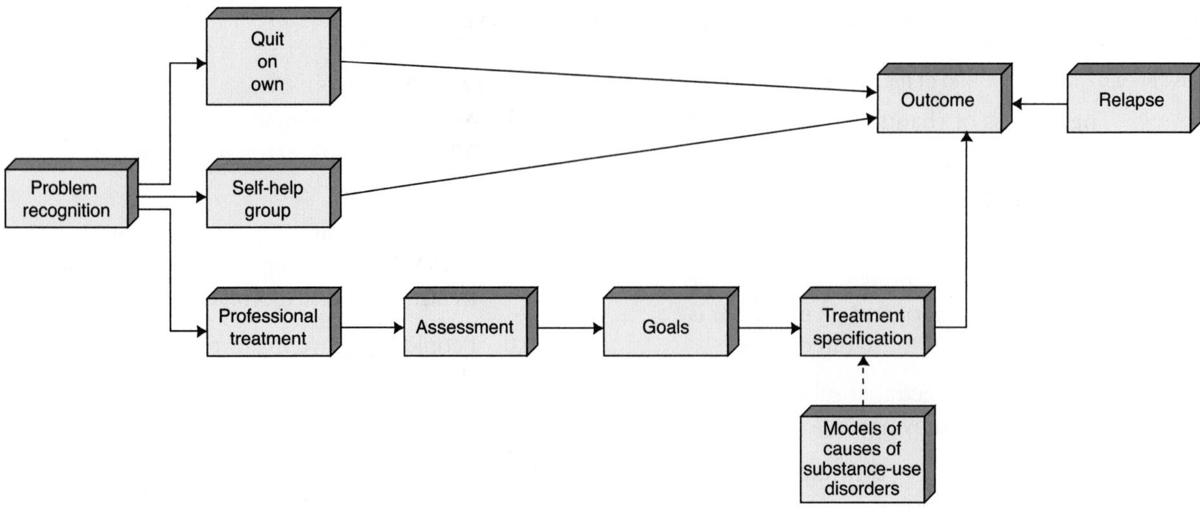

FIGURE 15.1
A model of events that occur in the course of treatment of substance-use disorders.

If individuals initiate professional treatment, some type of assessment of their problems usually occurs first. Assessment leads to the specification of treatment goals, which contribute to placement in a specific treatment setting or activity. The content and structure of treatments are influenced by models and theories of alcohol and drug problems, reflected by the broken line in Figure 15.1.

The result, or outcome, of these change options is of primary interest. Outcomes can take a variety of forms, especially over a long period of time. Following treatment for alcohol and other drug use, individuals may relapse after some time of substance-use problem reduction or resolution. If that happens, the person "goes back" to any of the preceding points in Figure 15.1, including back to the step of considering whether the person has a commitment to change.

With this framework, we can begin our presentation on treatment of the substance-use disorders. Like Figure 15.1, we start with a discussion of problem recognition and motivation to change.

Motivation to Change

"One way or another, with professional help or without, with friendly advice from uncle or neighbor or without it, with constant nagging from wife or husband or without it, the individual . . . makes a decision [to change]."

J. Orford, 1980 (Orford, 1985, p. 272)

Terms like *motivation* have been around as long as human behavior has been observed and interpreted. Motivation to change has been considered essential if individuals have any hope that treatment of a behavioral or psychological problem will be effective. In the context of substance-use disorders, motivation to change is discussed often and sometimes heatedly. For example, it frequently is asserted that the major barrier to change is a person's denial of a problem with alcohol or drugs. Denial may persist even with evidence of a problem that is blatant to everybody but the person who has the problem.

Despite all the discussion of motivation, it has not been as fruitful as we might expect in helping us to understand change in behavior like alcohol and drug use. Part of the problem is the many different ways to define a motivation to change and to measure it when conducting research or in clinical practice. One solution to this problem that has proved productive in addictions (smoking, alcohol, and other drug use) research is to look at "readiness" (or commitment) to change instead of grappling with the abstract idea of motivation. There have been several attempts to do this, but the one that has the greatest influence is the stages of change model (Prochaska, DiClemente, & Norcross, 1992). This model is thought to apply to people who change on their own or who use outside resources to change. The model has five stages: precontemplation, contemplation, preparation, action, and maintenance. A person may cycle through the stages to various points several times before reaching problem resolution. You can connect this idea to what we said both about self-quitters "quitting" smoking or drinking several times before it seems permanent and about the difficult problem of relapse.

People in the precontemplation stage of the change model are not aware of the problem or, if they are, have no interest in change. Precontemplators are those who often are said to be in "denial." It appears that progression in the change cycle requires acknowledgment of the problem and its negative consequences, and an accurate evaluation of change possibilities and how they might occur (for example, with or without professional treatment). Contemplators vacillate between the pros and cons of their problem behavior and between the pros and cons of making changes in it. So, they are deciding whether to change, but they have taken no steps to do so. People in the preparation stage are on the edge of taking action to change and may have made a try in the recent past. To progress, a commitment to take action and to set goals is needed. Individuals in the action stage already are engaged in explicit activities to change. Maintenance, the last stage, involves the continued use of behavior-change activities for as long as three years after the action stage began. After that time, the problem might be considered resolved. People are thought to progress through each of these stages in the process of change. The rate of progression and the amount of recycling differ from person to person and from problem to problem for a given person, but going through the stages applies generally. We should add here that identification of a person's stage is problem specific. For example, a person's stage of change for his or her drinking may not be indicative of that person's stage of change for smoking.

"We must use the carrot and stick of the criminal justice system to demand that drug-dependent offenders become involved in treatment."

Lee Brown, director of the U.S. Office of National Drug Control Policy (*The Alcoholism Report*, 1993, p. 6)

What this all means for us is that the stage of change helps us to identify a person's perception of the problem and readiness to change it. These factors may help us to determine the timing and content of treatment, or whether self-help groups or professional treatment is needed at all (Connors, Donovan, & DiClemente, 2001). Moreover, the stage may tell us what needs to be done to move the change process forward. For example, although coming to one's own conclusion that change is needed is the most effective foundation of long-term changes, external (to the individual) pushes to change (for example, from a spouse or employer) may help the person to progress from the precontemplation stage to a later stage that is characterized by a more internally based desire to change (Ryan, Plant, & O'Malley, 1995).

"Overcoming my addictions is the hardest thing I've ever done. I am still working on it. You have to want to learn it. It is a lot of change. You have to want to do it."

Recovering heroin addict

With problem recognition and a source of motivation to change, the next step is a decision about how change will occur. In turn, we consider problem resolution on one's own, the use of self-help groups, and the use of professional treatment services.

Change without Formal Treatment

We do not have sufficient space to discuss the research on spontaneous remission of alcohol and other drug-use problems, but suffice it to say that it happens. In fact, it is generally agreed that more people with such problems resolve them on their own than by using self-help groups or professional treatment. How such changes are initiated is of interest and has been studied most extensively with alcohol problems. Sobell et al. (1993) reported the best study methodologically of this question to date. Most of the people these researchers studied (57%) said their change resulted from weighing the benefits and costs of continuing their current alcohol-use pattern. When the disadvantages seemed to grow in number and importance, change occurred. Notice how similar this is to what people in the contemplation stage are thought to do. Another 29% of the study participants reported that change was immediate, and they either could not recall what triggered the change or said it was a major event, such as a serious alcohol-related health problem.

It is worth saying more about the 29% of Sobell et al.'s (1993) research participants who reported that change was immediate. This group is poorly represented in current ideas and theories about behavior change and its maintenance. Yet, as the Sobell et al. study suggests, immediate change is far from rare; we see this theme in fiction (Charles Dickens's Scrooge) and often in our own experiences or those of family members and friends. William Miller and Janet C'de Baca published a book called *Quantum Change* in 2001 about sudden-change experiences. The book describes the "quantum change" experiences of people from all walks of life and what happened to them in the years afterward. Miller and C'de Baca offer some ideas and questions to stimulate the scientific study of how sudden change occurs, in the hope of beginning to close an important gap in our knowledge of behavior change.

The most important point to take from this brief discussion is that spontaneous remission occurs and apparently occurs often. How often has not been determined; to specify the prevalence would be extremely costly and complex. Nevertheless, even with our limited knowledge of it, the phenomenon of change without treatment has taught us a lot about change processes in general, including change that occurs with the use of treatment resources. Many individuals with a diagnosis of substance-use disorder do eventually seek help from treatment resources (Kessler et al., 2001). We turn next to one of those resources: self-help groups.

Self-Help Groups

Peer self-help groups are a major part of the treatment of substance-use disorders. According to Emrick, Lassen, and Edwards (1977), members of peer self-help groups perform therapeutic functions without professional credentials. A member of a peer self-help group might have training pertinent to conducting therapy, but such credentials are not used in performing group functions. Members of these groups all have some identified problem that is the focus of the group's therapeutic activity. The term *peer self-help* distinguishes these groups from those in which therapeutic agents (the group leader, for example) are not identified as having the same problems as the clients. Therefore, through the peer self-help group, participants both give and receive help with their problems.

"The one thing I could never do is go to a formal rehab; for me to have to ask somebody else to help with a self-made problem, I would rather drink myself to death."

Individual who resolved his alcohol problem on his own (Tuchfeld, 1981, p. 631)

Although the peer self-help movement does not use professionally defined methods to help participants with their problems, professionals are not shunned. In fact, the professional community is welcome to join the peer self-help group in achieving common goals of helping people alleviate their problems (for example, Alcoholics Anonymous, 1972). Professionals and the self-help group have complementary functions. In practice, professionals who work in the treatment of alcohol and drug problems often use relevant self-help groups (such as Alcoholics Anonymous for alcohol problems and Narcotics Anonymous for other drug problems) in a professionally run rehabilitation program and as part of aftercare planning. Indeed, many alcohol and drug treatment programs are organized around principles of peer self-help groups.

In discussing treatment of the substance-use disorders, we must review peer self-help groups because of their popularity and influence. Peer self-help also has been a popular treatment of choice for other addictive behaviors: Weight Watchers and TOPS (Taking Off Pounds Sensibly) for treatment of obesity, Smokers Anonymous for treatment of cigarette smoking, and Gamblers Anonymous for treatment of compulsive gambling. One national survey estimates that, in 1990, close to 1.5 million people in the United States used self-help groups to treat addiction or other mental health problems (Regier et al., 1993).

Alcoholics Anonymous

In this section, we briefly describe the peer self-help movement organized for helping individuals identified as alcoholics—Alcoholics Anonymous (AA). Because of space limitations, we cannot describe in detail the major self-help groups for the treatment of drug problems, called Narcotics Anonymous (NA). NA is analogous to AA, however, and what we know about AA can be applied readily to NA.

Emrick, Lassen, and Edwards (1977) called AA the prototype self-help group because it is the oldest, established in 1935. It has been the basis for the development of other self-help movements for treatments in other problem areas. The AA movement began when an alcoholic surgeon (Dr. Bob) and an alcoholic stockbroker (Bill W.) helped each other to maintain sobriety. From Ohio, they spread their idea that alcoholics need to help each other. Today, AA is an international organization. A few alcohol self-help groups, such as Alateen and Al-Anon, have been derived from AA. Alateen's purpose is to help teenagers who have an alcoholic parent; Al-Anon generally is aimed at spouses and others close to those with alcoholism.

The bases of the AA "program" are self-help recovery through following the Twelve Steps and group participation. The core of AA is the model of recovery outlined in the Twelve Steps, which are listed in Table 15.1. In the first step, AA absolutely dismisses the notion that people with alcoholism can control their drinking or can ever reach that position. The beginning of recovery occurs when those with alcoholism admit to themselves as being powerless over alcohol, that without alcohol a return to health is possible, and that with it, the downward spiral to self-destruction continues. One cause of controversy is the frequent reference to God in the Twelve Steps. An immediate reaction to this is that AA is only for those with alcoholism who accept Western religious beliefs. However, AA takes pains to accent the phrase "God as we understood Him," which means people may interpret "God" or "Higher Power" as they wish. The importance of referring to a Supreme Being is to emphasize that people with alcoholism have lost control over alcohol and their lives and must enlist the assistance of a greater power in recovery. A final point is that the Twelve Steps recovery program is oriented toward action, both in self-examination and change and in behavior toward others.

"I am the black sheep of the family. I came to Alcoholics Anonymous and found the rest of the herd."

Quote from an AA meeting participant

The Twelve Steps are a guide designed for people to follow largely by themselves on the road to **recovery**. In addition to the bases of the steps, there are other parts to the AA program. One of these is group participation. Two major types are discussion meetings and speakers' meetings. In a discussion meeting, the chairperson of the group tells his or her personal history of alcoholism and recovery from it, and then the meeting is opened for members' discussion of alcoholism and related matters. In a speakers' meeting, a couple of members recite their personal histories of alcoholism and recovery. In open speakers' meetings, anyone who is interested may attend; closed meetings are for alcoholics only.

recovery
In the addictions field, changes back to health in physical, psychological, spiritual, and social functioning. It generally is believed that recovery is a lifetime process that requires total abstinence from alcohol and nonprescribed drugs.

One purpose of group meetings is to aid recovery through peer identification and learning from the experience of others. Building social relationships that do not revolve around alcohol represents an entirely new social life. The importance of forming sober social relationships may be seen in various AA functions such as "Sober Anniversaries" (the first day of a member's current episode of continuous sobriety) and "Sober Dances" (dances without alcohol or drugs).

TABLE 15.1 The Twelve Steps of Alcoholics Anonymous

1. We admitted we were powerless over alcohol—that our lives had become unmanageable.
2. Came to believe that a Power greater than ourselves could restore us to sanity.
3. Made a decision to turn our will and our lives over to the care of God as we understood Him.
4. Made a searching and fearless moral inventory of ourselves.
5. Admitted to God, to ourselves, and to another human being the exact nature of our wrongs.
6. Were entirely ready to have God remove all these defects of character.
7. Humbly asked Him to remove our shortcomings.
8. Made a list of all persons we had harmed, and became willing to make amends to them all.
9. Made direct amends to such people wherever possible, except when to do so would injure them or others.
10. Continued to take personal inventory and when we were wrong promptly admitted it.
11. Sought through prayer and meditation to improve our conscious contact with God as we understood Him, praying only for knowledge of His will for us and the power to carry that out.
12. Having had a spiritual awakening as the result of these steps, we tried to carry this message to other addicts, and to practice these principles in all our affairs.

Note: The Twelve Steps are reprinted with permission of Alcoholics Anonymous World Services, Inc. Permission to reprint the Twelve Steps does not mean that AA has reviewed or approved the contents of this publication, nor that AA agrees with the views expressed herein. AA is a program of recovery from alcoholism *only*—use of the Twelve Steps in connection with programs and activities which are patterned after AA, but which address other problems, or in any other non-AA context, does not imply otherwise.

Other major activities in the AA program are "Twelfth Stepping" and sponsorship. Twelfth Stepping refers to the twelfth of the Twelve Steps, which involves members reaching out to other alcoholics in a time of need. A member may help active alcoholics begin the AA program or help current AA members return to sobriety after they have begun drinking again. Sponsorship is similar to Twelfth Stepping, but there are important differences. First, sponsorship involves a stable one-to-one relationship between a member with more sobriety (the sponsor) and one with less (the sponsee). To quote, "[T]he process of sponsorship is this: An alcoholic who has made some progress in the recovery program shares that experience on a continuous, individual basis with another alcoholic who is attempting to attain or maintain sobriety through AA" (Alcoholics Anonymous, 1983, p. 5). Another important difference is that the sponsor helps the sponsee in ways such as taking the newer member's "inventory" (looking at what is behind a person's behavior) when asked; guiding an individual to AA literature, such as the *Big Book* and *Twelve Steps and Twelve Traditions*; and explaining the AA program to family and others close to the sponsee. The sponsor–sponsee relationship is more varied and more enduring than that involved in Twelfth Stepping. AA members view both types of activities as essential to their continued sobriety.

What has been described for AA is directly applicable to Narcotics Anonymous (NA). NA's organization and program of recovery are derived directly from AA's, including the use of the Steps to Recovery Program, group meetings, and the sponsor–sponsee relationship. As the name implies, NA evolved to help people addicted to opiate drugs, usually heroin. However, people who identify their primary problem as addiction to drugs of any type other than alcohol use NA instead of AA.

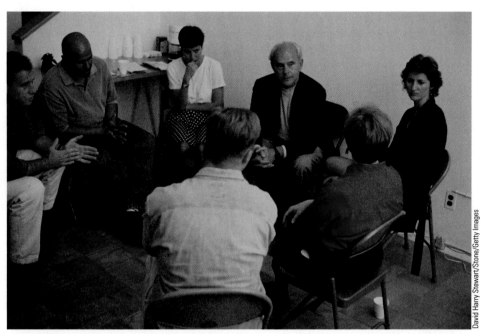
David Harry Stewart/Stone/Getty Images

Attendance at Alcoholics Anonymous meetings is the most popular self-help method for changing drinking behaviors in the United States.

In summary, the AA program of recovery has been the cornerstone of a self-help movement that has been of value to many and that is reaching increasing numbers of people. It is worth mentioning again that both AA and NA may be, and are, used alone as programs of treatment, but many members of these organizations began treatment or concurrently are receiving treatment from professional sources.

"God grant me the serenity to accept the things I cannot change, the courage to change the things I can, and the wisdom to know the difference."

"The Serenity Prayer," a guidepost to living along with the Twelve Steps, in AA and other 12-step programs

Other Self-Help Groups

We have spent so much space on AA and its "relatives" because they are by far the most prevalent and influential self-help treatments for alcohol- and drug-use disorders. Perhaps stimulated by AA's success, other types of self-help groups for alcohol and drug problems have been organized. One important example is Women for Sobriety (WFS), which began in 1975 (Women for Sobriety, 1985). WFS groups are now available throughout the United States and in other countries as well.

WFS agrees with AA that alcohol- and drug-use disorders are progressive illnesses. Complete abstinence from these substances is required to arrest the illnesses, but they cannot be cured. Also similar to AA, WFS members meet in groups (weekly) that a moderator leads. The WFS "program" that is the core topic of the discussion groups consists of 13 statements about spiritual and emotional change and growth.

So far, it is not clear why WFS required a new name, because it seems like a slight variant of AA. The focus of WFS is the special psychological and social needs and concerns that women face in achieving and maintaining sobriety. However, AA in general does not share this focus. WFS suggests that its program may be used alone to maintain sobriety, in conjunction with professional services, or in conjunction with AA.

A self-help group that claims to be based on methods that are scientifically validated is Self-Management and Recovery Training (SMART) (Rajacic, 1997). SMART groups usually have 4 to 12 members and are led by a "coordinator," someone who has maintained sobriety for an appreciable amount of time and who believes in SMART principles. Coordinators also may be individuals who have never had an alcohol problem (Fletcher, 2001). SMART groups are conducted to make people aware in four key areas: (1) motives for using alcohol and other drugs and for stopping such use, (2) beliefs that can help or be irrational and hinder a person's attempt to stop drinking, (3) emotions, and (4) behavior. SMART helps people combat irrational beliefs that are obstacles in quitting drinking, after Albert Ellis's system of psychotherapy called rational emotive behavior therapy. Then SMART helps people cope with feelings like fear and anger without drinking. Work on thoughts and feelings must be followed by changes in behavior for success in addressing an alcohol problem. Behavior change is said to occur by engaging in activities that are enjoyable that do not involve alcohol use.

SMART had been aligned with a former self-help movement called Rational Recovery (Trimpey, 1992). On January 1, 1999, however, Rational Recovery stopped holding self-help group meetings and, in fact, now condemns the self-help group movement. Rational Recovery considers itself an educational movement based on cognitive-behavioral principles (similar to rational emotive behavior therapy) and the addictive voice recognition technique (AVRT). AVRT is said to be a way to stop and take control of the "inner voice" that tells people to drink. Rational Recovery principles are disseminated via the Internet, videotapes and CDs, and books.

The last self-help group we discuss is SOS, which stands for Secular Organizations for Sobriety or, as an alternative, Save Our Selves. This self-help support group began in 1986, as an alternative to AA. As in SMART, the SOS alternative has no emphasis on spirituality or higher powers in staying sober. Instead, individuals are viewed as being in charge of making rational decisions about their use of alcohol and drugs. SOS's popularity is increasing rapidly and, as of 1990, had more than 200 sites in the United States where groups meet. SOS also is international, with groups in Europe as well as in the United States (http://www.cfiwest.org/sos/index.htm/).

Like AA, SOS uses peer support group meetings as the vehicle for staying sober. Groups generally have 10 to 12 members and meet weekly for 1 to $1\frac{1}{2}$ hours, but other procedures are possible, as the parent organization is flexible regarding the schedule and format of individual support group meetings. These meetings have a rotating leader, who is a group member. Groups are free, but members may make donations to sustain the group financially.

The core principle of SOS is that sobriety—abstinence from alcohol and drugs—is maintained "one day at a time," an expression well known to AA members. The "Sobriety Priority" program is the philosophy that underlies SOS, with these major points: (1) acknowledgment of one's addiction as a disease and a habit; (2) acceptance of one's problem; and (3) placement of sobriety as the number-one priority, separate from other problems or concerns in life. These three points may be viewed as analogous to AA's Twelve Steps. In SOS, groups are seen as safe places where members can discuss their concerns and ways that they stay sober. No limit is placed on how long people may stay in a group or on the number of meetings they attend.

Self-help groups are an extremely important resource that people use to change their patterns of alcohol or other drug use. Self-help groups may be used alone or in conjunction with professional treatment services, which is our next topic. Before we go into our discussion of what happens in such treatment, however, it is important for you to know something about the ideas (models and theories) behind it. You have seen in our review of self-help groups how beliefs about the causes of alcohol and drug problems greatly influenced the content of the self-help group and what participation in it involved. The same is true for professional treatments.

Models of Substance-Use Disorders

In Chapter 9, we discussed at length how many different models and theories have been championed to explain the causes of alcohol dependence. These conceptual views have spanned biological, psychological, and social/environmental domains of variables; tended to be heavy on one of the three variable domains and light or silent on the other two; and often explained something about the development of alcohol dependence, but not everything (Miller & Hester, 1995).

To make learning about these models and theories easier, we have organized them into five major categories (with specific variations within the categories): moral model, American disease model, biological model, social learning model, and sociocultural model. Each model has implications for designing treatment of the substance-use disorders. Our discussion is based heavily on chapters by Miller and Hester (1989; 2002).

"Society and its agencies have always had a consistent response, in that in the same breath they are able to say the homeless alcoholic is 'sad, mad, and bad.'"

Timothy Cook, 1975 (Orford, 1985, p. 292)

Five Model Categories

The first category is the moral model, in which individuals are seen as personally responsible for problems they may incur from their use of drugs and alcohol. That is, the development of a substance-use disorder is seen as the product of a series of personal decisions or choices to use those substances in a way that is harmful. This perspective implies that choices other than to use alcohol and drugs were available to the person but were not taken. Depending on the variation of the model, treatment consists of either spiritual or legal intervention.

The American disease model is especially important because of its widespread prevalence and prominence in the United States. It also is the foundation of Alcoholics Anonymous and other self-help groups. In the American disease model (it is called American because it is not nearly so popular in other countries), dependence on alcohol and drugs is viewed as the product of a progressive, irreversible disease. The disease is described as a merging of physical, psychological, and spiritual causes. The treatment that follows from the disease model is to identify people who have the disease, confront them with it, help them to accept that they have it, and persuade them to abstain from alcohol and other drugs.

In the biological model, dependence on alcohol or other drugs is viewed as the result of genetic or physiological processes. Theories about how the pharmacological action of drugs themselves in the brain can lead to dependence also fall under the biological umbrella. The treatment most clearly implied from biological models is to advise biologically at-risk people of their risk for developing a disorder, and perhaps to counsel those who are at risk to avoid alcohol and other drugs altogether.

Social learning theory is the position that alcohol and drug disorders are the result of complex learning from an interaction of individuals with their environments. Situations and psychological processes are most important. For example, harmful substance-use patterns may develop from direct experiences in using alcohol and drugs, from modeling the behavior of other individuals when they drink or use drugs in a harmful way, from false beliefs about the powers of alcohol and drugs in helping to get through difficult times, or from a failure to learn ways to cope with stress without alcohol or drug use. Treatment follows straightforwardly from this conception: Arrange the person's environment so that nonabuse of psychoactive substances is reinforced and abuse is not, or is punished (Higgins et al., 1991); display individuals ("models") engaging in desirable alcohol-use patterns (use of psychoactive drugs other than for medical purposes never is viewed positively by the greater society); teach facts about the actions of alcohol and drugs on the body and how humans experience their effects; and teach nondrug ways to cope with stress.

According to the sociocultural model, subcultures and societies shape alcohol- and drug-use patterns and consequences. Examples are norms and rules that a subculture has for alcohol use (such as when it is appropriate, as at adult dinner parties, and when it is not, as at work) and laws about substance use (such as what drugs are legal and what drugs are not). The treatment that follows from this perspective is interventions that affect large groups of people or society in general. For example, taxing sales of alcoholic beverages is an effort in part to control their availability and accessibility. Another example of a sociocultural intervention is the classification of drugs by "schedule" status (see Chapter 2).

You can see that the five major models and theories of substance-use disorder reflect a wide array of perspectives. You also might notice that, in general, the models do not overlap much. A summary of the five models and their implications for treatment is presented in Table 15.2.

Biopsychosocial Model

If no one model or theory of causes of substance-use disorders proves adequate, as is the case, then there must be some way of proceeding with treatment design. We could be atheoretical in our efforts, but that approach tends not to be too productive. Instead,

TABLE 15.2 The Five Major Models of the Causes of Substance-Use Disorders and Their Implications for Treatment

Model	Cause(s)	Treatment
Moral	The making of personal choices to use alcohol and drugs in a harmful way, when other choices could have been made	Punish legally or intervene spiritually.
American disease	Progressive, irreversible diseases that are the products of a mix of physical, psychological, and spiritual causes	Identify those with the disease, confront them with it, and persuade them to abstain from drugs and alcohol.
Biological	Genetic or physiological processes	Advise people at risk for problems of their risk status, and counsel them to avoid alcohol and drugs.
Social learning	Complex learning based on the interaction of the individuals with their environments	Arrange the environment to reinforce nonabuse of substances; do not reinforce, or punish, abuse; provide models of appropriate substance use; debunk myths about alcohol and drugs; teach nondrug alternatives for coping with stress.
Sociocultural	Practices and rules of subcultures and societies	Intervene in ways that affect large groups or society in general (e.g., drug-use laws and alcohol taxes).

Source: From R. K. Hester and W. R. Miller, *Handbook of Alcoholism Treatment Approaches Effective Alternatives*, 2nd ed., ©1995. Published by Allyn and Bacon, Boston, MA. Copyright ©1995 by Pearson Education. Reprinted by the permission of the publisher.

we can combine the disciplines (biological/medical–psychological–social/environmental) into one perspective. As you saw in Chapter 9, the term *biopsychosocial* reflects an attempt to simultaneously take into account three major variable domains that are known to influence human health and behavior. You will recognize again that this combined perspective follows from the theme of the drug experience and its determinants that we have articulated and developed since the first chapter of this text.

It is no secret that taking a biopsychosocial perspective of the causes of the substance-use disorders leads us to a new level of complexity. But drugs and human behavior is a complex subject that requires complex analysis for its understanding. Because of its complexity and recency, the biopsychosocial viewpoint is just that, a viewpoint, at this time—it is not precise or developed enough to be called a theory. Our premise is that this perspective has been providing and will continue to provide a guide for the kind of research that will find explanations of the causes of substance-use disorders.

Professional Treatment: Assessment and Goals

When individuals go to professionals for help to change their substance use, a process of assessment and treatment goal setting typically is initiated. Actually, models of etiology influence this part of the treatment experience as they do the treatment content. We also should note that discussing assessment and goals here is not meant to imply they are not relevant for self-change or self-help groups. Although no systematic, formally structured assessment occurs in those contexts, there has been some type of appraisal, however unsystematic or subtle, that a problem exists. Furthermore, goals are set that define the desired end of the change process. Again, such goals may not be explicitly documented or articulated, but they direct change. Note how this general concept of the need to set goals to direct change is incorporated in the stages of change model.

An overarching assumption in professional settings is that good assessment underlies good treatment. When we say *assessment* in this context, we mean the use of mostly formal (e.g., standard psychological tests) but sometimes informal (e.g., casual observation of a patient's behavior on a treatment unit) procedures to measure some aspect of a person's functioning. Assessment of people who appear for drug and alcohol treatment may include several different procedures.

Measuring qualities or characteristics of a person to design treatment means that treatment is tailored to the person. This is the same as matching the treatment to the individual. Matching concerns decisions about what treatment choices are preferred for different individuals to produce the best results. Along these lines, a major task of assessment and matching is to help define or specify treatment goals. Treatment goals refer to the purposes or aims of a treatment, which in general are to "get better"; however, that is too general to be of much use in guiding a treatment. We can be more specific. For example, in drug and alcohol treatment, everybody agrees that the person's use of drugs and alcohol must change. In the United States, that typically means a change to complete abstinence from these substances, although we will see that there has been some controversy over whether all people require a goal of total abstinence from alcohol.

There may be goals of alcohol and drug treatment besides a person's substance use. It may be important for changes to occur in an individual's family, work, and social functioning. This is because in virtually all people who appear for substance-abuse treatment, their use of alcohol or other drugs has affected other parts of their lives. Those changes in turn may affect a person's use of alcohol and drugs. It is important to see that the influences of substance use on different areas of life, and the reverse, are consistent with a biopsychosocial model. Substance use may be affected by multiple and varied factors, and the use of alcohol or other drugs may have multiple and varied consequences. These consequences may in turn affect future substance use.

How these multiple influences work in the development, maintenance, and change in substance use tends to differ for each person. As a result, a person's goals for treatment must be tailored to that person's specific, unique circumstances. Professionals working in drug and alcohol treatment call this "individualizing" treatment goals.

"Wouldn't stick to goals if they were forced on me; you have to make up your own mind."

Patient involved in "guided self-change" treatment (Sobell & Sobell, 1993, p. 159)

Abstinence or Moderation?

Before we leave the topic of treatment goals, it is important to discuss a specific question about goals relating to alcohol use. Traditionally, and still predominantly in the United States and Canada, the assumption is that the goal of treatment for alcohol problems is abstinence from alcohol. This applies to self-help treatments as well as to professional treatment services; indeed, AA and other self-help groups are adamant that abstinence is essential to a person's long-term improved functioning. However, a number of reports in the literature both on self-change and on treatment have stated that individuals identified as alcohol abusers or alcohol dependent can modify their alcohol use to a stable, moderate level.

These findings have created and still create heated controversy. The controversy stems from the disease model of alcohol problems, which implies that lifelong abstinence is the only safe course toward amelioration of alcohol problems. The need for abstinence typically is not questioned in the treatment of other drug problems, however. It is likely that abstinence from nonprescribed use of drugs is the only acceptable goal because the drugs are illegal, and society has a strong reaction against illicit drug use.

The question of moderation as a drinking goal is of more than academic importance. Knowledge about different drinking outcomes would increase our understanding of the causes and course of alcohol problems and improve the results of our treatment efforts through better individualization of treatment goals. We do know that moderate drinking outcomes happen, but knowledge beyond that is sketchier. It seems to make the most sense to frame this question the same way we framed treatment goals in general: They should reflect the individual's specific, unique circumstances.

Research does help somewhat in telling us what are the best "circumstances" for a goal of moderate drinking. Overall, it seems that less severe alcohol dependence (in DSM-IV terms, or in terms of physical dependence on alcohol), an individual's belief that moderate drinking is possible, younger age, employment, and psychological and social stability provide the "backdrop" for the feasibility of a moderate drinking outcome (Rosenberg, 1993). Some of these factors are not static (such as beliefs about moderate drinking), however, and it would be essential to monitor them closely over time to make sustained moderate drinking most likely.

"Complete abstinence is easier than perfect moderation."

St. Augustine

Moderate drinking outcomes will continue to stimulate debate and research for years to come. The best result of this activity would be a better understanding of the course of alcohol problems and the creation of better treatment service delivery. This result is assuming greater practical importance as programs that support moderate drinking outcome goals become more common and accessible. For example, the World Wide Web now has announcements and descriptions of moderate drinking programs in the United States.

Harm Reduction

In our discussion of the treatment of cigarette smoking in Chapter 7, we introduced the idea of harm reduction. To remind you of the definition, *harm reduction* refers to an emphasis on reducing the negative consequences of using a substance rather than on reducing the quantity or frequency of its consumption. In practice, harm reduction programs may encourage lighter consumption, but the focus is on reducing the harmful consequences that may ensue from substance use (Single, 1995). Common examples of applying the harm reduction idea to substance use among the general public are using a designated driver when social occasions involve alcohol consumption and training bartenders to recognize signs of intoxication in their patrons and to stop serving them alcohol accordingly.

Harm reduction is an idea that originally was applied in the treatment of illicit drug users. For example, offering addicts clean syringes to avoid the transmission of HIV or other viruses follows directly from a harm reduction approach. This idea also is relevant to alcohol treatment and stands in contrast to zero-tolerance or abstinence-only approaches. Harm reduction in some cases offers advantages over an abstinence-only goal. For instance, a harm reduction approach may be valuable in encouraging college students or other young adults to consider modifying the circumstances or quantity of their alcohol consumption, whereas an abstinence-only approach would be far less likely to have that result (Baer et al., 2001). Similarly, harm reduction approaches are useful for bringing into treatment drug addicts who claim they do not want to stop using drugs entirely but who may be interested in reducing the problems that their drug use causes them.

"We're all allowed to deal with the issue of drinking the way each of us wants to. If a guy wants to reduce his drinking, so let him try; AA stands for unconditional abstinence only; but with us, everyone makes his own program. I do recommend abstinence for all of those who have reached an advanced stage of alcoholism. That way you certainly get away with less distress and damage."

Member of the Tampere A-Guild, a Finnish self-help organization (Alasuutari, 1992, p. 130)

As in the application of the harm reduction model to the treatment of cigarette smoking, there is considerable resistance in the United States to widespread application of the model to the treatment of the substance-use disorders. As you might have guessed, the resistance is based at least in part in the reluctance to "condone" the use of alcohol or other drugs, even in individuals who show no signs of physical dependence on them. It is essential to recognize that the harm reduction model neither condones nor censures substance use. Rather, it takes the pragmatic view that some individuals in a society will use alcohol or other drugs, and the most important goal for these individuals and the society they live in is to reduce the frequency and severity of any negative consequences that may follow from such use.

After assessment and specification of treatment goals, the next step in professional treatment is to make the best use of that information to place individuals in the best treatment environment to meet their needs. Two levels of such matching may be considered: the treatment setting and the services that are delivered within a setting. We turn now to review both of these, first for alcohol treatment and then for other drug treatment. We also comment on how effective alcohol and drug treatments are. When we say drug treatment, we mean treatment for drugs of abuse, such as the opiates, stimulants, and depressant drugs. Nicotine is not covered in this chapter because we discussed the treatment of nicotine dependence in Chapter 7.

Alcohol Treatment Settings and Services

Types of Settings and Services

The settings and services of treatment for alcohol problems could be classified in a number of ways. We use the classification that Armor, Polich, and Stambul published in their well-known 1976 Rand Corporation study of alcoholism treatment in the United States. The settings that Armor et al. described are still widely used (American Psychiatric Association, 2000b).

Armor, Polich, and Stambul (1976, p. 102) identified the general treatment settings of hospital setting, intermediate setting, and outpatient setting. Within each of these settings, specific treatment services are offered. Inpatients in the hospital setting live there for the duration of their treatment, and their care is similar to that given to people hospitalized for physical problems. For example, nurses play a large role in treatment,

psychological treatment
Treatment geared to changing emotions, thoughts, or behavior without the use of medications or other physical or biological means.

and much weight is given to the medical aspects of alcohol problems. On the other hand, many of the specific alcohol rehabilitation methods followed in hospital-based programs are **psychological treatment** in origin. The emphasis of these nonmedical treatment methods is on learning about the self and the environment we live in, how they alter the development of alcohol problems, and how people can change both their self and their environment to produce desired changes in psychoactive substance use. (Similar treatment methods are followed in inpatient "free-standing" alcohol programs. These programs do not operate within the hospital setting and typically are "for profit"; that is, they need to make a profit to stay in business.) Partial hospital care occurs in the hospital setting, but the patient[1] is not in the setting for 24 hours a day. Typically, treatment programs of this type are designed for four- to eight-hour schedules, usually in the daytime or evening. The last type of service in the hospital setting is detoxification, mainly involving the medical management of alcohol withdrawal symptoms. Care mostly consists of the management of medications given to treat withdrawal, although counseling is available, especially referral to additional treatment services.

milieu treatment
Treatment in which the organization and structure of a setting are designed to change behavior.

counseling
In alcohol and drug treatment, counselors are specially trained professionals who perform a variety of treatment activities, including assessment, education, and individual, marital, and family counseling.

psychotherapy
Typically, conversation between a specially trained individual (therapist) and another person (or family) that is intended to change patterns of behavior, thoughts, or feelings in that person (or family).

Within the intermediate treatment setting are halfway house services. Halfway houses usually are designed as **milieu treatment** settings. (In milieu treatment, the organization and structure of a setting are designed to be therapeutic.) These settings are the patients' residence during treatment. Other treatment services usually available include **counseling**, **psychotherapy**, and a strong orientation toward the use of self-help groups, usually Alcoholics Anonymous (AA).

The outpatient setting is perhaps the most idiosyncratic of the three that Armor, Polich, and Stambul (1976) described. Two general distinctions of treatment services are made: individual and group. In individual treatment, patients work with a professional in a one-to-one relationship. Similarly, "individual" couples or families may work with a professional in a planned course of treatment. Hester and Delaney (1997) described an outpatient program that was designed for individuals whose drinking is relatively heavy (compared to population norms) but who are not dependent on alcohol. The intervention is called Behavioral Self-Control Program for Windows (BSCPWIN) and involves delivery of a drinking moderation program over eight weekly sessions by interaction with a personal computer program. This individual treatment program is based on both social learning theory and motivational enhancement principles; it differs from the typical outpatient program in its use of a personal computer to deliver the intervention and the consequent use of minimal therapist time. Because therapist time is greatly reduced, the potential for reducing treatment costs is considerable.

Hester and Delaney's (1997) work is an early example of how outpatient alcohol treatment is becoming more and more idiosyncratic as computer technology becomes more advanced. Prominent in this regard is the growing number of outpatient treatments being evaluated that present the content of the intervention on the Internet (Cunningham, 2009). These methods have the potential of being acceptable to people who, for various reasons, are not receptive to face-to-face, in-person (with a counselor or therapist) treatment. Furthermore, they have the potential of reducing the costs of delivering treatment considerably.

Group outpatient treatment usually involves 5 to 10 individuals meeting together in regular sessions led by a professional. Much of what helps group members to change theoretically stems from the way they interact with each other and form relationships.

[1]In the treatment of psychiatric disorders, including addictions, professionals are inconsistent in their use of the words *patient* and *client* to refer to individuals who present themselves for treatment. Underlying this disagreement are beliefs about the utility of a medical model as a guide to understanding the psychiatric disorders. In addition, often what term is chosen depends on the setting of treatment. For example, individuals in hospital inpatient settings are more likely to be referred to as patients, as compared with people who receive treatment in outpatient clinics. In this chapter, we use the terms *patient* and *client* as synonyms to refer to individuals who are in formal treatment for their alcohol or drug problems.

The leader's job is to guide this process and to keep group members on productive tracks of discussion. Groups often are organized around specific themes, which govern the types of people who join each group and what they discuss. Examples of themes are adults whose parents were alcoholic and ways to prevent a recurrence (relapse) of alcohol problems once they are treated. Other groups are general and have only the theme of maintaining abstinence from substance use. Interestingly, in this context, some Internet-based interventions also involve a "support network," not unlike a therapy group, that may or may not have a network moderator or "leader" (Cunningham, 2009).

Individual and group treatments may be conducted by workers with different types of mental health training. They may be "paraprofessionals," working in direct patient care and not possessing a formal degree, and they may be professionals, who are physicians (typically psychiatrists), clinical psychologists, social workers, clinical nurse specialists, and certified alcohol (or other drug) counselors. Actually, people in any of the professional disciplines also may earn certification as alcohol and drug counselors.

Outpatient care also varies in intensity; that is, some patients may have program contact only monthly or less often, with little structure in schedule, and other outpatient programs may be similar to what we described for the partial hospital setting. When such programs are not in the hospital, they typically are called day (or evening) treatment programs.

It is somewhat artificial to assign the settings for treatment of alcohol (and, for that matter, drug) abuse to discrete categories because a treatment episode for many people involves participation in more than one treatment setting. A common course of treatment includes detoxification from alcohol and later referral to an inpatient or outpatient treatment program. Or, individuals may begin treatment by completing an inpatient intensive rehabilitation program and then engage in outpatient treatment as part of an **aftercare** plan. Other combinations are possible, each suited to individual needs. At the end of this chapter, we discuss how trends in health insurance coverage have led to a major shift to the outpatient setting for treatment of alcohol-use disorders, in contrast to earlier emphasis on inpatient treatment.

aftercare
In alcohol and drug treatment, therapeutic activities following the completion of a formal treatment program.

Categories of treatment settings and services can give only an outline of the actual treatment activities that occur in alcohol programs. It is difficult to characterize alcohol programs except in the broadest terms. What is called individual or group counseling or psychotherapy may refer to many specific activities. The activities can occur in any of the treatment settings described, with some settings having greater latitude than others. For example, the smallest range of treatment activities take place in settings devoted primarily to detoxification. In contrast, outpatient or inpatient treatment programs can include many different activities that are called treatment, including medical care to a limited degree and pharmacotherapy.

Pharmacological Treatment

Although our discussion of alcohol treatment has emphasized nonmedical interventions, drugs frequently are used in the treatment of alcohol problems. This practice is known as *pharmacotherapy*. In discussing pharmacotherapy, we distinguish between detoxification and postdetoxification treatment. Detoxification of people who are physically dependent on alcohol often involves the use of drugs in the medical management of withdrawal, although there are drug-free approaches to detoxification. These latter approaches, as noted in Chapter 9, are called "social detoxification," in which a person's withdrawal is monitored by professional staff in a treatment setting, but no drugs are administered, if at all possible. There is little controversy about using drugs in managing acute withdrawal (Mayo-Smith, 1997); however, there are some disagreements over the use of chemicals in treatment activities subsequent to detoxification.

The first type of pharmacotherapy for alcohol problems uses compounds that alter the metabolism of alcohol if it is consumed. Peachey and Annis (1985) reviewed these compounds, which they called the alcohol-sensitizing drugs. The most popular of these are disulfiram (trade name Antabuse) and carbimide (Temposil). Antabuse has been in use in the United States since 1948. Temposil, on the other hand, is not available in the United States and is used less frequently overall than Antabuse (NIAAA, 2000). In any case, use of both agents in treatment is based on similar assumptions regarding the psychological effects of their chemical action.

The chemical action of alcohol-sensitizing drugs results in an increase of acetaldehyde in the blood level after alcohol consumption (see Chapter 9 on the metabolizing of alcohol). The consequence of the increased acetaldehyde depends on how much alcohol is drunk. For people on therapeutic doses of disulfiram or carbimide, one or two drinks will produce flushing, tachycardia (excessively rapid heartbeat, usually a pulse rate of over 100 per minute), tachypnea (excessively rapid respiration), sensations of warmth, heart palpitations, and shortness of breath. These effects usually last about 30 minutes and are not life-threatening. If larger quantities of alcohol are consumed, however, the reaction may include intense palpitations, dyspnea (difficult or labored breathing), nausea, vomiting, and headache, all of which may last more than 90 minutes. In some people, this more severe reaction has induced shock, loss of consciousness, or death due to myocardial infarction (Peachey & Annis, 1985, p. 202).

The unpleasant effects of drinking while on a regimen of the alcohol-sensitizing drugs are the reason such drugs are used in treatment. The assumption is that fear of experiencing the unpleasant effects will deter people from drinking and will build a learned aversion to alcohol. If a person on disulfiram or carbimide tests out the effects of drinking, the same learned aversion will proceed more rapidly because of the addition of experiencing direct, as well as imagined, negative consequences. The learned aversion to alcohol underlies eventual avoidance of it. When alcohol-sensitizing drugs are used, they are applied as part of a rehabilitative program that is concerned with the physical, psychological, and social problems that tend to accompany abusive drinking patterns.

A second type of pharmacotherapy for alcohol problems is based in biological theories of etiology, which focus on abnormalities or changes in brain chemistry as causes or consequences of substance abuse. Such theories imply that a correction of the abnormal brain chemistry is essential to alleviating the substance-use problem. From a broader perspective, including a biological component to treatment is entirely compatible to the biopsychosocial approach to drug use and its modification that this text takes. Pharmacological agents also may be applied as part of programs that are not derived from any particular model of alcohol dependence, simply if it is believed that such agents are effective (Brewer, 1996).

In recent years, the major advances that have been made in understanding the biological bases of addiction have resulted in the development and evaluation of pharmacotherapies for alcohol-use disorders. Table 15.3 shows the drugs that have current FDA approval in the United States for the treatment of alcohol-use disorders. You can see that the pharmacological agents have diverse biological actions, and some of the drugs are thought to act on the brain in different ways. Besides the FDA-approved compounds highlighted in Table 15.3, drugs currently showing promise in clinical trials for treatment of alcohol-use disorder include topiramate, baclofen, ondansetron, olanzepine, and quetiapine (Swift & Leggio, 2009).

Effectiveness of Alcohol Treatment

After reading about a variety of settings and methods that fall into the category of alcohol treatment, you probably are wondering whether any of the effort is worth it; that

TABLE 15.3 FDA-Approved Pharmacotherapies for Alcohol-Use Disorders

Pharmacotherapy	Hypothesized Action
Naltrexone	Works as an opiate antagonist
Acamprosate	Indirect partial agonist of the NMDA receptor and antagonist of metabotropic glutamate receptors
Disulfiram (Antabuse)	Interferes with the metabolism of alcohol

Source: Based on Koob, Lloyd, & Mason (2009); Lingford-Hughes, Welch, & Nutt (2004), NIAAA (2000), Swift & Leggio (2009).

is, you probably are wondering about the effectiveness of alcohol treatment. When we talk about treatment effectiveness, we refer to the relationship between participating in some treatment and achieving some treatment goal. Therefore, treatment effectiveness concerns whether and how treatment participation causes different outcomes. Evaluations of the effectiveness of treatment are called **treatment outcome research**.

treatment outcome research Research designed to show a causal relationship between undergoing a treatment and some physical, psychological, or social change.

In this section, we do not cover detoxification services because they are not considered rehabilitation. Rather, they should be viewed as effective in managing safe alcohol withdrawal but not in providing rehabilitation beyond that. When we discuss the effectiveness of treatment aimed at rehabilitation, we must take into account the rate of spontaneous remission of alcohol problems. As you might guess, to show that a treatment is worth its cost requires a demonstration that it helps significantly beyond the rate of spontaneous remission. This reasoning is sound, but it is extremely difficult to determine the rates of spontaneous remission. People who resolve their problems without treatment are the ones with whom clinicians and researchers are least likely to have contact. Professionals instead tend to see people who are referred to a formal treatment setting. We noted earlier in this chapter that making a credible effort to determine the prevalence of spontaneous remission of alcohol problems would be complex and costly.

Despite this problem, estimates of spontaneous remission have been made for alcohol-use disorders, mostly through studies of people who entered a formal treatment program but dropped out of it prematurely and could say they received "no treatment." Another method to estimate spontaneous remission involves rates of improvement in "no treatment" or similar control groups in treatment outcome studies. The estimates of spontaneous remission of alcohol problems that have been made vary with the definition of remission, the comparison groups used, and the length of the interval during which functioning is measured. Miller and Hester (1980) suggested that the spontaneous remission (abstinence or improvement in drinking patterns) in one year for individuals not treated for their alcohol problems is 19%, and Emrick (1975) calculated 13% for abstinence and 28% for abstinence plus "improved." "Improved" in this case means drinking is not as severe in amount or frequency compared to before treatment, but the person is not always abstinent.

Nonpharmacological Professional Treatment

As you can tell from this discussion about spontaneous remission and treatment outcome, the main criterion considered is drinking behavior, even though earlier you saw that other criteria could be used. Questions about the effectiveness of nonpharmacological professional treatment have been studied for many years. We can offer some general conclusions about the effectiveness of nonpharmacological treatments. First, a long-standing finding is that no single alcohol treatment type or setting is consistently better than others, but staying in any kind of treatment increases the chances of long-term improvement, even with rates of spontaneous remission taken into account (McKay, Murphy, & Longabaugh, 1991; NIAAA, 1993).

Some may find little positive in this overall conclusion about the effectiveness of alcohol treatment, but these findings should not be taken lightly. Studies have shown that the amount of money saved in, say, health care and business expenses as a result of improvements in people undergoing treatment is greater than the amount of money the treatment costs. Similarly, research that insurance companies completed suggests that substance abusers (and their families) use significantly fewer health care services after treatment than before. This shows the benefits of alcohol treatment in financial terms; the more important, but more difficult to measure, gains in human welfare are considerable.

The downside of our conclusion about alcohol treatment effectiveness is that it does not leave us with much of a guideline about placing a person in a specific treatment based on our assessment and the person's goals for change. Alcohol treatment research has advanced to emphasize patient–treatment matching, however, and this seems to be a productive direction for the field. Although our knowledge about matching is still not too sophisticated, there is some research on matching patients to some treatment settings and services. For example, inpatient or residential treatment settings may be best reserved for individuals whose alcohol problems are more severe, or who have other drug problems, or who have less social stability (for example, are not employed, not married, not living in a permanent residence), or who have psychiatric disorders. For other individuals, outpatient treatment likely will do just as well as inpatient and at far less cost. Another example is that psychotherapy works best if patients' conceptual level (defined by preference for rules, dependence on authority, and abstractness of thinking) is matched to their therapist's (McKay, Murphy, & Longabaugh, 1991). Finally, a major study of patient–treatment matching suggests that the severity of patients' psychiatric problems should be taken into account in assigning individuals to treatments implemented in the outpatient setting (Project MATCH Research Group, 1997).

It seems that the accumulation of findings such as these would take alcohol treatment to a level of more efficient service delivery. McCrady and Langenbucher (1996) substantiated this conclusion and reaffirmed in a later review of the American Psychiatric Association's practice guidelines for the treatment of substance-use disorders (McCrady & Ziedonis, 2001; McGovern and Carroll, 2003). McCrady and Langenbucher (1996) identified several specific nonpharmacological treatments for alcohol-use disorder that have been shown to be effective in well-done evaluations. The treatments that McCrady and Langenbucher identified are listed and briefly described in Table 15.4. You can see that most of the treatments listed in the table are based broadly on social learning principles. Motivational enhancement therapy also uses principles of social learning theory (also called social cognitive theory) but combines them with psychotherapy methods designed to help clients arrive at their own conclusions about the need to change rather than the therapist imposing change on clients. These promising treatment techniques and approaches would seem to be the best candidates for outcome research on patient–treatment matching.

Self-Help Treatment

What we have said so far about treatment effectiveness was pertinent to professional services. Because of its importance, self-help group treatment also should be evaluated. Almost all of the research on this question concerns AA, and we focus on that organization.

CONTEMPORARY ISSUE BOX 15.1

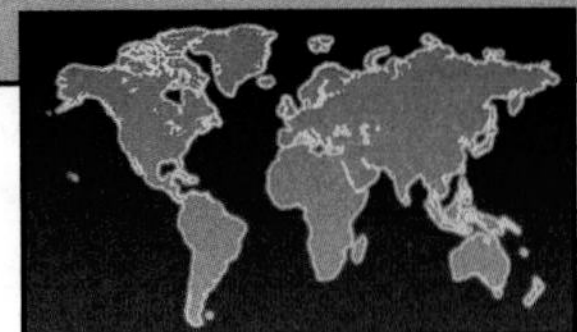

Brief Interventions for Alcohol Problems

Traditional ideas about alcohol treatment have been challenged by increased awareness and discussion of "brief" interventions for alcohol problems. What is called brief is relative to traditional alcohol treatment. Brief interventions average one to three sessions, and each session lasts up to 45 minutes, but much less time is often spent in a session. Traditional alcohol treatment has far more sessions that usually last about an hour. Brief interventions have been applied in several different settings, including college campuses, but perhaps the most important is the general medical care setting. Patients in that setting tend to have higher rates than the general population of unidentified alcohol problems of varying degrees of severity because of the correlation between heavy alcohol use and physical problems. Accordingly, if some type of intervention could be done in these settings to thwart the development of more severe alcohol problems, then there is the potential to save society billions of dollars. Fleming et al.'s (1997) study, showing that a physician-delivered brief intervention for alcohol problems detected in primary medical care settings can be effective, attracted a lot of attention among health care professionals. Since then, other studies also have shown that brief interventions are effective for treating alcohol problems (NIAAA, 1999; 2005). Furthermore, the success of brief interventions in treating alcohol problems has led more recently to evaluations of their effectiveness in treating people who have problems with other drugs, such as marijuana and amphetamines (Baker, Boggs, & Lewin, 2001; Stephens, Roffman, & Curtin, 2000).

Brief interventions can be as simple as feedback about the consequences of heavy alcohol use for a person (for example, "You have some liver problems, and we can trace it to your drinking") or advice to cut down or stop drinking. They are based on the idea that alcohol problems exist on a continuum of severity and that interventions can occur at any point along that continuum. The research has shown that, for the most part, brief interventions have been used with people who have mild to moderate alcohol problems; they are effective compared to no treatment in reducing alcohol consumption to below "risk" levels. There is some speculation about who is most helped by brief interventions and why they work. These clearly are topics for future research.

The findings about brief interventions have great practical implications for alcohol treatment providers and for saving society a lot of money and suffering. They also have implications for theories of the causes of alcohol problems. For example, what do you think disease or biological model adherents might say about brief interventions?

The question of how effective AA is can be difficult to answer. One reason for the difficulty is the AA emphasis on the anonymity of its members. The principle of anonymity is a major part of the "Twelve Traditions" of AA, which are a set of principles or guidelines adopted in 1950 for the operations of AA (Leach & Norris, 1977). The twelfth tradition, anonymity, "is the spiritual foundation of our traditions, ever reminding us to place principles before personalities." This tradition is strictly adhered to in AA groups and makes outcome research very difficult because it often requires identification of those receiving treatment.

Nevertheless, some research has been done. In their review of research related to AA's effectiveness, Emrick (1989) and Emrick et al. (1993) concluded:

> (a) it is not possible to predict who will affiliate with AA, except that it seems that people who have more severe alcohol problems are more likely to join; (b) among people who do join AA, it is not clear who will do well and who will not; (c) people who go to AA before, during, or after receiving other forms of treatment do as well as if not better than people who do not volunteer to go to AA; (d) AA participation is associated with relatively high abstinence rates but with average overall improvement in drinking rates; (e) people who achieve abstinence seem to participate in AA more than those who moderate their drinking or who continue to drink at a problem level. (Emrick, 1989, pp. 48–49)

TABLE 15.4 Effective Nonmedical Treatments for Alcohol-Use Disorders

Treatment	Brief Description
Motivational enhancement	Use of verbal psychotherapy, including feedback about the connection between alcohol use and negative consequences, to encourage individuals to "move forward" in the stages of changing their alcohol use patterns
Classical conditioning–based treatments	Application of principles of classical conditioning (see Chapter 5) either (1) to condition a negative reaction to alcohol cues such as sight, taste, or smell, or (2) to extinguish or eliminate urges to use alcohol in the presence of cues related to it
Conjoint treatments	Involvement of significant others (e.g., spouse or other family members) in a therapy approach that follows social learning principles (see Table 15.2)
Social learning–based treatments	Application of social learning principles to reduce or eliminate alcohol consumption; specific treatments include relapse prevention (discussed later in this chapter), community reinforcement, and social skills training (SST)—teaching individuals to use nonalcohol ways of coping with interpersonal situations

Source: Based on McCrady and Langenbucher (1996).

People's success in AA may be related to processes such as ways to cope with stress, beliefs that one can cope effectively in different situations without alcohol, and commitment to abstinence from alcohol (Morgenstern et al., 1997).

Emrick's (1989) review, confirmed by subsequent research (Humphreys et al., 2004), concludes that AA seems to help some but not all people. So, making blanket referrals to AA as part of a treatment plan, which is common, is not warranted. With the growth of groups such as SMART and SOS, other self-help options are available. Of course, currently we do not have clear evidence about the effectiveness of participation in these alternative groups, but studies are in progress. It is essential that matching research be aimed at discovering which individuals fit best with which self-help group participation.

As difficult as it is, well-controlled treatment outcome research on self-help groups is important. Emrick (1989) cited a few such studies on AA, but they involved individuals who were mandated by the legal system to attend treatment. This is not the best patient population for evaluation of a treatment's effectiveness because of its dubious commitment to change. Furthermore, future outcome studies of AA should include enough AA participants to make it likely that researchers will be able to detect any beneficial effects that AA might have (Tonigan, Toscova, & Miller, 1995). Controlled treatment outcome studies on self-help groups would go a long way toward helping clinicians to use such groups in ways that are best for their patients.

Effectiveness of Pharmacological Treatments

With the exception of disulfiram, pharmacotherapies for alcohol-use disorders have been developed only in recent years, and therefore we have relatively little outcome data on them. Furthermore, it is believed that all pharmacotherapies should be accompanied by psychological and social treatments if they are to have longer-term effectiveness (O'Brien, 1996). (Can you relate this to the nicotine replacement therapies discussed in Chapter 7?) The first pharmacotherapy to consider is disulfiram. When disulfiram became available, it was thought to be the long-sought answer to alcohol treatment. Unfortunately, the results of more than 50 years of research show that disulfiram has fallen far short of this mark. One problem in interpreting the research on disulfiram is that it has not been done well. The clinical trials on disulfiram that have been well controlled show modest effects on number of drinking days, but they also have yielded inconsistent findings (Garbutt et al., 1999).

One factor to keep in mind when evaluating disulfiram is that its effects may be enhanced considerably if its use is combined with a behavioral program that in part consists of supervised administration of the disulfiram (e.g., by the patient's spouse) to the patient (Hughes & Cook, 1997). This apparently addresses a major practical problem with using disulfiram clinically: It typically requires daily administration of the prescribed dose, and patients tend to show poor compliance with such a regimen. Disulfiram implants have been tried as another way to solve the compliance problem, but their effectiveness has not been shown clearly, and the bioavailability of the implanted disulfiram has not been demonstrated in clinical trials. Additional well-controlled studies of supervised disulfiram therapy would allow us to specify the conditions under which its administration is most likely to enhance outcomes.

As noted earlier, the FDA approved the use of naltrexone (in 1994) for the treatment of alcohol-use disorders. This approval was based largely on the results of two relatively small-scale clinical studies showing that naltrexone helped to reduce the craving for alcohol and the severity of any relapses to alcohol use that occurred after a period of abstinence (O'Malley et al., 1992; Volpicelli et al., 1992). As a result, the evaluation of naltrexone in the treatment of alcohol-use disorders has been an active research topic since the mid-1990s.

Kranzler and Van Kirk (2001) reviewed controlled clinical trials of naltrexone that have been conducted and compared its effects to placebo on outcomes such as percentage of days drinking alcohol and percentage of patients who "relapsed" (we discuss relapse later in this chapter). Their review showed only modest effects of naltrexone as well as inconsistency among the studies in their findings on naltrexone's effectiveness. Therefore, the promise that naltrexone showed in earlier research has been reduced somewhat by the results of later studies. On the other hand, we have learned more about what factors enhance naltrexone's effectiveness. For example, not surprisingly, compliance with taking the medication is extremely important for naltrexone, and for that reason, the FDA approved a sustained-release, injectible version of the medication in 2005. In addition, patients who report a greater degree of craving for alcohol and who have a family history of alcoholism tend to do better with naltrexone treatment (Swift & Leggio, 2009).

Kranzler and Van Kirk's (2001) review, as well as later reviews (Swift & Leggio, 2009), reveal modest results for acamprosate. As we noted earlier, this medication has received FDA approval for use in the United States and is used and studied widely in the rest of the world. The studies of acamprosate to date show, like naltrexone, modest effectiveness overall and inconsistency in findings from different studies. Interestingly, acamprosate has shown to be most effective in clinical trials conducted in Europe, but has shown far more modest effects in trials conducted in the United States. The reason(s) for this discrepancy are yet to be specified.

All trials testing the efficacy or effectiveness of naltrexone and acamprosate have involved their use in conjunction with some type of behavioral counseling or therapy.

The question of which medication is the more effective when used with some kind of nondrug therapy—acamprosate or naltrexone—may have occurred to you. A recently major study that was conducted in 11 academic treatment settings in the United States and included almost 1,400 adult patients diagnosed with alcohol dependence was designed to address just this question (Anton et al., 2006). The findings were complex, and we will just briefly describe those relevant to the general question of which drug therapy was the more efficacious when used in combination with either or both of two types of behavioral treatment ("medical management" and cognitive-behavior therapy). In this regard, patients taking naltrexone who had either medical management alone or medical management and cognitive-behavior therapy had outcomes that were superior to patients who received medical management only and placebo. On the other hand, patients receiving acamprosate with any combination of behavioral treatments did no better than patients receiving the same behavioral treatments and placebo. It also is notable that patients who received cognitive-behavior therapy and medical management and placebo (a nondrug treatment) did as well as the groups taking naltrexone with medical management only or with medical management and cognitive-behavior therapy.

In summary, the research on pharmacotherapy for alcohol-use disorders is still considered to be in its early stages. We already have increased our knowledge on this topic considerably, however, and have learned that the questions are complex. Future research needs not only to identify promising medications but also to determine more precisely how they work and what characterizes individuals who benefit most from different medications (notice the similarity of this conclusion to the concept of matching patients to treatment). In addition, because alcohol affects multiple neurotransmitters, simultaneous use of more than one medication may be needed to help some people. Research on this possibility is just beginning.

Other Drug Treatment Settings and Services

A wide array of treatment services is available for those who abuse drugs. Allison and Hubbard (1985) noted:

> Treatment programs may involve outpatient, residential, or day treatment and may take place in a hospital, clinic, mental health center, prison, or group home environment. Treatment may be drug-free or use chemical aids. Counseling, job training, physical health care, and a variety of other services may or may not be part of the treatment program. The staff may be highly trained professionals or the program may be of the self-help type. (p. 1322)

The traditional classification of drug-abuse treatments includes detoxification, methadone maintenance, residential, and outpatient. Our discussion of other drug treatment will make clear that this classification combines treatment setting with treatment services. Like alcohol treatment, the primary goal of detoxification is a medically managed withdrawal from physical dependence on drugs. Managing detoxification often involves the use of medications but could be drug-free. As with alcohol withdrawal treatment, detoxification services may include some counseling directed in part at guiding the patient to additional treatment services.

A major modality of drug treatment is the therapeutic community (TC). Drug TCs are run mostly by ex-addicts, who work as peer counselors and administrators. In recent years, however, TC staff members have included more health professionals (DeLeon, 1995). There is heavy reliance on self-help groups. The TC is a highly structured program, especially at the beginning of treatment, and clients gain more responsibilities and independence as they progress through the program by meeting certain requirements. In TCs, the emphasis is on group counseling and therapy, which often are confrontational. The essential agent of social and psychological change in TCs is purported to be the community itself (Ibid.). Earlier in this chapter, we referred to this idea as milieu treatment. One well-known example of a drug TC is Phoenix House in New York City.

The final drug-abuse treatment modality is outpatient. The outpatient setting may or may not have a policy prohibiting pharmacotherapies. Outpatient drug treatment is the most varied of the treatment types and includes a wide range of programs and services. Almost half of the drug abusers in treatment receive their treatment in this setting (Center for Substance Abuse Treatment, 1997).

Treatment of Nonopiate Drug Abusers

In general, the classification of drug-abuse treatment refers to services that have been available for the treatment of heroin abuse. In this regard, the great expansion in drug-abuse treatment services over the last 40 years was largely due to public alarm over increasingly widespread use and abuse of heroin, with its highly visible and well-publicized negative social effects. For example, a sharp increase in violent crime in some urban areas, such as the later (late 1980s) experience with crack use, was attributed to heroin use. In recent years, however, there has been an increase in the number of individuals appearing for drug-abuse treatment who primarily abuse drugs other than alcohol or the opiates. For example, in 1977, 33.4% of the clients admitted to drug-abuse treatment programs were nonopiate abusers, and this proportion had increased to 54.9% by 1980 (USDHHS, 1984). This trend continued throughout the 1980s, with a high number of people presenting themselves for treatment of cocaine dependence.

Like abusers of heroin and alcohol, nonopiate abusers may appear in treatment settings other than those designed specifically to treat the substance-use disorders. These include hospital emergency rooms, physicians' offices, and general psychiatric treatment settings. They currently also appear in settings traditionally created for those who abuse heroin, such as the therapeutic community (Center for Substance Abuse Treatment, 1997). In general, little is known about any unique problems and characteristics of those who abuse nonopiate drugs that might be important for their treatment, although there has been some discussion of this question (Washton, 1990; also see Schuckit's [1994] discussion of the treatment of stimulant dependence).

Pharmacotherapy of Other Drug Problems

Lingford-Hughes, Welch, and Nutt (2004), Litten and Allen (1999), McLellan et al. (2000), and Swift and Leggio (2009) summarized the major pharmacotherapies available for the treatment of drug-use disorders other than alcohol. Pharmacotherapies have received FDA approval only for the treatment of opioid and nicotine dependence; we discussed the latter in Chapter 7 and therefore do not review them again here. Table 15.5 presents a list of the pharmacotherapies that have FDA approval for the treatment of opioid dependence.

Methadone maintenance is the pharmacotherapy for drug-use disorders other than alcohol that has received the most attention—probably more than any other drug treatment, for that matter—from researchers and the popular press. The attention centers on the conflict in treating dependence on a chemical substance (heroin, an opiate) with an opiate agonist (methadone). Proponents of this approach say that if

CONTEMPORARY ISSUE BOX 15.2

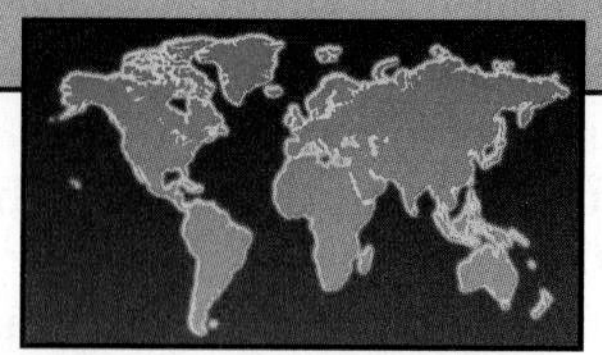

Factors Influencing the Expansion of Drug Treatment

Political and social forces currently contribute to the demand for drug treatment, just as these same forces pushed the growth of treatment of heroin abuse in the 1960s. These trends reaffirm the importance of social and political factors in how U.S. society deals with alcohol and other drug use.

In 1986, the surge in demand for drug treatment, particularly in the residential or inpatient setting, arose from two major sources: crack and AIDS. These worked in a political climate that was strongly in favor of eradicating drugs and drug abuse.

As you saw in Chapter 6, crack is the highly addictive, cheaper form of cocaine. People who start using it are quickly hooked on it, and in the mid-1980s, people from a wide range of social classes became addicted to crack. The variety of people affected, along with social consequences such as large increases in drug-related criminal activity and flagrant selling of crack in public places, lighted the public's torch for getting those who abuse crack off the streets and into treatment. Further, the media devoted much time to the crack epidemic, just as they have to other diseases or medical problems in the past.

The AIDS epidemic has sent those who abuse drugs, particularly individuals who take their drugs intravenously, to treatment programs to help them stop their drug abuse. The reason: fear of catching the deadly disease of AIDS through the use of contaminated needles. The fear of AIDS sent people looking for treatment when it is unlikely they otherwise would have done so. Again, the media attention to AIDS and the general public alarm and fears about AIDS supported the increased demands for more accessible drug treatment.

These two examples show how political and social forces, and not just an actual increase in drug use or in the valuing of a drug-free society, affect the demand for drug and alcohol treatment.

heroin addicts' desire for heroin is prevented by methadone, then they will be more likely to break out of the destructive lifestyle associated with drug addiction and engage in rehabilitation leading to a socially acceptable and productive way of living. The major opposition to methadone treatment is that it perpetuates individuals' dependence on an opiate drug. Interestingly, evidence against this fear has come recently from a study conducted with heroin addicts in Canada who failed in methadone treatment, but who were successful in treating their addiction if they were treated with heroin, in prescription form (Oviedo-Joekes et al., 2009). Although this approach to treating people with severe heroin addiction has been used in Europe for years, it had not been tried in North America because of the great resistance to using heroin to treat heroin addiction (recall from Chapter 7 how some felt once about using nicotine to treat nicotine addiction).

Methadone maintenance treatment typically involves administration of a daily, prescribed dose of methadone to block addicts' cravings for heroin. Usually, methadone maintenance programs are outpatient so that individuals may pursue activities that build a socially productive life. Furthermore, many programs (and state or federal regulations) require patients to receive some kind of counseling while enrolled in methadone

TABLE 15.5 FDA-Pharmacotherapies for Opioid Dependence

Methadone	Long-acting opioid
Levo-alpha-acetylmethadol (LAAM)	Opiate agonist or partial agonist
Buprenorphine	Partial agonist at different opioid receptors
Naltrexone (naloxone)	Opiate antagonist

maintenance, and patients are required to adhere to a formal set of rules for continued participation in methadone treatment.

As you might have guessed, one problem with the use of methadone is its potential for abuse; that is, addicts may use their methadone in nonprescribed ways just as they used heroin. Methadone programs have tried to handle this problem by requiring patients to swallow the methadone dose on the program premises while observed by the medical staff. In fact, one measure of progress in this program is whether the individuals come to the clinic less often than daily to get the methadone dose. As progress is made, people may earn the privilege of taking two to several days' worth of methadone home at a time. Another way to handle the problem of compliance is to administer **levo-alpha-acetylmethadol (LAAM)**, which is similar in pharmacological action to methadone but has longer-lasting effects. The advantage of a longer-lasting methadone substitute is that patients are more likely to comply with the regimen for taking the drug.

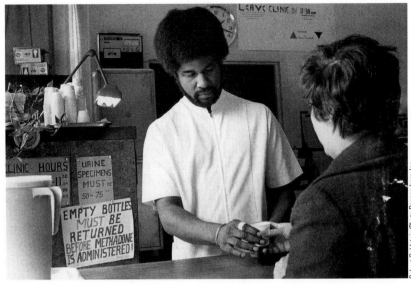

Methadone maintenance remains a controversial treatment for opiate dependence.

Robert Goldstein/Photo Researchers, Inc.

levo-alpha-acetylmethadol (LAAM) A drug used in treating heroin addiction that is similar in action to methadone but has longer-lasting effects.

Methadone maintenance involves replacing one opiate, say, heroin, with another, methadone. Another pharmacotherapy for heroin use involves blockade of opiate receptors by the use of naltrexone, which we discussed in the section on alcohol treatment. Naltrexone or its shorter-acting analogue drug, naloxone, is used most commonly with patients who have been maintained for long periods on methadone and then choose to become drug-free. The naltrexone may help these patients bridge the gap between methadone maintenance and a drug-free life. Naltrexone works, theoretically, because the abused opiate cannot achieve its effect in the brain (also see the discussion earlier in this chapter on the use of naltrexone in the treatment of alcohol dependence). The result is that the individual loses a major reason for using the opiate—its psychoactive effects. Along these same lines, buprenorphine, a mixed opiate agonist–antagonist, blocks the effects of heroin and has FDA approval for use in treatment of opiate drug dependence.

Effectiveness of Drug Treatment

The history of research on the effectiveness of drug treatment is not nearly as long as that for alcohol, but a number of good studies has appeared in the last few decades. Our summary of what is known about drug treatment effectiveness, like that of alcohol treatment, excludes detoxification.

The literature on drug treatment effectiveness has profited from the completion of several large, multisite (i.e., different programs), multimodal (i.e., different settings, like outpatient and methadone maintenance) studies (Ball, Meyers, & Friedman, 1988; DeLeon, 1984; Hubbard et al., 1989) and reviews of treatment research (Institute of Medicine, 1990b). Findings from the most recent large-scale, multisite drug treatment evaluation, called the Drug Abuse Treatment Outcome Study (DATOS) (Fletcher, Tims, & Brown, 1997), provided data that were largely consistent with the results of earlier research. Compared to the literature on alcohol, less attention is given in the drug treatment evaluation literature to individual treatment techniques or services. Instead, research tends to focus on the treatment settings, as we have organized them in this chapter.

Nonpharmacological Professional Treatment

Table 15.6 presents major conclusions about the effectiveness of therapeutic community and outpatient drug treatment. Note that conclusions about treatment are based on drug use as well as on correlated events such as social productivity and criminal behavior. The research on drug treatment reflects society's interest not only in whether a person has stopped illicit drug use but also in whether social disruption and disorder have stopped. Table 15.6 shows that, overall, two of the three major drug settings (the other is methadone maintenance) seem to be associated with improved functioning, if the person stays in treatment. Unfortunately, dropping out of drug treatment is a chronic problem that is difficult to solve. One of methadone maintenance's great advantages in this regard is that it is correlated with better treatment retention. Similarly, even though more good research is needed on this topic (French & McGeary, 1997), it seems that if people stay in drug treatment, it is cost-effective (Franey & Ashton, 2002). That is, society gets more back from the reduced drug use and the social and financial productivity that are associated with treatment than it pays to deliver the treatment services.

The overall summary of nonpharmacological drug treatment effectiveness is encouraging, but we should add there is considerable individual variation in patient outcomes. The big gap in this treatment literature pertains to patient–treatment matching research. Although several excellent studies done some time ago have matched patients to drug treatments (e.g., McLellan et al., 1983), more studies guided by the matching question would advance drug treatment (Franey & Ashton, 2002).

Self-Help Treatment

We can say very little on this topic because, as we noted earlier, virtually all the research on self-help groups has concerned AA. We know essentially nothing about the effectiveness of drug self-help groups like Narcotics Anonymous or Cocaine Anonymous,

TABLE 15.6 Effectiveness of Therapeutic Community and Outpatient Drug Treatment

Setting	Conclusions
Therapeutic community	Drug use and criminal behavior end while in residence; associated with a more productive life following discharge if length of stay in residence was sufficient (at least several months)
	High treatment attrition rates
	Treatment is cost-effective
Outpatient treatment	Associated with improved functioning compared to no treatment or detoxification only
	Benefits of treatment greater with longer involvement in treatment
	Treatment is cost-effective for people who stay in treatment longer than six months

Source: Adapted from Institute of Medicine (1990b).

DRUGS AND CULTURE BOX 15.3

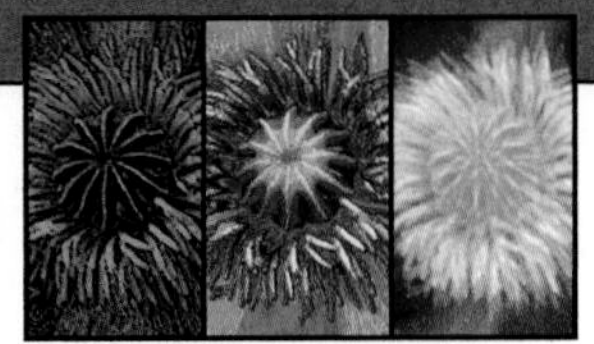

"Special Populations" and Alcohol and Drug Treatment

In Chapter 1, we examined substance use prevalence by gender and racial/ethnic subgroups. The idea behind doing this is that any subgroup differences in prevalence likely are due to biological or, more prominently, social and cultural factors that distinguish the subgroups. This same idea can be applied to assessment and treatment, although research on "special populations" (that is, subgroups) has lagged far behind other treatment research. For example, much of this chapter's content is based on research and clinical experiences with adults because a lot more information is available on adults compared to adolescents. Nevertheless, treatment research on special populations is important because subgroup differences can influence assessment and diagnosis, treatment accessibility and content, and treatment retention.

To cite several examples, studies show that, for adolescents, assessment of social factors in substance use, such as patterns of use and attitudes about use that peers have, is critical. Similarly, social skills training to resist peer pressure to use substances may be an emphasis in treatment. For the elderly, sensitive assessment and diagnostic practices incorporate knowledge about the interaction of alcohol and prescribed medications, and the interaction of alcohol with the aging body. In women, substance-use problems tend to develop faster than they do in men and tend to be more strongly related to psychological and familial variables. Failure to use this information precludes sensitive diagnosis and effective treatment. For all defined subgroups, learned aspects of substance use underlie beliefs and expectations about its effects and attitudes toward its use in different situations. Without sensitivity to these group differences, assessment and treatment are not adequate.

Special population differences could be viewed as corollaries of the idea that patient–treatment matching improves treatment. How? What models of the etiology of the substance-use disorders seem most flexible to you in incorporating gender, developmental (age), and racial/ethnic differences?

because the research simply has not been done. Like AA, however, drug self-help groups are popular, and their effectiveness is an important research question. Also similar to alcohol treatment, involvement in self-help groups following an episode of drug treatment is associated with improved outcomes (Fiorentine, 1997).

Pharmacological Treatments

As we showed earlier, for treatment of drug use besides alcohol and nicotine, the FDA has issued approval for agents used in pharmacotherapy of opiate addiction only. The first and most important of these agents is methadone. The Institute of Medicine (1990b), which was the source of the information in Table 15.6, also covered methadone. Its review of the literature through the 1980s on methadone's effectiveness showed positive findings. First, methadone treatment is associated with reduced drug use and criminal behavior compared to no treatment, detoxification alone, or methadone treatment terminators. Second, methadone, as we noted earlier, is effective in bringing reluctant addicts into treatment and keeping them there. Third, methadone is a cost-effective treatment of opioid dependence. These conclusions, which are based on clinical research done over almost three decades, have been supported and extended in more recent studies (Leshner, 1999; McLellan et al., 2000; Vocci, Acri, & Elkashef, 2005).

"The advantages of ethnically oriented programs appear not so much that something particularly efficacious happens in treatment, but rather the attraction to treatment is greater when one can join peers in a familiar setting."

Joseph Westermeyer, professor of psychiatry (Institute of Medicine, 1990a, p. 372)

The other pharmacotherapies for opioid dependence listed in Table 15.5 also have fared well in clinical trials. LAAM's effectiveness convinced the FDA in 1993 to approve it as a treatment for heroin dependence, although LAAM is not used often today because of problems with side effects on the heart (Swift & Leggio, 2009). Buprenorphine also has been shown to be effective in several clinical trials with heroin

CONTEMPORARY ISSUE BOX 15.4

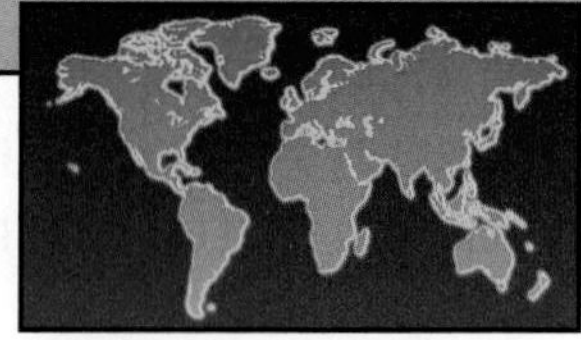

Treatment Research and Clinical Practice

Through the first half of the 20th century, treatment of the substance-use disorders was not informed by scientific research designed to identify the most effective treatment methods. Simply put, up to the 1960s, there were few treatment research studies in the substance-use disorders area that met high standards of scientific rigor so that we could have confidence in the validity of their findings. As a result, consumers had to take on faith anyone's claims that a given treatment method worked. But the picture began to change in the 1970s, and today we are fortunate to have a considerable amount of high-quality treatment research on the substance-use disorders. This means that alcohol and drug treatment that most people receive today is "empirically supported" (based on research findings of what methods are "effective" or is "evidence-based"). Right?

Unfortunately, wrong. Although research findings have had some influence on what happens in the clinical practice of alcohol and drug treatment, it is not as much influence as one might hope for or even expect. That is because it has become apparent to many that it is one thing to have built an impressive foundation of knowledge, but it is another thing to consistently apply that knowledge to enhance the quality of care that patients receive. Therefore, knowledge *diffusion* (another commonly used term is *dissemination,* and in the treatment area, *translation*) poses its own set of formidable challenges.

In this regard, we have learned in recent years that barriers of different types must often be overcome if knowledge is to be applied consistently, that is, if empirically supported methods of assessment and treatment are to become the standard of care in a given setting. These barriers may exist on multiple levels and could include factors related to the provider of the services (the clinician), to the patient who is to be the recipient of the services, or to the system in which treatment is delivered. For example, if a new treatment method is found through clinical trials (the same model of testing that the FDA requires in the evaluation of new drugs, as we reviewed in Chapter 5) to be effective, then clinicians must learn the new methods, become skilled in their use, and perhaps abandon familiar and comfortable ways of doing things. Or, patients may resist the new service or treatment method because it is different from what they have heard others claim works best. The system itself may resist going against long-held beliefs about treatment or simply may not provide the resources needed to support its clinicians in learning and mastering the delivery of a new treatment method.

The new awareness of the knowledge–practice gap in alcohol and drug treatment has resulted in studies that concern ways of overcoming the barriers to dissemination of treatment research. Can you think of some methods directed at clinicians, their patients, or the treatment system to shrink the knowledge–practice gap that could be tested?

addicts (Litten & Allen, 1999). Therefore, the data show that the clinician has the option of prescribing three opiate agonist or partial agonist drugs in the treatment of opioid dependence, according to the clinician's or the client's preferences.

The final drug for the treatment of opioid dependence is antagonist therapy with naltrexone. Although earlier clinical trials suggested that this drug is effective, clinicians do not use it often. One problem is that those with addictions tend not to prefer this drug initially in their treatment, perhaps because naltrexone does not have mild psychoactive effects as, for example, methadone does. Naltrexone therefore has found greater application among those with addictions who are highly motivated to change their drug use and those making the transition from methadone to drug-free maintenance (see the discussion earlier in this chapter).

Promising Treatment Techniques

In one sense, designating treatments as pharmacological or nonpharmacological misrepresents clinical practice because, especially in recent years, treatment for illicit drug use often combines pharmacological and psychosocial therapies. In fact, rarely is a medication prescribed without some sort of psychological or social therapy addition, although the latter treatments may be used without the adjunct of medication. In this section, we discuss nonpharmacological treatment techniques or methods that have shown some promise in clinical trials with illicit drug-use disorders. In these trials, the techniques were often used as part of a broad rehabilitation program that included pharmacotherapy or were used explicitly to complement pharmacotherapy.

Perhaps the strongest evidence for using nonmedical interventions in the treatment of illicit drug-use disorders comes from studies of structured behavioral contracting programs. These programs follow a social learning model and use explicit contingencies of consequences for, typically, maintenance of sobriety. The most effective of these programs apply positive reinforcers for desired behavior (for example, abstinence from drugs) rather than punishment for undesired behavior. For example, Stitzer, Iguchi, and Felch (1992) found that the privilege of receiving take-home doses of methadone by submitting drug-free urines resulted in four times as many patients reducing their illicit drug use compared to the number of patients who reduced such use when no contingencies were attached to receiving take-home methadone.

Iguchi et al. (1997) extended the idea of contracting with such a contingency by showing that contingent reinforcement of completing treatment plan tasks developed by the counselor and patient was more effective in reducing illicit drug use among opioid-dependent men and women enrolled in a methadone maintenance clinic than was contingent reinforcement of submitting clean urine. The contribution of this study is the idea that reinforcement of abstinence (indicated by clean urine) is essential for treatment progress, but gains are more likely to be maintained if the drug-dependent individual's psychosocial problems are addressed more broadly (indicated by goals and related tasks in the treatment plan). Reinforcement of achieving goals that are not compatible with drug use also tends to support abstinence from drugs. Carroll et al. (2002) showed the value of contingency contracting procedures as a complement to naltrexone treatment of individuals dependent on opioid drugs. Contingent abstinent programs implemented through the use of vouchers also have shown promise in treating individuals for their cocaine dependence (Katz, Robles-Sotelo, et al., 2002).

As we discussed earlier, the broadest application of contingent reinforcement principles is represented by the community reinforcement approach, which includes the patient's social and environmental network in the contingency program. The effectiveness of this program first was demonstrated in the treatment of alcohol-use disorders (Hunt & Azrin, 1973; Sisson & Azrin, 1989). Higgins and his colleagues (1991; 1993) showed that community reinforcement procedures also are effective in treating individuals who are dependent on cocaine. Moreover, this same research group showed that adding community reinforcement to a program of opioid detoxification by use of buprenorphine-enhanced abstinence from opioid drugs (Bickel, Amass, Higgins, Badger, & Esch, 1997).

Another technique that seems to be effective in treating users of illicit drugs is couples or family treatment (Stanton & Shadish, 1997). It is notable that the community reinforcement approach includes a family/couples (conjoint) component that is based in social learning principles (see Table 15.4).

In conclusion, structured programs that are based in social learning theory, as well as conjoint treatment, are nonmedical interventions that seem to enhance outcomes in the treatment of drug-use disorders. Our earlier discussion showed that treatment of alcohol-use disorders also is improved with these interventions. This seems to warrant their continued application and study in alcohol and drug treatment programs.

Special Topics in Alcohol and Drug Treatment

In this section, we discuss three topics that we think are important and that apply to both alcohol and drug treatment. The first is treatment of polysubstance abusers, or people who use more than one drug. We then briefly review the treatment of dual-diagnosis patients and especially how such treatment involves the use of psychotropic medication. The last topic is relapse (see Figure 15.1), which has challenged alcohol and drug treatment providers for many years.

Treatment of Polysubstance Abusers

In the traditional and common way of viewing treatment, people who have an alcohol-use disorder do not have trouble with or abuse other drugs. Similarly, the traditional view gives the impression that people who have drug-use disorders have no patterns of abusive alcohol use. However, it has been known for some time that it may be a mistake to designate programs as either alcohol treatment or drug treatment.

Sokolow et al. (1981) surveyed multiple substance use among patients arriving for treatment at New York state–funded alcoholism rehabilitation programs. The total sample of 1,340 men and women selected for this study represented wide ranges in age and educational background. Most (57.3%) of the patients were between 31 and 50 years old. In addition to their alcohol use, which was their reason for beginning treatment, patients were asked about their licit and illicit use in the past 30 days of minor and major tranquilizers, sedatives, amphetamines, antidepressants, opiates, hallucinogens, marijuana, and cocaine.

Almost half of the patients reported using at least one drug other than alcohol during the 30 days before their treatment began. About 20% of these patients used combinations of drugs. The single drug class reported most frequently was the tranquilizers (12.7% of the patients), which is notable because tranquilizers are cross-tolerant with alcohol and are the drugs most abused by those identified as alcoholics. We should also note that people identified as drug abusers often abuse alcohol, too, according to Carroll, Malloy, and Kenrick (1977). Today, it is widely recognized among treatment personnel that their patients may use multiple substances (Etheridge et al., 1997).

Studies of multiple substance use have important implications for treatment. As we have said, treatment programs have a strong tendency to focus on alcohol treatment or drug treatment, which have major differences in practice. Furthermore, some treatment providers object to treating substance abuse other than what had been identified as the patient's primary substance of abuse. Such reactions were found especially in alcohol programs, and they restrict treatment, given the prevalence of multiple substance use. In this respect, two points quickly emerge about treatment effects. First, if treatment programs concentrate on only alcohol use, for example, then the abuse of other drugs may result in poorer, shorter-lasting **treatment effects** than if the person's substance-use patterns were treated in a more unified way. Second, people seeking alcohol or drug treatment who are multiple substance abusers may have more severe social, legal, and psychiatric difficulties than those in treatment whose patterns of abuse are limited to single drug categories (Carroll et al., 1977). Beginning treatment with more severe problems predicts poorer functioning following treatment. So, failing to address patterns of multiple substance use because of program philosophy and policy could mean inadequate treatment planning.

treatment effects The results of experiencing a treatment, usually measured in different areas of functioning, such as substance use, family functioning, and vocational functioning.

Treatment of abusers of multiple substance relates to more general questions about treatment. One of these is the need to view substance use as part of a person's total pattern of behavior to achieve an understanding of drug and alcohol use. Those who take this approach suggest that effective treatment can be planned only if connections are made among all of a person's different problems. Similarly, some clinicians and researchers believe addictive behavior patterns have a lot in common in what causes them, what maintains them, and how they are treated. It is thought these commonalities should underlie treatment programming instead of the traditional emphasis on single addiction patterns. According to this viewpoint, behaviors identified as addictive, including, for example, alcohol and other drug abuse, overeating, and compulsive gambling, have common factors that may be addressed in "generic" treatment programs. The DSM-IV recognizes this approach in addressing the substance-use disorders as a diagnostic class rather than addressing alcohol and other drug diagnoses in a nonintegrated way. Nonetheless, it should be remembered that the properties of the various drugs of abuse vary, as might the characteristics of the users, and there is no guarantee that a program that works well for individuals with alcohol-use disorder would be successful with people whose primary drug problem is heroin.

Treatment of Dual-Diagnosis Patients

An important topic for alcohol and drug treatment providers is patients who have major psychiatric problems to go along with their substance-use problems. Such patients have been called dual-diagnosis patients. Dual-diagnosis patients, as you might imagine, typically have more complex and extensive treatment needs than do patients without major psychiatric problems, and dual-diagnosis patients tend to do more poorly in and following treatment.

Psychotropic medication may be part of the treatment of alcohol or drug abuse when a person has an alcohol or drug problem plus another psychiatric disorder. These psychiatric disorders include depression and manic depression, especially among individuals who have alcohol-use disorder. A relationship exists between alcohol- or drug-use disorders characterized by a high degree of anxiety and the **personality disorders**, particularly what is commonly called **sociopathy**. Psychotropic agents usually are used in the treatment of alcohol or drug problems on the premise that patients use alcohol and other drugs for **self-medication**. This means the individuals act as their own physician and self-prescribe alcohol and other drugs to lessen troubling psychological symptoms such as anxiety or depression. When used, psychotropic agents generally are administered in combination with nonmedical techniques in treating the substance-use disorder (Schuckit, 1996).

personality disorders
Long-standing patterns of behavior that frequently create distress for individuals due to their personal or social consequences; usually recognizable from adolescence or earlier.

sociopathy
Personality disorder characterized by a lack of concern for social obligations or rules, a lack of feelings for others, and a tendency toward violence.

self-medication
The idea that some people prescribe their own medication, in the form of alcohol or illicit drugs, to alleviate psychological difficulties such as anxiety or depression.

Relapse

Any discussion of alcohol and drug treatment is incomplete without including relapse. Defining and measuring relapse are not as simple as you might think, but in concept, it means the reappearance of some problem after a period of its remission. With physical diseases such as cancer, which is where the term *relapse* comes from, its measurement is more straightforward.

You have seen that arriving at a definition of alcohol and drug problems that has general consensus is no easy matter, however. This difficulty carries through to defining relapse, as reflected by the different operational definitions that have been used in research on this topic.

In spite of these complexities in definition, relapse has been studied extensively in the addictions field for the last 30 years. You might remember that we mentioned the problem of relapse in Chapter 7, when we discussed the treatment of smoking. Actually, alcohol and drug treatment providers have grappled with the problem of relapse for much longer than 30 years, and today, many people refer to alcohol and other drug abuse and dependence as "chronic relapsing conditions" (McLellan et al., 2000). The classic paper by Hunt, Barnett, and Branch (1971) illustrates this point. Their review of the literature at that time showed that about 70% of individuals treated for alcohol, tobacco, or heroin abuse in abstinence-oriented programs had returned to using their primary substance by the time they were out of treatment for three months. Today the problem is the same, and much treatment research is directed at discovering ways to help individuals maintain the changes they might make as a result of completing treatment.

The research on relapse and the substance-use disorders has generated several models and theories, summarized in Table 15.7. As you can see, the six models and theories make few distinctions among different drugs in the mechanisms of relapse. Another point is the emphasis on relapse precipitants, or the events immediately preceding the relapse. Events more removed from the immediate relapse environment

TABLE 15.7 Major Models and Theories of Relapse

Model/Theory	Mechanism(s) of Relapse
Cognitive-behavioral model (Marlatt & Gordon, 1985; Marlatt & Witkiewitz, 2005)	Interaction between "high risk" (for substance use) and the individual's self-efficacy to cope with those situations without substance use determines relapse. Expectations about the utility of drugs and alcohol in a situation also are important.
Person–situation interaction model (Litman, 1986)	Relapse is determined by an interaction among three factors: situations that the individual perceives as threatening ("high risk"), availability of an adequate repertoire of coping strategies, and the individual's perception of the effectiveness of available coping strategies.
Self-efficacy and outcome expectancies (Annis, 1986; Rollnick & Heather, 1982)	Initial substance use occurs from the mislabeling of negative affect and negative physical states as craving. After the first substance use, expectations of control over such use decrease along with self-efficacy. This process leads to a more severe relapse.
Opponent process (Solomon, 1980)	Through conditioning, formerly neutral internal and external stimuli become connected with various "A" and "B" states. Reexposure or reexperiencing these states may increase the individual's motivation to use drugs following a period of abstinence.
Craving and loss of control (Ludwig & Wikler, 1974)	Internal and external stimuli associated with drug withdrawal are labeled as craving. Drugs are sought as a way to relieve craving.
Urges and cravings (Tiffany, 1990; 1992; Wise, 1988)	Drug use and drug urges and cravings have occurred often enough to be "automatic cognitive processes." In the abstinent substance abuser, these processes can be triggered by various internal and external stimuli. Relapse may occur if an adequate "action plan" not to use drugs, a nonautomatic cognitive process, is impeded or not used. Wise adds that use of one drug may trigger urges to use another as a result of action in the brain.

Source: Adapted in part from Connors, Maisto, and Donovan (1996).

are given less attention. Examples of these are the social support a person has for nonproblem substance use, the period of time a person has been unemployed, and the level of tension among members of a family. Finally, the models and theories can be divided into two general categories: psychological and biological. The psychological theories emphasize cognitions, whereas the biological theories emphasize learned motivation to use drugs and cravings.

"Patient living alone, no job, complained of feeling bored and useless; could see no reason why he should not take a drink."
"Patient reported that everything was going so well for him that he wanted to celebrate by having a drink."

Reasons two patients gave for their alcohol-use relapses following treatment (Marlatt & Gordon, 1985, p. 74)

At this point, no one theory of relapse has emerged as superior to the others, so it makes sense to look across the theories to discern what may be the important ingredients of relapse. First are the internal (e.g., mood) and external (e.g., drinking setting) stimulus conditions that precede relapse. Cravings to use drugs also are important. Two types of expectancies may be relevant to relapse. The first is a person's beliefs about the effects of a drug in a given situation, and the second is a person's self-efficacy, which is an individual's estimation that he or she can successfully enact a behavior in a given situation. Finally, a person's coping responses or skills may be important in relapse.

Research and theory about relapse have generated treatment applications, known as relapse prevention methods (Marlatt, Bowen, & Witkiewitz, 2009; Marlatt & Witkiewitz, 2005). Relapse prevention methods first have focused on assessing "high-risk" situations, or those situations associated with abuse of alcohol or drugs in the past. High-risk situations may be negative moods such as anxiety or depression, positive moods, the presence of people the patient used to drink with, or some combination of internal and external precipitants. After high-risk situations have been identified, the next step is to look at the person's ways to cope with the situation without resorting to undesired levels of substance use, and the person's self-efficacy to do so. Coupled with this is an examination of the person's beliefs about how alcohol or drug use would help in different situations. For example, people may believe that drinking at a party would help them to talk with the other people present. Assessment of these elements then determines what might be done in treatment: teaching alternative coping skills to substance use (for example, using communication skills instead of alcohol to help a person enjoy a party), improving self-efficacy, or educating the person about the actual effects of alcohol and drugs. In practice, all of these elements typically are covered, and there is a correlation among them. For example, teaching people coping skills may elevate their self-efficacy about using that skill.

You can see that much of what is done in relapse prevention work follows from psychological models of relapse. The major method from the biological models is cue exposure. This method essentially involves presenting (exposing) the person with cues (for example, a bottle of a favorite brand of whiskey or drug-use paraphernalia like a syringe) that might elicit cravings to use a substance, without allowing its actual use. With repeated exposure, the cravings theoretically reduce in number and intensity. So, as a person's

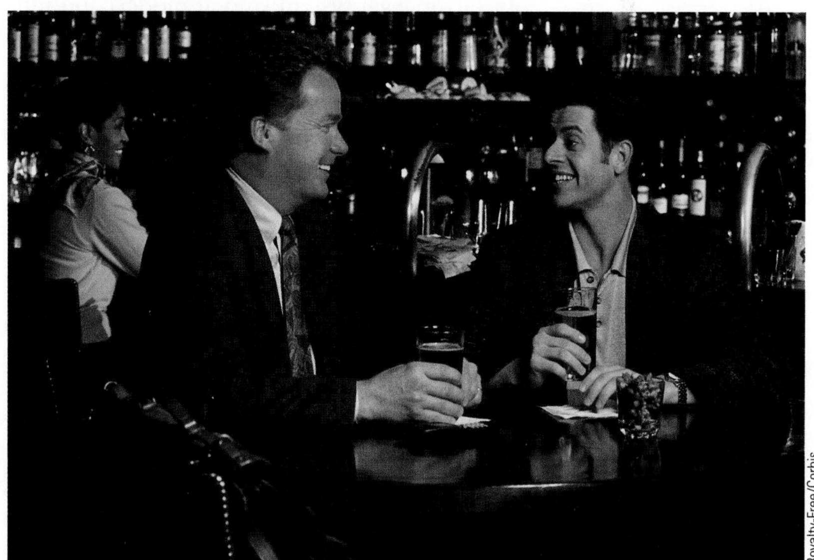
Royalty-Free/Corbis

Settings such as taverns that are associated with a person's heavy use of alcohol in the past may pose a risk of that person relapsing or drinking heavily after a period of abstinence from or moderate use of alcohol.

repeated association of these "stimulus conditions" with drug use resulted in the stimuli eliciting a strong desire to use drugs or alcohol, repeated pairing of the stimuli with nonuse of substances will decrease the power of the stimuli to elicit cravings.

The work on relapse has stimulated substantial advances in alcohol and drug treatment (Carroll, 1996; Stephens, Roffman, & Simpson, 1994). However, it also brings up an important point about relapse research and prevention, and about treatment more generally. What has been absent to a large degree in theories of relapse is more serious study of conditions in the "broader backdrop" of relapse, such as the person's social environment (family functioning, job satisfaction) or general level of stress (recent job change, recent divorce). Immediate relapse precipitants obviously are important, but so are these more remote factors. In fact, we know this from research on the long-term effects of alcohol and drug treatment, which seems highly relevant to relapse. Perhaps it would help to understand this more easily if you do not think of alcohol or drug treatment as a specific entity that "acts on" a person to produce some lasting outcome. Instead, treatment is one event in the life of people who are trying to change the way they use alcohol or drugs. Furthermore, individuals and the treatment interact in a social context that strongly contributes to the course of change. Fortunately, more recent extensions of models of relapse, such as those of Witkiewitz and Marlatt (2004), have attempted to integrate immediate and more distal relapse determinants.

Models of Causes and Treatment Methods

So far we have presented a lot of information about alcohol and drug treatment, although space limitations prevented us from going into great detail. You may have noticed the influence of each of the models of causes that we reviewed at the beginning of this chapter. We can cite several instances. Placing substance-abuse treatment programs in the hospital setting—a common practice—is broadly based in a disease model of thought. Indeed, the great achievement that came years ago with wide acceptance of the disease model was to take the treatment of alcohol and drug problems out of the legal system (moral model) and into the hands of physicians and medical settings—an apparently more useful means of rehabilitating people with addictions.

"The treatment setting of prime significance for recovery from alcohol (and other drug problems) is not a hospital, a clinic, a doctor's or minister's office, a social agency or a jail, or any other specialized institution or place. The prime setting of significance is the social, interpersonal setting of—daily life. And, equally important, it is that setting through time."

Seldon Bacon, 1973 (Orford, 1985, p. 246)

Another example is Alcoholics Anonymous, rooted in both the disease and moral models. Pharmacological treatments, like methadone maintenance, are most clearly linked to the biological model. Within most treatment settings, psychological and social interventions are consistent with the social learning and sociocultural models. The most explicit example of this merging of models is the community reinforcement approach (Budney & Higgins, 1998; Higgins et al., 1991; Hunt & Azrin, 1973), which centers on modifying the person's environment to reinforce nonabuse of substances and not to reinforce substance abuse.

We can trace individual parts of alcohol and drug treatment to a particular model of etiology, but virtually all treatment programs combine practices that are derived from two or more of the causes models. This is the result in part of the many clinical, social, political, and economic forces that influence substance-abuse treatment programs and that affect their evolution. Another force is the current scientifically based thought that the substance-use disorders are multifaceted problems, so treatment must relate to the person's biological, psychological, and social makeup. This thinking is implemented in the collection of activities that constitute many treatment programs.

So far, we have discussed treatment freely—that is, free from concerns about how available or accessible it is. We conclude this chapter by discussing this all-important question, especially as it pertains to economic forces and alcohol and drug treatment.

Economic Factors in Alcohol and Drug Treatment

An issue of great controversy and consequence that is not likely to be resolved soon is the influence of health insurance coverage on whether a person gets treatment and, if so, what kind (Holder & Blose, 1991). A brief history of the role of finances and insurance will help you to appreciate the current controversy (Rawson, 1990–1991).

In the early 1970s, alcohol and drug treatment was not considered in the mainstream of psychiatry, clinical psychology, and social work. By 1990, however, alcohol and drug treatment was a central concern. The change was due mostly to cocaine, AIDS, and adjustments in health care financing.

In the middle to late 1970s, interest in drug treatment had been quelled considerably because the heroin scare of the 1960s and early 1970s had quieted down. At the same time, 28-day inpatient programs became the standard alcohol treatment because of agreements among care providers, typically hospitals and health insurance companies. These 28-day programs proliferated during the 1980s, with legislation passed in many states that required insurers to cover alcohol and drug treatment. The cost to the insurance company was high; the price of completing an inpatient program varied, but it always was in the thousands of dollars. The term *chemical dependence treatment* was spawned in the 1980s, because the 28-day programs were also accommodating large numbers of individuals who abused drugs other than alcohol, especially cocaine. Treatment availability and accessibility (with an expanding economy) were rising rapidly. Another force in the treatment expansion was a social-political climate that encouraged people with alcohol and drug problems to get into treatment.

Therefore, by the late 1980s, treatment was accessible in an unprecedented way, at least for those who had health insurance or independent wealth. Typically, this trend is viewed as good, but a counterforce was operating. With increased expansion of and expectations for alcohol and drug treatment, employers' health insurance premiums were rising quickly. Quietly at first in the unbounded economy of the mid-1980s, then loudly as the economy recessed, came "managed" mental health and alcohol and drug treatment services. Managed care is a movement based on the goal of controlling the costs of health care, including alcohol and drug treatment. The term *cost-effectiveness* became popular: Is the benefit of a treatment worth what it costs?

Cost consciousness has led to a far more restricted use of inpatient alcohol and drug treatments, at least those that are paid for by health insurers. When inpatient stays are covered, they are often much shorter than 28 days. Instead, outpatient treatment is the insurer's preference. This policy is based on research that suggests that, on average, inpatient treatment is no more effective than the much cheaper outpatient treatment (Miller & Hester, 1986).

It seems that the trend to less inpatient and more outpatient care is here to stay. Many treatment providers, however, are concerned that this prescription for care is based too much on money and not enough on proven differences (or lack thereof) in

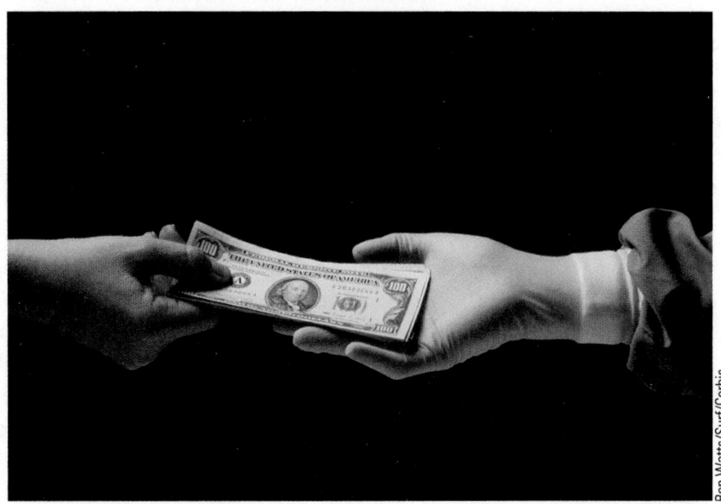
Ron Watts/Surf/Corbis

As in other areas of health care, economics is a driving force in the treatment of the substance-use disorders.

treatment benefits. Some treatment providers ask: What does a lack of difference in benefits overall tell us? What is outpatient treatment anyway? (We saw earlier in this chapter that what constitutes outpatient alcohol and drug treatment is highly variable.) Is the finding of no difference true for everybody? When is the more structured, more intense inpatient treatment indicated, and when is it not?

These and similar questions became more salient for alcohol treatment in the report of a study by Walsh et al. (1991). A total of 227 individuals who were newly identified as alcohol abusers were randomly assigned to one of three treatments through their employee assistance program (thus all these people had jobs). The treatments were compulsory inpatient treatment, compulsory AA attendance, and choice of treatment option. Two years after treatment, the three groups did not differ in measures of job performance. However, a major finding was that, overall, the cost of treatment for the compulsory inpatient group was only 10% more than it was for the AA and choice groups (remember that AA is free in that any financial contribution is voluntary). The small cost difference was particularly true for study participants who had used cocaine in the six months before they began treatment. The overall cost results occurred because the choice and AA groups had a much higher inpatient treatment admission rate during the two-year follow-up period than did the group who initially received compulsory inpatient care. One implication of the small cost difference that was confirmed during the follow-up assessments was that, at least for some of the time after treatment, the compulsory inpatient group used less alcohol and drugs than did the other two groups.

In summary, finances and insurance have played and do play a major role in the accessibility of alcohol and drug treatment and in what treatment options are available. In this regard, as the Walsh et al. (1991) study suggests, it may be that more intense treatments are less costly in the long run for some people, especially those who have more severe psychiatric or social difficulties (Washton, 1995). Therefore, we have a lot to learn about the effects of the strong current trend toward less intense, less expensive treatment. And we have focused in this discussion on people who rely on health insurance to pay for part or all of their health care. A serious concern is individuals who do not have health insurance—a major problem in the United States, and one that the United States must face squarely in its current push for health care reform legislation. Because of the current decreased availability of publicly funded treatment, those without insurance may find it impossible to get any professional care. This is a significant point when you remember that, overall, completing alcohol and drug treatment is associated with improved functioning in multiple areas.

The Stepped Care Approach

Our discussion in this chapter has focused on changes in patterns of alcohol and drug use and how they happen. Several main points have emerged from the discussion. Change may occur in many different ways and may or may not involve the use of professional treatment resources. Treatment itself consists of several different ways to help people reach different goals that relate to how they function in different parts of their lives, and it occurs in several different settings. Some treatment approaches or techniques have a stronger scientific base to support their effectiveness than do others. Therefore, people follow numerous pathways to change; some pathways involving professional treatment have more scientific support than others, and some seem better suited to the needs and goals of any given person. Finally, we have learned that, when we discuss professional treatment, what is accessible to individuals depends partly on their personal income and insurance coverage. Economics has been a major factor driving the pronounced trend toward briefer and less intense treatments conducted in outpatient settings.

This summary reflects major recent changes in alcohol and drug treatment services in the United States. Until the middle to late 1980s, professional alcohol and drug treatment was delivered with a "one-size-fits-all" approach. Insurance companies typically covered an episode of 28-day inpatient treatment with few questions asked. That era is over, but what is next? Is there a general approach to follow that offers the most effective and efficient treatment to people at any given time that they seek it? When individuals seek professional treatment, one model to follow in finding the services needed is called the "stepped care approach," which has been an effective heuristic in guiding the treatment of other medical disorders such as hypertension (Sobell & Sobell, 2000).

According to Sobell and Sobell (2000, 573–574), in the stepped care approach, the selection of any treatment is guided by three principles: (1) Treatment should be individualized with regard to the client's needs and problems; (2) the treatment selected should be consistent with the current knowledge about effectiveness; and (3) the treatment that is chosen should be the least restrictive (considering the physical effects of treatment on the client and the client's lifestyle and resources). A consequence of the third principle is that more intensive treatments are reserved for more severe problems.

These three principles apply to the selection of both initial treatment and subsequent treatments. What happens after the initial treatment is selected and begun is based on monitoring the clients' progress toward achieving their goals. If clients show improvement, then a treatment may be continued, decreased in frequency or intensity, or stopped. If there is no change or the clients show a decreased level of functioning, then a treatment may be changed in frequency or intensity, or a new treatment may be tried. Decisions about treatment are based mainly on clients' performances relevant to their treatment goals.

The stepped care approach seems simple in principle but may be complex in application. To use this approach in real clinical settings, several questions have to be considered. Are any scientifically supported treatments available for an individual's needs at a given time? Will an individual accept the treatment indicated by the stepped care approach? Will the individual be able to afford it? What is "improvement"? When is behavior "stable"?

Despite these and other difficult questions, the stepped care approach fits well with our current knowledge about change in patterns of alcohol and drug use and about the economics of treatment delivery. Stepped care fits what we know because it fosters a scientifically based, individualized delivery of effective treatment in the most efficient, least restrictive, and least expensive way. Indeed, major forces in addiction treatment, represented by the model of "addiction treatment matching" of the American Society of Addiction Medicine (Gastfriend, 2003), and the substance-abuse treatment guidelines of the U.S. Department of Veterans Affairs Health Care System, take a stepped care approach.

Summary

- Readiness or commitment to change is an important consideration in treatment. One model of this process is the stages of change model.
- As with nicotine dependence, people with substance-use disorders change these problem behaviors on their own quite frequently. This is known as spontaneous remission of the substance-use patterns.
- The self-help groups Alcoholics Anonymous and Narcotics Anonymous are major resources in helping people who have alcohol- and drug-use disorders, respectively.
- Other self-help groups, presented as alternatives to AA, also are becoming more popular. Two examples are SMART and Secular Organizations for Sobriety (SOS).

- The model of etiology of alcohol- and drug-use disorder that a treatment is based on affects its design. We review five models in this chapter: moral, American disease, biological, social learning, and sociocultural.
- The biopsychosocial model of etiology addresses the inadequacy of single-factor models by combining the major types of factors that seem to influence the development of alcohol- and drug-use disorders.
- Treatments have aims or goals. In alcohol and drug treatment, goals typically follow from a thorough assessment and refer to a person's use of alcohol and drugs and to other areas of life functioning.
- It has been standard practice to specify abstinence from alcohol or other drugs as the major outcome goal for a treatment. However, some argue that moderate, nonproblem use of alcohol is a reasonable outcome goal for some patients.
- Alcohol treatment can be classified broadly into three categories of settings: hospital, intermediate, and outpatient. Within each setting, a wide variety of services may be offered.
- FDA-approved pharmacological treatment of alcohol problems includes medication to manage withdrawal from alcohol, alcohol-sensitizing drugs, drugs that alter the reinforcing properties of alcohol, and drugs that manage alcohol craving.
- Overall, no one treatment for alcohol problems seems to be superior to others, but staying in treatment is associated with better outcomes. Individual treatments may be more effective if they are matched to patients' characteristics.
- It has proved difficult to conduct controlled outcome research on self-help groups. What research has been done suggests that AA helps some people but not everybody.
- Settings of drug treatment traditionally have been defined by treatment of heroin abuse, but abusers of other drugs now also appear in most of these settings. Traditionally, drug treatment settings include detoxification, methadone maintenance, residential, and outpatient. As with alcohol treatment, a wide variety of treatment services may be offered in a given setting.
- FDA-approved pharmacotherapy of dependence on opiate drugs includes managing drug withdrawal, replacing one opiate (e.g., heroin) with another one that is less addictive (methadone), and using antagonist drugs (e.g., naltrexone for opioids).
- Research shows that staying in residential or nonmethadone outpatient drug treatment is associated with reduced substance use and a more socially productive lifestyle. Drug treatment research would benefit from more studies of patient–treatment matching.
- Structured contingency reinforcement programs, including community reinforcement, are promising nonpharmacological treatments of illicit drug-use disorders. Conjoint therapies also seem to be effective.
- Drug and alcohol treatment providers have found that a large percentage of their patients abuse multiple substance. This has caused a change in the thinking that drug and alcohol treatment are independent efforts. Rather, there is wide recognition of the need for settings that can accommodate users of multiple substances and for understanding common aspects of the addictive behaviors.
- There has been a major increase in recognition that individuals who show up for alcohol or drug treatment may have major psychiatric disorders. One approach to treating these individuals uses psychotropic medications.
- The challenging problem of relapse has received a lot of research attention in the last 30 years. This work has resulted in treatment applications called relapse prevention.
- Financial factors, especially health insurance coverage, have had and are having great influence on the type and accessibility of alcohol and drug treatment.
- Stepped care is one approach to professional treatment selection that integrates current knowledge about alcohol and drug treatment effectiveness and the conditions under which it is delivered.

Answers to *"What Do You Think?"*

1. The process of changing a problem behavior seems to be different for everyone.
   F *According to one model, called the stages of change, self-change and change resulting from treatment can be characterized by progression through discrete steps or stages.*
2. Treatment is needed to change patterns of alcohol and drug abuse or dependence.

F *Research shows that spontaneous remission of the substance-use disorders occurs, and it seems to be the most common way that change in problem substance use occurs.*

3. Alcoholics Anonymous was created more than 100 years ago, and its influence is predominantly in the United States.
   F *Alcoholics Anonymous was created in 1935 and its influence spans the world.*
4. It is generally agreed that substance-use disorders are caused by psychological problems.
   F *Psychological theories are one explanation of the etiology of substance-use disorders, but there also are biological and sociocultural theories. A theory that incorporates all three approaches seems to have the best chance of providing an adequate explanation of etiology.*
5. Assessment typically is thought to be essential to good treatment.
   T *It is virtually universal in professional treatment contexts that assessment of the individual precedes any formally defined treatment activities.*
6. The only goal of any importance in alcohol and drug treatment is the reduction of substance use.
   F *Substance-use goals indeed are important, but goals that relate to other areas of life functioning, such as psychological or occupational, also are important.*
7. Abstinence from alcohol is a mandatory goal of alcohol treatment.
   F *Although the predominant assumption in U.S. and Canadian treatment programs is that abstinence is mandatory, there is evidence that certain individuals can modify their drinking patterns to stable, moderate, nonproblem use.*
8. Methadone maintenance seems to be an effective treatment for heroin dependence.
   T *You might not think this is true given all the controversy surrounding methadone maintenance; however, a lot of research has shown that staying in methadone treatment results in reduced opiate use and other related problem behaviors such as criminal activity.*
9. Today, there are good reasons for rigid boundaries between what we call alcohol treatment and drug treatment.
   F *With the large percentage of individuals presenting for treatment who abuse more than one substance, the reasons for segregating at least some settings of alcohol and drug treatment are not compelling.*
10. People who have major psychiatric problems are rarely seen in settings where alcohol and drug treatment are provided.
   F *Individuals who have major psychiatric disorders do appear for alcohol and drug treatment. The prevalence of such dual-diagnosis patients varies with the treatment setting.*
11. Relapse is such a long-standing problem in alcohol and drug treatment that we can do little about it.
   F *Relapse is a long-standing problem, but as a result of research and theory over the last 30 years or so, methods to prevent relapse have been developed and are in use.*
12. Professional treatment for substance-use disorders is freely available to anyone who wants it.
   F *Treatment is as available today as it ever has been, but major economic barriers come between treatment and some of the people who need and want it. Therefore, treatment is not always accessible.*

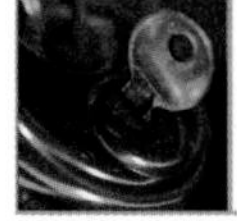

Key Terms

aftercare
counseling
levo-alpha-acetylmethadol (LAAM)
milieu treatment
personality disorders
psychological treatment
psychotherapy
recovery
self-medication
sociopathy
spontaneous remission
treatment
treatment effects
treatment outcome research

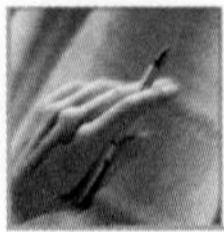

Essays/Thought Questions

1. What implications does the phenomenon of spontaneous remission of alcohol-use disorders have for designing formal treatments for them?
2. What do you think are some of the reasons that self-help groups might aid some people in their efforts to change their alcohol or other drug use?
3. Why do you think some people have argued that harm reduction approaches to changing alcohol and drug use might be especially applicable to adolescents and young adults?
4. If no one treatment for alcohol- or other drug-use disorders has been found to be effective for everyone, do the available formal treatments for these disorders have any value?

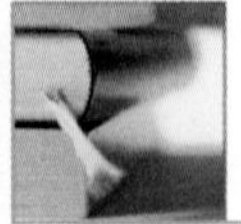

Suggested Readings

Fletcher, A. M. (2001). *Sober for good*. Boston: Houghton Mifflin Co.

Leshner, A. I. (1999). Science-based views of drug addiction and its treatment. *Journal of the American Medical Association, 282,* 1314–1318.

Miller, W. R., & C'de Baca, J. (2001). *Quantum change*. New York: Guilford Press.

Rogers, E. M. (2003). *Diffusion of information* (5th ed.). New York: Free Press.

Wagner, E. F., & Waldron, H. B. (Eds.). (2001). *Innovations in adolescent substance abuse interventions*. New York: Pergamon.

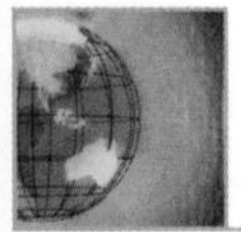

Web Resources

Visit the Book Companion Website at www.cengage.com/psychology/maisto to access study tools including a glossary, flashcards, and web quizzing. You will also find links to the following resources:

- Addiction Alternatives: Self-help groups have been an extremely important resource for the treatment of substance-use disorders in the United States and around the world. This website offers links to major non–12 step self-help groups in the addictions (and other) areas.
- U.S. Substance Abuse and Mental Health Services Administration

CHAPTER 16

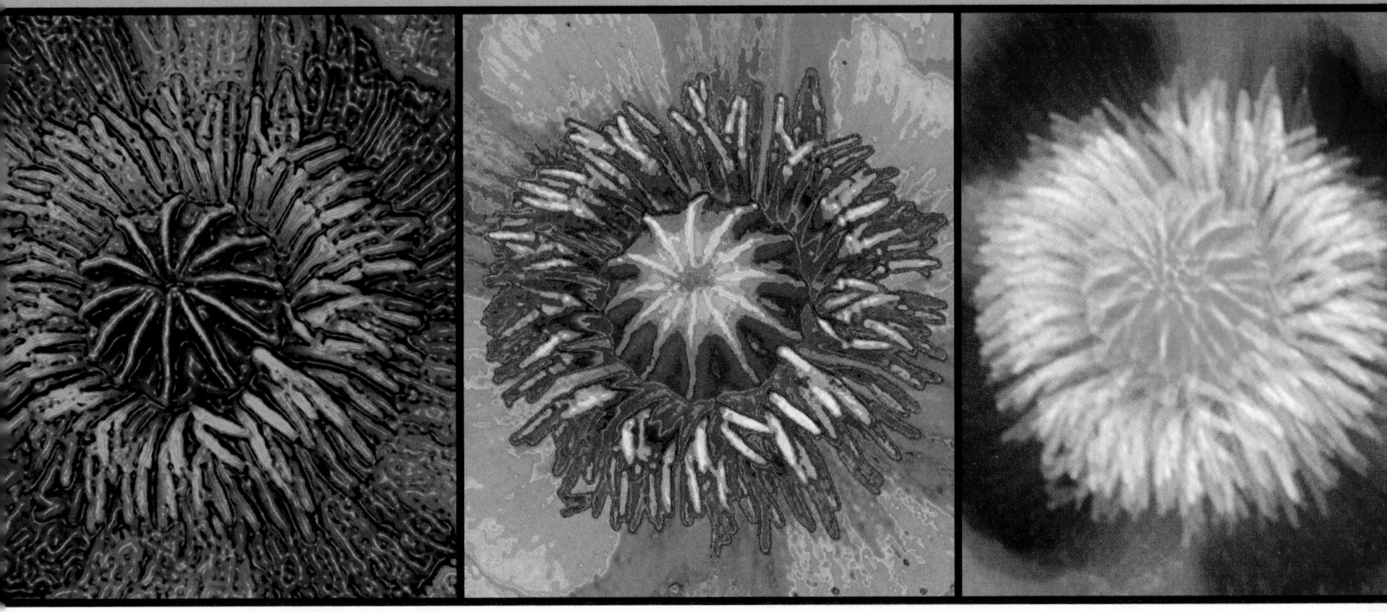

Prevention of Substance Abuse

What Do You Think? True or False?

Answers are given at the end of the chapter.

___ 1. Primary prevention includes interventions to treat people who are beyond the early stages of substance abuse or dependence.

___ 2. One strength of the sociocultural model of prevention is its emphasis on reducing the physical problems associated with alcohol consumption.

___ 3. Raising the price of alcohol relative to disposable income and limiting the hours of operation for bars are examples of prevention strategies based on the distribution of consumption model.

___ 4. The proscriptive model of prevention, which involves prohibiting the availability of drugs and promoting abstention from use, has proven to be the most effective of the three major models of prevention.

___ 5. The main proponents of warning labels on alcoholic beverages have been the manufacturers of these beverages.

___ 6. Research evidence indicates that mass media prevention strategies do not result in significant changes in patterns of alcohol or drug use.

___ 7. The primary goal of affect-oriented prevention programs is to increase the individual's knowledge base regarding drugs and alcohol.

___ 8. Research evidence has documented the effectiveness of DARE, the most popular school-based drug prevention program.

___ 9. The focus of most workplace prevention programs is primary prevention.

___ 10. One disadvantage of workplace prevention programs is their cost.

___ 11. The idea of holding people who serve alcohol responsible for the patrons' behavior if they become intoxicated is a recent development in drinking moderation strategies.

The preceding chapters included a great amount of information on alcohol and drugs, their actions, and their use and abuse. The previous chapter concerned the treatment of problems associated with substance use. This brings us to our final chapter, which focuses on the prevention of substance-use problems.

It may seem curious that we discuss preventing drug misuse in the last and not the first chapter of this text. After all, you might say, if the focus of society and government were on prevention, might material on drug abuse be unnecessary? Unfortunately, professionals and funding sources historically have not made prevention a high priority. The reasons for this are not certain, but two possibilities stand out. First is that past prevention efforts have tended to yield only modest influences in changing patterns of drug use. Second is that current, ongoing substance abuse is dramatically visible and thus receives a more rapid response in personnel and financial resources. Whether this approach is shortsighted is a question that is often and strongly debated.

Although prevention traditionally has received less attention than treatment, we nevertheless are now in a period when prevention research and development are on the rise. One of the leading reasons for this increased focus on prevention is that substance use has contributed to the spread of AIDS. Intravenous drug users are one of the largest groups to have contracted AIDS in the United States and in Europe. Furthermore, being under the influence of alcohol or other drugs in some cases may lead users to engage in unsafe sexual practices, increasing the risk of HIV transmission. Accordingly, federal and state resources have been increasingly used over the past decade to fund projects designed to prevent substance use.

Most people agree that prevention efforts should—indeed must—be an important component of any comprehensive approach to treating substance abuse. In this chapter, we first provide an overview of definitions of prevention. The major models of prevention and their implications are then discussed. We also provide examples of several types of prevention projects and their outcomes. The chapter closes with some comments on the prospects for future work in prevention.

Defining Prevention

Prevention in this context pertains broadly to the avoidance or alleviation of problems associated with substance use. This relatively straightforward definition opens the door to a variety of potential goals for prevention efforts. For example, the goal of prevention efforts aimed at illegal drug use generally is to stop its occurrence. An alternative or additional goal of such activities might be to minimize the effects of any illegal drug use that does occur (a harm reduction approach; see Drugs and Culture Box 16.5). Then the approaches chosen for implementation probably would be different. Therefore, when we speak of prevention, it is important to identify what is being prevented, whether it is onset of use, continued use, negative effects on society, health problems, or something else.

Prevention of substance abuse traditionally has been divided into three types of intervention. The first is **primary prevention**, which pertains to the avoidance of substance abuse before it has a chance to occur. One goal of primary prevention is to preclude the initial use of a substance. Never starting to use a drug, it is argued, means that you will not have any problems with it. This thinking in part underlies the "Just Say No" advertising effort used to encourage young people to turn down invitations to use drugs. Another goal of primary prevention for some substances is the development of responsible attitudes and substance-use behaviors, such as responsible drinking behaviors. A number of posters and television spots have emphasized, for example, the need not to drive after drinking or not to let friends drive drunk.

primary prevention
Attempts to avoid substance use or abuse before it has a chance to occur.

Secondary prevention refers to interventions applied when substance-use problems already have begun to appear. This type of prevention is analogous to early treatment in that interventions are used when problems are first surfacing. Secondary prevention frequently is used in the legal response to substance misuse. For example, people arrested for driving under the influence of alcohol often are referred to alcohol education courses designed to decrease the likelihood of the people drinking and driving again. Similarly, in some parts of the country, educational programs are used with youthful offenders first arrested for drug possession. In each case, the emphasis is on nipping the problem in the bud, as it first appears. Central to such efforts, of course, is the early identification of these drug problems.

secondary prevention
Interventions designed to prevent substance-use problems just as the early signs of abuse begin to appear.

The third form of prevention, called **tertiary prevention**, includes interventions used in treating people who are beyond the early stages of substance abuse or dependence. The goals of tertiary prevention essentially are to terminate use of the substance and thus avoid further deterioration in the person's functioning. Tertiary prevention and substance-abuse treatment (see Chapter 15) are comparable activities, and prevention efforts are more appropriately viewed as being either primary or secondary in nature. In the remainder of this chapter, we accordingly emphasize primary and secondary prevention activities.

tertiary prevention
Treatment interventions with people well beyond the early stages of substance abuse or dependence.

"It's easier to stop a moving bus than to stop doing drugs. Don't start and you won't have to stop."

Poster displayed in buses, subways, and bus shelters by the Partnership for a Drug-free Greater New York

Models of Prevention

Over years of much debate and some research, three major prevention models have evolved. In reading about these models, you will notice that the philosophy underlying each model has diverse implications for what approaches are recommended to prevent substance-use problems.

Sociocultural Model

The sociocultural, or social science, framework to understanding prevention posits that social norms directly influence the use and abuse of psychoactive substances. This model has been used primarily in efforts to prevent alcohol abuse, although the model also has implications for the prevention of other substance abuse, which we describe later in this section. When applied to drinking behavior, the model consists of three basic components (Blane, 1976): (1) an emphasis on the culture's normative structure, (2) a need to integrate drinking into socially meaningful activities, and (3) a focus on providing for the gradual socialization of drinking behavior. As you can see, prevention efforts derived from this model strive to influence the entire climate of drinking within the culture.

One of the strongest proponents of the sociocultural model is Rupert Wilkinson (1970), who argues that alcohol use can be affected by planned policy measures. Wilkinson notes identifiable patterns of alcohol consumption that correspond to low rates of problematic drinking, and he thinks these patterns can be used as guides for ingraining altered drinking patterns in the culture.

In his 1970 seminal work, which remains applicable today, Wilkinson identified five proposals for modifying drinking patterns culturally. First is the need to have within the culture a low level of emotionalism about drinking and at the same time a lack of ambivalence about alcohol use. Emotionalism surrounding drinking, according to Wilkinson, merely creates tension and produces an environment in which discussion and change in drinking behavior cannot occur. A more measured and nonreactive approach will have the added benefit of reducing societal ambivalence about drinking and thus provide more clarity about drinking norms.

A second proposal of Wilkinson's sociocultural model is that there must be a distinction between drinking per se and drunkenness. The notion here is that acceptable drinking and unacceptable drinking (drunkenness) both should be clearly defined. Unfortunately, arriving at such definitions is not easy.

Wilkinson's third point is that after identifying what drunkenness is, there should be firm taboos on its occurrence.

A fourth and central proposal is that drinking should be integrated into a broader social context; that is, alcohol consumption should not be the focus of activity at any given gathering but instead should be adjunctive to other activities.

Finally, Wilkinson proposes that society should allow the serving of alcohol only when food is also available. The belief here is that when food is available, alcohol consumption will not necessarily be the sole focus of activity. Furthermore, food slows the body's absorption of alcohol and potentially reduces the rate of drunkenness.

Taken together, these proposals designate acceptable and unacceptable forms of drinking and thus clearly identify desired patterns of responsible drinking. These patterns of drinking then should be integrated into routine family and other social activities. It is noteworthy that the goal of the sociocultural approach is not the cessation of drinking but rather changes in social norms regarding drinking. Therefore, the approach is not a prohibitionist strategy, and some have argued that a fault of the sociocultural approach is that it may encourage drinking.

A major criticism of the sociocultural model is that it may not be widely applicable. Many countries, such as the United States and Canada, have diverse cultures and subcultures, and customs and values that fit one of them may not be amenable to or accepted by another. A second criticism is that the sociocultural approach, while

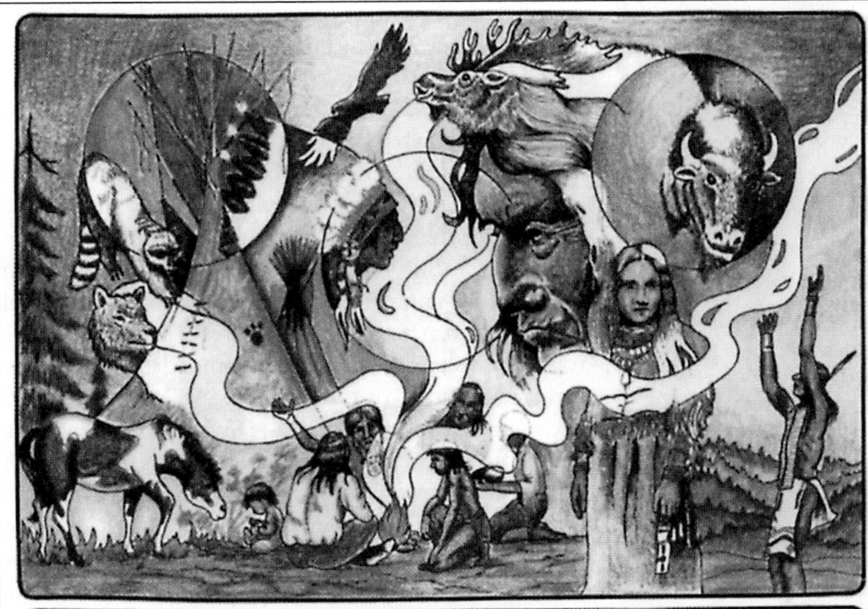
INHALANTS...
(Sprays / Aerosols / Glues)
EVIL SPIRITS THAT BREAK THE BONDS BETWEEN OURSELVES AND OUR ELDERS, DISRUPT THE CIRCLE OF OUR FAMILY SYSTEM, DESTROY THE HARMONY BETWEEN US AND ALL CREATION.
FOR OUR OWN SURVIVAL, THE SURVIVAL OF OUR FAMILY, OUR TRIBE AND THE INDIAN NATION, WE MUST RESIST THESE SPIRITS OF DEATH.

U.S. Dept. of Health and Human Services

Posters are widely used to communicate messages about the dangers of alcohol and drug abuse. Sometimes these posters deal with specific drugs and are directed at specific groups that might be at risk for drug use. This poster focuses on inhalants and is directed at Native American youths and young adults. Copies of similar posters are available from the U.S. Office of Substance Abuse Prevention, P.O. Box 2345, Rockville, MD 20852.

emphasizing moderate consumption, fails to account for the value and pleasure many people attach to heavier drinking. A third concern with the model is that it assumes attitudinal changes in the culture will result in the desired behavioral changes. There is no specification of the mechanisms by which that change will occur, however, and past research has provided no strong indication that attitudinal change leads to behavioral change. Finally, it is argued that the sociocultural model does not adequately consider physical problems associated with alcohol consumption (for example, cancers and liver and stomach ailments). In fact, some think that use of the sociocultural model may result in a greater prevalence of such physical problems, even if social problems are eliminated, simply by virtue of the widespread use of alcohol (Blane, 1976; Nirenberg & Miller, 1984; Skirrow & Sawka, 1987).

Despite these concerns, the sociocultural model remains an influential and frequently used strategy. When it is applied, the strategy has a broad scope. Examples of its applications include the advertising and education approaches to the problem of driving after drinking.

The sociocultural model has been applied predominantly in the context of alcohol-use problems, but it also has been a cornerstone to many prevention efforts geared toward problems associated with other drug use. As noted earlier, an example is the "Just Say No" campaign, which encourages people nationwide, but particularly young people, to refuse offers or temptations to use drugs. Another example is the advertising efforts of the Partnership for a Drug-Free America. The partnership's campaign, which focuses especially on marijuana, cocaine, and crack, seeks to decrease the social acceptance of drug use among young people and alert users or potential users to the risks of using drugs. Most of its communications are presented on television. To date, the effectiveness of these programs has not been documented. Furthermore, they may be limited in scope in that they generally are geared toward youth of middle and upper socioeconomic status. The only major difference between using the sociocultural model with drugs as opposed to alcohol is that the former application focuses on inculcating in society a norm of no use, as opposed to responsible use.

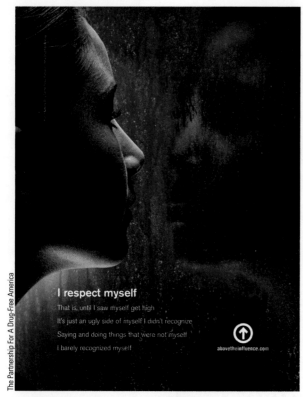

I respect myself
That is, until I saw myself get high
It's just an ugly side of myself I didn't recognize
Saying and doing things that were not myself
I barely recognized myself

The Partnership For A Drug-Free America

This poster is part of a series distributed through the AboveTheInfluence.com website, a program of the Office of National Drug Control Policy. According to the website, "Our goal is to help you stay above the influence. The more aware you are of the influences around you, the better prepared you will be to stand up to the pressures that keep you down."

"There is still a misguided notion that people can experiment with drugs with impunity. But we can't predict who will go on to develop dependence, and neither can the individual. It's essential that we get a consistent message across to young people that experimentation has its great risks."

Dr. Charles Schuster, National Institute on Drug Abuse Addiction Research Center (*The Journal*, October 1993)

Distribution of Consumption Model

The second major model of prevention is the distribution of consumption approach. This model has been studied predominantly in the context of prevention or reduction of alcohol problems, although efforts have been directed at extending it to other drugs (Skirrow & Sawka, 1987). The model is based on research showing a fairly consistent statistical distribution of alcohol consumption across cultures. The pioneering work in the development of the model was conducted by the French mathematician Sully Ledermann in the 1950s.

The distribution of consumption model has three central propositions (Rush & Gliksman, 1986; Schmidt & Popham, 1978). The first is that the proportion of heavy alcohol users in a given population is positively correlated with the mean level of alcohol consumption in that population. That is, the number of heavy drinkers in a society increases with the society's per capita consumption. Given this relationship, it is predicted that a decrease in average alcohol consumption within a given culture will be accompanied by a corresponding decrease in the proportion of heavy alcohol consumers.

The second proposition of the distribution of consumption model is that heavy alcohol consumption increases the probability of negative alcohol-related consequences, such as mental/emotional, physical, and social problems. If the population's mean consumption increases, and thus raises the number of heavy drinkers, a corresponding increase in these negative consequences is anticipated.

Finally, the model's third proposition is that societies should attempt to reduce the negative consequences of alcohol consumption by restricting the availability of alcohol. It is assumed that restricting alcohol availability, especially but not exclusively through procedures designed to raise the price of alcohol relative to disposable income, will lower per capita consumption and, correspondingly, the damages associated with alcohol use. Other approaches are limiting the hours that bars and taverns can be open, controlling retail sales of alcohol, and raising the minimum drinking age.

Although it is a well-regarded approach to prevention, the distribution of consumption model has its critics. Some think the model is purely descriptive and does not provide any insights into the reasons why people drink or how a person's drinking environment may contribute to drinking behavior. Skog (1985) has addressed this problem in more detail and noted that sociocultural variables such as the drinking environment actually can be incorporated into the distribution of consumption model. Whitehead (1975) has gone further in his discussion of the ways in which the sociocultural and distribution of consumption models might be used together.

Of more concern to critics is that "normal" drinkers in a population may react differently than "heavy" or "alcoholic" drinkers to efforts to reduce or restructure alcohol availability (Nirenberg & Miller, 1984). Again, the concern is that sociocultural and psychological variables are not included in the distribution of consumption model. For example, differences between normal drinkers and alcohol abusers may be crucial in predicting drinking behavior, with alcohol abusers perhaps being less likely to respond to price increases and other policies designed to decrease per capita consumption. Also, there may be a point at which these policies on restructuring alcohol use have no benefit. If, for example, the price of alcohol rises too much, the result may be an increase in bootlegging and home production of alcohol and in the mystique surrounding alcohol use (Skirrow & Sawka, 1987). As you can see, the task of reducing per capita consumption is complex.

The Partnership For A Drug-Free America

The "Check Yourself" media campaign, which includes this poster, encourages a self-evaluation of whether one is in control . . . or not. The campaign is operated through the Partnership for a Drug-Free America.

Proscriptive Model

This third prevention model is the most basic in principle. It takes a moral stance in addressing substance-use problems. The guiding theme is that if there is no use of the substance, then there can be no problem. If a person does use the substance, that use is not seen as a societal problem but instead as a product of a person's character flaw. The goals of the proscriptive model are prohibition of availability and abstention from use (Ibid., 1987).

The proscriptive model has been applied to both alcohol and other drug use. The most important application to alcohol use was Prohibition in the United States from 1920 to 1933. The model has been applied more consistently in the context of drug use, however. For decades, there has been a strong proscriptive approach to drug use, generally focused on marijuana and heroin and more recently on cocaine. The

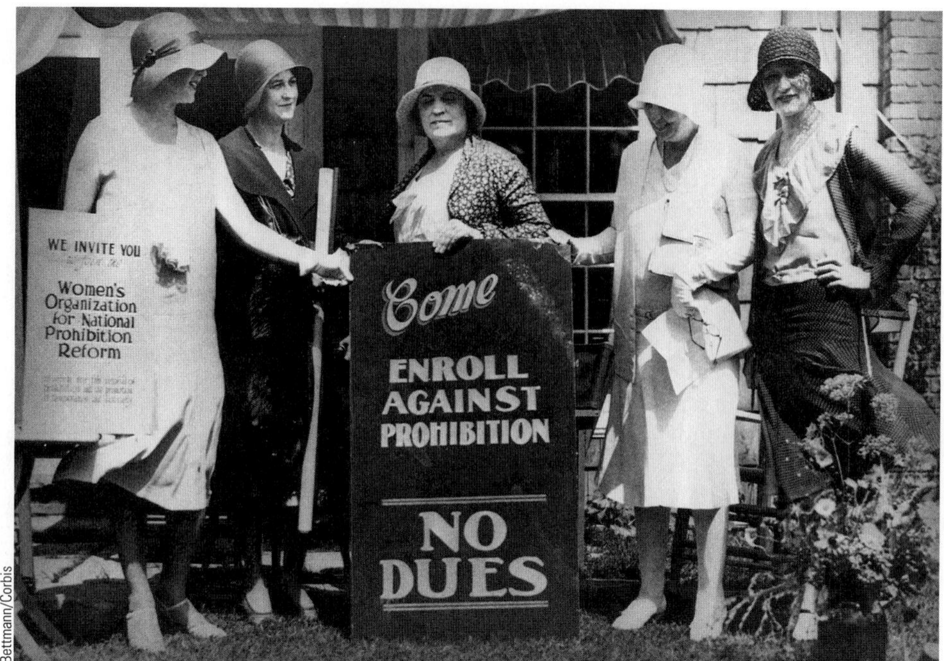
WE INVITE YOU
Women's Organization for National Prohibition Reform
Come
ENROLL AGAINST PROHIBITION
NO DUES

Bettmann/Corbis

An example of the application of the proscriptive model of prevention in the United States was Prohibition (1920–33). Public reaction to Prohibition was mixed. In this picture, taken in the 1920s, a group of women stand outside a house with signs inviting others to join their anti-Prohibition club.

proscriptive model in the 1930s and 1940s was most evident in films and newspaper and magazine articles aimed at mass audiences. Sensationalized stories about marijuana-induced crime sprees commonly were found in newspapers, and similar themes are evident in films from that era, such as *Reefer Madness, Assassin of Youth*, and *Marijuana: Weed with Roots in Hell*. Then, as now, the key to such campaigns has been that "good" people do not use drugs (Ibid.).

Although the proscriptive model remains popular with some, it has not made any significant contribution to the prevention of substance-abuse problems. It is well known that Prohibition was less than successful in alleviating problems associated with alcohol use, and other substance-use problems also have continued. Perhaps the major difficulty with the model is that it is too simple to tackle a complex problem.

Principles of Drug Abuse Prevention

The National Institute on Drug Abuse (NIDA) has developed a series of "prevention principles" relevant to the implementation of prevention programs for children and adolescents. The 16 principles, which are outlined in Table 16.1, were based on numerous research studies on the origins of drug-abuse behaviors and the common elements found in effective prevention programs. NIDA issued these principles for parents, educators, and community leaders to use in their thinking, planning, selection, and delivery of drug-abuse prevention programs.

As can be seen in Table 16.1, the principles fall under several broad domains. The first domain focuses on risk factors and protective factors, the second on the planning of prevention programs (including family programs, school-based programs, or broader community programs), and the third on the actual delivery of prevention programs.

CONTEMPORARY ISSUE BOX 16.1

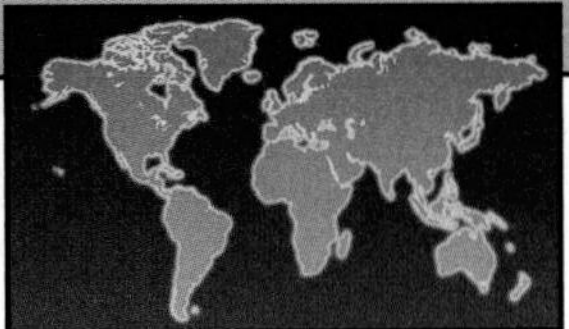

The Amethyst Initiative: Lowering the Legal Drinking Age to Decrease Alcohol Problems?

The Amethyst Initiative, launched in 2008, represents a movement by over 100 college presidents across the country to foster "an informed and dispassionate debate" (The Amethyst Initiative, www.amethystinitiative.org) on lowering the drinking age from 21 to 18 years of age as a strategy for reducing binge drinking on college campuses. The Initiative, which we discussed briefly in Chapter 9, also invites "new ideas about the best ways to prepare young adults to make responsible decisions about alcohol." (The word *amethyst*, by the way, is derived from the ancient Greek words meaning "not" [a-] and "intoxicated" [methustos]. According to legend, amethysts protected their owners from drunkenness.)

The foundation of the Amethyst Initiative is the argument that the minimum drinking age of 21, established in the mid-1980s by the National Minimum Drinking Age Act, has not served to decrease drinking- or alcohol-related problems among college students. According to their statement, the following were offered as premises:

> A culture of dangerous, clandestine "binge-drinking"—often conducted off-campus—has developed.
>
> Alcohol education that mandates abstinence as the only legal option has not resulted in significant constructive behavioral change among our students.
>
> Adults under 21 are deemed capable of voting, signing contracts, serving on juries, and enlisting in the military, but are told they are not mature enough to have a beer.
>
> By choosing to use fake IDs, students make ethical compromises that erode respect for the law. (The Amethyst Initiative, www.amethystinitiative.org)

A number of organizations and individuals are strongly opposed to the Amethyst Initiative, including Mothers Against Drunk Driving (MADD), the Governors Highway Safety Association, and several university presidents. The primary point they argue is that lowering the drinking age will result in greater alcohol consumption, more alcohol-related injuries, and more alcohol-related fatalities among those aged between 18 and 21.

There is no question, of course, that binge drinking on college campuses is a significant public health concern, and there should be focused debate on strategies for decreasing binge drinking. The specific proposal to lower the drinking age from 21 to 18 is understandably controversial. In pondering this issue, consider the following questions and issues.

First, raising the drinking age from 18 to 21 has been associated with significant decreases in alcohol-related motor vehicle accidents and fatalities in this age group (Fell et al., 2009; Wagenaar & Toomey, 2002). It is likely that lowering the drinking age from 21 to 18 will be associated with an increase in such accidents and fatalities. Relevant to this prediction, a study from New Zealand found that alcohol-related crashes rose 12% among 18- to 19-year-olds and 14% among 15- to 17-year-olds when the drinking age was lowered to 18 (Kypri et al., 2006).

Second, it is not clear that lowering the drinking age will decrease binge drinking among college students. In fact, there is the possibility that binge drinking will increase. For example, one potential scenario is that the rate of binge drinking remains unchanged among those who already are drinkers. At the same time, those currently between 18 and 20 who are not binge drinking might show an initiation of drinking, and of binge drinking, as a function of alcohol consumption becoming legal for their age group.

Third, it is likely that many college students who engage in binge drinking arrived at college with a previously established pattern of binge drinking. Changing the drinking age will not impact those individuals, who would have established this pattern prior to age 18.

Fourth, the debate would need to consider the impact of lowering the minimum drinking age on youth under the age of 18. A minimum drinking age of 18 would mean that high school seniors, who typically turn 18 during their senior year, would be able to purchase and consume alcohol (and illegally purchase it for younger high school students). This could have the unintended effect of facilitating alcohol consumption by younger adolescents. This has implications for the development of alcohol dependence, as research indicates that individuals who begin drinking prior to the age of 15 are four times more likely to meet the criteria for alcohol dependence at some point in their lives than are those who initiate drinking at an older age (Grant & Dawson, 1998).

Taken together, there should be strong encouragement of debate on strategies that have the potential for reducing binge drinking (and more generally facilitating responsible drinking decisions). It is not clear that lowering the drinking age will reduce binge drinking. Further, lowering the drinking age likely will result in an increase in alcohol-related motor vehicle accidents and fatalities and overall alcohol consumption in the 18- to 20-year-old age group.

TABLE 16.1 Principles of Drug Abuse Prevention

Risk Factors and Protective Factors

Principle 1: Prevention programs should enhance protective factors and reverse or reduce risk factors.

Principle 2: Prevention programs should address all forms of drug abuse, alone or in combination, including the underage use of legal drugs (e.g., tobacco or alcohol); the use of illegal drugs (e.g., marijuana or heroin); and the inappropriate use of legally obtained substances (e.g., inhalants), prescription medications, or over-the-counter drugs.

Principle 3: Prevention programs should address the type of drug-abuse problem in the local community, target modifiable risk factors, and strengthen identified protective factors.

Principle 4: Prevention programs should be tailored to address risks specific to population or audience characteristics, such as age, gender, and ethnicity, to improve program effectiveness.

Prevention Planning

Family Programs

Principle 5: Family-based prevention programs should enhance family bonding and relationships and include parenting skills; practice in developing, discussing, and enforcing family policies on substance abuse; and training in drug education and information.

School Programs

Principle 6: Prevention programs can be designed to intervene as early as *preschool* to address risk factors for drug abuse, such as aggressive behavior, poor social skills, and academic difficulties.

Principle 7: Prevention programs for *elementary school children* should target improving academic and social-emotional learning to address risk factors for drug abuse, such as early aggression, academic failure, and school dropout. Education should focus on the following skills: self-control; emotional awareness; communication; social problem solving; and academic support, especially in reading.

Principle 8: Prevention programs for *middle or junior high and high school students* should increase academic and social competence with the following skills: study habits and academic support; communication; peer relationships; self-efficacy and assertiveness; drug-resistance skills; reinforcement of antidrug attitudes; and strengthening of personal commitments against drug abuse.

Community Programs

Principle 9: Prevention programs aimed at general populations at key transition points, such as the transition to middle school, can produce beneficial effects even among high-risk families and children. Such interventions do not single out risk populations and therefore reduce labeling and promote bonding to school and community.

Principle 10: Community prevention programs that combine two or more effective programs, such as family-based and school-based programs, can be more effective than a single program alone.

Principle 11: Community prevention programs reaching populations in multiple settings—for example, schools, clubs, faith-based organizations, and the media—are most effective when they present consistent, communitywide messages in each setting.

Prevention Program Delivery

Principle 12: When communities adapt programs to match their needs, community norms, or differing cultural requirements, they should retain core elements of the original research-based intervention, which include: *structure* (how the program is organized and constructed); *content* (the information, skills, and strategies of the program); and *delivery* (how the program is adapted, implemented, and evaluated).

Principle 13: Prevention programs should be long-term with repeated interventions (e.g., booster programs) to reinforce the original prevention goals. Research shows that the benefits from middle school prevention programs diminish without follow-up programs in high school.

Principle 14: Prevention programs should include teacher training on good classroom management practices, such as rewarding appropriate student behavior. Such techniques help foster students' positive behavior, achievement, academic motivation, and school bonding.

Principle 15: Prevention programs are most effective when they employ interactive techniques, such as peer discussion groups and parent role-playing, that allow for active involvement in learning about drug abuse and reinforcing skills.

Principle 16: Research-based prevention programs can be cost-effective. Similar to earlier research, recent research shows that each dollar invested in prevention will bring about a savings of up to $10 in treatment for alcohol or other substance abuse.

Source: NIDA (2003).

The release of these prevention principles has been described as a landmark event in prevention science (Bukoski, 2003). In this regard, the principles summarized in practical terms what years of scientific study reveals about the nature of substance use and abuse and how to prevent it. As such, these principles have been influential in the development and implementation of a variety of prevention interventions.

Current Topics in Prevention

Prevention efforts are being implemented on a number of fronts, and in this section, we provide an overview of several contemporary topics and programs in primary and secondary prevention. (Notice that most of these prevention activities are derived predominantly from the sociocultural model.) We preface this section by highlighting the most noteworthy trends in prevention activities today:

- Increasing focus on having family (especially parental) involvement in prevention programs.
- Including attention to resistance-skills development, specifically strategies to use in avoiding pressures to use drugs.
- Developing programs in conjunction with more broad-based communitywide strategies—for example, a school-based intervention presented in conjunction with messages communicated through mass media outlets.
- Identifying subgroups of individuals most at risk for alcohol and other drug misuse and developing programs specifically for them—for example, inner-city youths, Native American youths, minority youths, and college students.
- Focusing attention on the "gateway" drugs. Almost all programs emphasize abstinence from all illegal substances, but some programs focus on not initiating the use of tobacco, alcohol, and marijuana in particular. These are viewed as "gateway" drugs, in that their use typically precedes the use of the so-called harder drugs such as cocaine, heroin, and LSD.
- Increasing attention to programs designed to minimize risk or negative consequences associated with any substance use that does occur. These risk-reduction programs do not sanction drug use but instead seek to minimize the negatives associated with such use for the individual and for society.
- Decreasing advertising geared toward (or readily accessible to) children and teenagers. Associated with this are efforts to reduce the positive portrayal of substance use (including smoking) in television shows and movies.

"Drug users must be seen as human beings and not as criminals."

Dr. Pat Erickson, criminologist with the Toronto Addiction Research Foundation (*The Journal*, October 1993)

You will observe these trends in many of the programs described next.

Education and Mass Media Efforts

mass media Communications designed for widespread distribution, such as advertisements, films, and printed materials.

By far the most common and pervasive approaches to substance-misuse prevention have been education and **mass media** efforts. Traditionally, these programs have been aimed at adolescents and young adults, two of the more visible groups at risk for substance abuse. More recently, efforts have been made to extend these interventions to children.

The school system has been touted as an ideal setting for providing educational materials on substance use and misuse. Indeed, most states now require education about alcohol and other drugs in the school curricula, although state laws unfortunately have not been translated in any systematic way into comprehensive instructional programs. In the past, programs were hampered by teachers who had not been sufficiently trained in alcohol and drug education materials. Major improvements have occurred in recent years, however, and programs have gradually become more and more systematized.

What happens when alcohol and drug education courses are implemented? The results have been mixed. The general outcome is that students presented with educational materials do increase their knowledge about the topics covered; however, there has not been much indication that patterns of substance use change (Bangert-Drowns, 1988; Botvin, 1999; Botvin & Griffin, 2003; Cellucci, 1984; Larimer & Cronce, 2007; Tobler, 1986). Indeed, in some cases (see Kinder, Pape, & Walfish, 1980; Stuart, 1974), students who were exposed to the education program were actually found in the short run to escalate their drug use! These findings should be viewed with caution until more systematic research on education programs has been conducted, especially research on the long-term effects of these interventions. Tentatively, though, increased knowledge about alcohol and other drugs does not necessarily translate into modifications in their use.

One factor that may contribute to these discouraging results is the age at which youths are exposed to the intervention. As a result of data indicating that young children have already begun to form ideas about intoxication, drinking behavior, and alcohol effects (Dunn & Goldman, 1996; Jahoda & Cramond, 1972; Zucker et al., 1996), more attention is being placed on educational materials geared toward children in early elementary school. Presenting materials for that level of development may be more successful than trying to modify beliefs at a later age when they are more firmly established. An example is research on smoking beliefs and behavior. Chen and Winder (1986) wanted to determine the best time to apply a smoking intervention program. They surveyed more than 500 6th, 9th, and 12th graders in a Massachusetts school system. The results showed that students are likely to respond best to a smoking education program in the 6th grade for several reasons. One is that fewer 6th graders (6.5%) described themselves as occasional or regular smokers than did 9th graders (21%) or 12th graders (32%). Sixth graders also reported much less peer pressure to smoke than the 9th or 12th graders, less knowledge about smoking and its effects, and less familiarity with their parents' attitudes about smoking. In addition, there were indications that many of the 6th graders surveyed were planning to smoke within the next five years. Consequently, aiming an education program at 6th grade students appears to hold the most promise for engendering attitudes against personal smoking.

A related trend in the area of prevention education, starting in the 1980s, has been the use of parents serving as teachers of their children. According to DuPont (1980), a former director of the National Institute on Drug Abuse, "It is ironic that after a decade of parent put-downs that we are today rediscovering that parents, who were written off as ignorant and meddlesome at best and as 'the problem' at worst, are now 'the solution' to drug problems" (p. 2). This statement might be overstating the point, but it does appear that parents can be an important—perhaps crucial—element in prevention activities. Much of this growing emphasis on parents during the last decade derives from the view that substance use is a family concern. These parent-focused programs seek to enhance family communication about alcohol and other drugs, to have parents model or foster either abstinence or responsible use of accepted substances (generally alcohol), and to encourage abstinence from other substances (Botvin & Botvin, 1992; Kimmel, 1976). One such program, called "The Power of Positive Parenting," includes a curriculum designed to make parents aware of the profound influence their behavior has on their children's behavior (Richmond, 1977). Children, especially in their preschool years, turn primarily to their parents when looking for models of appropriate behavior. The program aims to make parents aware of the ways they influence their children's beliefs about drugs and to help them determine what constitutes "responsible modeling" of, for example, drinking behavior. More recently, parents have been enlisted as agents in prevention efforts designed for incoming college freshmen students. In one application, parents of incoming freshmen students were provided with materials on talking to their teenage children about alcohol (Ichiyama et al., 2009). The parents implemented the intervention during the summer preceding their child's departure for college. The results showed that this parent-based intervention was associated with a decrease in the likelihood of transition into drinker status during the freshman academic year and, among the women, a slower growth in drinking over the freshman year.

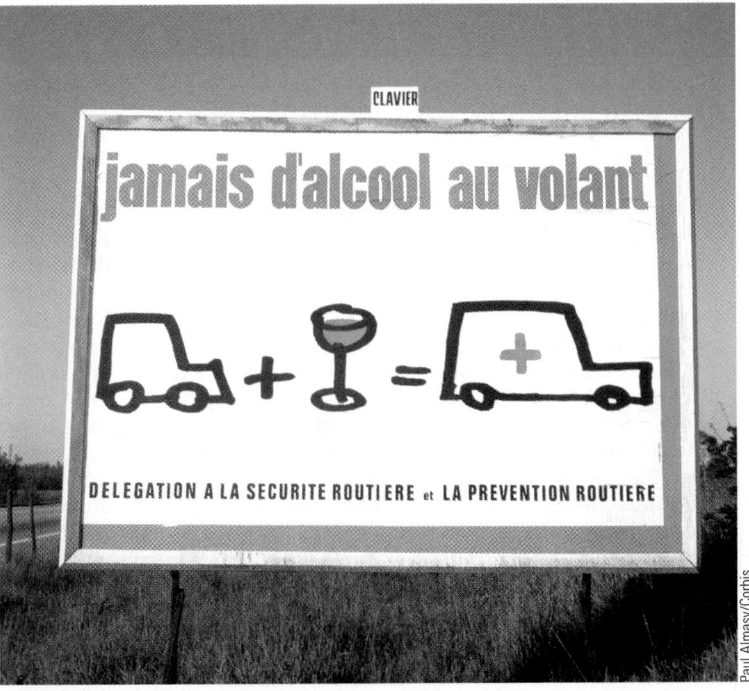

Billboards are an example of mass media prevention efforts. This roadside sign in France reminds motorists of the dangers of drinking and driving.

Broader educational efforts have been implemented using mass media technology. *Mass media* in this context refers to the widespread distribution of communications using such vehicles as television, radio, billboards, films, and printed material (including magazines). The most frequently used media, however, are television and radio, typically through what are called public service announcements (PSAs). Because mass media campaigns often involve frequent presentations of a relatively brief message (for example, a 15-second television spot), developers of these campaigns generally create a slogan that unites the material in the various spots. Slogans of some recent campaigns are "Just Say No" and "Cocaine: The Big Lie" for drugs and "Know When to Say When" and "Friends Don't Let Friends Drive Drunk" for alcohol. Most of the campaigns in recent years regarding alcohol abuse have focused on decreasing the incidence of driving under the influence.

Although research on mass media campaigns has not yielded a clear picture of their effects, the programs do succeed in raising knowledge levels and increasing awareness about the use of drugs (Blane, 1988; Botvin & Botvin, 1992; Gorman, 1995; Palmgreen & Donohew, 2003). Of particular note is the finding that campaigns on drunk driving consistently change the knowledge level (for example, knowing the legal definition of intoxication). As with other prevention approaches, attitude change has been found less consistently. There is no evidence, however, that general patterns of alcohol or drug use change significantly as a function of these mass media strategies. These approaches

CONTEMPORARY ISSUE BOX 16.2

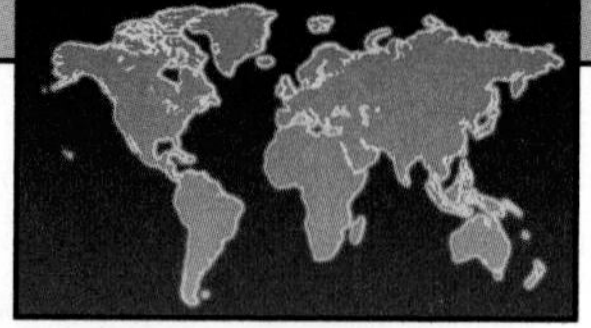

Warning Labels on Alcoholic Beverages

A form of education/mass media intervention directed at preventing alcohol-related problems is the placement of warnings at alcohol sales outlets and on alcoholic beverage containers. The idea behind the strategy is analogous to the reason labels are placed on cigarette packages.

For years, efforts to pass legislation to require alcohol warning labels had been unsuccessful, despite the endorsement of approximately a hundred health and public interest groups. However, such legislation became law in 1989. A bill passed by Congress now requires this warning on all alcohol beverage containers:

> Government Warning: (1) According to the Surgeon General, women should not drink alcoholic beverages during pregnancy because of the risk of birth defects. (2) Consumption of alcoholic beverages impairs your ability to drive a car or operate machinery and may cause health problems.

Research on warning labels suggests that consumers notice the labels (Mazis, Morris, & Swasy, 1991; Scammon, Mayer, & Smith, 1991). There has been little evidence that the labels have an effect on actual drinking behavior, however (Hilton, 1993; MacKinnon, 1995). It has been proposed that efforts be taken to evaluate the potential usefulness of warning labels in conjunction with other targeted prevention endeavors, such as specific television advertisements or programs with young adult drinkers.

Alcoholic beverage producers are less than supportive of warning labels. They argue that the information on the labels is common knowledge and unlikely to produce changes in drinkers' behavior. More basic, however, to their reservations is the issue of product liability. Some producers fear the use of the labels will open the door to lawsuits for drinkers' previous use of alcohol. On the other hand, argue proponents of the labeling, not placing the labels now, at a time when research supports the warnings, may result in even more lawsuits later.

The passage of the national labeling legislation goes beyond policies that already had been in place on a smaller scale in several cities. Since 1983, New York City, Philadelphia, Washington, DC, and Columbus, Ohio, among others, have passed city ordinances requiring posting of a sign where alcohol is sold indicating the relationship between drinking during pregnancy and the incidence of birth defects. Not all alcohol producers are against warning labels. For more than 25 years, Walter Stephen Taylor, a winemaker at Bully Hill Vineyards in upstate New York, placed warning labels on his products. He also testified at congressional hearings in favor of such labeling.

will more likely be successful if they are directed at particular substance-using groups. One example is the Montana Meth Project, designed to reduce methamphetamine use among children aged 12 to 17 (Montana Meth Project, 2008). Using graphic radio, television, and print/billboard advertisements, backed by increased enforcement and treatment availability, the state of Montana witnessed a dramatic decrease in meth use. In addition, Montana teenagers as a group had become much more wary of meth, relative to teens nationwide. The advertisement that was found to have greatest impact was a close-up picture of rotting teeth ("meth mouth"), often exhibited by chronic meth users.

Taken together, education and mass media approaches continue to command the majority of resources available for prevention. Their benefits appear to be primarily in the areas of knowledge and, to a lesser extent, attitude change. Their effectiveness is likely to increase as they tailor the campaign messages and efforts to target these campaigns to particular populations of drug users. And, of course, more work is needed to increase the likelihood that these approaches will result in actual changes in substance use.

Affect-Oriented Programs

Many prevention programs, and particularly those geared toward youths, incorporate what is called an "affective" component. This affective feature typically involves

values clarification and decision making. Values clarification activities include self-exploration, life values assessment, and strategies for fulfilling needs that are part of those values (Hewitt, 1982). These programs provide students with general strategies for making life choices and for applying these techniques to situations that involve alcohol or other drugs. The overall goal of the affect-oriented material is to have participants be aware of their own feelings and attitudes regarding drugs, so they can deal effectively with drug-use situations according to their individual value structures.

values clarification A common component of affect-oriented prevention programs; typically involves exploration of one's own needs and beliefs regarding drugs.

The logic behind the use of an affective component is that thoughts, feelings, attitudes, and values regarding alcohol and drugs can be just as important in drug-use situations as knowledge, and perhaps more so. As yet, we do not know the extent to which affect-oriented programs are beneficial. Unfortunately, indications to date suggest that such approaches do not have an impact on drug-use behavior (Botvin, 1999; Botvin & Griffin, 2003; Larimer & Cronce, 2007). As with educational programs, there has not been much well-designed research on the effects of affect-oriented interventions. The research that has been conducted does suggest, though, that such interventions help to clarify personal views on substance use. Popular in the 1970s and 1980s, these programs are used less frequently today, although some components of the affect-oriented programs have been incorporated in modified forms into contemporary programs.

Alternative Behaviors and Resistance-Skills Training

In recent years, there has been a significant growth in prevention programs that focus on developing alternatives to drug use or on developing skills to recognize and resist drug-use pressures. In developing alternatives to drug use, the objective is to provide people with the opportunity to engage in various productive activities (for example, sports, vocational training, hobbies) that have the same or more appeal than drug use. Although this strategy makes sense in theory, evaluations of these programs have not revealed any particular benefits in terms of substance-use behavior (Botvin & Botvin, 1992; Botvin & Griffin, 2003).

Resistance-skills training interventions, on the other hand, have shown more promise. As described by Flay (1985), these interventions often include some combination of the following informational and skill-building strategies:

- Developing problem-solving and decision-making skills
- Developing cognitive skills for resisting interpersonal and media-based (e.g., pro-drinking or pro-smoking) drug-use messages
- Increasing self-awareness and self-esteem
- Learning nondrug-use skills for dealing with anxiety and stress
- Enhancing interpersonal skills such as the ability to initiate a conversation
- Developing assertiveness skills such as the ability to express displeasure and anger and to communicate needs
- Understanding the relationship between drug use and health concerns

Typically in these programs, participants learn to be aware of social influences that lead to drug use and to use skills to resist these influences. For example, participants are exposed to strategies for refusing drugs when peers offer them. Often the programs include peers and peer leaders or coleaders. In summarizing the evaluation of resistance-skills training, Botvin and colleagues (Botvin, 1999; Botvin & Botvin, 1992; Botvin & Griffin, 2003) note some positive indications for several substances, including alcohol, marijuana, and especially cigarette smoking.

The most widely used resistance-oriented program in use today is DARE (Drug Abuse Resistance Education). The DARE curriculum, historically targeted at 5th and 6th grade students before they enter junior high school, has been modified for use with a wider range of students. The program is based on the assumption that students must be educated to recognize the dangers of substance use and to resist subtle as well as direct pressures to use drugs. Accordingly, the program is designed to train students to recognize and resist peer and other influences to experiment with drugs. The curriculum includes 15 to 20 modules, each led by a law enforcement officer and lasting 45 to 60 minutes. Modules focus on topics such as refusal skills, risk assessment, decision making, interpersonal and communication skills, critical thinking, and alternatives to substance use. Despite its widespread use, the DARE program has not fared well in research evaluations (see review by Botvin & Griffin, 2003). In response, the DARE organization has been modifying the program to include components that may be more successful in curtailing drug use among students exposed to the program (see Contemporary Issue Box 16.3).

"We talk about high-risk youth and families in the U.S., but I do not know of any continent that is not threatened by drug and alcohol abuse or misuse or any country not affected. We have youth at risk on a worldwide basis, families at risk on a worldwide basis. We have communities and institutions at risk on a worldwide basis, and we have nations at risk."

Dr. Benson Bateman, President of Human Resources Development Institute (*The Journal*, May 1993)

Worksite Programs

Substance-use problems among employees can be costly for employers in lost production, accidents, absenteeism, and thefts to support drug habits. Indeed, the total cost to the U.S. economy attributable to substance abuse is estimated to be more than $246 billion a year, with approximately 60% due to alcohol abuse and the remainder to other substance abuse (Harwood, Fountain, & Livermore, 1998). It has made sense to many employers to provide for early identification and intervention when an employee begins to show impairments due to drug use. Although part of the employer's motivation may be humanitarian, a central incentive frequently is to avoid losses in company productivity. The majority of the *Fortune* 500 companies and many smaller companies as well are using worksite programs.

CONTEMPORARY ISSUE BOX 16.3

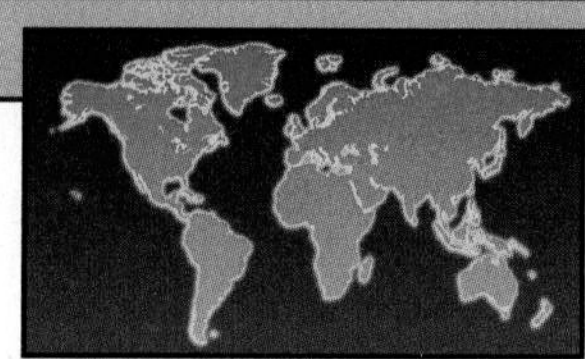

Dare We Question DARE?

Approximately three-quarters of the school systems in the United States have embraced the Drug Abuse Resistance Education (DARE) program, making it by far the most popular program in the nation. It has been endorsed by school officials, law enforcement agencies, and parents alike.

But is DARE getting the job done? Evaluations of the program over the past decade suggest probably not. The first strong indication appeared in 1994, when Ennett et al. published their summary of several DARE evaluation studies. Their conclusion: "DARE's short-term effectiveness for reducing or preventing drug use behaviors is small." Subsequent reports have provided a similar indication (Botvin & Griffin, 2003; West & O'Neal, 2004). In a 1999 study by Lynam et al., at a 10-year follow-up, it was found that students who had participated in DARE while in 6th grade did not have more successful outcomes than students not exposed to DARE.

If DARE is not the answer to helping students resist drugs, what is? The verdict there is still out, although encouraging results are emerging from evaluations of a program called Life Skills Training (LST). The LST program, developed by Gilbert Botvin of Cornell University Medical College, focuses on building students' drug-resistance abilities by helping them cope better with life's pressures. It keys on skills for being independent, gaining personal control, communicating effectively, relieving anxiety, overcoming shyness, and developing healthy friendships. The program has been found to curtail students' use of a variety of substances, including alcohol, cigarettes, and marijuana (e.g., Spoth et al., 2008).

It remains to be seen whether the current enthusiasm for DARE begins to wane and whether the program ultimately is markedly revamped or replaced by programs that have research support.

Worksite prevention programs have several potential advantages. One is their service to adults who still are functioning relatively well. As Nathan (1984) notes, these people still have their jobs and are more likely to be physically, psychologically, and economically healthy compared to those who have already lost jobs because of their substance abuse. Thus, they may be in a better position to respond to prevention opportunities. Other advantages, according to Nathan (1984), are that company employees are a captive audience, so it is easier to direct prevention-related messages to them. Employees do not have to travel outside the company to see or hear these messages. Finally, an employer implementing a program that benefits employees may improve employee morale, thus improving work performance.

One disadvantage to employers of worksite programs is the cost. Despite the possible payoff of enhanced employee functioning and reduced health care costs, some company executives are skeptical of the effectiveness of prevention programs or do not think program benefits outweigh program costs. Another problem is employees' concerns about confidentiality. Employees may hesitate to identify themselves as having problems with alcohol or other drugs for fear of being dismissed. A worksite prevention and intervention program is unlikely to be effective without stringent guidelines to protect the confidentiality of those the program is intended to help.

Prevention and intervention efforts, when they do occur, can take several forms. Primary prevention might include the use of posters and mailings that provide educational materials on drug problems. Some companies have used films and outside speakers to increase awareness of these problems. These strategies, which generally heighten awareness of substance use and its effects, also are intended to set the stage for employees who are abusing alcohol or drugs to decide to start treatment. This treatment phase represents a second tier of the prevention effort. It can take several forms. Frequently, the employee meets with an onsite counselor, who typically operates through

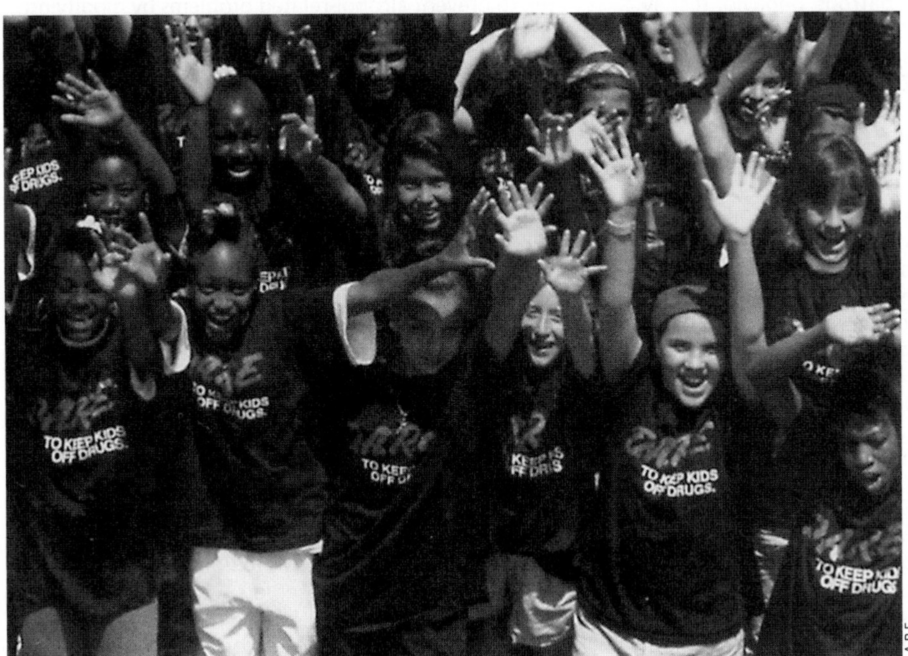

D.A.R.E.

The best-known resistance-oriented program in drug-use prevention is DARE (Drug Abuse Resistance Education). The program, traditionally targeted at fifth- and sixth-grade students, has been modified for use with a wider range of students.

what has been called an employee assistance program, or EAP. The counselor either works with the employee on the substance-use problem in that setting or arranges for the employee to participate in an outside treatment setting (for example, inpatient treatment or sessions with an outside counselor). Either separately or as part of one of these two treatment options, the counselor could encourage the employee to begin attending self-help groups, such as Alcoholics Anonymous or Cocaine Anonymous.

Although worksite programs have become increasingly prevalent in industrial settings (Lewis, 1991), their effectiveness rarely is evaluated. In addition, most current programs focus on secondary rather than primary prevention—that is, identifying alcohol or drug abusers and arranging for treatment. Only rarely is prevention a high priority within EAP programs or in the workplace more generally (Cook, 2003). When initiated, program approaches that appear to have particular potential include briefer interventions, interventions provided within a broader health and lifestyle program, psychosocial skills training, and peer referral (Webb et al., 2009).

Programs for College Students

Abuse of alcohol—whether chronic or sporadic—long has been a problem on college campuses. Studies on collegiate drinking practices have consistently documented a

CONTEMPORARY ISSUE BOX 16.4

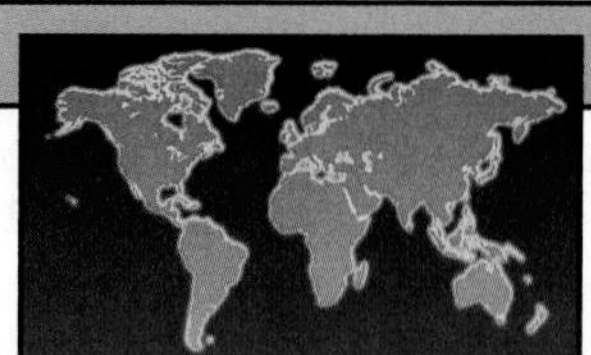

Server Interventions

Holding people who serve alcohol to patrons or guests responsible for the patrons' behavior if they become intoxicated is not a new idea. Its roots are in what are referred to as dram shop (an old English term for "taverns") laws. These laws, which in various forms are active and being upheld in courts today, have two implications. The first is that servers of alcohol, whether a bartender or the host of a private dinner party, can in some circumstances be held liable for the actions of intoxicated patrons or guests. The second implication, important in the context of prevention, is that servers and hosts can contribute to preventing alcohol-related problems through their decisions not to serve alcohol to people who are intoxicated. Indeed, the goal of model legislation for a uniform dram shop law is the prevention of alcohol-related injuries, deaths, and other damages (Mosher & Colman, 1986).

This model legislation has been enacted in a number of states and introduced in many others. Part of the legislation identifies practices that businesses and hosts may be able to use in preventing or limiting their liability in serving alcohol, such as encouraging patrons or guests not to become intoxicated if they consume alcohol, providing nonalcoholic beverages and food, and promoting the use of safe transportation alternatives to preclude intoxicated drinkers from driving home. These guidelines are derived from a sociocultural framework of drug misuse in that they seek to prevent alcohol-related problems by modifying the context of the drinking to encourage safer drinking practices.

One important outcome of the dram shop legislation is that a variety of education and training programs have been developed to help alcohol servers and hosts detect intoxication and stop serving alcohol to people who appear intoxicated. There are indications that these programs can have positive effects (see Geller, Russ, & Delphos, 1987; Gliksman et al., 1993), but there are obstacles to their implementation, especially in business situations. For example, one frustrating experience occurred in working with alcohol servers in Atlantic City gambling casinos (Nathan, 1984; Nathan & Niaura, 1987). Nathan and his colleagues were asked to provide information on how to detect intoxication among patrons and how to stop serving them drinks (most of which were served free to the patrons if they were at a gambling table). Although servers did acquire these skills, the program eventually broke down because casino owners did not want their servers to cut off intoxicated patrons who still were gambling. Thus, servers were in a true bind. According to Nathan and Niaura (1987), servers would refuse drinks to intoxicated patrons and avoid legal liability, but at the same time, they might antagonize their employer if the patrons stopped gambling!

higher prevalence of alcohol use than in the general population and an apparent increase in the number of alcohol-related problems over the course of the past 20 years. Problems associated with student drinking include relationship difficulties, driving under the influence, involvement in arguments or fights, vandalism and other property destruction, and lowered grades. Both male and female drinkers are candidates to experience alcohol-related problems. Estimates are that 40% of college students are heavy drinkers, defined as having five or more drinks in a row in the past two weeks (O'Malley & Johnston, 2002). A "snapshot" of the *annual* consequences of college student drinking was recently developed by the Task Force of the National Advisory Council on Alcohol Abuse and Alcoholism and is presented in Table 16.2. It provides an overview of the staggering consequences of alcohol misuse among college students.

In addition to reviewing the available studies on college student drinking, the task force identified three primary constituencies that need to be addressed to change the culture of drinking on college campuses. The first is college students as individuals,

TABLE 16.2 A Snapshot of Annual High-Risk College Drinking Consequences

Death: 1,700 college students between the ages of 18 and 24 die each year from alcohol-related unintentional injuries, including motor vehicle crashes (Hingson et al., 2005).

Injury: 599,000 students between the ages of 18 and 24 are unintentionally injured under the influence of alcohol (Ibid.).

Assault: More than 696,000 students between the ages of 18 and 24 are assaulted by another student who has been drinking (Ibid.).

Sexual abuse: More than 97,000 students between the ages of 18 and 24 are victims of alcohol-related sexual assault or date rape (Ibid.).

Unsafe sex: 400,000 students between the ages of 18 and 24 had unprotected sex, and more than 100,000 students between the ages of 18 and 24 report having been too intoxicated to know whether they consented to having sex (Hingson et al., 2002).

Academic problems: About 25% of college students report academic consequences of their drinking, including missing class, falling behind, doing poorly on exams or papers, and receiving lower grades overall (Engs, Diebold, & Hanson, 1996; Presley, Meilman, & Cashin, 1996; Presley et al., 1996; Wechsler et al., 2002).

Health problems/suicide attempts: More than 150,000 students develop an alcohol-related health problem (Hingson et al., 2002), and between 1.2% and 1.5% of students indicate that they tried to commit suicide within the past year due to drinking or drug use (Presley, Leichliter, & Meilman, 1998).

Drunk driving: 2.1 million students between the ages of 18 and 24 drove under the influence of alcohol last year (Hingson et al., 2002).

Vandalism: About 11% of college student drinkers report that they have damaged property while under the influence of alcohol (Wechsler et al., 2002).

Property damage: More than 25% of administrators from schools with relatively low drinking levels and over 50% from schools with high drinking levels say their campuses have a "moderate" or "major" problem with alcohol-related property damage (Wechsler et al., 1995).

Police involvement: About 5% of four-year college students are involved with the police or campus security as a result of their drinking (Wechsler et al., 2002), and an estimated 110,000 students between the ages of 18 and 24 are arrested for an alcohol-related violation such as public drunkenness or driving under the influence (Hingson et al., 2002).

Alcohol abuse and dependence: 31% of college students met criteria for a diagnosis of alcohol abuse and 6% for a diagnosis of alcohol dependence in the past 12 months, according to questionnaire-based self-reports about their drinking (Knight et al., 2002).

Source: From *A Call to Action: Changing the Culture of Drinking at U.S. Colleges* (National Advisory Council on Alcohol Abuse and Alcoholism, 2002, updated 2007).

including at-risk and alcohol-dependent drinkers. The second is the student population as a whole. Finally, the third constituency identified is the college and the surrounding community. It was argued that the needs of each of these constituencies require assessment and attention in the development and implementation of prevention programs on college campuses.

Colleges have taken or are taking a variety of steps to address drinking among their students. Many of these are designed to change social norms regarding drinking among college students. According to Perkins (2002), students generally view their peers as more permissive in their personal attitudes toward drinking than is actually the case. Similarly, students view their peers as consuming alcohol more frequently and more heavily than is the norm. The concern surrounding these exaggerated perceptions of one's peers is that students may feel pressure or license to conform to these incorrect expectations of their peers, and thus drink heavier and/or more frequently.

Applying what has been termed a "social norms approach," many campuses have begun to disseminate information about actual drinking norms (Perkins, 2002; 2007). The dissemination is as wide as possible to maximize the prospects for reaching as

DRUGS AND CULTURE BOX 16.5

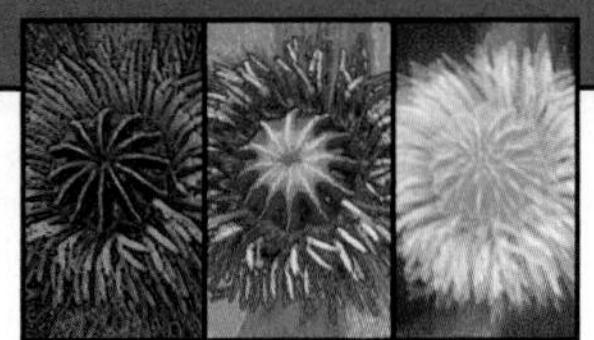

Harm-Reduction Social Policies

Countries vary widely in their social policies regarding substance use. You have read elsewhere in this book about the "war on drugs" and "zero-tolerance" policies in the United States. This stance is in striking contrast to another social policy strategy—called harm reduction or harm minimization—being implemented in some other countries, particularly the United Kingdom and the Netherlands. Harm-reduction policies focus on decreasing the negative consequences of drug use for individuals and the community, even if they endorse continued but safer drug use in the interim. According to Diane Riley at the Canadian Centre on Substance Abuse, "Harm reduction establishes a hierarchy of goals, with the more immediate and realistic ones to be achieved as first steps toward risk-free use or abstinence. It is a pragmatic approach, which recognizes that abstinence may be neither a realistic nor a desired goal for some, especially in the short term." Riley described two examples of harm-reduction policies. The first was in Merseyside in Great Britain. Health clinics collaborated with pharmacists and police officials to establish a "comprehensive approach [to drug abuse] involving prescription of drugs, provision of clean syringes and helping rather than criminalizing drug users." Among the reported benefits of the Merseyside collaboration were low incidence of HIV in drug users, continued employment for many drug abusers, and a decrease in thefts and robberies.

A second example is from Amsterdam, which sought to reduce drug-use harm by providing medical and social services to people who were continuing to use drugs. Among the strategies used were decreased police attention to marijuana possession and use and mobile methadone distribution stations. Prison terms apply only to dealers of hard drugs. An appreciation of the potential benefits of a harm-reduction orientation has been shown more recently in its use in school-based interventions to reduce harm associated with alcohol use (McBride et al., 2004) and smoking (Hamilton et al., 2005). In both cases, the use of a harm-reduction approach was superior to standard education/abstinence-based programs.

The policy of harm reduction has not been fully embraced in the United States (see Marlatt, Larimer, Baer, & Quigley, 1993), but some such strategies are being implemented. First was the introduction of methadone maintenance programs throughout the country in the 1960s. These programs were implemented in part to reduce crime rates among heroin users. A second strategy, more recently implemented, is needle-exchange programs designed to reduce the risk of HIV transmission among drug abusers. Both of these strategies have had their vocal opponents, however. There has been serious opposition to needle-exchange programs, despite research indicating that intravenous drug users who participate in such programs do not show an increase in the number of injections and that there has been no associated increase in the number of addictions. Nevertheless, a broad-based harm-reduction approach to the problems of drug use in the United States is gradually emerging.

many students as possible. Examples include publicizing the actual norms in orientation programs, student newspapers and websites, lectures, radio stations, and campus flyers and posters. The results from evaluations of such efforts have been very promising. Perkins (2002) reported that campuses with programs that have persistently communicated accurate norms about students' alcohol use have witnessed significant decreases in high-risk drinking, although the approach is not without its critics (Wechsler et al., 2003).

A second approach to tackling the problem of drinking among college students is exemplified in the work of Dr. Alan Marlatt and his colleagues at the University of Washington (Baer et al., 1994; Kivlahan et al., 1990). In contrast to the campuswide dissemination of information on real drinking norms, their focus has been on working with students (individually or in small groups) to develop skills that can be used to avoid the problematic use of alcohol. In this regard, their program includes four central components: (1) training in blood alcohol level–monitoring to acquire knowledge about specific alcohol effects, (2) developing coping skills to use in situations associated with risky or heavy drinking, (3) modifying expectations regarding alcohol use and alcohol effects, and (4) developing stress-management and other life-management skills.

Results from the University of Washington program have been impressive and encouraging. For example, from before to after the eight-week program, students in the skills-training program showed decreases on three measures of alcohol consumption: number of drinks per week, peak blood alcohol level reached per week, and hours per week with a blood alcohol level exceeding 0.055% (recall that a level of 0.08% is considered legally intoxicated in most of the United States). These decreases were not observed in other students who only participated in an assessment phase or only attended an alcohol education class that emphasized alcohol effects. Most important, the changes observed among the students who received the skills-training program were still evident 12 months after the intervention (Baer et al., 1994).

Closing Comments on Prevention

Prevention of alcohol and drug abuse is a topic that almost everyone acknowledges as being central to any coherent response to alcohol and drug problems in this country. Unfortunately, the area has been allocated few resources, at least in comparison to the monies spent annually on the treatment of alcohol and drug abuse. Although past efforts at prevention, especially education and mass media approaches, have increased relevant knowledge, they have had much less effect on alcohol and drug use. Especially critical in future research on prevention will be the design and evaluation of programs for specific cultural subgroups, the creation of programs geared toward the specific developmental levels of children and teenagers, parental involvement programs, and programs aimed at providing alternatives to alcohol and drug use. Full exploration of these possibilities requires more resources from state and federal agencies than have been available so far.

Summary

- Most people agree that prevention efforts should be an important component of any comprehensive approach to substance abuse, but professionals and funding sources have not made prevention efforts a high priority.
- Prevention traditionally has been divided into three types of intervention: primary, secondary, and tertiary.
- Primary prevention refers to efforts that focus on avoiding substance use or abuse before it occurs.

- Secondary prevention involves early interventions designed to address substance abuse just as problems are beginning to appear.
- Tertiary prevention, which actually is more treatment than prevention, includes intervention used to treat people beyond the early stages of substance abuse.
- The sociocultural model of prevention, probably the dominant approach in the United States, posits that social norms directly influence substance use. Prevention efforts derived from this model try to influence the entire climate of drinking within a culture.
- Another major prevention model is the distribution of consumption approach, which posits (1) that the proportion of heavy drinkers in a culture is positively related to the mean level of alcohol consumption, (2) that heavier alcohol consumption increases the probability of alcohol problems, and (3) that societies should attempt to reduce the negative consequences of drinking by reducing alcohol consumption across the culture.
- A third model of prevention is the proscriptive approach, which focuses on prohibiting the availability of substances and emphasizes abstention from drug use.
- The most common substance-abuse prevention interventions have been education and the use of mass media. Most states now require alcohol and drug education in school curricula.
- Alcohol and drug education courses generally have been shown to increase knowledge levels but have not been so successful in changing substance-use patterns.
- In recent years, there has been an increasing use of parents in prevention programs, especially in programs that focus on children.
- Mass media campaigns appear to succeed in raising levels of knowledge and awareness about drugs. Changes in attitudes and actual drug-use behavior have not been found so consistently.
- Prevention programs with a resistance-training approach have received much attention in recent years. These programs focus on training young people to recognize and resist pressures to use drugs.
- Prevention programs are sometimes located at worksites, where the goal is to identify drug abusers and to intervene when drug problems interfere with job performance. These programs, when established, generally concentrate more on secondary than on primary prevention.
- A variety of prevention programs, generally aimed at alcohol use, have been established on college campuses.
- The full potential of prevention interventions has not yet been tested. But before this potential can be assessed, more resources from state and federal agencies are needed.

Answers to "What Do You Think?"

1. Primary prevention includes interventions to treat people who are beyond the early stages of substance abuse or dependence.
   F *Primary prevention refers to the avoidance of substance abuse before it has the chance to occur. Tertiary prevention is the treatment of individuals already engaged in substance abuse.*
2. One strength of the sociocultural model of prevention is its emphasis on reducing the physical problems associated with alcohol consumption.
   F *This model has been criticized for not adequately taking these problems into account. Some believe that using the sociocultural model may result in a greater prevalence of such problems.*
3. Raising the price of alcohol relative to disposable income and limiting the hours of operation for bars are examples of prevention strategies based on the distribution of consumption model.
   T *This model posits that the proportion of heavy drinkers in a given population increases with the mean level of alcohol consumption in that population. Therefore, methods to lower per capita consumption should lead to a decrease in the prevalence of heavy drinking.*
4. The proscriptive model of prevention, which involves prohibiting the availability of drugs and promoting abstention from use, has proven to be the most effective of the three major models of prevention.

F *This model has not made any significant contribution to the prevention of substance abuse. One example of this approach was Prohibition, which was less than successful in alleviating problems associated with alcohol use.*

5. The main proponents of warning labels on alcoholic beverages have been the manufacturers of these beverages.

F *Most alcohol manufacturers have opposed these labels. They think that the information on the labels is common knowledge and that the labels may open the door to lawsuits associated with drinkers' previous use and abuse of alcohol.*

6. Research evidence indicates that mass media prevention strategies do not result in significant changes in patterns of alcohol or drug use.

T *Although evidence suggests that these programs do succeed in raising knowledge levels and increasing awareness about the use of drugs, there is no evidence that changes in patterns of use are occurring.*

7. The primary goal of affect-oriented prevention programs is to increase the individual's knowledge base regarding drugs and alcohol.

F *The goal of affect-oriented programs is to help participants be aware of their own feelings and attitudes regarding drugs so they can deal effectively with drug-use situations according to their individual value structures.*

8. Research evidence has documented the effectiveness of DARE, the most popular school-based drug prevention program.

F *Evaluations of DARE actually have not provided evidence that the program has had much impact on drug-use behaviors.*

9. The focus of most workplace prevention programs is primary prevention.

F *Most current programs focus on secondary rather than primary prevention. Prevention efforts are typically grafted onto treatment programs.*

10. One disadvantage of workplace prevention programs is their cost.

T *Many executives are skeptical of the efficacy and cost-effectiveness of these programs despite the potential of enhanced employee productivity.*

11. The idea of holding people who serve alcohol responsible for the patrons' behavior if they become intoxicated is a recent development in drinking moderation strategies.

F *This idea has its roots in what are referred to as dram shop (old English for "tavern") laws. Various forms of these laws have been enacted in several states and are being considered in many others.*

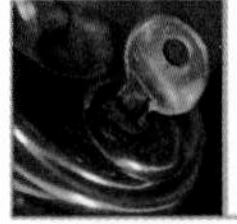

Key Terms

mass media
primary prevention
secondary prevention
tertiary prevention
values clarification

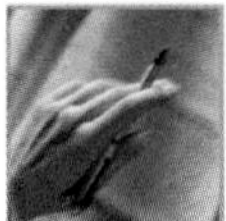

Essays/Thought Questions

1. Why do many prevention programs have modest, if any, effect on decisions by youths to use or not use drugs?
2. There has been increasing concern about "binge" drinking among college students. If you were designing a program to prevent or reduce binge drinking, what would be the most important elements you would include?
3. The Amethyst Initiative is intended to foster discussion on lowering the drinking age, among other approaches, to decrease alcohol-related problems among college students. Considering the arguments and implications on both sides of the issue, where do you stand and why?

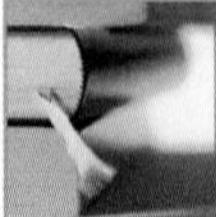

Suggested Readings

Ennet, S. T., Tobler, N. S., Ringwalt, C. L., & Flewelling, R. L. (1994). How effective is drug abuse resistance education? A meta-analysis of Project DARE outcome. *American Journal of Public Health, 84*, 1394–1401.

Larimer, M. E., & Cronce, J. M. (2007). Identification, prevention, and treatment revisited: Individual-focused college drinking prevention strategies 1999–2006. *Addictive Behaviors, 32*, 2439–2468.

National Advisory Council on Alcohol Abuse and Alcoholism. (2002). *A call to action: Changing the culture of drinking at U.S. colleges*. Bethesda, MD: National Institute on Alcohol Abuse and Alcoholism (NIH Publication No. 02-5010).

National Institute on Drug Abuse (NIDA). (2003). *Preventing drug abuse among children and adolescents: A research-based guide for parents, educators, and community leaders* (2nd ed.). NIDA: Bethesda, MD.

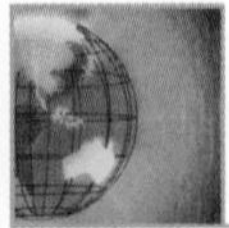

Web Resources

Visit the Book Companion Website at www.cengage.com/psychology/maisto to access study tools including a glossary, flashcards, and web quizzing. You will also find links to the following resources:

- Partnership for a Drug-Free America
- Center for Substance Abuse Prevention
- College drinking prevention
- Drug Abuse Resistance Education
- The Amethyst Initiative

GLOSSARY

Absorbed When drugs have entered the bloodstream (Chapter 4).

Acetaminophen (ə-'sē-tə-'mi-nə-fən) Aspirin-like analgesic (Chapter 14).

Acetylcholine (ə-'se-tᵊl-'kō-lēn) A neurotransmitter linked with memory processes that is found both in the brain and in the parasympathetic branch of the autonomic nervous system (Chapter 3).

Acetylsalicylic acid (ə-'sē-təl-'sa-lə-'si-lik) Chemical name for aspirin (Chapter 14).

Action potential The electrical impulse along the axon that occurs when a neuron fires (Chapter 3).

Acute tolerance A type of functional tolerance that occurs within a course of action of a single drug dose (Chapter 5).

Addiction In reference to drugs, overwhelming involvement with using a drug, getting an adequate supply of it, and having a strong tendency to resume use of it after stopping for a period (Chapter 1).

Addictive personality The hypothesis of a personality structure common to all people with substance-use disorders (Chapter 5).

Aftercare In alcohol and drug treatment, therapeutic activities following the completion of a formal treatment program (Chapter 15).

Agitated depression Depressed mood accompanied by a state of tension or restlessness. People with agitated depression show excessive motor activity, as they may, for example, be unable to sit still or may pace, wring the hands, or pull at their clothes (Chapter 13).

Agonist ('a-gə-nist) A substance that occupies a neural receptor and causes some change in the conductance of the neuron (Chapter 3).

Akinesia Slowness of movement and underactivity (Chapter 13).

Alzheimer's disease ('älts-'hī-mərz-) One of the most common forms of senility among the elderly; involves a progressive loss of memory and other cognitive functions (Chapter 3).

Amotivational syndrome Loss of effectiveness and reduced capacity to accomplish conventional goals as a result of chronic marijuana use (Chapter 11).

Amphetamines Central nervous system stimulants that act like naturally occurring adrenaline (Chapter 2).

Anabolic steroids Tissue-building drugs that produce masculinizing effects as well (Chapter 14).

Analgesia Pain relief produced without a loss of consciousness (Chapter 10).

Anandamide A lipid neurotransmitter mimicked by marijuana (Chapter 3).

Anorectic effects Causing one to lose appetite; suppression of eating (Chapter 6).

Antagonism The diminished or reduced effect of a drug when another drug is present (Chapter 4).

Antagonist A substance that occupies a neural receptor and blocks normal synaptic transmission (Chapter 3).

Anterograde amnesia Loss or limitation of the ability to form new memories (Chapter 13).

Anticholinergic hallucinogens A class of drugs including atropine and scopolamine (Chapter 12).

Antihistamines Common over-the-counter drugs with decongestant effects (Chapter 14).

Antitussives Cough-suppressant drugs (Chapter 14).

Anxiolytic Anxiety-reducing (Chapter 13).

Apothecary A pharmacist (Chapter 11).

As a function of A term expressing causality. In graphs of functional relationships between two variables, changes in one variable (for example, drug effect) associated with changes in another (drug dose) are represented (Chapter 4).

Atropine An anticholinergic hallucinogen found in certain plants (Chapter 12).

Attention deficit/hyperactivity disorder A disorder with features such as a greater-than-normal amount of activity, restlessness, difficulty concentrating or sustaining attention, and impulsivity (Chapter 5).

Autonomic nervous system (ANS) Part of the PNS; has two branches: sympathetic and parasympathetic (Chapter 3).

Avoirdupois Something sold or measured by weight based on 1 pound equaling 16 ounces (Chapter 2).

Axon ('ak-'sän) A long cylindrical extension of the cell body of the neuron; conducts an electrical charge from the cell body to the axon terminals (Chapter 3).

Axon terminals (or terminal buttons) Enlarged buttonlike structures at the ends of axon branches (Chapter 3).

Barbiturates Depressant drugs formerly used as sleeping pills; currently used in anesthesia and treatment for epilepsy (Chapter 13).

Basal ganglia ('bā-səl-'gaŋ-glē-ə) Forebrain structures important for motor control; include the caudate nucleus, the putamen, and the globus pallidus (Chapter 3).

Behavioral pharmacology The specialty area of psychopharmacology that concentrates on drug use as a learned behavior (Chapter 5).

Behavioral tolerance Adjustment of behavior through experience in using a drug to compensate for its intoxicating effects (Chapter 5).

Benzodiazepines Currently the most widely prescribed anxiolytic drugs (Chapter 13).

Beta-blockers Drugs that block beta-adrenergic receptors of the sympathetic system and thus act to relieve high blood pressure (Chapter 3).

Bioavailability The portion of the original drug dose that reaches its site of action or that reaches a fluid in the body that gives it access to its site of action (Chapter 4).

Blackout Failure to recall events that occurred while drinking even though there is no loss of consciousness (Chapter 9).

Blood-brain barrier The system that "filters" the blood before it can enter the brain (Chapter 3).

Brand name The commercial name given to a drug by its manufacturer (Chapter 5).

Cannabinoids The more than 60 chemical compounds present in cannabis. One is delta-9-tetrahydrocannabinol (better known as THC) (Chapter 11).

Cannabis sativa The Indian hemp plant popularly known as marijuana; its resin, flowering tops, leaves, and stem contain the plant's psychoactive substances (Chapter 2).

Causal relationship A relationship between variables in which changes in a second variable are due directly to changes in a first variable (Chapter 5).

Central nervous system (CNS) The brain and the spinal cord (Chapter 3).

Cerebellum ('ser-ə-'be-ləm) Hindbrain structure important in motor control and coordination (Chapter 3).

Chemical name The name given to a drug that represents its chemical structure (Chapter 5).

Combination pill Birth control pill that contains synthetic forms of both female sex hormones: progesterone and estrogen (Chapter 14).

Computerized axial tomography (CT) Technique that produces a three-dimensional X-ray image of the brain (Chapter 3).

Confabulation A fabrication of events, when asked questions concerning them, because of an inability to recall (Chapter 9).

Conflict paradigm A research procedure that concerns the effects on a behavior of a drug that has a history of both reinforcement and punishment (Chapter 5).

Control In research, to be able to account for variables that may affect the results of a study (Chapter 4).

Control group The reference or comparison group in an experiment. The control group does not receive the experimental manipulation or intervention whose effect is being tested (Chapter 5).

Cortex The outermost and largest part of the human brain (Chapter 3).

Counseling In alcohol and drug treatment, counselors are specially trained professionals who perform a variety of treatment activities, including assessment, education, and individual, marital, and family counseling (Chapter 15).

Crack A freebase cocaine produced by mixing cocaine salt with baking soda and water. The solution is then heated, resulting in brittle sheets of cocaine that are "cracked" into small smokable chunks or "rocks" (Chapter 6).

Craving A term that has been variously defined in reference to drug use; typically a strong or intense desire to use a drug (Chapter 1).

Cross-tolerance Tolerance to a drug or drugs never taken that results from protracted tolerance to another drug or drugs (Chapter 5).

Delta-9-tetrahydrocannabinol The principal active cannabinoid in marijuana responsible for the psychoactive effects (Chapter 11).

Dendrites ('den-'drīts) Spiny branchlike structures that extend from the cell body of a neuron; typically contain numerous receptor sites, and are thus important in neural transmission (Chapter 3).

Diffusibility A more diffusible substance is more easily entered into or "receptive" of another (Chapter 4).

Dispositional tolerance An increase in the rate of metabolizing a drug as a result of its regular use (Chapter 5).

Dissociative anesthetic A class of drugs including PCP and ketamine (Chapter 12).

Dissolved When a drug changes from solid to liquid by mixing it with a liquid (Chapter 4).

Distillation The process by which the heating of a fermented mixture increases its alcohol content (Chapter 9).

Distribution The transport of drugs by the blood to their site(s) of action in the body (Chapter 4).

Disulfiram A drug that interferes with the metabolism of alcohol so that people soon feel very ill if they drink while on a regimen of disulfiram. The drug may be used as part of a treatment program for alcohol dependence (Chapter 9).

Dopamine ('dō-pə-'mēn) A neurotransmitter in the brain that is involved with movement and reward (Chapter 3).

Drug Broadly defined as any chemical entity or mixture of entities not required for the maintenance of health but that alters biological function or structure when administered (Chapter 1).

Drug abuse Any use of drugs that causes physical, psychological, legal, or social harm to the individual user or to others affected by the drug user's behavior (Chapter 1).

Drug discrimination study A research procedure that primarily concerns the differentiation of drug effects (Chapter 5).

Drug dosage Measure of the quantity of drug consumed (Chapter 1).

Drug effects The action of a drug on the body. Drug effects are measured in different ways (Chapter 1).

Drug expectancy A person's anticipation of or belief about what he or she will experience upon taking a drug (Chapter 5).

Drug potency The minimum effective dose of a drug (Chapter 4).
Dyskinesia Disordered movements (Chapter 13).

Effective dose The dose at which a given percentage of individuals show a particular effect of a drug (Chapter 4).
Efficacy The most intense, or peak, level of a drug effect (Chapter 4).
Electroencephalography (EEG) Technique used to measure electrical activity in the brain (Chapter 3).
Emphysema Disease of the lung characterized by abnormal dilution of its air spaces and distension of its walls. Frequently, heart action is impaired (Chapter 7).
Endogenous Developed from within. When applied to depression, the term means that depressive symptoms seem to be due to genetic factors (Chapter 13).
Endorphins (en-'do˙r-fənz) Neurotransmitters in the brain that are mimicked by opiate drugs (Chapter 3).
Enzyme breakdown One process by which neurotransmitters are inactivated. Chemicals called enzymes interact with the transmitter molecule and change its structure so that it no longer is capable of occupying receptor sites (Chapter 3).
Estrogen ('es-trə-jən) One of the female sex hormones involved in the regulation of ovulation and the menstrual cycle (Chapter 14).
Exogenous Developed from without. When applied to depression, the term means that depressive symptoms seem to be in reaction to a particular situation or event (Chapter 13).
Extrapyramidal Outside the pyramidal tracts, with origin in the basal ganglia. These cell bodies are involved with starting, stopping, and smoothing out movements (Chapter 13).

Feedback In this context, in a series of events, what happens in a later event alters events that preceded it (Chapter 4).
Fermentation A combustive process in which yeasts interact with the sugars in plants such as grapes, grains, and fruits to produce an enzyme that converts the sugar into alcohol (Chapter 2).
Flashback A sudden recurrence of an LSD-like experience (Chapter 12).
Forebrain The largest part of the human brain; includes the cerebral cortex, thalamus, hypothalamus, and limbic system (Chapter 3).
Formication syndrome Symptoms of itching and feeling as if insects were crawling on skin, caused by cocaine and amphetamine (Chapter 6).
Freebase When a substance is separated, or "freed," from its salt base. The separated form of the substance is thus called "freebase" (Chapter 4).
Functional tolerance Decreased behavioral effects of a drug as a result of its regular use (Chapter 5).

GABA Short for gamma-aminobutyric acid; the most abundant inhibitory neurotransmitter in the brain (Chapter 3).
General anesthesia The reduction of pain by rendering the subject unconscious (Chapter 13).
Generalizable Applicability of a research finding from one setting or group of research participants to another (Chapter 5).
Generic name The general name given to a drug that is shorter (and easier for most people to say) than its chemical name (Chapter 5).
Glutamate An excitatory amino acid neurotransmitter (Chapter 3).
Grain As a measure, a unit of weight equal to 0.0648 gram (Chapter 1).
Group design A type of experimental design in which groups (as compared to individual cases) of subjects are compared to establish experimental findings (Chapter 5).
Guaifenesin (gwī-'fen-ə-sin) An over-the-counter expectorant (Chapter 14).

Half-life The amount of time that must pass for the amount of drug in the body to be reduced by half (Chapter 4).
Hash oil A potent distillate of marijuana or hashish. It first appeared in the United States in 1971 and can contain up to 60% THC (Chapter 11).
Hashish A drug produced from the resin that covers the flowers of the cannabis hemp plant. The resin generally contains a greater concentration of the drug's psychoactive properties (Chapter 2).
Heroin A drug produced by chemically processing morphine. It is more potent than morphine and has become the major opiate drug of abuse (Chapter 10).
Hindbrain The lower part of the brain, including the medulla, pons, and cerebellum (Chapter 3).
Hippocampus ('hi-pə-'kam-pəs) A structure of the limbic system thought to be important in the formation of memories (Chapter 3).
Homeostasis A state of equilibrium or balance. Systems at homeostasis are stable; when homeostasis is disrupted, the system operates to restore it (Chapter 5).
Hypothalamus ('hī-pō-tha-lə-məs) Forebrain structure that regulates eating, drinking, and other basic biological drives (Chapter 3).

Ibuprofen ('ī-byů-'prō-fən) Aspirin-like analgesic (Chapter 14).
Inferior colliculi (ko-'lik-yū-lī) Midbrain structures that control sound localization (Chapter 3).
Initial sensitivity The effect of a drug on a first-time user (Chapter 5).
Interact When the effects of one drug are modified by the presence of another drug (Chapter 4).

Intoxication A transient state of physical and psychological disruption caused by the presence of a toxic substance, such as alcohol, in the CNS (Chapter 9).

Ionotropic receptors Receptors that are coupled to ion channels and affect the neuron by causing those channels to open (Chapter 3).

Joint A hand-rolled marijuana cigarette (Chapter 11).

Ketamine A dissociative anesthetic (Chapter 12).

L-dopa ('el-'dō-pə) A chemical precursor of dopamine used in the treatment of Parkinson's disease (Chapter 3).

Lethal dose The dose of a drug at which a given percentage of individuals die within a specified time (Chapter 4).

Levo-alpha-acetylmethadol (LAAM) A drug used in treating heroin addiction that is similar in action to methadone but has longer-lasting effects (Chapter 15).

Limbic system Forebrain structures including the amygdala and hippocampus (Chapter 3).

Long-term memory Memory for remote events. According to one theory of memory, information enters long-term memory through short-term memory (Chapter 9).

Magnetic resonance imaging (MRI) Technique that creates a high-resolution, three-dimensional image of the brain (Chapter 3).

Manic Relating to mania, a mood disturbance that typically includes hyperactivity, agitation, excessive elation, and pressured speech (Chapter 13).

Mass media Communications designed for widespread distribution, such as advertisements, films, and printed materials (Chapter 16).

Medulla oblongata (mə-'də-lə-'ä-bl˙oŋ-gä-tə) The lowest hindbrain structure of the brain; important in the regulation of breathing, heart rate, and other basic life functions (Chapter 3).

Mescaline An LSD-like hallucinogen found in the peyote cactus (Chapter 12).

Mesolimbic dopaminergic pathway Pathway that is rewarding when stimulated (Chapter 3).

Metabolism The process by which the body breaks down matter into more simple components and waste (Chapter 4).

Metabotropic receptors Receptors that act through a second messenger system (Chapter 3).

Methylated amphetamines A class of drugs including MDA and MDMA (ecstasy) (Chapter 12).

Midbrain Part of the brain that includes the inferior and superior colliculi and the substantia nigra (Chapter 3).

Milieu treatment Treatment in which the organization and structure of a setting are designed to change behavior (Chapter 15).

Monoamines ('mä-nō-ə-'mēns) A class of chemicals characterized by a single amine group; includes the neurotransmitters norepinephrine, dopamine, and serotonin (Chapter 3).

Monoamine oxidase (MAO) inhibitors Drugs used to treat depressions that inhibit the activity of the enzyme monoamine oxidase, which degrades the neurotransmitters of norepinephrine and serotonin (Chapter 9).

Morphine A derivative of opium best known as a potent pain-relieving medication (Chapter 2).

Myelin ('mī-ə-lən) A fatty white substance that covers the axons of some neurons (Chapter 3).

Naloxone A short-acting opiate antagonist (Chapter 10).

Naproxen (nə-'prok-sən) Aspirin-like analgesic (Chapter 14).

Narcoleptic A state characterized by brief but uncontrollable episodes of sleep (Chapter 13).

Narcotic A central nervous system depressant that contains sedative and pain-relieving properties (Chapter 2).

Neuroleptics Tranquilizing drugs used to treat psychoses; a synonym is *major tranquilizer* (Chapter 13).

Neuromuscular junction Junction between neuron and muscle fibers where release of acetylcholine by neurons causes muscles to contract (Chapter 3).

Neurons ('nü-'räns) Individual nerve cells that are basic building blocks of the nervous system (Chapter 3).

Neuropsychological tests Formal ways of measuring behavioral functions that may be impaired by brain lesions (Chapter 9).

Neuroses Nonpsychotic emotional disturbance, pain, or discomfort beyond what is appropriate in the conditions of one's life (Chapter 13).

Neurotransmitters Chemical substances stored in the axon terminals that are released into the synapse when the neuron fires. Neurotransmitters then influence activity in postsynaptic neurons (Chapter 3).

Nicotine poisoning A consequence of nicotine overdose, characterized by palpitations, dizziness, sweating, nausea, or vomiting (Chapter 7).

Norepinephrine ('no˙r-'e-pə-'ne-frən) A neurotransmitter in the brain that is involved in activity of the sympathetic branch of the autonomic nervous system (Chapter 3).

Opium The dried sap produced by the poppy plant (Chapter 10).

Opium poppy A plant cultivated for centuries, primarily in Eurasia, for opium—a narcotic that acts as a central nervous system depressant (Chapter 2).

Orientation to time Awareness of temporal specification, such as time of day, day of the week, or year. Orientation to time is one of the functions assessed in a psychiatric mental status exam (Chapter 9).

Over-the-counter drugs Drugs that can be obtained legally without medical prescription (Chapter 1).

Paradoxical Contrary to what is expected. A paradoxical drug effect is opposite in direction to what is expected based on the drug's chemical structure (Chapter 5).

Paranoid schizophrenia A type of schizophrenia distinguished by systematic delusions or auditory hallucinations related to one theme (Chapter 13).

Parasympathetic branch Branch of the ANS that is responsible for lowering heart rate and blood pressure (Chapter 3).

Parkinson's disease A disease that primarily afflicts the elderly and involves a progressive deterioration of motor control (Chapter 3).

Patent medicines Products that were sold, most often in the 19th century, as medicines that would cure a host of illnesses and diseases (Chapter 2).

Peripheral nervous system (PNS) Sensory nerves, motor nerves, and the autonomic nervous system (Chapter 3).

Personality disorders Long-standing patterns of behavior that frequently create distress for individuals due to their personal or social consequences; usually recognizable from adolescence or earlier (Chapter 15).

Peyote (pā-'ō-tē) A cactus plant, the top of which (a "button") is dried and ingested for its hallucinogenic properties (Chapter 2).

Pharmacodynamics The branch of pharmacology that concerns the biochemical and physiological effects of drugs and their mechanisms of action (Chapter 4).

Pharmacokinetics The branch of pharmacology that concerns the absorption, distribution, biotransformation, and excretion of drugs (Chapter 4).

Pharmacology The scientific study of drugs; concerned with all information about the effects of drugs on living systems (Chapter 1).

Phencyclidine A dissociative anesthetic (Chapter 12).

Placebo In pharmacology, a chemically inactive substance (Chapter 1).

Placebo control A type of control originating in drug research. Placebo subjects have the same makeup and are treated exactly like a group of subjects who receive a drug, except that placebo subjects receive a chemically inactive substance (Chapter 5).

Polydrug use The same person's regular use of more than one drug (Chapter 1).

Pons ('pänz) Hindbrain structure important in the control of sleep and wakefulness (Chapter 3).

Positron emission transaxial tomography (PET) Technique used to measure activity in selected brain regions (Chapter 3).

Prevalence The general occurrence of an event, usually expressed in terms of percentage of some population. Another common statistic in survey studies is *incidence*, or the number of first-time occurrences of an event during some time period (Chapter 1).

Primary prevention Attempts to avoid substance use or abuse before it has a chance to occur (Chapter 16).

Progesterone (prō-'jes-tə-'rōn) One of the female sex hormones involved in the regulation of ovulation and the menstrual cycle (Chapter 14).

Progestin pill Birth control pill that contains only progestin, a synthetic progesterone (Chapter 14).

Prohibition The legislative forbidding of the sale of a substance, as in the alcohol Prohibition era in the United States, 1920–1933 (Chapter 2).

Proof The proportion of alcohol in a beverage, by volume. Proof typically is used in reference to distilled spirits and equals twice the percentage of alcohol (Chapter 9).

Prostaglandins ('präs-tə-'glan-dən) Naturally occurring chemicals blocked by aspirin and related analgesics (Chapter 14).

Protracted tolerance A type of functional tolerance that occurs over the course of two or more drug administrations (Chapter 5).

Pseudoephedrine ('sü-dō-i-'fed-rən) An over-the-counter decongestant (Chapter 14).

Psilocybin ('sī-lə-'sī-bən) An LSD-like hallucinogen found in mushrooms (Chapter 12).

Psychoactive Pertaining to effects on mood, thinking, and behavior (Chapter 1).

Psychological dependence The emotional state of craving a drug either for its positive effect or to avoid negative effects associated with its abuse (Chapter 1).

Psychological set An individual's knowledge, attitudes, expectations, and other thoughts about an object or event, such as a drug (Chapter 1).

Psychological treatment Treatment geared to changing emotions, thoughts, or behavior without the use of medications or other physical or biological means (Chapter 15).

Psychology The scientific study of behavior (Chapter 1).

Psychopharmacology The subarea of pharmacology that concerns the effects of drugs on behavior (Chapter 1).

Psychosis A severe mental disorder whose symptoms include disorganized thinking and bizarre behavior (Chapter 5).

Psychosurgery Surgery that entails the cutting of fibers connecting particular parts of the brain or the removal or destruction of areas of brain tissue with the goal of modifying severe behavioral or emotional disturbances (Chapter 13).

Psychotherapeutic Exerting a special or unique action on psychological functioning (Chapter 13).

Psychotherapy Typically, conversation between a specially trained individual (therapist) and another person (or family) that is intended to change patterns of behavior, thoughts, or feelings in that person (or family) (Chapter 15).

Punisher A consequence of a behavior that suppresses or decreases its future likelihood (Chapter 5).

Pylorospasm The shutting of the pylorus valve that occurs in some people when they drink very large quantities of alcohol (Chapter 9).

Qualitative The kind, as opposed to quantity, of effect (Chapter 4).

Rebound insomnia Inability to sleep produced as a withdrawal symptom associated with some depressant drugs (Chapter 13).

Receptor sites Specialized structures located on dendrites and cell bodies for neurons that are activated by neurotransmitters (Chapter 3).

Recovery In the addictions field, changes back to health in physical, psychological, spiritual, and social functioning. It generally is believed that recovery is a lifetime process that requires total abstinence from alcohol and nonprescribed drugs (Chapter 15).

Reinforcer A consequence of a behavior that increases its future likelihood (Chapter 5).

Relapse A term from physical disease; return to a previous state of illness from one of health. As applied to smoking, it means the smoker resumes smoking after having abstained for some amount of time (Chapter 7).

REM rebound An increase in the rapid eye movement or REM stage of sleep when withdrawing from drugs that suppress REM time (Chapter 13).

REM sleep Acronym for "rapid eye movements," which are associated with dream activity and are one stage in a cycle of sleep (Chapter 9).

Reticular activating system Pathway running through the medulla and pons that regulates alertness and arousal (Chapter 3).

Reuptake One process by which neurotransmitters are inactivated. Neurotransmitter molecules are taken back up into the axon terminal that released them (Chapter 3).

Reverse tolerance Increased sensitivity to a drug with repeated use of it (Chapter 5).

Route of drug administration The way that drugs enter the body (Chapter 1).

Scopolamine An anticholinergic hallucinogen found in certain plants (Chapter 12).

Secondary prevention Interventions designed to prevent substance-use problems just as the early signs of abuse begin to appear (Chapter 16).

Sedative-hypnotic effects The calming and sleep-inducing effects of some drugs (Chapter 13).

Self-administration study A study that involves testing whether research participants will "give themselves" a drug (Chapter 5).

Self-medication The idea that some people prescribe their own medication, in the form of alcohol or illicit drugs, to alleviate psychological difficulties such as anxiety or depression (Chapter 15).

Serotonergic hallucinogens A class of drugs that includes LSD and drugs with similar effects and mechanisms of action (Chapter 12).

Serotonin ('sir-ə-tō-nən) A neurotransmitter in the brain that is involved with sleep and mood (Chapter 3).

Short-term memory Memory for recent events; thought to differ from long-term memory in several important ways (Chapter 9).

Side effects Effects of a drug other than those of central interest; used most often in reference to the other-than-therapeutic effects of medications, such as the side effect of drowsiness for antihistamines. Note that what are considered a drug's side effects depend on what specifically the drug is being used for (Chapter 4).

Social detoxification Treatment of alcohol withdrawal without the use of medicine (Chapter 9).

Sociopathy Personality disorder that is characterized by a lack of concern for social obligations or rules, a lack of feelings for others, and a tendency toward violence (Chapter 15).

Solubility The ease with which a compound can be dissolved or entered into a solution (Chapter 4).

Solvent A substance, usually a liquid or gas, that contains one or more intoxicating components; examples are glue, gasoline, and nonstick–frying pan sprays (Chapter 2).

Speakeasy A slang expression used to describe a saloon operating without a license; popularly used during Prohibition (Chapter 2).

Spontaneous remission Resolution of a problem without the help of formal treatment (Chapter 15).

Standard drink The alcohol equivalent in a drink of beer, wine, or distilled spirits. A standard drink equals 0.5 ounce of alcohol—about the alcohol content in 12 ounces of beer, 4 ounces of table wine, or 1 ounce of 90- to 100-proof whiskey (Chapter 9).

State-dependent learning When learning under the influence of a drug is best recalled when one is in the same "state" (Chapter 6).

Stimulant psychosis Paranoid delusions and disorientation resembling the symptoms of paranoid schizophrenia, caused by prolonged use or overdose of cocaine and/or amphetamine (Chapter 6).

Substantia nigra (səb-'stan(t)-shē-ə-'nī-grə) Literally "black substance," this basal ganglia structure is darkly pigmented; produces dopamine. Damage to this area produces Parkinson's disease (Chapter 3).

Superior colliculi Midbrain structures that control visual localization (Chapter 3).

Suspended When a drug's particles are dispersed in solution but not dissolved in it (Chapter 4).

Sympathetic branch Branch of the ANS that is activated during emotional arousal and is responsible for such physiological changes as increased heart and respiratory rate, increased blood pressure, and pupil dilation (Chapter 3).

Sympathomimetic Drugs such as cocaine and amphetamine that produce the physiological effects of sympathetic activity (Chapter 3).

Synapse ('si-'naps) The junction between neurons (Chapter 3).

Syndrome In medicine, a number of symptoms that occur together and characterize a specific illness or disease (Chapter 1).

Synergism Any enhancing drug interaction (Chapter 4).

Synesthesia An effect sometimes produced by hallucinogens characterized by the perception of a stimulus in a modality other than the one in which it was presented (for example, a subject may report "seeing" music) (Chapter 12).

Tardive dyskinesia An extrapyramidal complication characterized by involuntary movements of the mouth and tongue, trunk, and extremities; a side effect of long-term (two or more years) use of antipsychotic drugs (Chapter 13).

Tea-pads Historically, places where people gathered to smoke marijuana. The sites could be anything from a rented room to a hotel suite (Chapter 11).

Teratogenic Producing abnormalities in the fetus (Chapter 13).

Teratology In biology, the study of monsters, or distortions in growth (Chapter 9).

Tertiary prevention Treatment interventions with people well beyond the early stages of substance abuse or dependence (Chapter 16).

Testosterone The male sex hormone. Anabolic steroids are basically synthetic versions of testosterone (Chapter 14).

Thalamus ('tha-lə-məs) Forebrain structure that organizes sensory input (Chapter 3).

Therapeutic index A measure of a drug's safety in medical care; it is computed as a ratio: LD 50/ED 50 (Chapter 4).

Tolerance Generally, increased amounts of a drug needed to achieve intoxication, or a diminished drug effect with its continued use (Chapter 1).

Treatment Planned activities designed to change some pattern of behavior(s) of individuals or their families (Chapter 15).

Treatment effects The results of experiencing a treatment, usually measured in different areas of functioning, such as substance use, family functioning, and vocational functioning (Chapter 15).

Treatment outcome research Research designed to show a causal relationship between undergoing a treatment and some physical, psychological, or social change (Chapter 15).

Values clarification A common component of affect-oriented prevention programs; typically involves exploration of one's own needs and beliefs regarding drugs (Chapter 16).

Vesicles ('ve-si-kəl) Tiny sacs in axon terminals that store neurotransmitters (Chapter 3).

Withdrawal A definable illness that occurs with a cessation or decrease in use of a drug (Chapter 1).

REFERENCES

Aaron, P., & Musto, D. (1981). Temperance and prohibition in America: A historical overview. In M. H. Moore & D. R. Gerstein (Eds.), *Alcohol and public policy* (pp. 127–181). Washington, DC: Academy Press.

Abbott, P. J. (1986). Caffeine: A toxicological overview. *The Medical Journal of Australia, 145,* 518–521.

Abel, E. L. (1971). Marihuana and memory: Acquisition or retrieval? *Science, 173,* 1038–1040.

Abel, E. L. (1980). *Marijuana: The first twelve thousand years.* New York: Plenum Press.

Abel, E. L. (1985). *Psychoactive drugs and sex.* New York: Plenum Press.

Abraham, H. D., Aldridge, A. M., & Gogia, P. (1996). The psychopharmacology of hallucinogens. *Neuropsychopharmacology, 14,* 285–298.

Abrahamov, A., Abrahamov, A., & Mechoulam, R. (1995). An efficient new cannabinoid anti-emetic in pediatric oncology. *Life Sciences, 56,* 2097–2102.

Abrams, D. I., Hilton, J. F., Leiser, R. J., Shade, S. B., Elbeik, T. A., Aweeks, F. T., Benowitz, N. L., Bredt, B. M., Korel, B., Aberg, J. A., Deeks, S. G., Mitchell, T. F., Mulligan, K., Baccheti, P., McCune, J. M., & Schambelan, M. (2003). Short-term effects of cannabinoids in patients with HIV-1 infection: A randomized placebo-controlled clinical trial. *Annals of Internal Medicine, 139,* 258–266.

Abrams, D. B., & Wilson, G. T. (1986). Habit disorders: Alcohol and tobacco dependence. In A. J. Frances & R. E. Hales (Eds.), *American Psychiatric Association annual review* (Vol. 5, pp. 606–626). Washington, DC: American Psychiatric Press.

Adams, I. B., & Martin, B. R. (1996). Cannabis: Pharmacology and toxicology in animals and humans. *Addiction, 91,* 1585–1614.

Adams, W. L., Yuan, Z., Barboriak, J. J., & Rimm, A. A. (1993). Alcohol-related hospitalizations of elderly people. *Journal of the American Medical Association, 270,* 1222–1225.

Adesso, V. J. (1985). Cognitive factors in alcohol and drug use. In M. Galizio & S. A. Maisto (Eds.), *Determinants of substance abuse* (pp. 179–208). New York: Plenum Press.

Adler, I., & Kandel, D. (1981). Crosscultural perspectives on developmental stages in adolescent drug use. *Journal of Studies on Alcohol, 42,* 701–715.

Agurell, S., Halldin, M., Lindgren, J. R., Ohlsson, A., Widman, M., Gillespie, H., & Hollister, L. (1986). Pharmacokinetics and metabolism of tetrahydrocannabinol and other cannabinoids with emphasis on man. *Pharmacological Reviews, 38,* 21–43.

Alasuutari, P. (1992). *A cultural theory of alcoholism.* Albany: State University of New York Press.

Alcoholics Anonymous. (1972). *If you are a professional, A. A. wants to work with you.* New York: Alcoholics Anonymous World Services.

Alcoholics Anonymous. (1983). *Questions and answers on sponsorship.* New York: Alcoholics Anonymous World Services.

Alda, M., Hajek, T., Calkin, C., & O'Donovan, C. (2009). Treatment of bipolar disorder: New perspectives. *Annals of Medicine, 41,* 186–196.

Aldrich, M. R. (1977). Tantric cannabis use in India. *Journal of Psychedelic Drugs, 9,* 227–233.

Allison, M., & Hubbard, R. L. (1985). Drug abuse treatment process: A review of the literature. *International Journal of the Addictions, 20,* 1321–1345.

Alvik, A., Haldorsen, T., & Lindermann, R. (2005). Consistency of reported alcohol use by pregnant women: Anonymous versus confidential questionnaires with item response differences. *Alcoholism: Clinical and Experimental Research, 29,* 1444–1449.

Amar, M. B. (2006). Cannabinoids in medicine: A review of their therapeutic potential. *Journal of Ethnopharmacology, 105,* 1–25.

American Psychiatric Association. (1987). *Diagnostic and statistical manual of mental disorders* (3rd ed., rev. ed.). Washington, DC: Author.

American Psychiatric Association (APA). (1994). *Diagnostic and statistical manual of mental disorders* (4th ed.). Washington, DC: Author.

American Psychiatric Association. (2000a). *Diagnostic and statistical manual of mental disorders* (4th ed., rev.). Washington, DC: Author.

American Psychiatric Association. (2000b). *Practice guidelines for the treatment of psychiatric disorders.* Washington, DC: Author.

Anderson, D., Beckerleg, S., Hailu, D., & Klein, A. (2007). *The khat controversy: Stimulating the debate on drugs.* Oxford: Berg Press.

Anderson, T. L., & Levy, J. A. (2003). Marginality among older injectors in today's illicit drug culture: Assessing the impact of aging. *Addiction, 98,* 761–770.

Andrain-McGovern, J., Tercyak, K. P., Shields, A. E., Bush, A., Espinel, C. F., & Leman, C. (2003). Which adolescents are most receptive to tobacco industry marketing? Implications for counter advertising campaigns. *Health Communication, 15,* 490–513.

Andrews, J. M., & Nemeroff, C. B. (1994). Contemporary management of depression. *American Journal of Medicine, 97*(Supplement 6A), 24S–32S.

Annis, H. M. (1986). A relapse prevention model for treatment of alcoholics. In W. R. Miller & N. Heather (Eds.), *Treating addictive behaviors* (pp. 407–433). New York: Plenum Press.

Anthosinen, N. R., Skeans, M. A., Wise, R. A., Manfreda, J., Kanner, R. E., & Connett, R. E., for the Lung Health Study Research Group. (2005). The effects of a smoking cessation intervention on 14.5-year mortality. *Annals of Internal Medicine, 142,* 233–239.

Anton, R. F., et al. (2006). Combined pharmacotherapies and behavioral interventions for alcohol dependence. *Journal of the American Medical Association, 295,* 2003–2017.

Arango, V., & Mann, J. J. (2009). Abnormalities of brain structure and function in mood disorders. In D. S. Charney & E. J. Nestler (Eds.), *Neurobiology of mental illness* (3rd ed., pp. 515–529). New York: Oxford University Press.

Armor, D. J., Polich, J. M., & Stambul, H. B. (1976). *Alcoholism and treatment.* Report prepared for the National Institute on Alcohol Abuse and Alcoholism (R-1739-NIAAA). Santa Monica, CA: Rand Corporation.

Ashley, R. (1975). *Cocaine: Its history, uses, and effects.* New York: Warner.

Ashton, R. (2002). *This is heroin.* London: Sanctuary Publishing LTD.

Austin, S. B., & Gortmaker, S. L. (2001). Dieting and smoking initiation in early adolescent girls and boys: A prospective study. *American Journal of Public Health, 91,* 446–450.

Australian Drug Law Reform Foundation. (1996). *Drug love: The questioning of our current drug law.* Canberra: Author.

Baer, J. S., Kivlahan, D. R., Blume, A. W., McKnight, P., & Marlatt, G. A. (2001). Brief intervention for heavy drinking college students: 4-year follow-up and natural history. *American Journal of Public Health, 91,* 1310–1316.

Baer, J. S., Kivlahan, D. R., Fromme, K., & Marlatt, G. A. (1994). Secondary prevention of alcohol abuse with college student populations: A skills-training approach. In G. Howard & P. E. Nathan (Eds.), *Alcohol use and misuse by young adults* (pp. 83–108). Notre Dame, IN: Notre Dame University Press.

Bak, A. A., & Grobbee, D. E. (1989). The effect on serum cholesterol levels of coffee brewed by filtering or boiling. *New England Journal of Medicine, 321,* 1432–1437.

Baker, A., Boggs, T. G., & Lewin, T. J. (2001). Randomized controlled trial of brief cognitive-behavioral interventions among regular users of amphetamine. *Addiction, 96,* 1279–1287.

Balazs, R., Bridges, R. J., & Cotman, C. W. (2006). *Excitatory amino acid transmission in health and disease.* Oxford, UK: Oxford University Press.

Baldessarini, R. J. (1985). *Chemotherapy in psychiatry: Principles and practice* (rev. ed.). Cambridge, MA: Harvard University Press.

Ball, J. C., Meyers, C. P., & Friedman, S. R. (1988). Reducing the risk of AIDS through methadone maintenance treatment. *Journal of Health and Social Behavior, 29,* 214–226.

Bangert-Drowns, R. L. (1988). The effects of school-based substance abuse education: A meta-analysis. *Journal of Drug Education, 18,* 243–264.

Barkley, R. A. (2001). Foreword. In L. L. Weyandt (Ed.), *An ADHD primer* (pp. ix–x). Boston: Allyn & Bacon.

Barnes, G. E. (1979). The alcoholic personality: A reanalysis of the literature. *Journal of Studies on Alcohol, 40,* 571–634.

Baron, A., & Galizio, M. (2005). Positive and negative reinforcement: Should the distinction be preserved? *The Behavior Analyst, 28,* 85–99.

Barone, J. J., & Roberts, H. R. (1996). Caffeine consumption. *Food and Chemical Toxicology, 34,* 119–129.

Barr, H. M., & Streissguth, A. P. (2001). Identifying maternal self-reported alcohol use associated with fetal alcohol spectrum disorders. *Alcoholism: Clinical and Experimental Research, 25,* 283–287.

Barrett, R. J. (1985). Behavioral approaches to individual differences in substance abuse. In M. Galizio & S. A. Maisto (Eds.), *Determinants of substance abuse: Biological, psychological, and environmental factors* (pp. 125–175). New York: Plenum Press.

Barrett-Connor, E., Chang, J. C., & Edelstein, S. L. (1994). Coffee-associated osteoporosis offset by daily milk consumption. *Journal of the American Medical Association, 271,* 280–283.

Bartholow, B. D., & Heinz, A. (2006). Alcohol and aggression without consumption. *Psychological Science, 17,* 30–37.

Bartolet, J., & Levine, S. (2001). The holy men of heroin. In H. T. Wilson (Ed.), *Drugs, society and behavior* (pp. 85–86). Guilford, CT: McGraw-Hill/Dushkin.

Baur, J. A., & Sinclair, D. A. (2006). Therapeutic potential of resveratrol: The in vivo evidence. *Nature Reviews Drug Discovery, 5,* 493–506.

Bauman, M. H., Wang, X., & Rothman, R. B. (2007). 3,4-methylinedioxymethamphetamine (MDMA) neurotoxicity in rats: A reappraisal of past and present findings. *Psychopharmacology, 189,* 407–424.

Beardsley, P. M., Balster, R. L., & Harris, L. S. (1996). Evaluation of the discriminative stimulus and reinforcing effects of gammahydroxybutyrate (GHB). *Psychopharmacology, 127,* 315–322.

Becker, C. E., Roe, R. L., & Scott, R. A. (1975). *Alcohol as a drug.* New York: Medcom Press.

Becker, H. S. (1953). Becoming a marihuana user. *American Journal of Sociology, 59,* 235–242.

Becker, H. S. (1963). *Outsiders: Studies in the sociology of deviance.* New York: Free Press.

Belluzzi, J. D., Lee, A. G., Oliff, H. S., & Leslie, F. M. (2004). Age-dependent effects of nicotine on locomotor activity and conditioned place preference in rats. *Psychopharmacology, 174,* 389–395.

Benet, L. Z., Mitchell, J. R., & Sheiner, L. B. (1990a). General principles. In A. G. Gilman, T. W. Rall, A. S. Nies, & P. Taylor (Eds.), *Goodman and Gilman's The pharmacological basis for therapeutics* (8th ed., pp. 1–2). New York: Pergamon Press.

Benet, L. Z., Mitchell, J. R., & Sheiner, L. B. (1990b). Pharmacokinetics: The dynamics of drug absorption, distribution, and elimination. In A. G. Gilman, T. W. Rall, A. S. Nies, & P. Taylor (Eds.), *Goodman and Gilman's The pharmacological basis of therapeutics* (8th ed., pp. 3–32). New York: Pergamon Press.

Benowitz, N. L., Hall, S. M., & Modin, G. (1989). Persistent increase in caffeine concentrations in people who stop smoking. *British Medical Journal, 298,* 1075–1076.

Benowitz, N. L., Porchet, H., Sheiner, L., & Jacob, P. (1988). Nicotine absorption and cardiovascular effects with smokeless tobacco use: Companion with cigarettes and nicotine gum. *Clinical Pharmacology and Therapeutics, 44,* 23–28.

Berild, D., & Hasselbalch, H. (1981). Survival after a blood alcohol of 1127 mg/dl. *Lancet, 2*(8242), 363.

Berman, R. M., Sporn, J., Charney, D. S., & Matthew, S. J. (2009). Principles of the pharmacotherapy of depression. In D. S. Charney & E. J. Nestler (Eds.), *Neurobiology of mental illness* (3rd ed., pp. 491–514). New York: Oxford University Press.

Berridge, K. C., & Robinson, T. E. (1998). What is the role of dopamine in reward: Hedonic impact, reward learning or incentive salience? *Brain Research Reviews, 28,* 309–369.

Bhana, N., Foster, R. H., Olney, R., & Plosker, G. L. (2001). Olanzapine: An updated review of its use in the management of schizophrenia. *Drugs, 61,* 111–161.

Bickel, W. K., Amass, L., Higgins, S. T., Badger, G. J., & Esch, R. A. (1997). Effects of adding behavioral treatment to opioid detoxification with buprenorphine. *Journal of Consulting and Clinical Psychology, 65,* 803–810.

Bickel, W. K., & DeGrandpre, R. J. (1995). Price and alternatives: Suggestions for drug policy from psychology. *International Journal of Drug Policy, 6,* 93–105.

Bickel, W. K., DeGrandpre, R. J., & Higgins, S. T. (1995). The behavioral economics of concurrent drug reinforcers: A review and reanalysis of drug self-administration research. *Psychopharmacology, 118,* 250–259.

Bina, C. (1998). Drug testing 101: Detecting tainted samples. *Corrections Today, 60,* 122–128.

Bishara, D., & Taylor, D. (2008). Upcoming agents for the treatment of schizophrenia. *Drugs, 68,* 2269–2292.

Blane, H. T. (1976). Education and the prevention of alcoholism. In B. Kissin & H. Begleiter (Eds.), *The biology of alcoholism: Vol. 4. Social aspects of alcoholism* (pp. 519–578). New York: Plenum Press.

Blane, H. T. (1988). Research on mass communications and alcohol. *Contemporary Drug Problems, 15,* 7–20.

Bloomquist, E. R. (1971). *Marijuana: The second trip* (rev. ed.). Beverly Hills, CA: Glencoe Press.

Blum, K. (1984). *Handbook of abusable drugs.* New York: Gardner Press.

Bofetta, P., Hecht, S., Gray, N., Gupta, P., & Staif, K. (2008). Smokeless tobacco and cancer. *Lancet Oncology, 9,* 667–675.

Bonham, C., & Abbott, C. (2008). Are second generation antipsychotics a distinct class? *Journal of Psychiatric Practice, 14,* 225–231.

Borelli, B., Spring, B., Niaura, R., Hitsman, B., & Papandonatos, G. (2001). Influences of gender and weight gain on short-term relapse to smoking in a cessation trial. *Journal of Consulting and Clinical Psychology, 69,* 511–515.

Botvin, G. J. (1999). Adolescent drug abuse prevention: Current findings and future directions. In M. D. Glantz & C. R. Hartel (Eds.), *Drug abuse: Origins and interventions* (pp. 285–308). Washington, DC: American Psychological Association.

Botvin, G. J., & Botvin, E. M. (1992). School-based and community-based prevention approaches. In J. H. Lowinson, P. Ruiz, & R. B. Millman (Eds.), *Substance abuse: A comprehensive textbook* (2nd ed., pp. 910–927). Baltimore, MD: Williams & Wilkins.

Botvin, G. J., & Griffin, K. W. (2003). Drug abuse prevention curricula in schools. In Z. Sloboda & W. J. Bukoski (Eds.), *Handbook of drug abuse prevention: Theory, science, and practice* (pp. 45–74). New York: Kluwer Academic/Plenum Publishers.

Bouso, J. C., Boblin, R., Farre, M., Alcazar, M. A., & Gomez-Jarabo, G. (2008). MDMA-assisted psychotherapy using low doses in a small sample of women with chronic posttraumatic stress disorder, *Journal of Psychoactive Drugs, 40,* 225–236.

Boutros, N. N., & Bowers, M. B. (1996). Chronic substance-induced psychotic disorders: State of the literature. *Journal of Neuropsychiatry and Clinical Neurosciences, 8,* 262–269.

Boys, A., Marsden, J., & Strang, J. (2001). Understanding reasons for drug use amongst young people: A functional perspective. *Health Education Research, 16,* 457–469.

Bozarth, M. A. (Ed.). (1987). *Methods of assessing the reinforcing properties of drugs.* New York: Springer-Verlag.

Bozarth, M. A., & Wise, R. A. (1985). Toxicity associated with long-term intravenous heroin and cocaine self-administration in the rat. *Journal of the American Medical Association, 254,* 81–83.

Bradley, K. A., Donovan, D. M., & Larson, E. B. (1993). How much is too much? Advising patients about safe levels of alcohol consumption. *Archives of Internal Medicine, 153,* 2734–2740.

Brandon, T. H., Juliano, L. M., & Copeland A. L. (1999). Expectancies for tobacco smoking. In I. Kirsch (Ed.), *How expectancies shape experience* (pp. 263–300). Washington, DC: American Psychological Association.

Brands, B., Sproule, B., & Marshman, J. (Eds.). (1998). *Drugs and drug abuse* (3rd ed.). Toronto: Addiction Research Foundation.

Brecher, E. M. (1972). *Licit and illicit drugs.* Boston: Little, Brown.

Brecher, E. M. (1986). Drug laws and drug law enforcement: A review and evaluation based on 111 years of experience. *Drugs and Society, 1,* 1–27.

Breggin, P. R. (2001). Questioning the treatment for ADHD. *Science, 291,* 595.

Breslau, N., & Peterson, E. L. (1996). Smoking cessation in young adults: Age at initiation of cigarette smoking and other suspected influences. *American Journal of Public Health, 86,* 214–220.

Brewer, C. (1996). On the specific effectiveness and under-valuing of pharmacological treatments for addiction: A comparison of methadone, naltrexone and disulfiram with psychosocial interventions. *Addiction Research, 3,* 297–313.

Brick, J. (1990). *Marijuana.* New Brunswick, NJ: Rutgers University Center of Alcohol Studies.

Brody, A. L., Mandelkern, M. A., Cosyello, M. R., Abrams, A. L., Scheibal, D. Farahi, J., London, E. D., Olmstead, R. E., Rose, J. E., & Mukhin, A. G. (2008). Brain nicotinic acetylcholine receptor occupancy: Effect of smoking a denicotinized cigarette. *The International Journal of Neuropsychopharmacology,* DOI: 10.1017/S146114570800922X.

Brody, A. L., Mandelkern, M. A., London, E. D., Olmstead, R. E., Farahi, J., Scheibal, D., Jou, J., Allen, V., Tiongson, E., Chefer, S. I., Koren, A. O., & Mukhin, A. G. (2006). Cigarette smoking saturates brain α4β2 nicotinic acetylcholine receptors. *Archives of General Psychiatry, 63,* 907–915.

Brown, B. A., Christiansen, B. A., & Goldman, M. S. (1987). The Alcohol Expectancy Questionnaire: An instrument for the assessment of adolescent and adult alcohol expectancies. *Journal of Studies on Alcohol, 48,* 483–491.

Brown, L., Kroon, P. A., Das, D. K., Samarjit, D., Tosaki, A., Chan, V., Singer, M. V., & Feick, P. (2009). The biological responses to resveratrol and other polyphenols from alcoholic beverages. *Alcoholism: Clinical and Experimental Research, 33,* 1–11.

Brown, R. T., Amler, R. W., Freeman, W. S., Perrin, J. M., Stein, M. T., Feldman, H. M., et al. (2005). Treatment of attention-deficit disorder: Overview of the evidence. *Pediatrics, 115,* 749–757.

Bruce, M., Scott, N., Shine, P., & Lader, M. (1992). Angiogenic effect of caffeine in patients with anxiety disorders. *Archives of General Psychiatry, 49,* 867–869.

Budney, A. J., & Higgins, S. T. (1998, April). *A community reinforcement approach to treating cocaine addiction.* NIDA publication No. 98–4309.

Budney, A. J., Hughes, J. R., Moore, B. A., & Vandrey, R. (2004). Review of the validity and significance of cannabis withdrawal syndrome. *The American Journal of Psychiatry, 161,* 1967–1977.

Budney, A. J., Moore, B. A., & Vandrey, R. (2004). Health consequences of marijuana use. In J. Brick (Ed.), *Handbook of the medical consequences of alcohol and drug abuse* (pp. 171–217). New York: The Haworth Press.

Bukoski, W. J. (2003). The emerging science of drug abuse prevention. In Z. Sloboda & W. J. Bukoski (Eds.), *Handbook of drug abuse prevention: Theory, science, and practice* (pp. 3–24). New York: Kluwer Academic/Plenum Publishers.

Burke, L. M. (2008). Caffeine and sports performance. *Applied Physiology, Nutrition, and Metabolism, 33,* 1319–1334.

Burroughs, W. S. (1953). *Junky.* Middlesex, England: Penguin Books.

Burstein, S. H., Karst, M., Schneider, U., & Zurier, R. B. (2004). Ajulemic acid: A novel cannabinoid produces analgesia without a "high." *Life Sciences, 75,* 1513–1522.

Bushman, B. J., & Cooper, H. M. (1990). Effects of alcohol on human aggression: An integrative research review. *Psychological Bulletin, 107,* 341–354.

Butelman, E. R., Prisinzano, T. E., Deng, H., Rus, S., & Kreek, M. J. (2009). *The Journal of Pharmacology and Experimental Therapeutics, 328,* 588–597.

Byck, R. (Ed.). (1974). *Cocaine papers by Sigmund Freud.* New York: Stonehill Publishing Company.

Cairney, S., Maruff, P., Burns, C., & Currie, B. (2002). The neurobehavioral consequences of petrol (gasoline) sniffing. *Neuroscience and Biobehavioral Reviews, 26,* 81–89.

Cairney, S., Maruff, P., Burns, C. B., Currie, J., & Currie, B. J. (2005). Neurological and cognitive recovery following abstinence from petrol sniffing. *Neuropsychopharmacology, 30,* 1019–1027.

Caldwell, A. E. (1970). *Origins of psychopharmacology—From CPZ to LSD.* Springfield, IL: Charles Thomas.

Caldwell, A. E. (1978). History of psychopharmacology. In W. G. Clark & J. del Guidice (Eds.), *Principles of psychopharmacology* (2nd ed., pp. 9–30). New York: Academic Press.

Caligiuri, M. P., & Buitenhuys, C. (2005). Do preclinical findings of methamphetamine-induced motor abnormalities translate to an observable clinical phenotype? *Neuropsychopharmacology, 30,* 2125–2134.

Cappell, H. D., Sellers, E. M., & Busto, U. (1986). Benzodiazepines as drugs of abuse and dependence. In H. D. Cappell, F. B. Glaser, Y. Israel, H. Kalant, W. Schmidt, E. M. Sellers, & R. C. Smart (Eds.), *Research advances in alcohol and drug problems* (Vol. 9, pp. 53–126). New York: Plenum Press.

Carlin, A. S., Bakker, C. B., Halpern, L., & Post, R. D. (1972). Social facilitation of marijuana intoxication: Impact of social set and pharmacological activity. *Journal of Abnormal Psychology, 80,* 132–140.

Carlson, N. R. (2001). *Physiology of behavior* (7th ed.). Boston: Allyn & Bacon.

Carlson, N.R. (2008). *Foundations of physiological psychology* (7th ed.). Boston: Pearson.

Carroll, J. F. X., Malloy, T. E., & Kenrick, F. M. (1977). Drug abuse by alcoholics and problem drinkers: A literature review and evaluation. *American Journal of Drug and Alcohol Abuse, 4,* 317–341.

Carroll, K. M. (1996). Relapse prevention as a psychosocial treatment: A review of controlled clinical trials. *Experimental and Clinical Psychopharmacology, 4,* 46–54.

Carroll, K. M., Sinha, R., Nich, C., Babuscio, T., & Rounsaville, B. (2002). Contingency management to enhance naltrexone treatment of opioid dependence: A randomized clinical trial of reinforcement magnitude. *Experimental and Clinical Psychopharmacology, 10,* 54–63.

Carroll, M. E. (1990). PCP and hallucinogens. *Advances in Alcohol and Substance Abuse, 9,* 167–190.

Carter, W. E. (1980). *Cannabis in Costa Rica.* Philadelphia: Institute for the Study of Human Issues.

Carter, W. E., & Doughty, P. L. (1976). Social and cultural aspects of cannabis use in Costa Rica. *Annals of the New York Academy of Sciences, 282,* 2–16.

Cellucci, T. (1984). The prevention of alcohol problems: Conceptual and methodological issues. In P. M. Miller & T. D. Nirenberg (Eds.), *Prevention of alcohol abuse* (pp. 15–53). New York: Plenum Press.

Center for AIDS Prevention Studies. (1998). *Does needle exchange work?* Chicago: American Medical Association.

Center for Disease Control and Prevention. (1993). Mortality trends for selected smoking-related and breast cancer in the United States, 1950–1990. *Morbidity and Mortality Weekly Report, 42,* 857, 863–866.

Center for Disease Control and Prevention. (2006). *Unintended Pregnancy Prevention: Contraception.* Retrieved February 26, 2006, from http://www.cdc.gov/reproductivehealth/UnintendedPregnancy/Contraception.htm

Center for Substance Abuse Treatment. (1997). *The National Treatment Improvement Evaluation: Final report.* Washington, DC: Author.

Cepada-Benito, A., Reynoso, J. T., & Erath, S. (2004). Meta-analysis of the efficacy of nicotine replacement therapy for smoking cessation: Differences between men and women. *Journal of Consulting and Clinical Psychology, 72,* 712–722.

Chait, L. D., & Pierri, J. (1992). Effects of smoked marijuana on human performance: A critical review. In L. Murphy & A. Bartke (Eds.), *Marijuana/cannabinoids: Neurobiology and neurophysiology* (pp. 387–423). Boca Raton, FL: CRC Press.

Chakos, M. H., Mayerhoff, D. I., Loebel, A. D., Alvir, J. M., & Lieberman, J. A. (1992). Incidence and correlates of acute extrapyramidal symptoms in first episode of schizophrenia. *Psychopharmacology Bulletin, 28,* 81–86.

Charness, M. E. (1993). Brain lesions in alcoholics. *Alcoholism: Clinical and Experimental Research, 17,* 2–11.

Chen, T. T. L., & Winder, A. E. (1986). When is the critical moment to provide smoking education at schools? *Journal of Drug Education, 16,* 121–134.

Cherek, D. R., Roache, J. D., Egli, M., Davis, C., Spiga, R., & Cowan, K. (1993). Acute effects of marijuana smoking on aggressive, escape, and point-maintained responding of male drug users. *Psychopharmacology, 111,* 163–168.

Childress, A. R., Mozley, P. D., McElgin, W., Fitzgerald, J., Reivich, M., & O'Brien, C. P. (1999). Limbic activation during cue-induced cocaine craving. *American Journal of Psychiatry, 156,* 11–18.

Chou, S. P., Grant, B. F., Dawson, D. A., Stinson, F. S., Saha, T., & Pickering, R. P. (2006). Twelve-month prevalence and changes in drinking after driving. *Alcohol Research and Health, 29,* 143–151.

Cicero, T. J. (1980). Alcohol self-administration, tolerance, and withdrawal in humans and animals: Theoretical and methodological issues. In H. Rigter & J. Crabbe Jr. (Eds.), *Alcohol tolerance and dependence* (pp. 1–50). Amsterdam: Elsevier/North-Holland Biomedical Press.

Cicero, T. J., Inciardi, J. A., & Munoz, A. (2005). Trends in abuse of Oxycontin and other opioid analgesics in the United States: 2002–2004. *Journal of Pain, 6,* 662–672.

Ciraulo, D. A., Barnhill, J. G., Greenblatt, D. J., Shader, R. I., Ciraulo, A. M., Tarmey, M. F., et al. (1988). Abuse liability and clinical pharmacokinetics of alprazolam in alcoholic men. *Journal of Clinical Psychiatry, 49,* 333–337.

Clapton, E. (2007). *Clapton: The autobiography.* New York: Random House.

Clark, W. G., Brater, D. C., & Johnson, A. R. (Eds.). (1988). *Goth's medical pharmacology* (12th ed.). St. Louis: C. V. Mosby.

Clinger, O. W., & Johnson, N. A. (1951). Purposeful inhalation of gasoline vapors. *Psychiatric Quarterly, 25,* 557–567.

Cobain, K. (2002). *Journals.* New York: Riverhead Books.

Cohen, L. J. (1997). Rational drug use in the treatment of depression. *Pharmacotherapy, 17,* 45–61.

Cohen, M. M., & Marmillo, M. J. (1967). Chromosome damage in human leukocytes induced by lysergic acid diethylamide. *Science, 155,* 1417–1419.

Cohen, R. S. (1998). *The love drug: Dancing to the beat of ecstasy.* Binghamton, NY: Haworth Press.

Cohen, S. (1981). *The substance abuse problems.* Binghamton, NY: Haworth Press.

Cohen, S., & Andrysiak, T. (1982). *The therapeutic potential of marijuana's components.* Rockville, MD: American Council on Marijuana and Other Psychoactive Drugs.

Colder, C. R., Mehta, P., Balanda, K., Campbell, R. T., Mayhew, K. P., Stanton, W. R., et al. (2001). Identifying trajectories of adolescent smoking: An application of latent growth mixture modeling. *Health Psychology, 20,* 127–135.

Collins, J. J., Jr. (Ed.). (1980). *Alcohol use and criminal behavior: An empirical, theoretical, and methodological overview.* New York: Guilford Press.

Colpaert, F. C. (1987). Drug discrimination: Methods of manipulation, measurement, and analysis. In M. A. Bozarth (Ed.), *Methods of assessing the reinforcing properties of drugs* (pp. 341–372). New York: Springer-Verlag.

Comer, S. D., Haney, M., Foltin, R. W., & Fischman, M. W. (1997). Effects of caffeine withdrawal on humans living in a residential laboratory. *Experimental and Clinical Psychopharmacology, 5,* 399–403.

Comer, S. M., & Zacny, J. P. (2005). Subjective effects of opioids. In M. Earlywine (Ed.), *Mind-altering drugs: The science of subjective experience* (pp. 217–239). London: Oxford Press.

Comitas, L. (1976). Cannabis and work in Jamaica: A refutation of the amotivational syndrome. *Annals of New York Academy of Sciences, 282,* 24–32.

Community Epidemiology Work Group (2009). *Epidemiological trends in substance abuse: Highlights and executive summary.* Bethesda, MD: National Institute on Drug Abuse. http://www.drugabuse.gov/PDF/CEWG/CEWGJan09508Compliant.pdf

Compton, D. R., Harris, L. S., Lichtman, A. H., & Martin, B. R. (1996). Marijuana. In C. R. Schuster & M. J. Kuhar (Eds.), *Pharmacological aspects of drug dependence: Toward an integrated neurobehavioral approach* (pp. 83–158). New York: Springer-Verlag.

Compton, W. M., & Volkow, N. D. (2006). Major increases in opioid analgesic abuse in the United States: Concerns and strategies. *Drug and Alcohol Dependence, 81,* 103–107.

Connecticut Clearing House. (2001). *Qs and As on drug testing.* Plainville, CT: Author.

Connors, G. J., Donovan, D. M., & DiClemente, C. C. (2001). *Substance abuse treatment and the stages of change.* New York: Guilford Press.

Connors, G. J., Maisto, S. A., & Donovan, D. M. (1996). Conceptualization of relapse: A summary of psychological and psychobiological models. *Addiction, 91* (Supplement), S5–S14.

Cook, R. F. (2003). Drug abuse prevention in the workplace. In Z. Sloboda & W. J. Bukoski (Eds.), *Handbook of drug abuse prevention: Theory, science, and practice* (pp. 157–172). New York: Kluwer Academic/Plenum Publishers.

Cooper, Z. D., & Haney, M. (2009). Comparison of subjective, pharmacokinetic, and physiological effects of marijuana smoked as joints and blunts. *Drug and Alcohol Dependence, 103,* 107–113.

Cooperrider, C. (1988). Antidepressants. In G. W. Lawson & C. A. Cooperrider (Eds.), *Clinical psychopharmacology* (pp. 91–108). Rockville, MD: Aspen Publishers.

Coplan, J. D., Wolk, S. I., & Klein, D. F. (1995). Anxiety and the serotonin 1A receptor. In F. E. Bloom & D. J. Kupfer (Eds.), *Psychopharmacology: The fourth generation of progress* (pp. 1301–1310). New York: Raven Press.

Cornelis, M. C., El-Sohemy, A., Kabagambe, E. K., & Campos, H. (2006). Coffee, CYP1A2 genotype, and risk of myocardial infarction. *Journal of the American Medical Association, 295,* 1135–1141.

Coryell, W., & Winokur, G. (1982). Course and outcome. In E. S. Paykel (Ed.), *Handbook of affective disorders.* New York: Guilford Press.

Cose, E. (2009). Closing the gap: Obama could fix cocaine sentencing. *Newsweek,* July 20, pp. 25.

Costa, E., Guidotti, A., & Mao, C. C. (1975). Evidence for involvement of GABA in the action of benzodiazepines. Studies on rat cerebellum. In E. Costa & P. Greengard (Eds.), *Mechanism of action of benzodiazepines* (pp. 113–130). New York: Raven Press.

Cotton, P. (1993). Low tar cigarettes come under fire. *Journal of the American Medical Association, 270,* 1399.

Coultas, D. B., Stidley, C. A., & Samet, J. M. (1993). Cigarette yields of tar and nicotine and markers of exposure to tobacco smoke. *American Review of Respiratory Disease, 148,* 435–440.

Council on Scientific Affairs. (1984). Caffeine labeling. *Journal of the American Medical Association, 252,* 803–806.

Cox, E. R., Halloran, D. R., Homan, S. M., Welliver, S. & Mager, D. E. (2008). Trends in the prevalence of chronic medication use in children: 2002–2005. *Pediatrics, 122,* 1053–1061.

Cox, W. M. (1986). *The addictive personality.* New York: Chelsea.

Craft, R. M., & Lee, D. A. (2005). NMDA antagonist modulation of morphine antinociception in female vs. male rats. *Pharmacology, Biochemistry & Behavior, 80,* 639–649.

Croft, R. J., Mackay, A. J., Mills, A. T. D., & Gruzelier, J. G. H. (2001). The relative contributions of ecstasy and cannabis to cognitive impairment. *Psychopharmacology, 153,* 373–379.

Crowley, T. J. (1981). The reinforcers for drug abuse: Why people take drugs. In H. Shaffer & M. E. Burglass (Eds.), *Classic contributions in the addictions* (pp. 367–381). New York: Brunner/Mazel.

Cunningham, J. A. (2009). Internet evidence-based treatments. In P. M. Miller (Ed.), *Evidence-based addiction treatment* (pp. 379–398). Boston: Elsevier.

Cunningham, J. K., & Liu, L. M. (2005). Impacts of federal precursor chemical regulations on methamphetamine arrests. *Addiction, 100,* 479–488.

Curatolo, P. W., & Robertson, D. (1983). The health consequences of caffeine. *Annals of Internal Medicine, 98,* 641–653.

Curry, S. J., Wagner, E. H., & Grothaus, L. C. (1990). Intrinsic and extrinsic motivation for smoking cessation. *Journal of Consulting and Clinical Psychology, 58,* 310–316.

Dackis, C. A., & Gold, M. S. (1985). New concepts in cocaine addiction: The dopamine depletion hypothesis. *Neuroscience and Biobehavioral Reviews, 9,* 469–477.

Dafters, R. I. (2006). Chronic ecstasy (MDMA) use is associated with deficits in task-switching but not inhibition or memory updating executive functions. *Drug and Alcohol Dependence, 83,* 181–184.

Dafters, R. I., Hoshi, R., & Talbot, A. C. (2004). Contribution of cannabis and MDMA ("ecstasy") to cognitive changes in long-term polydrug users. *Psychopharmacology, 173,* 405–410.

Dal Cason, T. A., & Franzosa, E. S. (2003). Occurrences and forms of the hallucinogens. In R. Laing (Ed.), *Hallucinogens: A forensic drug handbook* (pp. 37–66). London: Academic Press.

Daly, J. W., & Fredholm, B. B. (2004). Mechanisms of action of caffeine on the nervous system. In A. Nehlig (Ed.), *Coffee, tea, chocolate, and the brain* (pp. 1–11). Boca Raton, FL: CRC Press.

Damasio, A. R. (1994). *Descartes' error: Emotion, reason and the human brain.* New York: Avon Books.

D'Amicis, A., & Viani, R. (1993). The consumption of coffee. In S. Garattini (Ed.), *Caffeine, coffee, and health* (pp. 1–16). New York: Raven Press.

Daumann, J., Fischermann, T., Heekeren, K., Henke, K., Thron, A., & Gouzoulis-Mayfrank, E. (2005). *Psychopharmacology, 180,* 607–611.

Daumann, J., Hensen, G., Thimm, B., Rezk, M., Till, B., & Gouzoulis-Mayfrank, E. (2004). *Psychopharmacology, 173,* 398–404.

David, G. L., Koh, W.-P., Lee, H.-P., Yu, M. C., & London, S. J. (2005). Childhood exposure to environmental tobacco smoke and chronic respiratory symptoms in nonsmoking adults: The Singapore Chinese health study. *Thorax,* DOI: 10.1136/thx.2005.042960.

Davis, J. M., & Schlemmer, R. F. (1980). The amphetamine psychosis. In J. Caldwell & S. J. Mule (Eds.), *Amphetamines and related stimulants: Chemical, biological, clinical, and sociological aspects* (pp. 161–174). Boca Raton, FL: CRC Press.

Davis, W. (1988). *Passage of darkness: The ethnobiology of the Haitian zombie.* Chapel Hill: University of North Carolina Press.

Davis, W. R., Johnson, B. D., Randolph, D., & Liberty, H. J. (2006). Risks for HIV infection among users and sellers of crack, powder cocaine and heroin in central Harlem: Implications for interventions. *AIDS Care, 18,* 158–165.

Dawson, D. A. (2000). U.S. low-risk drinking guideline: An examination of four alternatives. *Alcoholism: Clinical and Experimental Research, 2000,* 1820–1829.

Day, N. L., & Richardson, G. A. (1991). Prenatal marijuana use: Epidemiology, methodological issues, and infant outcome. *Chemical Dependency and Pregnancy, 18,* 77–91.

Deahl, M. (1991). Cannabis and memory loss. *British Journal of Addiction, 86,* 249–252.

De Fonseca, F. R., & Schneider, M. (2008). The endogenous cannabinoid system and drug addiction: 20 years after the discovery of the CBI receptor. *Addiction Biology, 13,* 143–146.

DeGrandpre, R. J., Bickle, W. K., Hughes, J. R., & Higgins, S. T. (1992). Behavioral economics of drug self-administration, III. A reanalysis of the nicotine regulation hypothesis. *Psychopharmacology, 108,* 1–10.

DeLeon, G. (1984). *The therapeutic community: Study of effectiveness.* NIDA Treatment Research Monograph 84. Rockville, MD: National Institute on Drug Abuse.

DeLeon, G. (1995). Therapeutic communities for addictions: A theoretical framework. *International Journal of the Addictions, 30,* 1603–1645.

DeLisi, L. E. (2008). The effect of cannabis on the brain: can it cause brain anomalies that lead to increased risk for schizophrenia? *Current Opinion in Psychiatry, 21,* 140–150.

DeLong, F. L., & Levy, B. I. (1974). A model of attention describing the cognitive effects of marijuana. In L. L. Miller (Ed.), *Marijuana: Effects on human behavior* (pp. 103–120). New York: Academic Press.

Deniker, P. (1983). Discovery of the clinical use of neuroleptics. In M. J. Parnham & J. Bruinvels (Eds.), *Discoveries in pharmacology (Vol. 1): Psycho- and neuropharmacology* (pp. 163–180). New York: Elsevier.

Denissenko, M. F., Pao, A., Tang, M., & Pfeiffer, G. P. (1996). Preferential formation of benzo[*a*]pyrene adducts at lung cancer mutational hotspots in *P53. Science, 274,* 430–432.

de Sola, S., Tarancon, T., Pena-Casanova, J., Espadaler, J. M., Langohr, K., Poudevida, S., Farre, M., Verdejo-Garcia, A., & de la Torre, R. (2008). Auditory event-related potentials (P3) and cognitive performance in recreational ecstasy polydrug users: Evidence from a 12-month longitudinal study. *Psychopharmacology, 200,* 425–437.

Deutsch, A. Y., & Roth, R. H. (2009). Neurochemical systems in the central nervous system. In D. S. Charney & E. J. Nestler (Eds.), *Neurobiology of mental illness* (3rd ed., pp. 12–28). New York: Oxford University Press.

Devane, W. A., Dysarz, F. A., Johnson, R., Melvin, L. S., & Howlett, A. C. (1988). Determination and characterization of a cannabinoid receptor in the rat brain. *Molecular Pharmacology, 34,* 605–613.

Devane, W. A., Hanus, L., Breuer, A., Pertwee, R. G., Stevenson, L. A., Griffin, G., et al. (1992). Isolation and structure of a brain constituent that binds to the cannabinoid receptor. *Science, 258,* 1946–1949.

Dews, P. B., Curtis, G. L., Hanford, K. J., & O'Brien, C. P. (1999). The frequency of caffeine withdrawal in a population-based survey and in a controlled, blinded experiment. *Journal of Clinical Pharmacology, 39,* 1221–1232.

Dews, P. B., O'Brien, C. P., & Bergman, J. (2002). Caffeine: Behavioral effects of withdrawal and related issues. *Food and Chemical Toxicology, 40,* 1257–1261.

Diem, S. J., Blackwell, T. L., Stone, K. L., Yaffe, K., Haney, E. M., Bliziotes, M. M., & Ensrud, K. E. (2007). Use of antidepressants and rates of hip bone loss in older women: The study of osteoporotic fractures. *Archives of Internal Medicine, 167,* 1240–1245.

Di Forti, M., Morrison, P. D., Butt, A., & Murray, R. M. (2007). Cannabis use and psychiatric and cognitive disorders: The chicken or the egg? *Current Opinion in Psychiatry, 20,* 228–234.

Djousse, L., Lee, I-M., Buring, J. E., & Gaziano, J. M. (2009). Alcohol consumption and risk of cardiovascular disease and death in women. Potential mediating mechanisms. *Circulation, 120,* 237-244.

Dolan, K., Rouen, D., & Kimber, J. (2004). An overview of the use of urine, hair, sweat, and saliva to detect drug use. *Drug and Alcohol Reviews, 23,* 213–217.

Doll, R. (1998). The benefit of alcohol in moderation. *Drug and Alcohol Review, 17,* 353–363.

Droomers, M., Schrijvers, C. T. M., & Mackenbach, J. P. (2002). Why do lower educated people continue smoking? Explanations from the longitudinal GLOBE study. *Health Psychology, 21,* 263–272.

Drug Abuse Warning Network. (1996). Retrieved from http://www.samhsa.gov

Duman, R. S. (2004). Depression: A case of neuronal life and death? *Biological Psychiatry, 56,* 140–145.

Duman, R. S. (2009). Neurochemical theories of depression: Preclinical studies. In D. S. Charney & E. J. Nestler (Eds.), *Neurobiology of mental illness* (3rd ed., pp. 413–434). New York: Oxford University Press.

Duman, R. S., Nakagawa, S., & Malberg, J. (2001). Regulation of adult neurogenesis by antidepressant treatment. *Neuropsychopharmacology, 25,* 836–844.

Duncan, D. F. (1987). Lifetime prevalence of "amotivational syndrome" among users and nonusers of hashish. *Psychology of Addictive Behaviors, 1,* 114–119.

Dunn, M. E., & Goldman, M. S. (1996). Empirical modeling of an alcohol expectancy network in elementary-school children as a function of grade. *Experimental and Clinical Psychopharmacology, 4,* 209–217.

DuPont, R. L. (1980). The future of primary prevention: Parent power. *Journal of Drug Education, 10,* 1–5.

Durrant, R., & Thakker, J. (2003). *Substance use and abuse: Cultural and historical perspectives.* Thousand Oaks, CA: Sage Press.

Earleywine, M. (1994). Personality risk for alcoholism and alcohol expectancies. *Addictive Behaviors, 19,* 577–582.

Earleywine, M. (2002). *Understanding marijuana: A new look at the scientific evidence.* New York: Oxford University Press.

Ebmeier, K. P., Donaghey, C., & Steele, J. D. (2006). Recent developments and current controversies in depression. *The Lancet, 367,* 153–167.

Edwards, D. D. (1986). Nicotine: A drug of choice? *Science News, 129,* 44–45.

Eede, H. V., Montenij, L. J., Touw, D. J., & Norris, E. M. (2009). Rhabdomyolysis in MDMA intoxication: A rapid and underestimated killer. *Journal of Emergency Medicine,* June 3, [epub ahead of print].

Efron, S. (2005). Drug war fails to dent U.S. supply. *Los Angeles Times,* June 29.

Ehrenkranz, J. R. L., & Hembree, W. C. (1986). Effects of marijuana on male reproductive function. *Psychiatric Annals, 16,* 243–248.

Eissenberg, T., Ward, K. D., Smith-Simone, S., & Maziak, W. (2008). Waterpipe tobacco smoking on a U.S. college campus: Prevalence and correlates. *Journal of Adolescent Health, 42,* 526–529.

Eliopoulos, C., Klein, J., Phan, M., Knie, B., Greenwald, M., Chitayat, D., et al. (1994). Hair concentrations of nicotine and cotinine in women and their newborn infants. *Journal of the American Medical Association, 271,* 621–623.

El Sohly, M. A. (2002). Chemical constituents of cannabis. In F. Grotenhermen & E. Russo (Eds.), *Cannabis and cannabinoids: Pharmacology, toxicology and therapeutic potential* (pp. 27–36). London: Haworth Press.

El Sohly, M. A., Ross, S. A., Mehmedic, Z., Arafat, R., Yi, B., & Banahan, B. F. (2000). Potency trends of delta(9)-THC and other cannabinoids in confiscated marijuana from 1980–1997. *Journal of Forensic Sciences, 45,* 24–30.

Emrick, C. D. (1975). A review of the psychologically oriented treatment of alcoholism, II. The relative effectiveness of different treatment approaches and the effectiveness of treatment vs. no treatment. *Journal of Studies on Alcohol, 36,* 88–108.

Emrick, C. D. (1989). Alcoholics Anonymous: Membership characteristics and effectiveness as treatment. In M. Galanter (Ed.), *Recent developments in alcoholism* (Vol. 7, pp. 37–53). New York: Plenum Press.

Emrick, C. D., Lassen, C. L., & Edwards, M. T. (1977). Nonprofessional peers as therapeutic agents. In A. S. Gurman & A. M. Razin (Eds.), *Effective psychotherapy: A handbook of research* (pp. 120–161). New York: Pergamon Press.

Emrick, C. D., Tonigan, J. S., Montgomery, H., & Little, L. (1993). Alcoholics Anonymous: What is currently known? In B. S. McCrady & W. R. Miller (Eds.), *Research on Alcoholics Anonymous: Opportunities and alternatives* (pp. 41–76). New Brunswick, NJ: Rutgers Center of Alcohol Studies.

Endo, O., Matsumoto, M., Inaba, Y., Sugita, K., Nakajima, D., Goto, S., Ogata, H., & Susuki, G. (2009). Nicotine, tar, and mutagenicity of mainstream smoke generated by machine smoking with International Organization for Standardization and Health Canada Intense regimens of major Japanese cigarette brands. *Journal of Health Science, 55,* 421–427.

Engs, R. C., Diebold, B. A., & Hansen, D. J. (1996). The drinking patterns and problems of a national sample of college students, 1994. *Journal of Alcohol and Drug Education, 41,* 13–33.

Ennett, S. T., Tobler, N. S., Ringwalt, C. L., & Flewelling, R. L. (1994). How effective is drug abuse resistance education? A meta-analysis of Project DARE outcome. *American Journal of Public Health, 84,* 1394–1401.

Erenhart, C. B. (1991). Clinical correlations between ethanol intake and fetal alcohol syndrome. In M. Galanter (Ed.), *Recent developments in alcoholism* (Vol. 9, pp. 127–150). New York: Plenum Press.

Ernster, V. L. (1993). Women and smoking. *American Journal of Public Health, 83,* 1202–1203.

Eskelinen, M. H., Ngandu, T., Tuomilehto, J., Soininen, H., & Kivipelto, M. (2009). Midlife coffee and tea drinking and the risk of late-life dementia: A population-based CAIDE study. *Journal of Alzheimer's Disease, 16,* 85–91.

Etheridge, R. M., Hubbard, R. L., Anderson, J., Craddock, S. G., & Flynn, P. M. (1997). Treatment structure and program services in the Drug Abuse Treatment Outcome Study (DATOS). *Psychology of Addictive Behaviors, 11,* 244–260.

Evans, A. M., & Griffiths, R. R. (1999). Caffeine withdrawal: A parametric analysis of caffeine dosing conditions. *The Journal of Pharmacology and Experimental Therapeutics, 289,* 285–294.

Exum, M. L. (2006). Alcohol and aggression: An integration of findings from experimental studies. *Journal of Criminal Justice, 34,* 131–145.

Ezzati, M., & Lopez, A. D. (2003). Estimates of global mortality attributable to smoking in 2000. *The Lancet, 362,* 847–852.

Fainaru-Wada, M., & Williams, L. (2006). *Game of shadows.* New York: Gotham Books.

Fait, M. L., Wise, M. G., Jachna, J. S., Lane, R. D., & Gelenberg, A. J. (2002). Psychopharmacology. In M. Wise & J. R. Rundell (Eds.), *Textbook of consultation-liaison psychiatry* (2nd ed., pp. 939–987). Washington, DC: American Psychiatric Publishing.

Fallon, J. H., Keator, D., Mbgori, J., & Potkin, S. G. (2004). Hostility differentiates the brain metabolic effects of nicotine. *Cognitive Brain Research, 18,* 142–148.

Farre, M., Teran, M., & Cami, J. (1996). A comparison of the acute behavioral effects of flunitrazepam and triazolam in healthy volunteers. *Psychopharmacology, 125,* 1–12.

Federal Trade Commission. (2001). *"Tar," nicotine, and carbon monoxide of the smoke of 1294 varieties of domestic cigarettes for the year 1998.* Washington, DC: Author.

Fein, G., Torres, J., Price, L. J., & Sclafani, V. D. (2006). Cognitive performance in long-term abstinent alcoholic individuals. *Alcoholism: Clinical and Experimental Research, 30,* 1538–1544.

Feldman, H. W., Agar, M. H., & Beschner, G. M. (1979). *Angel dust.* Lexington, MA: Lexington Books.

Feldman, R. S., Meyer, J. S., & Quenzer, L. F. (1997). *Principles of neuropsychopharmacology.* Sunderland, MA: Sinauer Associates.

Fell, J. C., Fisher, D. A., Voas, R. B., Blackman, K., & Tippetts, A. S. (2009). The impact of underage drinking laws on alcohol-related fatal crashes of young drivers. *Alcoholism: Clinical and Experimental Research, 33,* 1208–1219.

Fergusson, D. M., Boden, J. M., & Horwood, L. J. (2006). Cannabis use and other illicit drug use: Testing the cannabis gateway hypothesis. *Addiction, 101,* 556–569.

Fergusson, D. M., & Horwood, L. J. (2000). Does cannabis use encourage other forms of illicit drug use? *Addiction, 95,* 505–520.

Ferreira, S. E., Tulio de Mello, M., Pompeia, S., & Oliveira de Souza-Formigoni, M. L. (2006). Effects of energy drink ingestion on alcohol intoxication. *Alcoholism: Clinical and Experimental Research, 30,* 598–605.

Field, T. (2008). Breastfeeding and antidepressants. *Infant Behavior and Development, 31,* 481–487.

Fieve, R. R. (1976). Therapeutic uses of lithium and rubidium. In L. L. Simpson (Ed.), *Drug treatment of mental disorders* (pp. 193–208). New York: Raven Press.

Fillmore, K. M., et al. (2006). Moderate alcohol use and reduced mortality risk: Systematic error in prospective studies. *Addiction Theory and Research, 14,* 101–132.

Fillmore, M. T., & Vogel-Sprott, M. (1996). Evidence that expectancies mediate behavioral impairment under alcohol. *Journal of Studies on Alcohol, 57,* 598–603.

Fiorentine, R. (1997). After drug treatment: Are 12-step programs effective in maintaining abstinence? *American Journal of Drug and Alcohol Abuse, 25,* 93–116.

Fiori, M. G., Keller, P. A., & Curry, S. J. (2007). Health system changes to facilitate the delivery of tobacco dependence treatment. *American Journal of Preventive Medicine, 33,* S349–S356.

Fischer, B. D., Miller, L. L., Henry, F. E., Picker, M. J., & Dykstra, L. A. (2008). Increased efficacy of micro-opioid agonist induced antinociception by metabotropic glutamate receptor antagonists in C57BL/6 mice: comparison with 6-phosphonomethyl-decahydroisoquinoline-3-carboxylic acid (LY235959). *Psychopharmacology, 198,* 271–278.

Fischman, M. W. (1984). The behavioral pharmacology of cocaine in humans. In J. Grabowski (Ed.), *Cocaine: Pharmacology, effects and treatment of abuse.* Research Monograph 50. Washington, DC: National Institute on Drug Abuse.

Fisher, L. M. (1992, October 6). New drugs by process of elimination. *The New York Times,* pp. D1, D13.

Fisone, G., Borgkvist, A., & Usiello, A. (2004). Caffeine as a psychomotor stimulant: Mechanism of action. *Cellular and Molecular Life Sciences, 61,* 857–872.

Flay, B. R. (1985). What we know about the social influences to smoking prevention: Review and recommendations. In C. Bell & R. Battjes (Eds.), *Prevention research: Deterring drug abuse among children and adolescents* (pp. 67–112). Rockville, MD: National Institute on Drug Abuse.

Fleming, M. F., Barry, K. L., Manwell, L. B., Johnson, K., & London, R. (1997). Brief physician advice for problem alcohol drinkers. *Journal of the American Medical Association, 277,* 1039–1045.

Fletcher, A. M. (2001). *Sober for good.* Boston: Houghton Mifflin.

Fletcher, B. W., Tims, F. M., & Brown, B. S. (1997). Drug Abuse Treatment Outcome Study (DATOS): Treatment evaluation research in the United States. *Psychology of Addictive Behaviors, 11,* 216–229.

Foltin, R. W., & Fischman, M. W. (1992). The cardiovascular and subjective effects of intravenous cocaine and morphine combinations in humans. *Journal of Pharmacology and Experimental Therapeutics, 261,* 623–632.

Foltin, R. W., & Fischman, M. W. (1993). Self-administration of smoked cocaine by humans. In L. Harris (Ed.), *Problems of drug dependence, 1992.* Research Monograph 132 (p. 63). Washington, DC: National Institute on Drug Abuse.

Foltin, R. W., Fischman, M. W., Brady, J. V., Bernstein, D. J., Capriotti, R. M., Nellis, M. J., et al. (1990). Motivational effects of smoked marijuana: Behavioral contingencies and low-probability activities. *Journal of the Experimental Analysis of Behavior, 53,* 5–19.

Foltin, R. W., Fischman, M. W., Brady, J. V., Kelly, T. H., Bernstein, D. J., & Nellis, M. J. (1989). Motivational effects of smoked marijuana: Behavioral contingencies and high-probability recreational activities. *Pharmacology, Biochemistry, and Behavior, 34,* 871–877.

Food and Drug Administration (FDA). (2002). FDA approves Xyrem for cataplexy attacks in patients with narcolepsy. FDA Talk Paper, July 17.

FDA. (2009). Organ-specific warnings; internal analgesic, antipyretic, and antirheumatic drug products for over-the-counter human use. *Federal Register,* 74, April 29, 2009.

Franck, P. H. (1983). "If you drink, don't drive" motto now applies to hangovers as well. *Journal of the American Medical Association, 250,* 1657–1658.

Franey, C., & Ashton, M. (2002). The grand design lessons from DATOS. *Drug and Alcohol Findings, 7,* 4–19.

Frary, C. D., Johnson, R. K., & Wang, M. Q. (2005). Food sources and intakes of caffeine in the diets of persons in the United States. *Journal of the American Dietetic Association, 105,* 110–113.

Fredholm, B. B., Battig, K., Holmen, J., Nehlig, A., & Zvartau, E. E. (1999). Actions of caffeine in the brain with special reference to factors that contribute to its widespread use. *Pharmacological Reviews, 51,* 83–133.

Freedman, R. R., Johanson, C., & Tancer, M. E. (2005). Thermoregulatory effects of 3,4-methylenedioxymethamphetamine (MDMA) in humans. *Psychopharmacology, 183,* 248–256.

French, M. T., & McGeary, K. A. (1997). Estimating the cost of substance abuse treatment. *Health Economics Letters, 6,* 1–6.

Frezza, M., di Padova, C., Pozzato, G., Terpin, M., Baraona, E., & Lieber, C. S. (1990). High blood alcohol levels in women: The role of decreased gastric alcohol dehydrogenase activity and first pass metabolism. *New England Journal of Medicine, 322,* 95–99.

Fried, P. A. (1986). Marijuana and human pregnancy. In I. J. Chasnoff (Ed.), *Drug use in pregnancy: Mother and child* (pp. 64–74). Lancaster, PA: MTP Press.

Fried, P. A., Watkinson, B., & Gray, R. (1992). A follow-up study of attentional behavior in 6-year-old children exposed prenatally to marijuana, cigarettes, and alcohol. *Neurotoxicology and Teratology, 14,* 299–311.

Friedl, K. E. (2000a). Effect of anabolic steroid use on body composition and physical performance. In C. E. Yesalis (Ed.), *Anabolic steroids in sport and exercise* (2nd ed., pp. 139–174). Champaign, IL: Human Kinetics Press.

Friedl, K. E. (2000b). Effects of anabolic steroid use on physical health. In C. E. Yesalis (Ed.), *Anabolic steroids in sport and exercise* (2nd ed., pp. 175–224). Champaign, IL: Human Kinetics Press.

Frunkel, E. N., Kanner, J., German, J. B., Parks, E., & Kinsella, J. E. (1993). Inhibition of oxidation of human low-density lipoprotein by phenolic substances in red wine. *Lancet, 341,* 454–457.

Galenberg, A. J. (1991). Psychoses. In A. J. Galenberg, E. L. Bussuk, & S. C. Schoonover (Eds.), *The practitioner's guide to psychoactive drugs* (3rd ed., pp. 125–178). New York: Plenum Medical Book Company.

Galenberg, A. J., & Schoonover, S. C. (1991). Depression. In A. J. Galenberg, E. L. Bussuk, & S. C. Schoonover (Eds.), *The practitioner's guide to psychoactive drugs* (3rd ed., pp. 23–89). New York: Plenum Medical Book Company.

Galizio, M., Keith, J. R., Mansfield, W., & Pitts, R. C. (2003). Repeated spatial acquisition: Effects of NMDA antagonists and morphine. *Experimental and Clinical Psychopharmacology, 11,* 79–90.

Galizio, M., & Maisto, S. A. (Eds.). (1985). *Determinants of substance abuse.* New York: Plenum Press.

Galloway, G. P., Frederick-Osborne, S. L., Seymour, R., Contini, S. E., & Smith, D. E. (2000). Abuse and therapeutic potential of gamma-hydroxybutyric acid. *Alcohol, 20,* 263–269.

Ganio, M. S., Klau, J. F., Casa, D. J., Armstrong, L. E., & Maresh, C. M. (2009). Effect of caffeine on sport-specific endurance performance: A systematic review. *Journal of Strength and Conditioning Research, 23,* 315–324.

Gaoni, Y., & Mechoulam, R. (1964). Isolation, structure, and partial synthesis of an active constituent of hashish. *Journal of the American Chemical Society, 86,* 1646–1647.

Garbutt, J. C., West, S. L., Carey, T. S., Lohr, K. N., & Crews, F. T. (1999). Pharmacological treatment of alcohol dependence: A review of the evidence. *Journal of the American Medical Association, 281,* 1318–1325.

Gardner, D. M., Baldessarini, R. J., & Waraich, P. (2005). Modern antipsychotic drugs: A critical overview. *CMAJ, 172,* 1703–1711.

Gastfriend, D. R. (Ed.). (2003). *Addiction treatment matching.* New York: Haworth Medical Press.

Gautier, T. (1844/1966). *Le club des hachichins.* In D. Solomon (Ed.), *The marijuana papers* (pp. 121–135). New York: Bobbs-Merrill.

Gauvin, D. V., Cheng, E. Y., & Holloway, F. A. (1993). Biobehavioral correlates. In M. Gallanter (Ed.), *Recent developments in alcoholism* (Vol. 11, pp. 281–304). New York: Plenum Press.

Gavaghan, C. (2009). "You can't handle the truth"; Medical paternalism and prenatal alcohol use. *Journal of Medical Ethics, 35,* 300–303.

Gay, G. R., & Way, E. L. (1972). Pharmacology of the opiate narcotics. In D. E. Smith & G. R. Way (Eds.), *It's so good, don't even try it once* (pp. 32–44). Englewood Cliffs, NJ: Prentice Hall.

Gaziano, J. M., et al. (1993). Moderate alcohol intake, increased levels of high-density lipoprotein and its subfractions, and decreased risk of myocardial infarction. *New England Journal of Medicine, 329,* 1829–1834.

Geller, E. S., Russ, N. W., & Delphos, W. A. (1987). Does server intervention training make a difference? *Alcohol Health and Research World, 11,* 64–69.

Ghatol, A., & Kazory, A. (2009). Ecstasy-associated acute severe hyponatremia and cerebral edema: A role for osmotic diuresis? *Journal of Emergency Medicine,* June 3, [epub ahead of print].

Gilbert, R. M. (1976). Caffeine as a drug of abuse. In R. J. Gibbins, Y. Israel, H. Kalant, R. E. Popham, W. Schmidt, & R. G. Smart (Eds.), *Research advances in alcohol and drug problems* (Vol. 3, pp. 49–176). New York: John Wiley.

Gilbert, R. M. (1984). Caffeine consumption. *Progress in Clinical Biological Research, 158,* 185–213.

Gitlin, M. J. (1990). *The psychotherapist's guide to psychopharmacology.* New York: Free Press.

Glantz, S. A., & Parmley, W. W. (1991). Passive smoking and heart disease. *Circulation, 83,* 1–12.

Gliksman, L., McKenzie, D., Single, E., Douglas, R., Brunet, S., & Moffatt, K. (1993). The role of alcohol providers in prevention: An evaluation of a server intervention programme. *Addiction, 88,* 1195–1203.

Golan, D. (2005, Summer 2005 Special Edition). Building better medicines. *Newsweek,* pp. 37–39.

Goldman, A. (1971). *Ladies and gentlemen, Lenny Bruce!* New York: Random House.

Goldman, M. S., Darkes, J., & Del Boca, F. K. (1999). Expectancy mediation of biopsychosocial risk for alcohol use and alcoholism. In I. Kirsch (Ed.), *How expectancies shape experience* (pp. 263–300). Washington, DC: American Psychological Association.

Goldschmidt, L., Day, N. L., & Richardson, G. A. (2000). Effects of prenatal marijuana exposure on child behavior problems at age 10. *Neurotoxicology and Teratology, 22,* 325–336.

Goldstein, A. (2001). *Addiction: From biology to social policy* (2nd ed.). New York: Oxford University Press.

Goldstein, A., & Wallace, M. E. (1997). Caffeine dependence in school children? *Experimental and Clinical Psychopharmacology, 5,* 388–392.

Goldstein, A. S., Kaizer, S., & Whitby, O. (1969). Psychotropic effects of caffeine in man. IV. Quantitative and qualitative differences associated with habituation to coffee. *Clinical and Pharmacological Therapeutics, 10,* 489–497.

Goldstein, J. W., & Sappington, J. T. (1977). Personality characteristics of students who became heavy drug users: An MMPI study of an avant garde. *American Journal of Drug and Alcohol Abuse, 4,* 401–412.

Goode, E. (1972). *Drugs in American society.* New York: Alfred A. Knopf.

Goode, E. (1993). *Drugs in American society* (4th ed.). New York: McGraw-Hill.

Gordon, B. (1979). *I'm dancing as fast as I can*. New York: Bantam Books.

Gorman, D. M. (1995). The changing role of mass media in preventing excessive alcohol use. *Drugs: Education, Prevention, and Policy, 2,* 77–84.

Gould, E., Reeves, A. J., Graziano, M. S., & Gross, C. G. (1999). Neurogenesis in the neocortex of adult primates. *Science, 286,* 548–552.

Government Printing Office (GPO). (1972). *Drug abuse: Games without winners.* Washington, DC: Author.

Graham, D. M. (1978). Caffeine: Its identity, dietary sources, intake and biological effects. *Nutrition Reviews, 36,* 97–102.

Graham, K., Leonard, K. E., Room, R., Wild, C., Pihl, R. O., Boiss, C., et al. (1998). Current directions in research on understanding and preventing intoxicated aggression. *Addiction, 93,* 659–676.

Grant, B. F., & Dawson, D.A. (1998). Age of onset of drug use and its association with DSM-IV drug abuse and dependence: Results from the National Longitudinal Alcohol Epidemiologic Survey. *Journal of Substance Abuse, 10,* 163–173.

Grant, I., Gonzalez, R., Carey, C.L., Natarajan, L., & Wolfson, T. (2003). Non-acute (residual) neurocognitive effects of cannabis use: a meta-analytic study. *Journal of the International Neuropsychological Society, 9,* 679–689.

Grant, S. G. (2005). Qualitatively and quantitatively similar effects of active and passive maternal tobacco smoke exposure on in utero mutagenesis at the HPRT locus. *BMC Pediatrics,* DOI:10.1186/ 1471-2431-5-20.

Greden, J. F. (1974). Anxiety or caffeinism: A diagnostic dilemma. *American Journal of Psychiatry, 131,* 1089–1092.

Greden, J. F., & Walters, A. (1992). Caffeine. In J. H. Lowinson, P. Ruiz, & R. B. Millman (Eds.), *Substance abuse: A comprehensive textbook* (2nd ed., pp. 357–370). Baltimore, MD: Williams & Wilkins.

Greeley, J., & Oei, T. (1999). Alcohol and tension reduction. In K. E. Leonard & H. T. Blane (Eds.), *Psychological theories of drinking and alcoholism* (2nd ed., pp. 14–53). New York: Guilford Press.

Green, T. C., Serrano, J. M. G., Licari, A., Budman, S. H., & Butler, S. (2009). Women who abuse prescription opioids: Findings from the Addiction Severity Index-Multimedia Version Connect prescription opioid database. *Drug and Alcohol Dependence, 103,* 65–73.

Griffiths, R. R., Bigelow, G. E., Liebson, I., & Kaliszak, J. E. (1980). Drug preference in humans: Double-blind choice comparison of pentobarbital, diazepam, and placebo. *Journal of Pharmacology and Experimental Therapeutics, 215,* 649–661.

Griffiths, R. R., McLeod, E. R., Bigelow, G. E., Liebson, I. A., & Roache, J. D. (1984). Relative abuse liability of diazepam and oxazepam: Behavior and subjective dose effects. *Psychopharmacology, 84,* 147–154.

Griffiths, R. R., McLeod, E. R., Bigelow, G. E., Liebson, I. A., Roache, J. D., & Nowowieski, P. (1984). Comparison of diazepam and oxazepam: Preference liking and extent of abuse. *Journal of Pharmacology and Experimental Therapeutics, 229,* 501–508.

Griffiths, R. R., & Woodson, P. P. (1988a). Caffeine physical dependence: A review of human and animal laboratory studies. *Psychopharmacology, 94,* 437–451.

Griffiths, R. R., & Woodson, D. P. (1988b). Reinforcing properties of caffeine: Studies in human and laboratory animals. *Pharmacology, Biochemistry, and Behavior, 28,* 419–427.

Grilly, D. M. (2002). *Drugs and human behavior.* Boston: Allyn & Bacon.

Grinspoon, L., & Bakalar, J. B. (1976). *Cocaine: A drug and its social evolution.* New York: Harper Books.

Grinspoon, L., & Bakalar, J. B. (1979). *Psychedelic drugs reconsidered.* New York: Basic Books.

Grinspoon, L., & Bakalar, J. B. (1983). *Psychedelic reflections.* New York: Human Sciences Press.

Gritz, E. R., Ksir, C., & McCarthy, W. J. (1985). Smokeless tobacco use in the United States: Present and future trends. *Annals of Behavioral Medicine, 7,* 24–27.

Grobbee, D., Rimm, E., Giovannucci, E., Colditz, G., Stampfer, M., & Willett, W. (1990). Coffee, caffeine, and cardiovascular disease in men. *New England Journal of Medicine, 323,* 1026–1032.

Grogan, F. J. (1987). *The pharmacist's prescription.* New York: Rawson Associates.

Gronbaek, M., Deis, A., Sorensen, T. I. A., Becker, U., Schnohr, P., & Jensen, G. (1995). Mortality associated with moderate intake of wine, beer, or spirits. *British Medical Journal, 310,* 1165–1169.

Grotenhermen, F. (2007). The toxicology of cannabis and cannabis prohibition. *Chemistry & Biodiversity, 4,* 1744–1769.

Grufferman, S., Schwartz, A. G., Ruymann, F. B., & Maurer, H. M. (1993). Parent's use of cocaine and marijuana and increased risk of rhabdomyosarcoma in their children. *Cancer Causes Control, 4,* 217–224.

Grunder, G., Hippius, H., & Carlsson, A. (2009). The 'atypicality' of antipsychotics: A concept re-examined and re-defined. *Nature Reviews, 8,* 197–202.

Gutjahr, E., Gmel, G., & Rehm, J. (2001). Relation between average alcohol consumption and disease: An overview. *Addiction Research, 7,* 117–127.

Hajek, P., West, R., Foulds, J., Nilsson, F., Burrow, S., & Meadow, A. (1999). Randomized comparative trials of nicotine polacrilex, a transdermal patch, nasal spray, and inhaler. *Archives of Internal Medicine, 159,* 2033–2038.

Halkitis, P. N. (2009). *Methamphetamine addiction: Biological foundations, psychological factors, and social consequences.* Washington: American Psychological Association Press.

Hall, K. M., Irwin, M. M., Bowman, K. A., Frankenberger, W., & Jewett, D. C. (2005). Illicit use of prescribed stimulant medication among college students. *Journal of American College Health, 53,* 167–174.

Hall, W. D., & Lynskey, M. (2005). Is cannabis a gateway drug? Testing hypotheses about the relationship between cannabis use and the use of other illicit drugs. *Drug and Alcohol Review, 24,* 39–48.

Halpern, J. H., & Pope, H. G. (1999). Do hallucinogens cause residual neuropsychological toxicity? *Drug and Alcohol Dependence, 53,* 247–256.

Halpern, J. H., & Pope, H. G. (2003). Hallucinogen persisting perception disorder: What do we know after 50 years? *Drug and Alcohol Dependence, 69,* 109–119.

Halpern, J. H., Pope, H. G., Sherwood, A. R., Barry, S., Hudson, J. I., & Yurgelin-Todd, D. (2004). Residual neuropsychological effects of illicit 3,4-methylenedioxymethamphetamine (MDMA) in individuals with minimal exposure to other drugs. *Drug and Alcohol Dependence, 75,* 135–147.

Hamilton, G., Cross, D., Resnicow, K., & Hall, M. (2005). A school-based harm minimization smoking intervention trial: Outcome results. *Addiction, 100,* 689–700.

Han, J. S., & Terenius, L. (1982). Neurochemical basis of acupuncture analgesia. *Annual Review of Pharmacology and Toxicology, 22,* 193–220.

Harris, G. (2004, December 6). At FDA, strong drug ties and less monitoring. *The New York Times,* pp. A1, A20.

Harris, G. (2007). Potentially incompatible goals at the FDA. *The New York Times,* June 11, 2007.

Harris, L. S., Dewey, W. L., & Razdan, R. K. (1977). Cannabis: Its chemistry, pharmacology, and toxicology. In W. R. Martin (Ed.), *Drug addiction II: Amphetamine, psychotogen, and marihuana dependence* (pp. 371–429). New York: Springer-Verlag.

Hart, C. L., Gunderson, E. W., Perez, A., Kirkpatrick, M. G., Thurmond, A., Comer, S. D., & Foltin, R. W. (2008). Acute physiological and behavioral effects of intranasal methamphetamine in humans. *Neuropsychopharmacology, 33,* 1847–1855.

Harvey, S. C. (1980). Hypnotics and sedatives. In A. G. Gilman, L. S. Goodman, & A. Gilman (Eds.), *Goodman and Gilman's The pharmacological basis of therapeutics* (6th ed., pp. 339–379). London: Macmillan.

Harwood, H., Fountain, D., & Livermore, G. (1998). *The economic costs of alcohol and drug abuse in the United States—1992.* Rockville, MD: U.S. Department of Health and Human Services.

Hatzidimitriou, G., McCann, U. D., & Ricaurte, G. A. (1999). Altered serotonin innervation patterns in the forebrain of monkeys treated with (1/2)-3, 4-methylenedioxymethamphetamine seven years previously: Factors influencing abnormal recovery. *Journal of Neuroscience, 19,* 5096–5107.

Hawks, R. L., & Chiang, C. N. (1986). *Urine testing for drugs of abuse.* Research Monograph 73. Washington, DC: National Institute on Drug Abuse.

Hecht, A. (1985). *Addictive behavior: Drug and alcohol abuse.* Englewood, CO: Morton Publishing.

Hegadoren, K. M., Baker, G. B., & Bourin, M. (1999). 3,4-methyl-enedioxy analogues of amphetamine: Defining the risks to humans. *Neuroscience and Biobehavioral Reviews, 23,* 539–553.

Heishman, S. J., Taylor, R. C., & Henningfield, J. E. (1994). Nicotine and smoking: A review of effects on human performance. *Experimental and Clinical Psychopharmacology, 2,* 345–395.

Henningfield, J. E., Lukas, S. E., & Bigelow, G. E. (1986). Human studies of drugs as reinforcers. In S. R. Goldberg & I. P. Stolerman (Eds.), *Behavioral analysis of drug dependence* (pp. 69–122). New York: Academic Press.

Henningfield, J. E., Santora, P. S., & Stillman, F. A. (2005). Exploitation by design—could tobacco industry documents guide more effective smoking prevention and cessation in women? *Addiction, 100,* 715–716.

Hepler, R. S., & Petrus, R. J. (1976). Experiences with administration of marijuana to glaucoma patients. In S. Cohen & R. C. Stillman (Eds.), *The therapeutic aspects of marijuana* (pp. 63–75). New York: Plenum Press.

Hepple, J., & Robson, P. (1996). The effect of caffeine on cue exposure responses in ex-smokers. *Addiction, 91,* 269–273.

Herkenham, M., Lynn, A. B., Little, M. D., Johnson, M. R., Melvin, L. S., deCosta, B. R., et al. (1990). Cannabinoid receptor localization in the brain. *National Academy of Science, 87,* 1932–1936.

Hester, R. K., & Delaney, H. D. (1997). Behavioral self-control program for Windows: Results of a controlled clinical trial. *Journal of Consulting and Clinical Psychology, 65,* 683–693.

Hester, R. K., & Miller, W. R. (Eds.). (1989). *Handbook of alcoholism treatment approaches: Effective alternatives.* Elmsford, NY: Pergamon Press.

Hewitt, L. E. (1982). Current status of alcohol education programs for youth. In *Special Population Issues,* Alcohol and Health Monograph 4 (pp. 227–260). Rockville, MD: National Institute on Alcohol Abuse and Alcoholism.

Higdon, J.V., & Frei, B. (2006). Coffee and health: A review of recent human research. *Critical Reviews in Food Science and Nutrition, 46,* 101–123.

Higgins, S. T., Budney, A. J., Bickel, W. K., Hughes, J. R., Foerg, F., & Badger, G. (1993). Achieving cocaine abstinence with a behavioral approach. *American Journal of Psychiatry, 150,* 763–769.

Higgins, S. T., Delaney, D. D., Budney, A. J., Bickel, W. K., Hughes, J. R., Foerg, F., et al. (1991). A behavioral approach to achieving initial cocaine abstinence. *American Journal of Psychiatry, 148,* 1218–1224.

Higgins, S. T., & Stitzer, M. L. (1988). Time allocation in a concurrent schedule of social interaction and monetary reinforcement: Effects of *d*-amphetamine. *Pharmacology, Biochemistry, and Behavior, 31,* 227–231.

Higuchi, S., Parrish, K. M., Dufour, M. C., Towle, L., & Harford, T. C. (1992). The relationship between three types of the flushing response and DSM-III alcohol abuse in Japanese. *Journal of Studies on Alcohol, 53,* 553–560.

Hill, S. Y., Wang, S., Kostelnik, B., Carter, H., Holmes, B., McDermott, M., Zezza, N., Stiffler, S., & Keshavan, M. S. (2009). Disruption of orbitofrontal cortex laterality in offspring from multiplex alcohol dependence families. *Biological Psychiatry, 65,* 129–136.

Hilton, M. E. (1993). An overview of recent findings on alcohol beverage warning labels. *Journal of Public Policy Marketing, 12,* 1–9.

Hindmarch, I., Rigney, U., Stanley, N., Quinlan, P., Rycroft, J., & Lane, J. (2000). A naturalistic investigation of the effects of daylong consumption of tea, coffee, and water on alertness, sleep onset, and sleep quality. *Psychopharmacology, 149,* 203–216.

Hingson, R. W., Heeren, T., Winter, M., & Wechsler, H. (2005). Magnitude of alcohol-related mortality and morbidity among U.S. college students ages 18–24. *Annual Review of Public Health, 26,* 259–279.

Hingson, R. W., Heeren, T., Zakocs, R. C., Kopstein, A., & Wechsler, H. (2002). Magnitude of alcohol-related mortality and morbidity among U.S. college students ages 18–24. *Journal of Studies on Alcohol, 63,* 136–144.

Hinson, R. E. (1985). Individual differences in tolerance and relapse: A Pavlovian conditioning perspective. In M. Galizio & S. A. Maisto (Eds.), *Determinants of substance abuse: Biological, psychological, and environmental factors* (pp. 101–124). New York: Plenum Press.

Ho, A. K. S., & Allen, J. P. (1981). Alcohol and the opiate receptor: Interactions with the endogenous opiates. *Advances in Alcohol & Substance Abuse, 1,* 53–75.

Hofmann, A. (1980). *LSD: My problem child.* New York: McGraw-Hill.

Hofmann, F. G. (1975). *A handbook on drug and alcohol abuse.* New York: Oxford University Press.

Hogan, E. H., Hornick, B. A., & Bouchoux, A. (2002). Communicating the message: Clarifying the controversies about caffeine. *Nutrition Today, 37,* 28–36.

Hogervorst, E., Bandelow, S., Schmitt, J., Jentjens, R., Oliveira, M., Allgrove, J., Carter, T., & Gleeson, M. (2008). Caffeine improves physical and cognitive performance during exhaustive exercise. *Medicine & Science in Sports & Exercise, 40,* 1841–1851.

Holder, H. D., & Blose, J. D. (1991). Typical patterns and cost of alcoholism treatment across a variety of populations and providers. *Alcoholism: Clinical and Experimental Research, 15,* 190–195.

Holland, J. (2001). The history of MDMA. In J. Holland (Ed.), *Ecstasy: The complete guide.* Rochester, VT: Park Street Press.

Hollis, J. F., et al. (2005). Teen Reach: Outcomes from a randomized, controlled trial of a tobacco reduction program for teens seen in primary medical care. *Pediatrics, 115,* 981–989.

Hollister, L. E., Richards, R. K., & Gillespie, H. K. (1968). Comparison of tetrahydrocannabinol and synhexyl in man. *Clinical Pharmacology and Therapeutics, 9,* 783–791.

Hopfer, C., Mendelson, B., Van Leeuwen, J. M., Kelly, S., & Hooks, S. (2006). Club drug use among youths in treatment for substance abuse. *American Journal on Addictions, 15,* 94–99.

House of Lords Select Committee on Science and Technology. (1988). *Cannabis: The scientific and medical evidence* (HL Paper 151). London: HMSO.

Howland, R. H. (2009). Prescribing psychotropic medications during pregnancy and lactation: Principles and guidelines. *Journal of Psychosocial Nursing, 47,* 19–23.

Hrobjartsson, A., & Gotzsche, P. C. (2001). Is the placebo powerless? An analysis of clinical trials comparing placebo with no treatment. *New England Journal of Medicine, 344,* 1594–1603.

Hser, Y-I., Hoffman, V., Grella, C. E., & Anglin, M. D. (2001). A 33-year follow-up of narcotics addicts. *Archives of General Psychiatry, 58,* 503–508.

Hubbard, R. L., Marsden, M. E., Rachal, J. V., Harwood, H. J., Cavanaugh, E. R., & Ginzburg, H. M. (1989). *Drug abuse treatment: A national study of effectiveness.* Chapel Hill: University of North Carolina Press.

Hudson, G. M., Green, J. M., Bishop, P. A., & Richardson, M. T. (2008). Effects of caffeine and aspirin on light resistance training performance, perceived exertion, and pain perception. *Journal of Strength and Conditioning Research, 22,* 1950–1957.

Hughes, C. E., Pitts, R. C., & Branch, M. N. (1996). Cocaine and food deprivation: Effects on food-reinforced fixed ratio performance in pigeons. *Journal of the Experimental Analysis of Behavior, 65,* 145–158.

Hughes, J. C., & Cook, C. H. (1997). The efficacy of disulfiram: A review of outcome studies. *Addiction, 92,* 381–395.

Hughes, J. R. (1993). Pharmacotherapy for smoking cessation: Unvalidated assumptions, anomalies, and suggestions for future research. *Journal of Consulting and Clinical Psychology, 61,* 751–760.

Hughes, J. R. (1996). The future of smoking cessation therapy in the United States. *Addiction, 91,* 1797–1802.

Hughes, J. R., & Carpenter, M. J. (2006). Does smoking reduction increase future cessation and decrease disease risk? A qualitative review. *Nicotine and Tobacco Research, 6,* 739–749.

Hughes, J. R., Goldstein, M. G., Hurt, R. D., & Shiffman, S. (1999). Recent advances in the pharmacotherapy of smoking. *Journal of the American Medical Association, 281,* 72–75.

Hughes, J. R., Grist, S. W., & Pechacek, T. F. (1987). Prevalence of tobacco dependence and withdrawal. *American Journal of Psychiatry, 144,* 205–208.

Hughes, J. R., & Hale, K. L. (1998). Behavioral effects of caffeine and other methylxanthines on children. *Experimental and Clinical Psychopharmacology, 6,* 87–95.

Hughes, J. R., Oliveto, A. H., Helzer, J. E., Higgins, S. T., & Bickel, W. K. (1992). Should caffeine abuse, dependence or withdrawal be added to DSM-IV or ICD-10? *American Journal of Psychiatry, 149,* 33–40.

Hull, J. G., & Bond, C. F. (1986). Social and behavioral consequences of alcohol consumption: A meta analysis. *Psychological Bulletin, 99,* 347–360.

Humphreys, K., Wing, S., McCarty, D., Chappel, J., Gallant, L., Haberle, B., et al. (2004). Self-help organizations for alcohol and drug problems: Toward evidence-based practice and policy. *Journal of Substance Abuse Treatment, 26,* 151–158.

Hunt, G. M., & Azrin, N. H. (1973). A community reinforcement approach to alcoholism. *Behavior Research and Therapy, 11,* 91–104.

Hunt, W. A., Barnett, L. W., & Branch, L. G. (1971). Relapse rates in addiction programs. *Journal of Clinical Psychology, 27,* 455–456.

Huxley, A. (1954). *The doors of perception.* New York: Harper.

Huxley, R., Jamrozik, T. H., Lam, T. H., Barzi, F., Ansary-Moghaddam, A., Jiamg, C. Q., Suh, I., & Woodward, M., on behalf of the Asia Pacific Cohort Studies Collaboration. (2007). Impact of smoking and smoking cessation on lung cancer mortality in the Asia-Pacific region. *American Journal of Epidemiology, 165,* 1280–1286.

Hyde, J. S., & DeLamater, J. D. (2006). *Understanding human sexuality* (9th ed.). New York: McGraw-Hill.

Hypericum Depression Trial Study Group. (2002). Effect of *Hypericum perforatum* (St. John's Wort) in major depressive disorder: A randomized controlled trial. *Journal of the American Medical Association, 287,* 1807–1814.

Ichiyama, M. A., Fairlie, A. M., Wood, M. D., Turrisi, R., Francies, D. P., Ray, A. E., & Stanger, L. A. (2009). A randomized trial of a parent-based intervention on drinking behavior among incoming college freshmen. *Journal of Studies on Alcohol and Drugs, Supplement, 16,* 67–76.

Iguchi, M. Y., Belding, M. A., Morral, A. R., Lamb, R. J., & Husband, S. D. (1997). Reinforcing operants other than abstinence in drug abuse treatment: An effective alternative for reducing drug use. *Journal of Consulting and Clinical Psychology, 65,* 421–428.

Inciardi, J. A. (2002). *The war on drugs III: The continuing saga of the mysteries and miseries of intoxication, addiction, crime, and public policy.* Boston: Allyn & Bacon.

Infante-Rivard, C., Fernandez, A., Gauthier, R., David, M., & Rivard, G. E. (1993). Fetal loss associated with caffeine intake before and during pregnancy. *Journal of the American Medical Association, 270,* 2940–2943.

Institute of Medicine. (1982). *Marijuana and health.* Washington, DC: National Academy Press.

Institute of Medicine. (1990a). *Broadening the base of treatment for alcohol problems.* Washington, DC: National Academy Press.

Institute of Medicine. (1990b). *Treating drug problems* (Vol. 1). Washington, DC: National Academy Press.

Institute of Medicine. (2001). *Caffeine for the sustainment of mental task performance: Formulations for military operations.* Washington, DC: National Academy of Sciences.

Iversen, L. L. (2000). *The science of marijuana.* New York: Oxford University Press.

Iversen, L. L. (2003). Cannabis and the brain. *Brain, 126,* 1252–1270.

Iversen, L. L. (2008). *Speed, ecstasy, Ritalin: The science of amphetamines.* Oxford: Oxford University Press.

Iversen, L. L., Iversen, S. D., Bloom, F. E., & Roth, R. H. (2009). *Introduction to neuropsychopharmacology.* New York: Oxford University Press.

Jacobs, B. L. (2004). Depression: The brain finally gets into the act. *Current Directions in Psychological Science, 13,* 103–106.

Jacobs, M. R., & Fehr, K. O'Brien. (1987). *Drugs and drug abuse: A reference text* (2nd ed.). Toronto: Addiction Research Foundation.

Jacobson, J. L., Jacobson, S. W., Sokol, R. J., Martier, S. S., Ager, J. W., & Kaplan-Estrin, G. (1993). Teratogenic effects of alcohol on infant development. *Alcoholism: Clinical and Experimental Research, 17,* 174–183.

Jaffe, J. H. (1990). Drug addiction and drug abuse. In A. G. Gilman, T. W. Rall, A. S. Nies, & P. Taylor (Eds.), *The pharmacological basis of therapeutics* (8th ed., pp. 522–573). New York: Pergamon Press.

Jaffe, J. H., & Martin, W. R. (1990). Opioid analgesics and antagonists. In A. G. Gilman, T. W. Rall, A. S. Nies, & P. Taylor (Eds.), *Goodman and Gilman's The pharmacological basis of therapeutics* (8th ed., pp. 485–521). New York: Pergamon Press.

Jahoda, G., & Cramond, J. (1972). *Children and alcohol.* London: HMSO.

James, J. E. (1991). *Caffeine and health.* New York: Academic Press.

James, W. H., & Johnson, S. L. (1996). *Doin' drugs: Patterns of African American addiction.* Austin: University of Texas Press.

Jansen, K. (2004). *Ketamine: Dreams and realities.* Sarasota, FL: Multidisciplinary Association for Psychedelic Studies.

Jarvik, M. E., Madsen, D. C., Olmstead, R. E., Iwamoto-Schapp, P. N., Elins, J. L., & Benowitz, N. L. (2000). Nicotine blood levels and subjective craving for cigarettes. *Pharmacology, Biochemistry, and Behavior, 66,* 553–558.

Jefferson, D. J. (2005, August). America's most dangerous drug. *Newsweek.*

Johanson, C. E. (1992). Biochemical mechanisms and pharmacological principles of drug action. In J. Grabowski & G. R. VandenBos (Eds.), *Master lecture series. Psychopharmacology: Basic mechanisms and applied interventions* (pp. 11–58). Washington, DC: American Psychological Association.

Johanson, C. E., & Uhlenhuth, E. H. (1978). Drug self-administration in humans. In N. A. Krasnegor (Ed.), *Self-administration of abused substances: Methods for study.* NIDA Research Monograph 20 (pp. 68–87). Washington, DC: U.S. Government Printing Office.

Johnson, B. D. (1973). *Marihuana users and drug subcultures.* New York: John Wiley.

Johnson, C., Drgon, T., Liu, O. R., Walther, D., Edenberg, H., Rice, J., Foroud, T., & Uhl, G. R. (2006). Pooled association genome scanning for alcohol dependence using 104,268 SNPs: Validation and use to identify alcoholism vulnerability lici in unrelated individuals from the collaborative study on the genetics of alcoholism. *American Journal of Medical Genetics. Part B, Neuropsychiatric Genetics, 141B,* 844–853.

Johnston, L. D., O'Malley, P. M., Bachman, J. G., & Schulenberg, J. E. (2009a). *Monitoring the future national results on adolescent drug use: Overview of key findings, 2008.* Bethesda, MD: National Institute on Drug Abuse.

Johnston, L. D., O'Malley, P. M., Bachman, J. G., & Schulenberg, J. E. (2009b). *Monitoring the future national results on adolescent drug use, 1975–2008. Volume 1: Secondary school students.* Bethesda, MD: National Institute on Drug Abuse.

Jones, G. (2008). Caffeine and other sympathomimetic stimulants: Modes of action and effects on sports performance. *Essays in Biochemistry, 44,* 109–123.

Jones, K. L., Smith, D. W., Ulleland, C. N., & Streissguth, P. (1973). Pattern of malformation in offspring of chronic alcoholic mothers. *Lancet, 1 (7815),* 1267–1271.

Jones, R. T. (1980). Human effects: An overview. In R. C. Peterson (Ed.), *Marijuana research findings: 1980* (pp. 54–80). Rockville, MD: National Institute on Drug Abuse.

Jones, R. T. (1987a). The psychopharmacology of cocaine. In A. M. Washton & M. S. Gold (Eds.), *Cocaine: A clinician's handbook* (pp. 55–72). New York: Guilford Press.

Jones, R. T. (1987b). Tobacco dependence. In H. Y. Meltzer (Ed.), *Psychopharmacology: The third generation of progress* (pp. 1589–1595). New York: Raven Press.

Joy, J. E., Watson, S. J., & Benson, J. A. (1999). *Marijuana and medicine: Assessing the science base.* Washington, DC: National Academy Press.

Juliano, L. M., & Brandon, T. H. (2002). Effects of nicotine dose, instructional set, and outcome expectancies on the subjective effects of smoking in the presence of a stressor. *Journal of Abnormal Psychology, 111,* 88–97.

Juliano, L. M., & Griffiths, R. R. (2001). Is caffeine a drug of dependence? *Psychiatric Times,* 18.

Juliano, L. M., & Griffiths, R. R. (2004). A critical review of caffeine withdrawal: Empirical validation of symptoms and signs, incidence, severity, and associated features. *Psychopharmacology, 176,* 1–29.

Julien, R. M. (1996). *A primer of drug action* (7th ed.). New York: W. H. Freeman.

Julien, R. M. (1998). *A primer of drug action* (8th ed.). New York: W. H. Freeman.

Julien, R. M. (2001). *A primer of drug action* (9th ed.). New York: W. H. Freeman.

Julien, R. M. (2005). *A primer of drug action* (10th ed.). New York: Worth Publishers.

Julien, R. M., Advokat, C. D., & Comaty, J. E. (2008). *A primer of drug action* (11th ed). New York: Worth Publishers.

Jung, J. (2001). *Psychology of alcohol and other drugs: A research perspective.* Thousand Oaks, CA: Sage Publications.

Kalant, H. (1996). Current state of knowledge about the mechanisms of alcohol tolerance. *Addiction Biology, 1,* 133–141.

Kalant, H., LeBlanc, A. E., & Gibbins, R. J. (1971). Tolerance to, and dependence on, some nonopiate psychotropic drugs. *Pharmacological Reviews, 23,* 135–191.

Kalat, J. W. (2009). *Biological psychology* (10th ed.). Belmont, CA: Wadsworth.

Kalivas, P. W., & Volkow, N. D. (2005). The neural basis of addiction: A pathology of motivation and choice. *American Journal of Psychiatry, 162,* 1403–1413.

Kalus, O., Asnis, G. M., & van Praag, H. M. (1989). The role of serotonin in depression. *Psychiatric Annals, 19,* 348–353.

Kanayama, G. Hudson, J. I., & Pope, H. G. (2008). Long-term psychiatric and medical consequences of anabolic-androgenic steroid abuse: A looming public health concern? *Drug and Alcohol Dependence, 98,* 1–12.

Kanayama, G. Hudson, J. I. & Pope, H. G. (2009). Features of men with anabolic-androgenic steroid dependence: A comparison with nondependent AAS users and with AAS nonusers. *Drug and Alcohol Dependence, 102,* 130–137.

Kandel, D. (1975). Stages in adolescent involvement in drug use. *Science, 190,* 912–914.

Kandel, D., & Yamaguchi, K. (1993). From beer to crack: Developmental patterns of drug involvement. *American Journal of Public Health, 83,* 851–855.

Kapoun, J. (1998). Teaching undergrads web evaluation: A guide for library instruction. *College and Research Library News, 59,* 522–523.

Karch, S. B. (2000). Ma huang and the ephedra alkaloids. In M. J. Cupp (Ed.), *Toxicology and clinical pharmacology of herbal products* (pp. 11–30). Totowa, NJ: Humana Press.

Karlmangla, A. S., Sarkisian, C. A., Kado, D. M., Dedes, H., Liao, D. H., Kim, S., Reuben, D. B., Greendale, G. A., & Moore, A. A. (2009). Light to moderate alcohol consumption and disability: Variable benefits by health status. *American Journal of Epidemiology, 169,* 96–104.

Karst, M., Salim, K., Burstein, S., Conrad, I., Hoy, L., & Schneider, U. (2003). Analgesic effect of the synthetic cannabinoid CT-3 on chronic neuropathic pain: A randomized controlled trial. *Journal of the American Medical Association, 290,* 1757–1762.

Katz, E. C., Robles-Sotelo, E., Correia, C. J., Silverman, K., Stitzer, M. L., & Bigelow, G. (2002). The brief abstinence test: Effects of continued incentive availability on cocaine abstinence. *Experimental and Clinical Psychopharmacology, 10,* 10–17.

Kawachi, I., Colditz, G. A., Speizer, F. E., Manson, J. E., Stampfer, M. J., Willett, W. C., et al. (1997). A prospective study of passive smoking and coronary heart disease. *Circulation, 95,* 2374–2379.

Keh-Ming, L., Smith, M., & Ortiz, V. (2001). Culture and psychopharmacology. *Cultural Psychiatry: International Perspectives, 24,* 523–538.

Keller, M. (1979). A historical overview of alcohol and alcoholism. *Cancer Research, 39,* 2822–2829.

Kelly, T. H., Foltin, R. W., & Fischman, M. W. (1993). Effects of smoked marijuana on heart rate, drug ratings and task performance by humans. *Behavioural Pharmacology, 4,* 167–178.

Kelly, Y., Sacker, A., Gray, R., Kelly, J., Wolke, D., & Quigley, M. A. (2009). Light drinking in pregnancy, a risk for behavioral problems and cognitive deficits at 3 years of age? *International Journal of Epidemiology, 38,* 129–140.

Kendler, K. S., Heath, A. C., Neale, M. C., Kessler, R. C., & Eaves, L. J. (1992). A population-based twin study of alcoholism in women. *Journal of the American Medical Association, 268,* 1877–1882.

Kennedy, J. (1985). *Coca exotica.* Cranbury, NJ: Associated University Presses.

Kenny, M., & Darragh, A. (1985). Central effects of caffeine in man. In S. D. Iversen (Ed.), *Psychopharmacology: Recent advances and future prospects* (pp. 278–288). Oxford: Oxford University Press.

Kerns, L. L., & Davis, G. P. (1986). Psychotropic drugs in pregnancy. In I. J. Chasnoff (Ed.), *Drug use in pregnancy: Mother and child* (pp. 81–93). Lancaster, PA: MTP Press.

Kesselheim, A. S., Misono, A. S., Lee, J. L., Stedman, M. R., Brookhart, M. A., Choudhry, N. K., & Shrank, W. H. (2008). Clinical equivalence of generic and brand-name drugs used in cardiovascular disease: A systematic review and meta-analysis. *Journal of the American Medical Association, 300,* 2514–2526.

Kessler, R. C., Aguilar-Gaxiola, S., Bergland, P., Caraveo-Anduaga, J. J., DeWit, D. J., Greenfield, S. F., et al. (2001). Patterns and predictors of treatment seeking after the onset of a substance use disorder. *Archives of General Psychiatry, 58,* 1065–1071.

Kessler, R. C., Berglund, P., Demler, O., Jin, R., & Walters, E. E. (2005). Lifetime prevalence and age-of-onset distributions of DSM-IV disorders in the national comorbidity survey replication. *Archives of General Psychiatry, 62,* 593–602.

Kessler, R. C., Chiu, W. T., Demler, O., & Walters, E. E. (2005). Prevalence, severity, and comorbidity of 12-month DSM-IV disorders in the national comorbidity survey replication. *Archives of General Psychiatry, 62,* 617–627.

Kimmel, C. K. (1976). A prevention program with punch: The national PTA's Alcohol Education Project. *Journal of School Health, 46,* 208–210.

Kinder, B. N., Pape, N. E., & Walfish, S. (1980). Drug and alcohol education programs: A review of outcome studies. *International Journal of the Addictions, 15,* 1035–1054.

King, M. B. (1994). Long-term benzodiazepine users—a mixed bag. *Addiction, 89,* 1367–1370.

Kirsch, I., & Sapirstein, G. (1999). Listening to Prozac but hearing placebo: A meta-analysis of antidepressant medications. In I. Kirsch (Ed.), *How expectancies shape experience* (pp. 303–320). Washington, DC: American Psychological Association.

Kirsch, M. M. (1986). *Designer drugs.* Minneapolis: Comp-Care Publications.

Kitano, H. H. L. (1989). Alcohol and the Asian American. In T. D. Watts & R. Wright, Jr. (Eds.), *Alcoholism in minority populations* (pp. 143–158). Springfield, IL: Charles C. Thomas.

Kivlahan, D. R., Marlatt, G. A., Fromme, K., Coppel, D. B., & Williams, E. (1990). Secondary prevention with college drinkers: Evaluation of an alcohol skills training program. *Journal of Consulting and Clinical Psychology, 58,* 805–810.

Klatsky, A. L., Morton, C., Udaltsova, N., & Friedman, G. D. (2006). Coffee, cirrhosis, and transaminase enzymes. *Archives of Internal Medicine, 166,* 1190–1195.

Knight, J. R., Wechsler, H., Kuo, M., Seibring, M., Weitzman, E. R., & Schuckit, M. (2002). Alcohol abuse and dependence among U.S. college students. *Journal of Studies on Alcohol, 63,* 263–270.

Kollins, S. (2005). Subjective effects of methylphenidate. In M. Earlywine (Ed.), *Mind-altering drugs: The science of subjective experience* (pp. 275–304), London: Oxford Press.

Kollins, S. H., & Rush, C. R. (2002). Sensitization to the cardiovascular but not subject-rated effects of oral cocaine in humans. *Biological Psychiatry, 51,* 143–150.

Koob, G. F., & Bloom, F. E. (1988). Cellular and molecular mechanisms of drug dependence. *Science, 242,* 715–723.

Koob, G. F., & Le Moal, M. (2006). *Neurobiology of addiction.* London: Academic Press.

Koob, G. F., Lloyd, G., & Mason, B. J. (2009). Development of pharmacotherapies for drug addiction: A Rosetta Stone approach. *Nature Reviews. Drug Discovery, 8,* 500–515.

Koslowski, L. T., Henningfield, R. M., Keenan, R. M., Lei, H., Leigh, G., Jelinek, L. C., et al. (1993). Patterns of alcohol, cigarette, and caffeine and other drug use in two drug-abusing populations. *Journal of Substance Abuse Treatment, 10,* 171–179.

Kramer, J. C. (1972). A brief history of heroin addiction in America. In D. E. Smith & G. R. Gay (Eds.), *It's so good, don't even try it once* (pp. 12–31). Englewood Cliffs, NJ: Prentice Hall.

Kranzler, H. R., & Van Kirk, J. (2001). Efficacy of naltrexone and acamprosate for alcoholism treatment: A meta-analysis. *Alcoholism: Clinical and Experimental Research, 25,* 1335–1341.

Krogh, D. (1991). *Smoking: The artificial passion.* New York: W. H. Freeman.

Kypri, K., Voas, R. B., Langley, J. D., Stephenson, S. C. R., Begg, D. J., Tippetts, A. S., & Davie, G. S. (2006). Minimum purchasing age for alcohol and traffic crash injuries among 15- to 19-year-olds in New Zealand. *American Journal of Public Health, 96,* 126–131.

Lacey, M. (2009). The Drug (Statistics) War: Is Cocaine Getting More Expensive? http://economix.blogs.nytimes.com/2009/04/17/the-drug-statistics-war-cocaine-prices/

LaCroix, A. Z., Lang, J., Scherr, P., Wallace, R. B., Cornoni-Huntley, J., Berkman, L., et al. (1991). Smoking and mortality among older men and women in three communities. *New England Journal of Medicine, 324,* 1619–1625.

Lakins, N. E., LaVallee, R., Williams, G. D., & Yi, H. (2008). Apparent per capita alcohol consumption: National, state, and regional trends, 1977–2006. *Surveillance Report #85,* National Institute on Alcohol Abuse and Alcoholism.

Lam, T. H., He, Y., Sun, L., Liang, L. S., He, F. S., & Liang, B. Q. (1997). Mortality attributable to cigarette smoking in China. *Journal of the American Medical Association, 278,* 1505–1508.

Lang, A. R., Searles, J., Lauerman, R., & Adesso, V. (1980). Expectancy, alcohol, and sex guilt as determinants of interest in and reaction to sexual stimuli. *Journal of Abnormal Psychology, 60,* 285–293.

Langenbucher, J. Hildebrandt, T. & Carr, S. J. (2008). Medical consequences of anabolic steroids. In J. Brick (Ed.), *Handbook of the medical consequences of alcohol and drug abuse* (pp. 385–421). New York: Haworth Press.

Langlieb, A. M., & Kahn, J. P. (2005). How much does quality mental health care profit employers? *Journal of Occupational and Environmental Medicine, 47,* 1099–1109.

Langston, J. W. (2002). The impact of MPTP on Parkinson's disease research: Past, present, and future. In S. A. Factor & W. J. Weiner (Eds.), *Parkinson's disease: Diagnosis and clinical management.* New York: Demos Medical Publishing.

Largent-Milnes, T. M., Guo, W., Wang, H. Y., Burns, L. H. & Vanderah, T. W. (2008). Oxycodone plus ultra-low-dose naltrexone attenuates neuropathic pain and associated mu-opioid receptor Gs coupling. *Journal of Pain, 9,* 700–713.

Larimer, M. E., & Cronce, J. M. (2007). Identification, prevention, and treatment revisited: Individual-focused college drinking prevention strategies 1999–2006. *Addictive Behaviors, 32,* 2439–2468.

Laties, V. G., & Weiss, B. (1981). The amphetamine margin in sports. *Federation Proceedings, 40,* 2689–2692.

Latimer, D., & Goldberg, J. (1981). *Flowers in the blood: The story of opium.* New York: Franklin Watts.

Lawvere, S., & Mahoney, M. C. (2005). St. John's wort. *American Family Physician, 72,* 2249–2254.

Leach, B., & Norris, J. L. (1977). Factors in the development of Alcoholics Anonymous (AA). In B. Kissin & H. Begleiter (Eds.), *The biology of alcoholism* (Vol. 5, pp. 441–544). New York: Plenum Press.

Leavitt, F. (1982). *Drugs and behavior* (2nd ed.). New York: John Wiley.

LeDain Commission. (1972). *A report of the Commission of Inquiry into the non-medical use of drugs.* Ottawa: Information Canada.

Lee, S. J., Sudore, R. L., Williams, B. A., Lindquist, K., Chen, H. L., & Covinsky, K. E. (2009). Functional limitations, socioeconomic status, and all-cause mortality in moderate alcohol drinkers. *Journal of the American Geriatric Society, 57,* 955–962.

Lender, M. E., & Martin, J. K. (1982). *Drinking in America.* New York: Free Press.

Leonard, T. K., Watson, R. R., & Mohs, M. E. (1987). The effects of caffeine in various body systems: A review. *Journal of the American Dietetic Association, 87,* 1048–1053.

Lerner, M., & Wigal, T. (2008). Long-term safety of stimulant medications used to treat children with ADHD. *Journal of Psychosocial Nursing, 46,* 38–48.

Leshner, A. I. (1999). Science-based views of drug addiction and its treatment. *Journal of the American Medical Association, 282,* 1314–1318.

Leuchter, A. F., Cook, I. A., Witte, E. A., Morgan, M., & Abrams, M. (2002). Changes in brain function of depressed subjects during treatment with placebo. *American Journal of Psychiatry, 159,* 122–129.

Levenson, H. S., & Bick, E. C. (1977). Psychopharmacology of caffeine. In M. E. Jarvic (Ed.), *Psychopharmacology in the practice of medicine* (pp. 451–463). New York: Appleton-Century-Crofts.

Levine, J. M., Kramer, G. G., & Levine, E. N. (1975). Effects of alcohol on human performance: An integration of research findings based on an abilities classification. *Journal of Applied Psychology, 89,* 644–653.

Lewin, L. (1964). *Phantastica— narcotic and stimulating drugs: Their use and abuse.* London: Routledge & Kegan Paul.

Lewine, R. R. J. (1988). Gender and schizophrenia. In M. T. Tsuang & J. C. Simpson (Eds.), *Handbook of schizophrenia (Vol. 3): Nosology, epidemiology, and genetics of schizophrenia.* Amsterdam: Elsevier.

Lewis, J. A. (1991). Alcohol abuse prevention in industrial settings. In B. Forster & J. C. Salloway (Eds.), *Preventions and treatments of alcohol and drug abuse* (pp. 137–152). Lewiston, NY: Edwin Mellen Press.

Lichtenstein, E. (1982). The smoking problem: A behavioral perspective. *Journal of Consulting and Clinical Psychology, 50,* 804–819.

Lieberman, J. A., Stroup, T. S., McEvoy, J. P., Swartz, M. S., Rosenheck, R. A., Perkins, D. O., et al. (2005). Effectiveness of antipsychotic drugs in patients with chronic schizophrenia. *New England Journal of Medicine, 353,* 1209–1223.

Liechti, M. E., Kunz, I., Greminger, P., Speich, R., & Kupferschmidt, H. (2006). Clinical features of gamma-hydroxybutyrate and gamma-butyrolactone toxicity and concomitant drug and alcohol use. *Drug and Alcohol Dependence, 8,* 323–326.

Liguori, A., Hughes, J. R., & Grass, J. A. (1997). Absorption and subjective effects of caffeine from coffee, cola, and capsules. *Pharmacology, Biochemistry, and Behavior, 58,* 721–726.

Lim, H. K., Pae, C. U., Joo, R. H, Yoo, S. S., Choi, B. G., Kim, D. J., et al. (2005). fMRI investigation on cue-induced smoking craving. *Journal of Psychiatric Research, 39,* 333–335.

Lin, K. M., & Poland R. E. (1995). Ethnicity, culture and psychopharmacology. In F. E. Bloom & D. J. Kupfer (Eds.), *Psychopharmacology: The fourth generation of progress* (pp. 1907–1917). NY: American College of Neuropsychopharmacology.

Linde, K., Berner, M. M., Kriston, L. (2008). St. John's wort for major depression. *Cochrane Database of Systematic Reviews,* Issue 4.

Linder, R. L., Lerner, S. E., & Burns, R. S. (1981). *PCP: The devil's dust.* Belmont, CA: Wadsworth.

Lingford-Hughes, A. R., Welch, S., & Nutt, D. J. (2004). Evidence-based guidelines for the pharmacological management of substance misuse, addiction, and co-morbidity: Recommendations from the British Association for Psychopharmacology. *Journal of Psychopharmacology, 18,* 293–335.

Linszen, D., & van Amelsvoort, T. (2007). Cannabis and psychosis: An update on course and biological plausible mechanisms. *Current Opinion in Psychiatry, 20,* 116–120.

Litman, G. K. (1986). Alcoholism survival: The prevention of relapse. In W. R. Miller & N. Heather (Eds.), *Treating addictive behaviors* (pp. 391–405). New York: Plenum Press.

Litten, R. Z., & Allen, J. P. (1999). Medications for alcohol, illicit drug, and tobacco dependence: An update of research findings. *Journal of Substance Abuse Treatment, 16,* 105–112.

Lloyd, T., Johnson-Rollings, N., Eggli, D. F., Kieselhorst, K., Mauger, E. A., & Cusatis, D. C. (2000). Bone status among postmenopausal women with different habitual caffeine intakes: A longitudinal investigation. *Journal of the American College of Nutrition, 19,* 256–261.

Lopez, A. D. (1998). Counting the dead in China. *British Medical Journal, 317,* 1399–1400.

Lorist, M. M., & Tops, M. (2003). Caffeine, fatigue, and cognition. *Brain and Cognition, 53,* 82–94.

Lowe, G. (1988). State-dependent retrieval effects with social drugs. *British Journal of Addiction, 83,* 99–103.

Luby, J. L., Si, X., Belden, A. C., Tandom, M., & Spitznagel, E. (2009). Preschool depression: Homotypic continuity and course over 24 months. *Archives of General Psychiatry, 66,* 897–905.

Luce, J. (1972). End of the road: A case study. In D. E. Smith & G. R. Gay (Eds.), *It's so good, don't even try it once* (pp. 143–147). Englewood Cliffs, NJ: Prentice Hall.

Ludlow, F. H. (1857/1979). *The hasheesh eater, being passages from the life of a Pythagorean.* San Francisco: City Lights Books.

Ludwig, A. M., & Wikler, A. (1974). "Craving" and relapse to drink. *Quarterly Journal of Studies on Alcohol, 35,* 108–130.

Lyketsos, C. G., Garrett, E., Liang, K. Y., & Anthony, J. C. (1999). Cannabis use and cognitive decline in persons under 65 years of age. *American Journal of Epidemiology, 149,* 794–800.

Lynam, D. R., Milich, R., Zimmerman, R., Novak, S. P., Logan, T. K., Martin, C., et al. (1999). Project DARE: No effects at 10-year follow-up. *Journal of Consulting and Clinical Psychology, 67,* 590–593.

MacAndrew, C., & Edgerton, R. B. (1969). *Drunken comportment.* Chicago: Aldine.

Mackay, A. V. P. (1982). Antischizophrenic drugs. In P. J. Tyrer (Ed.), *Drugs in psychiatric practice.* London: Butterworths.

MacKinnon, D. P. (1995). Review of the effects of the alcohol warning label. In R. R. Watson (Ed.), *Drug and alcohol abuse reviews: Vol. 7. Alcohol, cocaine, and accidents* (pp. 131–161). Totowa, NJ: Humana Press.

Magliozzi, J. R., & Schaffer, C. B. (1988). Psychosis. In J. P. Tupin, R. I. Shader, & D. S. Harnett (Eds.), *Handbook of clinical psychopharmacology* (2nd ed., pp. 1–48). Northvale, NJ: Jason Aronson.

Maitre, M., Andriamampandry, C., Kemmel, V., Schmidt, C., Hode, Y., Hechler, V., et al. (2000). Gamma-hydroxybutyric acid as a signaling molecule in brain. *Alcohol, 20,* 277–283.

Malberg, J. E., Eisch, A. J., Nestler, E. J., & Duman, R. S. (2000). Chronic antidepressant treatment increases neurogenesis in adult rat hippocampus. *Journal of Neuroscience, 20,* 9104–9110.

Malsch, U., & Kieser, M. (2001). Efficacy of kava-kava in the treatment of non-psychotic anxiety following pretreatment with benzodiazepines. *Psychopharmacology, 157,* 277–283.

Marks, V., & Kelly, J. F. (1973). Absorption of caffeine from tea, coffee, and Coca Cola. *Lancet, 3,* 827.

Marlatt, G. A., Bowen, S. W., & Witkiewitz, K. (2009). Relapse prevention: Evidence base and future. In P. M. Miller (Ed.), *Evidence-based addiction treatment* (pp. 215–232). Boston: Elsevier.

Marlatt, G. A., & Gordon, J. R. (Eds.). (1985). *Relapse prevention.* New York: Guilford Press.

Marlatt, G. A., Larimer, M. E., Baer, J. S., & Quigley, L. A. (1993). Harm reduction for alcohol problems: Moving beyond the controlled drinking controversy. *Behavior Therapy, 24,* 461–504.

Marlatt, G. A., & Witkiewitz, K. (2005). Relapse prevention for alcohol and drug problems. In G. A. Marlatt & D. M. Donovan (Eds.), *Relapse prevention* (2nd ed., pp. 1–44). New York: Guilford Press.

Marmot, M. G. (2001). Alcohol and coronary heart disease. *International Journal of Epidemiology, 30,* 724–729.

Marona-Lewicka, D., Thisted, R. A., & Nichols, D. E. (2005). Distinct temporal phases in the behavioral pharmacology of LSD: Dopamine D2 receptor-mediated effects in the rat and implications for psychosis. *Psychopharmacology, 180,* 427–435.

Marshal, M. P., Friedman, M. S., Stall, R. S., King, K. M., Miles, J., Gold, M. A., Bukstein, O. G., & Morse, J. Q. (2008). Sexual orientation and adolescent substance use: A meta-analysis and methodological review. *Addiction, 103,* 546–556.

Marshall, E. (1988). The drug of champions. *Science, 242,* 183–184.

Martin, B. R., Cabral, G., Childers, S. R., Deadwyler, S., Mechoulam, R., & Reggio, P. (1993). International Cannabis Research Society meeting summary, Keystone, CO (June 19–20, 1992). *Drug and Alcohol Dependence, 31,* 219–227.

Martin-Soelch, C., Leenders, K. L., Chevalley, A. F., Missemer, J., Kuenig, G., Magyar, S., et al. (2001). Reward mechanisms in the brain and their role in dependence: Evidence from neurophysiological and neuroimaging studies. *Brain Research Reviews, 36,* 139–149.

Mathew, S. J. (2008). Treatment-resistant depression: Recent developments and future directions. *Depression and Anxiety, 25,* 989–992.

Matsuda, L., Lolait, S. J., Brownstein, J. J., Young, A. C., & Bonner, T. I. (1990). Structure of a cannabinoid receptor and functional expression of the cloned cDNA. *Nature, 346,* 561–564.

Matthew, R. J., Wilson, W. H., Coleman, R. E., Turkington, T. G., & DeGrado, T. R. (1997). Marijuana intoxication and brain activation in marijuana smokers. *Life Sciences, 60,* 2075–2089.

Mayor LaGuardia's Committee on Marihuana. (1944). *The marihuana problem in the city of New York.* Lancaster, PA: Jacques Cattell Press. Reprinted by Scarecrow Reprint Corporation, Metuchen, NJ, 1983.

Mayo-Smith, M. F. (1997). Pharmacological management of alcohol withdrawal. *Journal of the American Medical Association, 278,* 144–151.

Maziak, W. (2008). The waterpipe: Time for action. *Addiction, 103,* 1763–1767.

Mazis, M. B., Morris, L. A., & Swasy, J. L. (1991). An evaluation of the alcohol warning label: Initial survey results. *Journal of Public Policy and Marketing, 10,* 229–241.

McBride, C. M., Pollak, K. L., Lyna, P., Lipkus, I. M., Samsa, G. P., & Beplor, G. (2001). Reasons for quitting smoking among low-income African American smokers. *Health Psychology, 20,* 334–340.

McBride, N., Farringdon, F., Midford, R., Meuleners, & Phillips, M. (2004). Harm minimization in school drug education: Final results of the School Health and Alcohol Harm Reduction Project (SHAHRP). *Addiction, 99,* 278–291.

McCann, U. D., Szabo, Z., Seckin, E., Rosenblatt, P., Mathews, W. B., Ravert, H. T., et al. (2005). Quantitative PET studies of the serotonin transporter in MDMA users and controls using [11C]McN5652 and [11C] DASB. *Neuropsychopharmacology, 30,* 1741–1750.

McCarthy, D. M., Kroll, L. S., & Smith, G. T. (2001). Integrating disinhibition and learning risk for alcohol use. *Experimental and Clinical Psychopharmacology, 9,* 389–398.

McCarty, D. (1985). Environmental factors in substance abuse: The microsetting. In M. Galizio & S. A. Maisto (Eds.), *Determinants of substance abuse: Biological, psychological, and environmental factors* (pp. 247–282). New York: Plenum Press.

McCloskey, J., & Bailes, J. (2005). *When winning costs too much: Steroids, supplements and scandal in today's sports.* Lanham, MD: Taylor Trade Publishing Group Inc.

McCrady, B. S., & Langenbucher, J. W. (1996). Alcohol treatment and health care system reform. *Archives of General Psychiatry, 53,* 737–746.

McCrady, B. S., & Ziedonis, D. (2001). American Psychiatric Association practice guideline for substance use disorders. *Behavior Therapy, 32,* 309–336.

McGlothlin, W. H., & West, L. J. (1968). The marihuana problem: An overview. *American Journal of Psychiatry, 125,* 370–378.

McGovern, M. P., & Carroll, K. M. (2003). Evidence-based practices for substance use disorders. *Psychiatric Clinics of North America, 26,* 991–1010.

McGregor, C., Srisurapanont, M., Jittiwutikarn, J., Laobhripatr, S., Wongtan, T., & White, J. (2005). The nature, time course, and severity of methamphetamine withdrawal. *Addiction, 100,* 1320–1329.

McKay, J. R., Murphy, R. T., & Longabaugh, R. (1991). The effectiveness of alcoholism treatment: Evidence from outcome studies. In S. M. Mirin, J. T. Gossett, & M. C. Grob (Eds.), *Psychiatric treatment: Advances in outcome research* (pp. 143–158). Washington, DC: American Psychiatric Press.

McKee, S. A., O'Malley, S. S., Salovey, P., Krishnan-Sarin, S., & Mazure, C. M. (2005). Perceived risks and benefits of smoking cessation: Gender-specific predictors of motivation and treatment outcome. *Addictive Behaviors, 30,* 423–435.

McKenna, T. (1992). *Food of the gods: The search for the original tree of knowledge.* New York: Bantam Books.

McKim, W. A. (2000). *Drugs and behavior* (4th ed.). Upper Saddle River, NJ: Prentice Hall.

McLaren, J., Swift, W., Dillon, P., & Allsop, S. (2008). Cannabis potency and contamination: A review of the literature. *Addiction, 10,* 1100–1109.

McLellan, A. T., Luborsky, L., Woody, G. E., O'Brien, C. P., & Druley, K. A. (1983). Increased effectiveness of substance abuse treatment: A prospective study of patient treatment matching. *Journal of Nervous and Mental Disease, 171,* 597–605.

McLellan, T., Lewis, D. C., O'Brien, C. P., & Kleber, H. D. (2000). Drug dependence, a chronic medical illness: Implications for treatment, insurance, and outcomes evaluation. *Journal of the American Medical Association, 284,* 1689–1695.

Mechoulam, R. (1973). Cannabinoid chemistry. In R. Mechoulam (Ed.), *Marijuana: Chemistry, pharmacology, metabolism, and clinical effects* (pp. 2–99). New York: Academic Press.

Mellaart, J. (1967). *Catal Huyuk: A Neolithic town in Anatolia.* New York: McGraw-Hill.

Mello, N. K. (1987). Alcohol abuse and alcoholism: 1978–1987. In H. Y. Meltzer (Ed.), *Psychopharmacology: The third generation of progress* (pp. 1515–1520). New York: Raven Press.

Mello, N. K., & Griffiths, R. R. (1987). Alcoholism and drug abuse: An overview. In H. Y. Meltzer (Ed.), *Psychopharmacology: The third generation of progress* (pp. 1511–1514). New York: Raven Press.

Mendelson, J. H., & Mello, N. K. (1985). *Alcohol: Use and abuse in America.* Boston: Little, Brown.

Mendelson, W. B. (1980). *The use and misuse of sleeping pills: A clinical guide.* New York: Plenum Press.

Merritt, J. C., Crawford, W. J., Alexander, P. C., Anduze, A. L., & Gelbart, S. S. (1980). Effect of marihuana on intraocular and blood pressure in glaucoma. *Ophthalmology, 87,* 222–228.

Messinis, L., Kyprianidou, A., Malefaki, S., & Papathanasopoulos, P. (2006). Neuropsychological deficits in long-term frequent cannabis users. *Neurology, 66,* 737–739.

Meyer, J. S., & Quenzer, L. F. (2005). Psychopharmacology: Drugs, the brain, and behavior. Sunderland, MA: Sinauer Associates Inc.

Meyer, R. E., & Mirin, S. M. (1979). *The heroin stimulus: Implications for a theory of addiction.* New York: Plenum Press.

Midanik, L. T., & Room, R. R. (1992). The epidemiology of alcohol consumption. *Alcohol Health and Research World, 16,* 183–190.

Miller, K. E. (2008). Energy drinks, race, and problem behaviors among college students. *Journal of Adolescent Health, 43,* 490–497.

Miller, L. G., & Greenblatt, D. J. (1996). Benzodiazepine discontinuation syndromes: Clinical and experimental aspects. In C. R. Schuster & M. J. Kuhar (Eds.), *Pharmacological aspects of drug dependence: Toward an integrated neurobehavioral approach* (pp. 53–82). Berlin: Springer-Verlag.

Miller, N. S. (1991). *The pharmacology of alcohol and drugs of abuse/addiction.* New York: Springer-Verlag.

Miller, W. R., & C'de Baca, J. (2001). *Quantum change.* New York: Guilford Press.

Miller, W. R., & Hester, R. K. (1980). Treating the problem drinker: Modern approaches. In W. R. Miller (Ed.), *The addictive behaviors: Treatment of alcoholism, drug abuse, smoking, and obesity* (pp. 11–141). New York: Plenum Press.

Miller, W. R., & Hester, R. K. (1986). Inpatient alcoholism treatment: Who benefits? *American Psychologist, 41,* 794–805.

Miller, W. R., & Hester, R. K. (1989). Treating alcohol problems: Toward an informed eclecticism. In R. K. Hester & W. R. Miller (Eds.), *Handbook of alcoholism treatment approaches* (pp. 3–14). New York: Pergamon Press.

Miller, W. R., & Hester, R. K. (1995). Treatment for alcohol problems: Toward an informed eclecticism. In R. K. Hester & W. R. Miller (Eds.), *Handbook of alcoholism treatment approaches* (2nd ed., pp. 1–11). Needham Heights, MA: Allyn & Bacon.

Miller, W. R., & Hester, R. K. (2002). Treating alcohol problems: Toward an informed eclecticism. In R. K. Hester & W. R. Miller (Eds.), *Handbook of alcoholism treatment approaches* (3rd ed., pp. 1–12). Boston: Allyn & Bacon.

Mills, J. L., Holmes, L. B., Aarons, J. H., Simpson, J. L., Brown, A. A., Jovanovic-Peterson, L. G., et al. (1993). Moderate caffeine use and the risk of spontaneous abortion on intrauterine growth retardation. *Journal of the American Medical Association, 269,* 593–597.

Mintzer, M. Z., Copersino, M. L., & Stitzer, M. L. (2005). Opioid abuse and cognitive performance. *Drug and Alcohol Dependence, 78,* 225–230.

Mintzer, M. Z., Guarino, J., Kirk, T., Roache, J. D., & Griffiths, R. R. (1997). Ethanol and pentobarbital: Comparison of behavioral and subjective effects in sedative drug abusers. *Experimental and Clinical Psychopharmacology, 5,* 203–215.

Modell, J. G. (1997). Protracted benzodiazepine withdrawal syndrome mimicking psychotic depression. *Psychosomatics, 38,* 160–161.

Möhler, H., & Okada, T. (1977). Benzodiazepine receptor: Demonstration in the central nervous system. *Science, 198,* 849–851.

Molarus, A., Parsons, R. W., Dobson, A. J., Evans, A., Fortmann, S. P., Jamrozik, K., et al. (2001). Trends in cigarette smoking in 36 populations from the early 1980s to the mid-1990s: Findings from the WHO MONICA project. *American Journal of Public Health, 91,* 206–212.

Moncrieff, J., & Kirsch, I. (2005). Education and debate. *BMJ, 331,* 155–159.

Montana Meth Project (2008, May 3). *The Economist,* 36.

Moore, T. H. M., Zammit, S., Lingford-Hughes, A., Barnes, T. R. E., Jones, P. B., Burke, M., & Lewis, G. (2007). Cannabis use and risk of psychotic or affective mental health outcomes: a systematic review. *The Lancet, 370,* 319–328.

Moreau, R. (2009, August 3). America's new nightmare. *Newsweek,* 38–42.

Morgan, C. J. A., Riccelli, M., Maitland, C. H., & Curran, H. V. (2004). Long-term effects of ketamine: Evidence for a persisting impairment of source memory in recreational users. *Drug and Alcohol Dependence, 75,* 301–308.

Morgan, H. W. (1981). *Drugs in America: A social history, 1800–1980.* Syracuse, NY: Syracuse University Press.

Morgenstern, J., Labouvie, E., McCrady, B. S., Kahler, C. W., & Frey, R. M. (1997). Affiliation with Alcoholics Anonymous after treatment: A study of its therapeutic effects and mechanisms of action. *Journal of Consulting and Clinical Psychology, 65,* 768–777.

Morral, A. R., McCaffrey, D. F., & Paddock, S. M. (2002). Reassessing the marijuana gateway effect. *Addiction, 97,* 1493–1504.

Mortimer, W. G. (1901). *Peru: History of coca, "the divine plant" of the Incas.* New York: J. H. Vail.

Morton, J. (2005). Ecstasy: Pharmacology and neurotoxicity. *Current Opinion in Pharmacology, 5,* 79–86.

Mosher, J. F., & Colman, V. J. (1986). Prevention research: The model Dram Shop Act of 1985. *Alcohol Health and Research World, 10,* 4–11.

Mumford, G. K., Rush, C. R., & Griffiths, R. R. (1995). Alprazolam and DN-2327 (Pazinaclone) in humans: Psychomotor, memory, subjective, and reinforcing effects. *Experimental and Clinical Psychopharmacology, 3,* 39–48.

Munro, S., Thomas, K. L., & Abu-Shaar, M. (1993). Molecular characterization of a peripheral receptor for cannabinoids. *Nature, 365,* 61–65.

Myrick, H., Anton, R. F., Li, X., Henderson, S., Drobes, D., Voronin, K. et al. (2004). Differential brain activity in alcoholics and social drinkers to alcohol cues: Relationship to craving. *Neuropsychopharmacology, 29,* 393–402.

Nace, E. P., & Isbell, P. G. (1991). Alcohol. In R. J. Francis & S. I. Miller (Eds.), *Clinical textbook of addictive disorders* (pp. 43–68). New York: Guilford Press.

Nadelmann, E. A. (1989). Drug prohibition in the United States: Costs, consequences, and alternatives. *Science, 245,* 939–947.

Nahas, G. G. (1973). *Marijuana—Deceptive weed.* New York: Raven Press.

Naqvi, N. H., Rudrauf, D., Demasioo, H., & Bechara, A. (2007). Damage to the insula disrupts addiction to cigarette smoking. *Science, 315,* 531–534.

Naranjo, C. (2001). Experience with the interpersonal psychedelics. In J. Holland (Ed.), *Ecstasy: The complete guide: A comprehensive look at the risks and benefits of MDMA* (pp. 208–221). Rochester, VT: Park Street Press.

Nathan, P. E. (1984). Alcoholism prevention in the workplace: Three examples. In P. M. Miller & T. D. Nirenberg (Eds.), *Prevention of alcohol abuse* (pp. 387–405). New York: Plenum Press.

Nathan, P. E., & Niaura, R. S. (1987). Prevention of alcohol problems. In W. M. Cox (Ed.), *Treatment and prevention of alcohol problems: A resource manual* (pp. 333–354). New York: Academic Press.

National Advisory Council on Alcohol Abuse and Alcoholism. (2002). *A call to action: Changing the culture of drinking at U.S. colleges.* (NIH Publication No. 02-5010). Bethesda, MD: National Institute on Alcohol Abuse and Alcoholism.

National Cancer Council of Australia. (2006). *National cancer prevention policy: 2004–2006.* New South Wales: Author.

National Institute on Alcohol Abuse and Alcoholism (NIAAA). (1993). *Eighth special report to the U.S. Congress on alcohol and health.* Washington, DC: U.S. Department of Health and Human Services.

NIAAA. (1999). Brief interventions for alcohol problems. *Alcohol Alert, No. 43.*

NIAAA. (2000). *Tenth special report to the U.S. Congress on alcohol and health.* Washington, DC: U.S. Department of Health and Human Services.

NIAAA. (2001, July). Cognitive impairment and recovery from alcoholism. *Alcohol Alert,* No. 53.

NIAAA. (2002). *A call to action: Changing the culture of drinking at U.S. colleges.* Washington, DC: U.S. Department of Health and Human Services.

NIAAA. (2005). *Helping patients who drink too much.* Bethesda, MD: National Institutes of Health.

NIAAA. (2008). *Research findings on college drinking and the minimum drinking age.* Bethesda, MD: Author.

National Institute on Drug Abuse (NIDA). (1982). *Marijuana and health: Ninth annual report to the U.S. Congress from the Secretary of Health and Human Services.* Rockville, MD: Author.

NIDA. (1991). *Annual emergency room data: 1990.* Washington, DC: Author.

NIDA. (2002). *Research report series: Nicotine addiction.* Bethesda, MD: Author.

NIDA. (2003). *Preventing drug abuse among children and adolescents: A research-based guide for parents, educators, and community leaders* (2nd ed.). Bethesda, MD: Author.

NIDA. (2005). *HIV/AIDS.* NIDA Research Report, Bethesda, MD.

National Institutes of Health. (2000, January). *Cirrhosis of the liver.* NIH Publication No. 00-1134.

Neal, D. J., & Fromme, K. (2007). Event-level covariation of alcohol intoxication and behavioral risks during the first year of college. *Journal of Consulting and Clinical Psychology, 75,* 294–306.

Nehlig, A. (2004). Dependence upon coffee and caffeine: An update. In A. Nehlig (Ed.), *Coffee, tea, chocolate, and the brain* (pp. 133–146). Boca Raton, FL: CRC Press.

Nestler, E. J. (2009). Cellular and molecular mechanisms of drug addiction. In D. S. Charney & E. J. Nestler (Eds.), *Neurobiology of mental illness* (3rd ed., pp. 775–786). New York: Oxford University Press.

Newsweek. (1989, January 16). A tide of drug killing.

Newsweek. (1993, December 12). Death on the spot: The end of a drug king.

Newsweek. (1996, March 18). Mother's little helper.

Newsweek. (1997a, March 31). White storm warning.

Newsweek. (1997b, October 27). Death of the party.

Newsweek. (2001, May 14). Painkiller crackdown.

Newton, T. F., De La Garza, R., Kalechstein, A. D., & Nestor, L. (2005). Cocaine and methamphetamine produce different patterns of subjective and cardiovascular effects. *Pharmacology, Biochemistry and Behavior, 82,* 90–97.

Nichols, D. E. (2004). Hallucinogens. *Pharmacology and Therapeutics, 101,* 131–181.

Nies, A. S. (2001). Principles of therapeutics. In J. G. Hardman & L. E. Limbird (Eds.), *Goodman & Gilman's The pharmacological basis of therapeutics* (10th ed., pp. 45–66). New York: McGraw-Hill.

Nirenberg, T. D., & Miller, P. M. (1984). History and overview of the prevention of alcohol abuse. In P. M. Miller & T. D. Nirenberg (Eds.), *Prevention of alcohol abuse* (pp. 3–14). New York: Plenum Press.

Nkondjock, A. (2009). Coffee consumption and the risk of cancer: An overview. *Cancer Letters, 277(Issue 2),* 121–125.

Nolen-Hoeksema, S. (2004). Gender differences in risk factors and consequences for alcohol use and problems. *Clinical Psychology Review, 24,* 981–1010.

O'Brien, C. (1995). *Nicotine dependence.* University of Pennsylvania Health System, Internet Alcohol Recovery Center.

O'Brien, C. P. (1996). Recent developments in the pharmacotherapy of substance abuse. *Journal of Consulting and Clinical Psychology, 64,* 677–686.

O'Brien, C. P. (2001). Drug addiction and drug abuse. In J. G. Hardman & L. E. Limbird (Eds.), *Goodman & Gilman's The pharmacological basis of therapeutics* (10th ed., pp. 621–643). New York: McGraw-Hill.

O'Brien, R., & Cohen, S. (1984). *The encyclopedia of drug abuse.* New York: Facts on File.

O'Hanlon, J. F., & de Gier, J. J. (1986). *Drugs and driving.* London: Taylor & Francis.

Olds, J., & Milner, P. (1954). Positive reinforcement produced by electrical stimulation of septal area and other regions of rat brains. *Journal of Comparative and Physiological Psychology, 47,* 419–427.

O'Loughlin, J., Gervais, A., Dugas, E., & Meshefedjian, G. (2009). Milestones in the process of cessation among novice adolescent smokers. *American Journal of Public Health, 99,* 499–504.

Olfson, M., & Marcus, S. C. (2009). National patterns in antidepressant medication treatment. *Archives of General Psychiatry, 66,* 848–856.

O'Malley, P. M., & Johnston, L. D. (2002). Epidemiology of alcohol and other drug use among American college students. *Journal of Studies on Alcohol,* Supplement 14, 23–39.

O'Malley, S. S., Jaffe, A. J., Chang, G., Schottenfeld, R. S., Meyer, R. E., & Rounsaville, B. (1992). Naltrexone and coping skills therapy for alcohol dependence. *Archives of General Psychiatry, 49,* 881–887.

Orcutt, J. D. (1987). Differential association and marijuana use: A closer look at Sutherland (with a little help from Becker). *Criminology, 25,* 341–358.

Orford, J. (1985). *Excessive appetites: A psychological view of addictions.* Chichester, England: John Wiley.

Oviedeo-Joekes, E., Brissette, S., Marsh, D. C., Lauzon, P., Guh, D., Anis, A., & Schechter, M. T. (2009). Diacetylmorphine versus Methadone for the treatment of opioid addiction. *The New England Journal of Medicine, 361,* 777–786.

Owen, F. (2007). *No speed limit: The highs and lows of meth.* New York: St. Martins Press.

Page, J. B. (1983). The amotivational syndrome hypothesis and the Costa Rica study: Relationship between methods and results. *Journal of Psychoactive Drugs, 15,* 261–267.

Palmgreen, P., & Donohew, L. (2003). Effective mass media strategies for drug abuse prevention campaigns. In Z. Sloboda & W. J. Bukoski (Eds.), *Handbook of drug abuse prevention: Theory, science, and practice* (pp. 27–43). New York: Kluwer Academic/Plenum Publishers.

Parrino, L., & Terzano, M. G. (1996). Polysomnographic effects of hypnotic drugs. *Psychopharmacology, 126,* 1–16.

Parrott, A. C. (1998). Nesbitt's paradox revisited? Stress and arousal modulation during cigarette smoking. *Addiction, 93,* 27–39.

Parrott, A. C. (2004). Is ecstasy MDMA? A review of the proportion of ecstasy tablets containing MDMA, their dosage levels, and the changing perceptions of purity. *Psychopharmacology, 173,* 234–241.

Parrott, A. C., Milani, R. M., Parmar, R., & Turner, J. J. D. (2001). Recreational ecstasy/MDMA and other drug users from the UK and Italy: Psychiatric symptoms and psychobiological problems. *Psychopharmacology, 159,* 77–82.

Parrott, D. J., & Giancola, P. R. (2004). A further examination of the relation between trait anger and alcohol-related aggression: The role of anger control. *Alcoholism: Clinical and Experimental Research, 28,* 855–864.

Parsons, O. A. (1986). Alcoholics' neuropsychological impairment: Current findings and conclusions. *Annals of Behavioral Medicine, 8,* 13–19.

Paton, W. D. M., & Pertwee, R. G. (1973). The actions of cannabis in man. In R. Mechoulam (Ed.), *Marijuana: Chemistry, pharmacology, metabolism, and clinical effects* (pp. 288–333). New York: Academic Press.

Peachey, J. E., & Annis, J. (1985). New strategies for using the alcohol-sensitizing drugs. In C. A. Naranjo & E. M. Sellers (Eds.), *Research advances in new psychopharmacological treatments for alcoholism* (pp. 199–216). Amsterdam: Elsevier Science Publishers.

Peele, S. (1996). Assumptions about drugs and the marketing of drug policies. In W. K. Bickel & R. J. DeGrandpre (Eds.), *Drug policy and human nature* (pp. 199–220). New York: Plenum Press.

Perez-Reyes, M., Hicks, R. E., Bumberry, J., Jeffcoat, A. R., & Cook, C. E. (1988). Interaction between marijuana and ethanol: Effect on psychomotor performance. *Alcoholism: Clinical and Experimental Research, 12,* 268–276.

Perkins, H. W. (2002). Social norms and the prevention of alcohol misuse in collegiate contexts. *Journal of Studies on Alcohol,* Supplement 14, 164–172.

Perkins, H. W. (2007). Misperceptions of peer drinking norms in Canada: Another look at the "reign of terror" and its consequences among college students. *Addictive Behaviors, 32,* 2645–2656.

Perkins, K. A. (1996). Sex differences in nicotine versus nonnicotine reinforcement as determinants of tobacco smoking. *Experimental and Clinical Psychopharmacology, 4,* 166–177.

Perkins, K. A., Fonte, C., Ashcom, J., Broge, M., & Wilson, A. (2001). Subjective responses to nicotine in smokers may be associated with responses to caffeine and to alcohol. *Experimental and Clinical Psychopharmacology, 9,* 91–100.

Perrine, D. M. (1996). *The chemistry of mind-altering drugs. History, pharmacology, and cultural context.* Washington, DC: American Chemical Society.

Pert, C., & Snyder, S. H. (1973). Opiate receptor: Demonstration in nervous system tissue. *Science, 179,* 1011–1014.

Pertwee, R. (2002). Sites and mechanism of action. In F. Grotenhermen & E. Russo (Eds.), *Cannabis and cannabinoids: Pharmacology, toxicology and therapeutic potential* (pp. 73–88). London: Haworth.

Petersen, R. C. (1977). History of cocaine. In R. C. Petersen & R. C. Stillman (Eds.), *Cocaine: 1977.* Research Monograph 13 (pp. 17–34). Washington, DC: National Institute on Drug Abuse.

Petersson, A., Garle, M., Holmgren, P., Druid, H., Krantz, P., & Thiblin, I. (2006). Toxicological findings and manner of death in autopsied users of anabolic androgenic steroids. *Drug and Alcohol Dependence, 81,* 241–250.

Petrovic, P., Kalso, E., Petersson, K. M., & Ingvar, M. (2002). Placebo and opioid analgesia: Imaging a shared neuronal network. *Science, 295,* 1737–1740.

Peugh, J., & Belenko, S. (2001). Alcohol, drugs, and sexual function: A review. *Journal of Psychoactive Drugs, 33,* 223–232.

Pierce, J. P., & Gilpin, E. A. (1995). A historical analysis of tobacco marketing and the uptake of smoking by youth in the United States: 1890–1977. *Health Psychology, 14,* 500–508.

Pijlman, F. T., Rigter, S. M., Hoek, J., Goldschmidt, H. M. J., & Niesink, R. J. M. (2005). Strong increase in total delta-THC in cannabis preparations sold in Dutch coffee shops. *Addiction Biology, 10,* 171–180.

Pisinger, C., & Godtfredsen, N. S. (2007). Is there a health benefit of reduced tobacco consumption? A systematic review. *Nicotine and Tobacco Research, 9,* 631–646.

Pittler, M. H., Verster, J. C., & Ernst, E. (2005). Interventions for preventing or treating alcohol hangover: Systematic review of randomized controlled trials. *British Medical Journal, 331,* 1515–1517.

Plasse, T. F., Gorter, R. W., Krasnow, S. H., Lane, M., Shepard, K. V., & Wadleigh, R. G. (1991). Recent clinical experience with Dronabinol. *Pharmacology, Biochemistry, and Behavior, 40,* 695–700.

Pliner, P., & Cappell, H. (1974). Modification of affective consequences of alcohol: A comparison of social and solitary drinking. *Journal of Abnormal Psychology, 89,* 224–233.

Poling, A., & Cross, J. (1993). State-dependent learning. In F. van Haaren (Ed.), *Methods in behavioral pharmacology* (pp. 245–256). Amsterdam: Elsevier.

Pomerleau, C. S. (1997). Co-factors for smoking and evolutionary psychobiology. *Addiction, 92,* 397–408.

Pomerleau, C. S., & Saules, K. (2007). Body image, body satisfaction, and eating patterns in normal-weight and overweight/obese women current smokers and never-smokers. *Addictive Behaviors, 32,* 2329–2334.

Pope, H. G., Jr., Gruber, A. J., Hudson, J. I., Huestis, M. A., & Yurgelun-Todd, D. (2001). Neuropsychological performance in long-term cannabis users. *Archives of General Psychiatry, 58,* 909–915.

Pope, H. G., Jr., & Katz, D. L. (1988). Affective and psychotic symptoms associated with anabolic steroid use. *American Journal of Psychiatry, 145,* 487–490.

Porjesz, B., & Begleiter, H. (1995). Event-related potentials and cognitive function in alcoholism. *Alcohol Health and Research World, 19,* 108–113.

Prasad, S., Arellano, J., Steer, C., & Libretto, S. E. (2009). Assessing the value of atomoxetine in treating children and adolescents with ADHD in the UK. *International Journal of Clinical Practice, 63,* 1031–1040.

Presley, C. A., Leichliter, M. A., & Meilman, P. W. (1998). *Alcohol and drugs on American college campuses: A report to college presidents: Third in a series, 1995, 1996, 1997.* Carbondale: Core Institute, Southern Illinois University.

Presley, C. A., Meilman, P. W., & Cashin, J. R. (1996). *Alcohol and drugs on American college campuses: Use, consequences, and perceptions of the campus environment, Vol. IV: 1992–1994.* Carbondale: Core Institute, Southern Illinois University.

Presley, C. A., Meilman, P. W., Cashin, J. R., & Lyerla, R. (1996). *Alcohol and drugs on American college campuses: Use, consequences, and perceptions of the campus environment, Vol. III: 1991–1993.* Carbondale: Core Institute, Southern Illinois University.

Primack, B. A., Gold, M. A., Land, S. R., & Fine, M. J. (2006). Association of cigarette smoking and media literacy about smoking among adolescents. *Journal of Adolescent Health, 39,* 465–472.

Prochaska, J. O., DiClemente, C. C., & Norcross, J. C. (1992). In search of how people change. Applications to addictive behaviors. *American Psychologist, 47,* 1102–1114.

Project MATCH Research Group. (1997). Matching alcoholism treatments to client heterogeneity: Project MATCH posttreatment drinking outcomes. *Journal of Studies on Alcohol, 58,* 7–29.

Quaglio, G., Lugoboni, F., Pattaro, C., Melara, B. Mezzelani, P., & Des Jarlais, D. C. (2008). Erectile dysfunction in male heroin users receiving methadone and buprenorphine maintenance treatment. *Drug and Alcohol Dependence, 94,* 12–18.

Quickfall, J., & Crockford, D. (2006). Brain neuroimaging in cannabis use: A review. *Journal of Neuropsychiatry and Clinical Neurosciences, 18,* 318–332.

Rajacic, N. (1997). Coordinator presents on SMART to social workers. *S.M.A.R.T. Recovery News and Views, III,* 4–5.

Rall, T. W. (1990a). Drugs used in the treatment of asthma. The methylxanthines, cromolyn sodium, and other agents. In A. G. Gilman, T. W. Rall, A. S. Niles, & P. Taylor (Eds.), *Goodman and Gilman's The pharmacological basis of therapeutics* (8th ed., pp. 618–637). New York: Pergamon Press.

Rall, T. W. (1990b). Hypnotics and sedatives; Ethanol. In A. G. Gilman, T. W. Rall, A. S. Nies, & P. Taylor (Eds.), *Goodman and Gilman's The pharmacological basis of therapeutics* (8th ed., pp. 345–382). New York: Pergamon Press.

Ranganathan, M., & D'Souza, D. C. (2006). The acute effects of cannabinoids on memory in humans: A review. *Psychopharmacology, 188,* 425–444.

Rasmussen, C. (2005). Executive functioning and working memory in fetal alcohol spectrum disorder. *Alcoholism: Clinical and Experimental Research, 29,* 1359–1367.

Raven, M. A., Necessary, B. D., Danluck, D. A., & Ettenberg, A. (2000). Comparison of the reinforcing and anxiogenic effects of intravenous cocaine and cocaethylene. *Experimental and Clinical Psycholopharmacology, 8,* 117–124.

Rawson, R. A. (1990–1991). Chemical dependency treatment: The integration of the alcoholism and drug addiction/use treatment systems. *International Journal of the Addictions, 25,* 1515–1536.

Ray, W. A., Chung, C. P., Murray, K. T., Hall, K., & Stein, M. (2009). Atypical antipsychotic drugs and the risk of sudden cardiac death. *New England Journal of Medicine, 360,* 225–235.

Ream, G. L., Benoit, E., Johnson, B. D., & Dunlap, E. (2008). Smoking tobacco along with marijuana increases symptoms of cannabis dependence. *Drug and Alcohol Dependence, 95,* 199–208.

Reed, S. C., Haney, M., Evans, S. M., Vadhan, N. P., Rubin, E. & Foltin, R. W. (2009). Cardiovascular and subjective effects of repeated smoked cocaine administration in experienced cocaine users. *Drug and Alcohol Dependence, 102,* 102-107.

Rees, V., & Connolly, G. N. (2006). Measuring air quality to protect children from second smoke in cars. *American Journal of Preventive Medicine, 31,* 363–368.

Regier, D. A., Narrow, W. E., Rae, D. S., Manderscherd, R. W., Locke, B. Z., & Goodwin, R. K. (1993). The de facto U.S. mental and addictive disorders service system. *Archives of General Psychiatry, 50,* 85–94.

Rehm, J., Mathers, C., Popova, S., Thavorncharoensap, M., Teerawattananon, Y., & Patra, J. (2009). Global burden of disease and injury and economic cost attributable to alcohol use and alcohol-use disorders. *Lancet, 373,* 2223–2233.

Reissig, C. J., Strain, E. C., & Griffiths, R. R. (2009). Caffeinated energy drinks—A growing problem. *Drug and Alcohol Dependence, 99,* 1–10.

Renaud, S., & deLorgerd, M. (1992). Wine, alcohol, platelets, and the French paradox for coronary heart disease. *The Lancet, 339,* 1523–1526.

Rezvani, A. H., Overstreet, D. H., Perfumi, M., & Massi, M. (2003). Plant derivatives in the treatment of alcohol dependency. *Pharmacology, Biochemistry & Behavior. 75,* 593–606.

Riba, J., Rodriguez-Fornells, A., Urbano, G., Morte, A., Antonijoan, R., Montero, M., et al. (2001). Subjective effects and tolerability of the South American psychoactive beverage Ayahuasca in healthy volunteers. *Psychopharmacology, 154,* 85–95.

Ricaurte, G., Bryan, G., Strauss, L., Seiden, L., & Schuster, C. (1985). Hallucinogenic amphetamine selectively destroys brain serotonin nerve terminals. *Science, 299,* 986–988.

Rich, J. D., McKenzie, M., Macalino, G. E., Taylor, L. E., Sanford-Colby, S., Wolf, F., et al. (2004). A syringe protection program to prevent infectious disease and improve health of injection drug users. *Journal of Urban Health, 81,* 122–134.

Richards, J. B., Papaioannou, A., Adachi, J. D., Joseph, L., Whitson, H. E., Prior, J. C., & Goltzman, D., for the Canadian Multicentre Osteoporosis Study (CaMos) Research Group. (2007). Effect of selective serotonin reuptake inhibitors on the risk of fracture. *Archives of Internal Medicine, 167,* 188–194.

Richmond, L. B. (1977, Winter). Decisions and drinking: A prevention approach. *Alcohol Health and Research World,* 22–26.

Ridenour, T. A., Bray, B. C., & Cottler, L. B. (2007). Reliability of use abuse, and dependence of four types of inhalants in adolescents and young adults. *Drug and Alcohol Dependence, 91,* 40–49.

Riedlinger, J., & Montagne, M. (2001). Using MDMA in the treatment of depression. In J. Holland (Ed.), *Ecstasy: The complete guide: A comprehensive look at the risks and benefits of MDMA* (pp. 261–272). Rochester, VT: Park Street Press.

Rimm, E. B. (2000). Moderate alcohol intake and lower risk of coronary heart disease: Meta-analysis of effects on lipids and homeostatic factors. *Journal of the American Medical Association, 319,* 1523–1528.

Rinaldi, R. C., Steindler, E. M., Wilford, B. B., & Goodwin, D. (1988). Clarification and standardization of substance abuse terminology. *Journal of the American Medical Association, 259,* 555–557.

Ritchie, J. M. (1985). The aliphatic alcohols. In A. G. Gilman, L. S. Goodman, T. W. Rall, & F. Murod (Eds.), *Goodman and Gilman's The pharmacological basis of therapeutics* (7th ed., pp. 372–386). New York: Macmillan.

Robins, L. N., Helzer, J. E., & Davis, D. H. (1975). Narcotic use in Southeast Asia and afterward. *Archives of General Psychiatry, 32,* 955–961.

Robinson, T. E., & Berridge, K. C. (2003). Addiction. *Annual Review of Psychology, 54,* 25–53.

Robison, L. L., Buckley, J. D., Daigle, A. E., Wells, R., Benjamin, D., Arthur, D. C., et al. (1989). Maternal drug use and risk of childhood non-lymphoblastic leukemia among offspring. *Cancer, 63,* 1904–1911.

Robson, P. (2001). Therapeutic aspects of cannabis and cannabinoids. *British Journal of Psychiatry, 178,* 107–115.

Roine, R., Gentry, R. T., Hernández- Muñoz, R., Baraona, E., & Leiber, C. S. (1990). Aspirin increases blood alcohol concentration in humans after ingestion of ethanol. *Journal of the American Medical Association, 264,* 2406–2408.

Roiser, J. P., & Sahakian, B. J. (2004). Relationship between ecstasy use and depression: A study controlling for poly-drug use. *Psychopharmacology, 173,* 411–417.

Roldan, M. (1999). Colombia: Cocaine and the "miracle" of modernity in Medellin. In P. Gootenberg (Ed.), *Cocaine: Global histories* (pp. 165–182). London: Routledge Press.

Rollnick, S., & Heather, N. (1982). The application of Bandura's self-efficacy theory to abstinence-oriented alcoholism treatment. *Addictive Behaviors, 7,* 243–250.

Rose, A. H. (1977). History and scientific basis of alcoholic beverage production. In A. H. Rose (Ed.), *Alcoholic beverages* (pp. 1–41). New York: Academic Press.

Rose, J. E. (1991). Transdermal nicotine and nasal nicotine administration as smoking cessation treatments. In J. A. Cocores (Ed.), *The clinical management of nicotine dependence* (pp. 196–207). New York: Springer-Verlag.

Rosenberg, H. (1993). Prediction of controlled drinking by alcoholics and problem drinkers. *Psychological Bulletin, 113,* 129–139.

Rosenberg, N. L., & Sharp, C. W. (1992). Solvent toxicity: A neurological focus. In C. W. Sharp, F. Beauvais, & R. Spence (Eds.), *Inhalant abuse: A volatile research agenda.* Research Monograph 129 (pp. 117–171). Rockville, MD: National Institute on Drug Abuse.

Ross, E. M., & Gilman, A. G. (1985). Pharmacodynamics: Mechanisms of drug action and the relationship between drug concentration and effect. In A. G. Gilman, L. S. Goodman, T. W. Rall, & F. Murod (Eds.), *Goodman and Gilman's The pharmacological basis of therapeutics* (7th ed., pp. 35–48). New York: Macmillan.

Rosso, A., Mossey, J., & Lippa, C. F. (2008). Caffeine: Neuroprotective functions in cognition and Alzheimer's disease. *American Journal of Alzheimer's Disease & Other Dementias, 23,* 417–422.

Rowberg, R. E. (2001). *Pharmaceutical research and development: A description and analysis of the process: A CRS report for Congress.* Washington, DC: Library of Congress.

Rush, B., & Gliksman, L. (1986). The distribution of consumption approach to the prevention of alcohol-related damage: An overview of relevant research and current issues. *Advances in Alcohol and Substance Abuse, 5,* 9–32.

Rush, C. R., & Griffiths, R. R. (1996). Zolpidem, triazolam, and temazepam: Behavioral and subject-rated effects in normal volunteers. *Journal of Clinical Psychopharmacology, 16,* 146–157.

Rush, C. R., & Griffiths, R. R. (1997). Acute participant-rated and behavioral effects of alprazolam and buspirone, alone and in combination with ethanol in normal volunteers. *Experimental and Clinical Psychopharmacology, 5,* 28–38.

Rush, C. R., Roll, J. M., & Higgins, S. T. (1998). Controlled laboratory studies on the effects of cocaine in combination with other commonly abused drugs in humans. In S. T. Higgins & J. L. Katz (Eds.), *Cocaine abuse: Behavior, pharmacology, and clinical applications* (pp. 239–264). San Diego: Academic Press.

Russell, M. A. H. (1976). Tobacco smoking and nicotine dependence. In R. J. Gibbins, Y. Israel, H. Kalant, R. E. Popham, W. Schmidt, & R. G. Smart (Eds.), *Research advances in alcohol and drug problems* (Vol. 3, pp. 1–47). New York: John Wiley.

Ryan, R. M., Plant, R. W., & O'Malley, S. S. (1995). Initial motivations for alcohol treatment: Relations with patient characteristics, treatment involvement, and dropout. *Addictive Behaviors, 20,* 279–297.

Sack, R. L., & DeFraites, E. (1977). Lithium and the treatment of mania. In J. D. Barchas, P. A. Berger, R. D. Ciaranello, & G. R. Elliott (Eds.), *Psychopharmacology: From theory to practice.* New York: Oxford University Press.

Saitz, R. (2005). Unhealthy alcohol use. *New England Journal of Medicine, 352,* 596–607.

Salzman, C. (1992). Behavioral side effects of benzodiazepines. In J. M. Kane & J. A. Lieberman (Eds.), *Adverse effects of psychotropic drugs* (pp. 139–152). New York: Guilford Press.

Sanchez-Craig, M., Wilkinson, A., & Davila, R. (1995). Empirically based guidelines for moderate drinking: 1-year results from three studies with problem drinkers. *American Journal of Public Health, 85,* 823–828.

Sanger, D., Willner, P., & Bergman, J. (2003). Applications of behavioral pharmacology in drug discovery. *Behavioral Pharmacology, 14,* 363–367.

Santarelli, L., Saxe, M., Gross, C., Surget, A., Battaglia, F., Dulawa, S., et al. (2003). Requirement of hippocampal neurogenesis for the behavioral effects of antidepressants. *Science, 301,* 805–809.

Saul, S. (2007). More generics slow the surge in drug prices. *The New York Times,* August 8, 2007.

Sawa, A., & Snyder, S. H. (2002). Schizophrenia: Diverse approaches to a complex disease. *Science, 296,* 692–695.

Sawyer, D. A., Julia, H. L., & Turin, A. C. (1982). Caffeine and human behavior: Arousal, anxiety, and performance effects. *Journal of Behavioral Medicine, 5,* 415–439.

Sayette, M. A., Kirchner, T. R., Moreland, R. L., Levine, J. M., & Travis, T. (2004). Effects of alcohol on risk-seeking behavior: A group-level analysis. *Psychology of Addictive Behaviors, 18,* 190–193.

Scammon, D. L., Mayer, R. N., & Smith, K. R. (1991). Alcohol warnings: How do you know when you have had one too many? *Journal of Public Policy and Marketing, 10,* 214–228.

Schama, K. F., Howell, L. L., & Byrd, L. D. (1998). Prenatal exposure to cocaine. In S. T. Higgins & J. L. Katz (Eds.), *Cocaine abuse: Behavior, pharmacology, and clinical applications* (pp. 159–180). San Diego: Academic Press.

Scheffler, R. M., Brown, T. T., Fulton, R. D., Hinshaw, S. P., Levine, P. & Stone, S. (2009). Positive association between attention-deficit/hyperactivity disorder medication use and academic achievement during elementary school. *Pediatrics, 123,* 1273–1279.

Schifano, F. (2004). A bitter pill. Overview of ecstasy (MDMA, MDA) related fatalities. *Psychopharmacology, 173,* 242–248.

Schivelbusch, W. (1992). *Taste of paradise.* New York: Pantheon Books.

Schlieffer, H. (1973). *Sacred narcotic plants of the New World Indians.* New York: Hafner Press.

Schmidt, W., & Popham, R. E. (1978). The single distribution theory of alcohol consumption. *Journal of Studies on Alcohol, 39,* 400–419.

Schneider Institute for Health Policy. (2001). *Substance abuse: The nation's number one health problem.* Waltham, MA: Heller Graduate School, Brandeis University.

Schuckit, M. A. (1987). Biology of risk of alcoholism. In H. Y. Meltzer (Ed.), *Psychopharmacology: The third generation of progress* (pp. 1527–1533). New York: Raven Press.

Schuckit, M. A. (1994). The treatment of stimulant dependence. *Addiction, 89,* 1559–1563.

Schuckit, M. A. (1995). *Drug and alcohol abuse: A clinical guide to diagnosis and treatment* (4th ed.). New York: Plenum Press.

Schuckit, M. A. (1996). Recent developments in the pharmacotherapy of alcohol dependence. *Journal of Consulting and Clinical Psychology, 64,* 669–676.

Schuckit, M. A. (2000). *Drug and alcohol abuse: A clinical guide to diagnosis and treatment* (5th ed.). New York: Kluwer Academic/ Plenum Publishers.

Schuckit, M. A., Smith, T. L., & Kalmijn, J. (2004). The search for genes contributing to the low level of response to alcohol: Patterns of findings across studies. *Alcoholism: Clinical and Experimental Research, 28,* 1449–1458.

Schultes, R. E. (1976). *Hallucinogenic plants.* New York: Golden Press.

Scott, J. M. (1969). *The white poppy: A history of opium.* New York: Funk & Wagnalls.

Seligman, J., & King, P. (1996). Roofies: The date rape drug. *Newsweek,* February 26, p. 54.

Selvaraj, S., Hoshi, R., Bhagwagar, Z., Murthy, N. V., Hinz, R., Cowen, P., Curran, H. V., & Grasby, P. (2009). Brain serotonin transporter binding in former users of MDMA (ecstasy). *British Journal of Psychiatry, 194,* 355–359.

Senate Special Committee on Illegal Drugs. (2002). *Cannabis: Our position for a Canadian public policy.* Ottawa: Senate of Canada.

Sevak. R. J., Stoops, W. W., Hays, L. R., & Rush, C. R. (2009). Discriminative-stimulus and subject-rated effects of methamphetamine, d-amphetamine, methylphenidate and triazolam in methamphetamine trained humans. *The Journal of Pharmacology and Experimental Therapeutics, 328,* 1007–1018.

Sharp, C. W. (1992). Introduction to inhalant abuse. In C. W. Sharp, F. Beauvais, & R. Spence (Eds.), *Inhalant abuse: A volatile research agenda.* Research Monograph 129 (pp. 1–12). Rockville, MD: National Institute on Drug Abuse.

Shelton, R. C., Keller, M. B., Gelenberg, A., Dunner, D., Hirschfeld, R., Thase, M. E., et al. (2001). Effectiveness of St. John's wort in major depression: A randomized controlled trial. *Journal of the American Medical Association, 285,* 1978–1986.

Shenfeld, H. (2006). The best high they've ever had. *Newsweek,* June 12.

Sher, K. J. (1987). Stress response dampening. In H. T. Blane & K. E. Leonard (Eds.), *Psychological theories of drinking and alcoholism* (pp. 227–271). New York: Guilford Press.

Sher, K. J., & Levenson, R. W. (1982). Risk for alcoholism and individual differences in the stress-dampening effect of alcohol. *Journal of Abnormal Psychology, 91,* 350–368.

Shiffman, S. (1993). Smoking cessation treatment: Any progress? *Journal of Consulting and Clinical Psychology, 61,* 718–722.

Shiffman, S., Gnys, M., Richards, T. J., Paty, J. A., Hickcox, M., & Kassel, J. D. (1996). Temptations to smoke after quitting: A comparison of lapsers and maintainers. *Health Psychology, 15,* 455–461.

Siegel, R. K. (1984). The natural history of hallucinogens. In B. L. Jacobs (Ed.), *Hallucinogens: Neurochemical, behavioral, and clinical perspectives* (pp. 1–19). New York: Raven Press.

Siegel, R. K. (1985). New patterns of cocaine use: Changing doses and routes. In N. J. Kozel & E. H. Adams (Eds.), *Cocaine use in America: Epidemiological and clinical perspectives* (pp. 204–220). NIDA Research Monograph 61.

Siegel, R. K. (1992). *Fire in the brain: Clinical tales of hallucination.* New York: Dutton.

Single, E. (1995). Harm reduction and alcohol. *International Journal of Drug Policy, 6,* 26–30.

Sisson, R., & Azrin, N. (1989). The community reinforcement approach. In R. K. Hester & W. R. Miller (Eds.), *Handbook of alcoholism treatment approaches* (pp. 242–258). New York: Pergamon Press.

Skirrow, J., & Sawka, E. (1987). Alcohol and drug abuse prevention strategies: An overview. *Contemporary Drug Problems, 14,* 147–241.

Skog, O. J. (1985). The collectivity of drinking cultures: A theory of the distribution of alcohol consumption. *British Journal of Addiction, 80,* 83–99.

Smit, H. J., & Rogers, P. J. (2000). Effects of low doses of caffeine on cognitive performance, mood, and thirst in low and higher caffeine consumers. *Psychopharmacology, 152,* 167–173.

Smith, A. (2002). Effects of caffeine on human behavior. *Food and Chemical Toxicology, 40,* 1243–1255.

Smith, D. E. (1968). Acute and chronic toxicity of marijuana. *Journal of Psychoactive Drugs, 2,* 37–47.

Smith, D. E., & Gay, G. R. (1972). *It's so good, don't even try it once.* Englewood Cliffs, NJ: Prentice Hall.

Smith, N. T. (2002). A review of the published literature into cannabis withdrawal symptoms in human users. *Addiction, 97,* 621–632.

Smith, P. (2004). The influence of St. John's wort on the pharmacokinetics of protein binding of imatinib mesylate. *Pharmacotherapy, 24,* 1508–1514.

Smith, T. C., Cooperman, L. H., & Wollman, H. (1980). The therapeutic gases. In A. G. Gilman, L. S. Goodman, & A. Gilman (Eds.), *Goodman and Gilman's The pharmacological basis of therapeutics* (6th ed., pp. 321–338). London: Macmillan.

Snel, J., Tieges, Z., & Lorist, M. M. (2004). Effects of cocaine on sleep and wakefulness: An update. In A. Nehlig (Ed.), *Coffee, tea, chocolate, and the brain* (pp. 13–33). Boca Raton, FL: CRC Press.

Snyder, S. H. (1989). *Brainstorming: The science and politics of opiate research.* Cambridge, MA: Harvard University Press.

Snyder, S. H., Burt, D. R., & Creese, I. (1976). Dopamine receptor of mammalian brain: Direct demonstration of binding to agonist and antagonist states. *Neuroscience Symposia, 1,* 28–49.

Snyder, S. H., & Largent, B. L. (1989). Receptor mechanisms in antipsychotic drug action: Focus on sigma receptors. *Journal of Neuropsychiatry, 1,* 7–15.

Snyder, S. H., & Sklar, P. (1984). Behavioral and molecular actions of caffeine: Focus on adenosine. *Journal of Psychiatric Research, 18,* 91–106.

Sobell, L. C., Sobell, M. B., Toneatto, T., & Leo, G. I. (1993). What triggers the resolution of alcohol problems without treatment? *Alcoholism: Clinical and Experimental Research, 17,* 217–224.

Sobell, M. B., & Sobell, L. C. (1981). *Alcohol abuse curriculum guide for psychology faculty.* Rockville, MD: U.S. Department of Health and Human Services.

Sobell, M. B., & Sobell, L. C. (1993). *Problem drinkers: Guided self-change treatment.* New York: Guilford Press.

Sobell, M. B., & Sobell, L. C. (2000). Stepped care as a heuristic approach to the treatment of alcohol problems. *Journal of Consulting and Clinical Psychology, 68,* 573–579.

Sokolow, L., Welte, J., Hynes, G., & Lyons, J. (1981). Multiple substance use by alcoholics. *British Journal of Addiction, 76,* 147–158.

Solomon, D. (Ed.). (1966). *The marijuana papers.* New York: Bobbs-Merrill.

Solomon, R. (1980). The opponent process theory of acquired motivation: The costs of pleasure and the benefits of pain. *American Psychologist, 35,* 691–712.

Solomon, R. L., & Corbit, J. D. (1974). An opponent-process theory of motivation: I. Temporal dynamics of affect. *Psychological Review, 81,* 119–145.

Solowij, N. (1998). *Cannabis and cognitive functioning.* Cambridge, England: Cambridge University Press.

Sommers, I., Baskin, D., & Baskin-Sommers, A. (2006). Methamphetamine use among young adults: Health and social consequences. *Addictive Behaviors, 31,* 1469–1476.

Sorer, H. (1992). *Acute cocaine intoxication: Current methods of treatment.* Research Monograph 123. Washington, DC: National Institute on Drug Abuse.

Spector, I. (1985). AMP: A new form of marijuana. *Journal of Clinical Psychiatry, 46,* 498–499.

Spiegel, R., & Aebi, H. (1983). *Psychopharmacology.* New York: John Wiley.

Spillane, J. F. (2000). *Cocaine: From medical marvel to modern menace in the United States, 1884–1920.* Baltimore, MD: Johns Hopkins Press.

Spinella, M. (2001). *The psychopharmacology of herbal medicine.* Cambridge, MA: MIT Press.

Spitzer, R. L., Gibbon, M., Skodol, A. E., Williams, J. B. W., & First, M. B. (1989). *DSM-III-R case book.* Washington, DC: American Psychiatric Press.

Spitzer, R. L., Skodol, A. E., Gibbon, M., & Williams, J. B. W. (1981). *DSM–III case book.* Washington, DC: American Psychiatric Press.

Spoth, R. L., Randall, G. K., Trudeau, L., Shin, C., & Redmond, C. (2008). Substance use outcomes 5 ½ years past baseline for partnership-based family-school preventive interventions. *Drug and Alcohol Dependence, 96,* 57–68.

Squires, R. F., & Braestrup, C. (1977). Benzodiazepine receptors in rat brain. *Nature, 266,* 732–734.

Stanton, M. D., & Shadish, W. R. (1997). Outcome, attrition, and family-couples treatment for drug abuse: A meta-analysis and review of controlled, comparative studies. *Psychological Bulletin, 122,* 170–191.

Steenland, K., Thun, M., Lally, C., & Heath, C., Jr. (1996). Environmental tobacco smoke and coronary heart disease in the American Cancer Society CPS-II cohort. *Circulation, 94,* 622–628.

Stephens, R. S., Roffman, R. A., & Curtin, L. (2000). Comparison of extended versus brief treatments for marijuana use. *Journal of Consulting and Clinical Psychology, 68,* 898–908.

Stephens, R. S., Roffman, R. A., & Simpson, E. E. (1994). Treating adult marijuana dependence: A test of the relapse prevention model. *Journal of Consulting and Clinical Psychology, 62,* 92–99.

Steptoe, A., & Wardle, J. (1999). Mood and drinking: A naturalistic diary study of alcohol, coffee, and tea. *Psychopharmacology, 141,* 315–321.

Sternbach, L. H. (1983). The discovery of CNS active 1,4-benzodiazepines. In E. Costa (Ed.), *The benzodiazepines: From molecular biology to clinical practice* (pp. 1–6). New York: Raven Press.

Stevens, J. (1987). *Storming heaven: LSD and the American dream.* New York: Atlantic Monthly Press.

Stewart, G. C. (1967). A history of the medical use of tobacco. *Medical History, 11,* 228–268.

Stewart, O. C. (1987). *Peyote religion: A history.* Norman: University of Oklahoma Press.

Stinson, F. S., Grant, B. F., & Dufour, M. C. (2001). The critical dimension of ethnicity in liver cirrhosis mortality statistics. *Alcoholism: Clinical and Experimental Research, 25,* 1181–1187.

Stitzer, M. L., Iguchi, M. Y., & Felch, L. J. (1992). Contingent take-home incentive: Effects on drug use in methadone maintenance patients. *Journal of Consulting and Clinical Psychology, 60,* 927–934.

Stock, S. H. (1986). Synthetic drugs: A history of ups and downs—Part 2. *PharmChem Newsletter, 15–5,* 1–6.

Strain, E. C., Mumford, G. K., Silverman, K., & Griffiths, R. R. (1994). Caffeine dependence syndrome: Evidence from case histories and experimental evaluations. *Journal of the American Medical Association, 272,* 1043–1048.

Strassman, R. (2005). Hallucinogens. In M. Earlywine (Ed.), *Mind-altering drugs: The science of subjective experience* (pp. 49–85), Oxford, UK: Oxford University Press.

Streatfeild, D. (2001). *Cocaine: An unauthorized biography.* New York: St. Martins Press.

Stuart, R. B. (1974). Teaching facts about drugs: Pushing or preventing. *Journal of Educational Psychology, 66,* 189–201.

Subramaniam, G. A., & Stitzer, M. A. (2009). Clinical characteristics of treatment-seeking prescription opioid vs. heroin-using adolescents with opioid use disorder. *Drug and Alcohol Dependence, 101,* 13–19.

Substance Abuse and Mental Health Services Administration (SAMHSA). (2008). *National Survey on Drug Use & Health.* Retrieved from http://www.oas.samhsa.gov/NSDUHlatest.htm

Substance Abuse and Mental Health Services Administration (SAMHSA). (2008). *Results from the 2007 National Survey on Drug Use and Health: National findings.* Rockville, MD: SAMHSA Office of Applied Studies.

Sugiura, T., Kondo, S., Kishimoto, S., Miyashita, T., Nakan, S., Kodaka, T., et al. (2000). Evidence that 2-arachidonoylglycerol but no *N*-palmitoylethanolamine or anandamide is the physiological ligand for the cannabinoid CB2 receptor. Comparison of the agonistic activities of various cannabinoid receptor ligands in HL-60 cells. *Journal of Biological Chemistry, 275,* 605–612.

Sullivan, E. V., Rosenbloom, M. J., & Pfefferbaum, A. (2000). Pattern of motor and cognitive deficits in detoxified alcoholic men. *Alcoholism: Clinical and Experimental Research, 24,* 611–621.

Sussman, S., Stacy, A. W., Dent, C. W., Simon, T. R., & Johnson, C. A. (1996). Marijuana use: Current issues and new research directions. *Journal of Drug Issues, 26,* 695–733.

Suter, P. M., Schutz, Y., & Jequier, E. (1992). The effect of ethanol on fat storage in healthy subjects. *New England Journal of Medicine, 326,* 983–987.

Swift, R., & Leggio, L. (2009). Adjunctive pharmacotherapies in the treatment of alcohol and drug dependence. In P. M. Miller (Ed.), *Evidence-based addiction treatment* (pp. 287–310). Boston: Elsevier.

Syed, I. B. (1976). The effects of caffeine. *Journal of the American Pharmaceutical Association, 16,* 568–572.

Tancer, M., & Johanson, C. (2003). Reinforcing, subjective, and physiological effects of MDMA in humans: A comparison with d-amphetamine and mCPP. *Drug and Alcohol Dependence, 72,* 33–44.

Taylor, P. (2001). Anticholinesterase agents. In J. G. Hamilton & L. E. Limbird (Eds.), *Goodman & Gilman's The pharmacological basis of therapeutics* (10th ed., pp. 175–192). New York: McGraw-Hill.

Temple, J. L. (2009). Caffeine use in children: What we know, what we have left to learn, and why we should worry. *Neuroscience and Biobehavioral Reviews, 33,* 793–806.

The Alcoholism Report. (1993). Drug czar calls for treatment of drug addicted criminals. *The Alcoholism Report, 21,* 6–7.

Thompson, H. S. (1971). *Fear and loathing in Las Vegas.* New York: Random House.

Ticku, M. K., Burch, T. P., & Davis, W. C. (1983). The interactions of ethanol with the benzodiazepine-GABA receptor-ionophore complex. *Pharmacology, Biochemistry, and Behavior, 18,* 15–18.

Tiffany, S. T. (1990). A cognitive model of drug urges and drug use behavior: Role of automatic and nonautomatic processes. *Psychological Review, 97,* 147–168.

Tiffany, S. T. (1992). A critique of contemporary urge and craving research: Methodological, psychometric, and theoretical issues. *Advances in Behavior Research and Therapy, 14,* 123–139.

Tilashalski, K., Rodu, B., & Cole, P. (2005). Seven-year follow-up of smoking cessation with smokeless tobacco. *Journal of Psychoactive Drugs, 37,* 105–108.

Time. (1993). Cyberpunk. *Time, 141*(6), pp. 58–65.

Tobler, N. S. (1986). Meta-analysis of 143 adolescent drug prevention programs: Quantitative outcome results of program participants compared to a control or comparison group. *Journal of Drug Issues, 16,* 537–567.

Todd, M. (2004). Daily processes in stress and smoking: Effects of negative events, nicotine dependence, and gender. *Psychology of Addictive Behaviors, 18,* 31–39.

Tolman, S. A. (2005). The Oxycontin epidemic. *The Boston Globe,* June 30.

Tolstrup, J., Jensen, M. K., Tjanneland, A., Overvad, K., Mukamel, M. J., & Granbaak, M. (2006). Prospective study of alcohol drinking and coronary heart disease in women and men. *British Medical Journal, 332,* 1244–1248.

Tonigan, J. S., Toscova, R., & Miller, W. R. (1995). Meta-analysis of the literature on Alcoholics Anonymous: Sample and study characteristics moderate findings. *Journal of Studies on Alcohol, 57,* 65–72.

Trimpey, J. (1992). *Rational recovery from alcoholism* (4th ed.). New York: Delacorte Press.

Troisi, J. R., II, Critchfield, T. S., & Griffiths, R. R. (1993). Buspirone and lorazapam abuse liability in humans: Behavioral effects, subjective effects, and choice. *Behavioural Pharmacology, 4,* 217–230.

Tuchfeld, B. (1981). Spontaneous remission in alcoholics: Empirical observation and theoretical implications. *Journal of Studies on Alcohol, 42,* 626–641.

Tunnicliff, G., Eison, A., & Taylor, D. (1991). *Buspirone: Mechanisms and clinical aspects.* Orlando, FL: Academic Press.

Tyler, L. (2000). *Understanding alternative medicine: New health paths in America.* New York: Haworth Herbal Press.

Tyre, P. (2005). A problem in the brain. *Newsweek,* October 17.

Tyrer, P. J. (1982a). Evaluation of psychotropic drugs. In P. J. Tyrer (Ed.), *Drugs in psychiatric practice* (pp. 31–44). London: Butterworths.

Tyrer, P. J. (Ed.). (1982b). *Drugs in psychiatric practice.* London: Butterworths.

Tyrer, S., & Shaw, D. M. (1982). Lithium carbonate. In P. J. Tyrer (Ed.), *Drugs in psychiatric practice.* London: Butterworths.

Uhl, G. R., Liu, Q-R., Drgon, T., Johnson, C., Walther, D., Rose, J. E., David, S. P., Niaura, R., & Lerman, C. (2008). Molecular genetics of successful smoking cessation. *Archives of General psychiatry, 65,* 683–693.

United Nations Office on Drugs and Crime. (2009a). *Global illicit drug trends: 2009.* Vienna: Author.

United Nations Office on Drugs and Crime. (2009b). *World drug report: 2009.* Vienna: Author.

U.S. Department of Health and Human Services (USDHHS). (1984). *Drug abuse and drug abuse research.* Washington, DC: U.S. Government Printing Office.

USDHHS. (1987a). *Alcohol and health.* Rockville, MD: Author.

USDHHS. (1987b). *Smoking, tobacco, and health. A fact book.* Rockville, MD: U.S. Public Health Service.

USDHHS. (1989). *Reducing the health consequences of smoking: 25 years of progress.* Rockville, MD: U.S. Public Health Service.

USDHHS. (1990). *Alcohol and health.* Rockville, MD: Author.

USDHHS. (1993). *Alcohol and health.* Bethesda, MD: National Institutes of Health.

USDHHS (2001). *Women and smoking: A report to the Surgeon General.* Rockville, MD: Author.

USDHHS (2008). *Treating tobacco use and dependence: 2008 update.* Rockville, MD: Author.

U.S. Drug Enforcement Agency (2009). Meth clandestine laboratory incidents. http://www.usdoj.gov/dea/concern/map_lab_seizures.html

U.S. National Highway Traffic Safety Administration (USNHTSA). (1997). Setting limits, saving lives. The case for .08 BAC laws. Washington, DC: U.S. Department of Transportation.

University of California–Irvine Transdisciplinary Tobacco Use Research Center (UCI TTURC). (2005). Closing the gap on youth tobacco use. Irvine, CA: Author.

Urgert, R., Meyboom, S., Kuilman, M., Rexwinkel, H., Vissers, M. N., Klerk, M., et al. (1996). Comparison of effect of cafetiere and filtered coffee on serum concentrations of liver aminotransferases and lipids: A six-month randomized controlled trial. British Medical Journal, 313, 1362–1366.

Uttal, W. R. (2001). *The new phrenology.* Cambridge, MA: MIT Press.

Valenstein, E. S. (2005). *The war of the soups and the sparks: The discovery of neurotransmitters and the dispute over how nerves communicate.* New York: Columbia University Press.

Van Amsterdam, J. G. C., van der Laan, J. W., & Slangen, J. L. (1996). *Residual effects of prolonged heavy cannabis use.* National Institute of Public Health and the Environment, Report No. 318902003. Bilthoven, Netherlands.

van Dam, R. M. (2008). Coffee consumption and risk of type 2 diabetes, cardiovascular diseases, and cancer. *Applied Physiology, Nutrition, and Metabolism, 33,* 1269–1283.

van Laar, M., van Dorsselaer, S., Monshouwer, K., & de Graaf, R. (2007). Does cannabis use predict the first incidence of mood and anxiety disorders in the adult population? *Addiction, 102,* 1251–1260.

Vastag, B. (2005). Ibogaine therapy: A "vast uncontrolled experiment." *Science, 308,* 345–346.

Vega, W. A., et al. (2002). Prevalence and age of onset for drug use in seven international sites: Results from the international consortium of psychiatric epidemiology. *Drug and Alcohol Dependence, 68,* 285–297.

Viscusi, W. K. (1992). *Smoking: Making the risky decision.* New York: Oxford University Press.

Vocci, F. J., Acri, J., & Elkashef, A. (2005). Medication development for addictive disorders: The state of the science. *American Journal of Psychiatry, 162,* 1432–1440.

Vogel-Sprott, M. (1992). *Alcohol tolerance and social drinking: Learning the consequences.* New York: Guilford Press.

Vogel-Sprott, M., & Fillmore, M. T. (1999). Expectancy and behavioral effects of socially used drugs. In I. Kirsch (Ed.), *How expectancies shape experience* (pp. 215–232). Washington, DC: American Psychological Association.

Volkow, N. D., Chang, L., Wang, G. J., Fowler, J. S., Leonido-Yee, M., Franceschi, D., Sedler, M., Gatley, R., Hitzemann, R., & Ding, Y. S (2001). Association of dopamine transporter reduction with psychomotor impairment in methamphetamine abusers. *American Journal of Psychiatry, 158,* 377–382.

Volpicelli, J. R., Alterman, A. I., Hayashida, M., & O'Brien, C. P. (1992). Naltrexone in the treatment of alcohol dependence. *Archives of General Psychiatry, 49,* 876–880.

Vuchinich, R. E., & Tucker, J. A. (1988). Contributions from behavioral theories of choice to an analysis of alcohol abuse. *Journal of Abnormal Psychology, 97,* 181–195.

Wagenaar, A. C., & Toomey, T. L. (2002). Effects of minimum drinking age laws: Review and analyses of the literature from 1960 to 2000. *Journal of Studies on Alcohol, Supplement No. 14,* 206-225.

Walker, D. J., & Zacny, J. P. (2005). Subjective effects of nitrous oxide. In M. Earlywine (Ed.). *Mind-altering drugs: The science of subjective experience* (pp. 305–337). Oxford, UK: Oxford University Press.

Walsh, B. T., Seidman, S. N., Sysko, R., & Gould, M. (2002). Placebo response in studies of major depression: Variable, substantial, and growing. *Journal of the American Medical Association, 287,* 1840–1847.

Walsh, D. C., Hingson, R. W., Merrigan, D. M., Levenson, S. M., Cupples, A., Heeren, T., et al. (1991). A randomized trial of treatment options for alcohol abusing workers. *New England Journal of Medicine, 325,* 775–782.

Walters, P. G. (1992). FDA's new drug evaluation process: A general overview. *Journal of Public Health and Dentistry, 52,* 333–337.

Wang, P. S., Berglund, P., Olfson, M., Pincus, H. A., Wells, K. B., & Kessler, R. C. (2005). Failure and delay in initial treatment contact after first onset of mental disorders in the national comorbidity survey replication. *Archives of General Psychiatry, 62,* 603–613.

Wang, P. S., Lane, M., Olfson, M., Pincus, H. A., Wells, K. B., & Kessler, R. C. (2005). Twelve-month use of mental health services in the United States. *Archives of General Psychiatry, 62,* 629–640.

Wansink, B., & van Ittersum, K. (2005). Shape of glass and amount of alcohol poured: Comparative study of effect of practice and concentration. *British Medical Journal, 331,* 1512–1514.

Ward, A. S., Haney, M., Fischman, M. W., & Foltin, R. W. (1997). Binge cocaine self-administration in humans: Intravenous cocaine. *Psychopharmacology, 132,* 375–381.

Warner, J. (1997). Shifting categories of the social harms associated with alcohol: Examples from late medieval and early modern England. *American Journal of Public Health, 87,* 1788–1797.

Warner, K. E., Slade, J., & Sweanor, L. L. B. (1997). The emerging market for long-term nicotine maintenance. *Journal of the American Medical Association, 278,* 1087–1092.

Washton, A. M. (1990). Structured outpatient treatment of alcohol vs. drug dependence. In M. Galanter (Ed.), *Recent developments in alcoholism* (Vol. 8, pp. 285–304). New York: Plenum Press.

Washton, A. M. (Ed.). (1995). *Psychotherapy and substance abuse.* New York: Guilford Press.

Wasson, R. G. (1979). Fly agaric and man. In D. H. Efron, B. Holmstedt, & N. S. Kline (Eds.), *Ethnopharmacologic search for psychoactive drugs* (pp. 505–514). New York: Raven Press.

Webb, G., Shakeshaft, A., Sanson-Fisher, R., & Havard, A. (2009). A systematic review of work-place interventions for alcohol-related problems. *Addiction, 104,* 365–377.

Webster, L. R. (2007). Oxytrex: An oxycodone and ultra-low-dose naltrexone formulation. *Expert Opinions and Investigations on Drugs, 16,* 1277–1283.

Wechsler, H., Lee, J. E., Kuo, M., Seibring, M., Nelson, T. F., & Lee, H. P. (2002). Trends in college binge drinking during a period of increased prevention efforts: Findings from four Harvard School of Public Health study surveys, 1993–2001. *Journal of American College Health, 50,* 203–217.

Wechsler, H., Moeykens, B., Davenport, A., Castillo, S., & Hansen, J. (1995). The adverse impact of heavy episodic drinkers on other college students. *Journal of Studies on Alcohol, 56,* 628–634.

Wechsler, H., Nelson, T. F., Lee, J. E., Seibring, M., Lewis, C., & Keeling, R. P. (2003). Perception and reality: A national evaluation of social norms marketing interventions to reduce college students' heavy alcohol use. *Journal of Studies on Alcohol, 64,* 484–494.

Weil, A., & Rosen, W. (1983). *From chocolate to morphine.* Boston: Houghton Mifflin.

Weiss, K. J., & Greenfield, D. P. (1986). Prescription drug abuse. *Psychiatric Clinics of North America, 9,* 475–490.

Weiss, R. D., & Mirin, S. M. (1987). *Cocaine.* Washington, DC: American Psychiatric Press.

Welte, J. W., & Barnes, G. M. (1985). Alcohol: The gateway to other drug use among secondary-school students. *Journal of Youth and Adolescence, 14,* 487–498.

West, R. J., & Russell, M. A. H. (1985). Nicotine pharmacology and smoking dependence. In S. D. Iverson (Ed.), *Psychopharmacology: Recent advances and future prospects* (pp. 303–314). Oxford, UK: Oxford University Press.

West, S. L., & O'Neal, K. K. (2004). Project D.A.R.E. outcome effectiveness revisited. *American Journal of Public Health, 94,* 1027–1029.

Wester, R. C., & Maibach, H. I. (1983). Cutaneous pharmacokinetics: 10 steps to percutaneous absorption. *Drug Metabolism Reviews, 14,* 169–205.

Wetter, D. W., Kenford, S. L., Welsch, S. K., Smith, S. S., Fouladi, R. T., Fiori, M. C., et al. (2004). Prevalence and predictors of transitions in smoking behavior among college students. *Health Psychology, 23,* 168–177.

Wexler, B. E., Gottschalk, C. H., Fulbright, R. K., Prohovnik, I., Lacadie, C. M., Rounsaville, R. J., et al. (2001). Functional magnetic resonance imaging of cocaine craving. *American Journal of Psychiatry, 158,* 86–95.

Whitaker, B. (1987). *The global connection: The crisis of drug addiction.* London: Jonathan Cade.

White, J. M. (1991). *Drug dependence.* Englewood Cliffs, NJ: Prentice Hall.

Whitehead, P. C. (1975). Prevention of alcoholism: Divergences and convergences of two approaches. *Addictive Diseases, 7,* 431–443.

Wiegand, T., Thai, D., & Benowitz, N. (2008). Medical consequences of the use of hallucinogens: LSD, mescaline, PCP and MDMA (ecstasy). In J. Brick (Ed.), *Handbook of the medical consequences of alcohol and drug abuse* (2nd ed., pp. 461–490). New York: Haworth Press.

Wilens, T. E., Faraone, S. V., Biederman, J., & Gunawardene, S. (2003). Does stimulant therapy of attention-deficit/hyperactivity disorder beget later substance abuse? A meta-analytic review of the literature. *Pediatrics, 111,* 179–185.

Wilkinson, J. (1986). *Tobacco: The facts behind the smoke screen.* Middlesex, England: Penguin Books.

Wilkinson, R. (1970). *The prevention of drinking problems: Alcohol control and cultural influences.* New York: Oxford University Press.

Williams, G. C., Gagne, M., Ryan, R. M., & Deci, E. L. (2002). Facilitating autonomous motivation for smoking cessation. *Health Psychology, 21,* 40–50.

Williams, N. (1996). How the ancient Egyptians brewed beer. *Science, 273,* 432.

Wilsnack, S. C., Klassen, A. D., & Wilsnack, R. W. (1984). Drinking and reproductive dysfunction among women in a 1981 national survey. *Alcoholism: Clinical and Experimental Research, 8,* 451–458.

Windle, M., Barnes, G. M., & Welte, J. (1989). Causal models of adolescent substance use: An examination of gender differences using distribution-free estimators. *Journal of Personality and Social Psychology, 56,* 132–142.

Winickoff, J. P., Friebely, J., Tanski, S. E., Sherrod, C., Matt, G. E., Hovell, M. F., & McMillen, R. C. (2009). Beliefs about the health effects of "third hand" smoke and home smoking bans. *Pediatrics, 123,* e74-e79.

Winkelmayer, W. C., Stampfer, M. J., Willett, W. C., & Curhan, G. C. (2005). Habitual caffeine intake and the risk of hypertension in women. *Journal of the American Medical Association, 294,* 2330–2335.

Wise, R. A. (1988). The neurobiology of craving: Implications for the understanding and treatment of addiction. *Journal of Abnormal Psychology, 97,* 118–132.

Witkiewitz, K., & Marlatt, G. A. (2004). Relapse prevention for alcohol and drugs: That was Zen, this is Tao. *American Psychologist, 59,* 224–235.

Wolfe, T. (1969). *The electric Kool-Aid acid test.* New York: Bantam Books.

Woloshin, S., Schwartz, L. M., & Welch, H. G. (2002). Risk charts: Putting cancer in context. *Journal of the National Cancer Institute, 94,* 799–804.

Women for Sobriety. (April 1985). *Sobering thoughts.* Quakertown, PA: Author.

Woods, J. H., & Winger, G. (1997). Abuse liability of flunitrazepam. *Journal of Clinical Psychopharmacology, 17* (Supplement 2), 1–57.

Woodward, B. (1984). *Wired: The short life and fast times of John Belushi.* New York: Pocket Books.

Workshop on the Medical Utility of Marijuana. (1997). *Report to the Director, National Institutes of Health, by the Ad Hoc group of experts.* Washington, DC: National Institutes of Health.

World Health Organization (WHO). (1981). Nomenclature and classification of drugs and alcohol-related problems: A WHO memorandum. *Bulletin of the World Health Organization, 59,* 225–242.

WHO. (1999). Press releases 1999. *Cigars and pipes as lethal as cigarettes, says new European study.* Geneva, Switzerland: Author.

Wray, L. A., Herzog, A. R., Willis, R. J., & Wallace, R. B. (1998). The impact of education and heart attack on smoking cessation among middle-aged adults. *Journal of Health and Social Behavior, 39,* 271–294.

Wu, L., Pilowsky, D. J., & Patkar, A. A. (2008). Non-prescribed use of pain relievers among adolescents in the United States. *Drug and Alcohol Dependence, 94,* 1–11.

Yang, S. (2005). Researchers find that passive smoking kills as many women as active smoking in China. Retrieved October 2005, from http://www.berkeley.edu/news/media/releases/2005/09/04_smoking.shtml

Yesalis, C. E., Bahrke, M. S., Kopstein, A. M., & Barsukiewicz, C. K. (2000). Incidence of anabolic steroid use: A discussion of methodological issues. In C. E. Yesalis (Ed.), *Anabolic steroids in sport and exercise* (2nd ed., pp. 73–116). Champaign, IL: Human Kinetics Press.

Young, A. M., & Herling, S. (1986). Drugs as reinforcers: Studies in laboratory animals. In S. R. Goldberg & I. Stolerman (Eds.), *Behavioral analysis of drug dependence* (pp. 9–68). Orlando, FL: Academic Press.

Young, A. M., McCabe, S. E., & Boyd, C. J. (2007). Adolescents' sexual inferences about girls who consume alcohol. *Psychology of Women Quarterly, 31,* 229–240.

Young, C. R. (1997). Sertraline treatment of hallucinogen persisting perception disorder. *Journal of Clinical Psychiatry, 58,* 85.

Young, T., Lawson, G. W., & Gacono, C. B. (1987). Clinical aspects of phencyclidine (PCP). *The International Journal of the Addictions, 22,* 1–15.

Yuan J., Hatzidimitriou, G., Suthar, P., Mueller, M., McCann, U., & Ricaurte, G. (2006). Relationship between temperature, dopaminergic neurotoxicity, and plasma drug concentrations in methamphetamine-treated squirrel monkeys. *Journal of Pharmacology and Experimental Therapeutics, 316,* 1210–1218.

Zacny, J. P. (1995). A review of the effects of opioids on psychomotor and cognitive functioning in humans. *Experimental and Clinical Psychopharmacology, 3,* 432–466.

Zador, P. L. (1991). Alcohol-related relative risk of fatal driver injuries in relation to driver age and sex. *Journal of Studies on Alcohol, 52,* 302–310.

Zhdanova, I. V., & Friedman, L. (2002). Melatonin for sleep disorders. In D. Mischoulon & J. F. Rosenbaum (Eds.), *Natural medications for psychiatric disorders* (pp. 147–171). Philadelphia: Lippincott, Williams & Wilkins.

Zimmer, L., & Morgan, J. P. (1997). *Marijuana myths, marijuana facts.* New York: Lindesmith Center.

Zinberg, N. E. (1984). *Drug, set, and setting.* New Haven, CT: Yale University Press.

Zubieta, J. K., Bueller, J. A., Jackson, L. R., Scott, D. J., Xu, Y., Koeppe, R. A., et al. (2005). Placebo effects mediated by endogenous opioid activity on μ-opioid receptors. *The Journal of Neuroscience, 25,* 7754–7762.

Zubieta, J. K., & Stohler, C. S. (2009). Neurobiological mechanisms of placebo responses. *Annals of the New York Academy of Sciences, 1156,* 198–210.

Zucker, R. A., Kincaid, S. B., Fitzgerald, H. E., & Bingham, R. C. (1996). Alcohol schema acquisition in preschoolers: Differences between children of alcoholics and children of nonalcoholics. *Alcoholism: Clinical and Experimental Research, 19,* 1011–1017.

Zuckerman, B., Frank, D. A., & Mayes, L. (2002). Cocaine-exposed infants and developmental outcomes. *Journal of the American Medical Association, 287,* 1990–1991.

Zuckerman, M. (1979). *Sensation seeking: Beyond the optimal level of arousal.* New York: John Wiley.

Zusy, A. (1987). For smokers, ways to quit are many, but the goal is elusive. *The New York Times,* July 15, pp. C1, C10.

Note: Photographs are indicated by page numbers in italic type. Figures or tables are indicated by "f" or "t" following the page number.